Dietary Supplements

Special Issue Editors

Johanna T. Dwyer
Paul M. Coates

MDPI • Basel • Beijing • Wuhan • Barcelona • Belgrade

MDPI

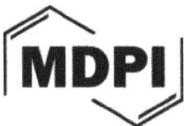

Special Issue Editors
Johanna T. Dwyer
Office of Dietary Supplements, National Institutes of Health
USA

Paul M. Coates
Office of Dietary Supplements, National Institutes of Health
USA

Editorial Office
MDPI
St. Alban-Anlage 66
Basel, Switzerland

This edition is a reprint of the Special Issue published online in the open access journal *Nutrients* (ISSN 2072-6643) from 2017–2018 (available at: http://www.mdpi.com/journal/nutrients/special_issues/dietary_supplements).

For citation purposes, cite each article independently as indicated on the article page online and as indicated below:

Lastname, F.M.; Lastname, F.M. Article title. *Journal Name* **Year**, *Article number, page range.*

First Edition 2018

ISBN 978-3-03842-921-0 (Pbk)
ISBN 978-3-03842-922-7 (PDF)

Table of Contents

About the Special Issue Editors

Johanna T. Dwyer is Senior Nutrition Scientist (contractor) at the Office of Dietary Supplements, National Institutes of Health. She is a Professor of Medicine (Nutrition) and Community Health at the Tufts University Medical School and the Friedman School of Nutrition Science and Policy. She is senior scientist at the Jean Mayer/USDA Human Nutrition Research Center on Aging at Tufts University and director of the Frances Stern Nutrition Center at Tufts Medical Center, Boston. Dwyer received her D.Sc. and M.Sc. from the Harvard School of Public, where she served as an adjunct professor for many years, her MS from the University of Wisconsin, and the BS with distinction from Cornell University. She is the author or coauthor of more than 300 research articles and 375 review articles in scientific journals on topics including the health effects of flavonoids, the dietary treatment of end-stage renal disease, preventing diet-related disease in children and adolescents, maximizing the quality of life and health in the elderly, vegetarian and other lifestyles, and databases and outcome studies for flavonoids. She serves as the editor of Nutrition Today and as co-editor of the "Handbook of Nutrition and Food". She is an elected member of the National Academy of Medicine and past president of both the American Institute of Nutrition (now American Society for Nutrition) and the Society for Nutrition Education (now the Society for Nutrition Education and Behavior.

Paul M. Coates directs the Office of Dietary Supplements (ODS) at the National Institutes of Health in its mission to strengthen knowledge and understanding of dietary supplements. Through a range of initiatives made possible by an energetic and knowledgeable staff, he has established the ODS as a strong and authoritative voice for rigorous science in dietary supplements and related areas of nutrition. The ODS addresses many of the issues in dietary supplements, from the evaluation of the literature to supporting and conducting science, and translating the results of that work into reliable and effective information for the public. Dr. Coates served as Acting Director of the NIH Office of Disease Prevention (ODP) from December 2010 through September 2012. Dr. Coates also served from 1996 to 1999 as Deputy Director of the Division of Nutrition Research Coordination (DNRC) at the National Institute of Diabetes and Digestive and Kidney Diseases (NIDDK). In that role, Dr. Coates helped to coordinate human nutrition research efforts, both at the NIH and between the NIH and other government agencies. Dr. Coates acted as Co-Chair of the joint DHHS/USDA Steering Committee, overseeing plans for the National Nutrition Summit that was held in Washington in May 2000. He is a member of the Federal Steering Committee that oversees the development of the Dietary Reference Intakes. He is Co-Executive Secretary of the Interagency Committee on Human Nutrition Research and Chair of the Federal Working Group on Dietary Supplements. Prior to joining the DNRC, Dr. Coates was NIDDK's Program Director for the Type 2 Diabetes Research Program (1993–1996) and Project Officer for the multicenter clinical study called Epidemiology of Diabetes Interventions and Complications (1994–1996). From 1994 until his departure from NIDDK, he maintained an active role in career development and fellowship training in the Division of Diabetes, Endocrinology, and Metabolic Diseases. In 2011, he received the Conrad A. Elvehjem Award from the American Society for Nutrition (ASN) for public service in nutrition. In 2013, he became a Fellow of the ASN and currently serves on the ASN Board of Directors. He is lead editor of the Encyclopedia of Dietary Supplements, now in its second edition, and associate editor of the American Journal of Clinical Nutrition. Prior to his career at NIH, he was on the faculty of the Children's Hospital of Philadelphia and the University of Pennsylvania School of Medicine. His Ph.D. in human genetics was awarded by Queen's University in Canada, followed by postdoctoral training in the Department of Human Genetics and Biometry at University College London.

Preface to "Dietary Supplements"

We are pleased to introduce this volume based on the Special Issue of Nutrients on Dietary Supplements, which we edited. We undertook it to advance the study of dietary supplement science, a goal that is shared by our institution, the Office of Dietary Supplements (ODS) at the US National Institutes of Health (NIH).

The thirty papers presented in this volume cover a very wide range of studies on a broad variety of dietary supplement ingredients. The book begins with a brief description of some of the regulatory challenges and research resources that are available [1]. It is followed by two very thoughtful papers on specific regulatory considerations involving sports [2,3].

The remaining chapters advance dietary supplement science by discussing scientific issues and current developments in the field. The overviews we commissioned drew heavily upon the work of the ODS staff and collaborators, focusing on ingredients of particular public health interest today: omega-3 fatty acids [4], vitamin D [5], iodine [6], and iron [7]. The contributions from other authors on a broad range of topics have enriched the volume. They include the health effects of nutrients, both positive and negative, with an emphasis on human studies, and human clinical trials of dietary supplement use. Many contributions discussed biomarkers of nutritional status, especially those measured in human samples, which are so essential for monitoring and evaluating health effects. Others were devoted to mechanisms of action and the development and application of analytical tools for the measurement of nutrients and other bioactive components of dietary supplements. Highlights include these areas:

- Omega-3 Fatty Acids: A systematic evidence-based review of omega-3 fatty acids and cardiovascular disease [4] is followed by the developmental outcomes of a randomized double-blind clinical trial in young children [8] and new data on their effects on metabolic and inflammatory pathways [9] . Precision nutrition and omega-3 supplements are discussed [10]. The effects of altered fatty acid ratios on bone turnover [11] in humans and other in vitro effects [12,13] are also discussed. The fact that seven of the contributed papers address various aspects of omega-3 fatty acids underscores the broad interest in understanding the health effects of these ingredients.
- Vitamin D: An overview of recent human studies of vitamin D [5] is followed by a report on the evaluation of vitamin D status in obese persons with different skin color and sun exposure [14]. The section concludes with new information from a large cohort on the association between vitamin D genetic risk score and cancer risk [15].
- Iron: Recent work on human studies of iron [7] is presented. The effects of protein hydrolysates on non-heme iron absorption are summarized [16]. Another contribution describes the effects of amino acid supplements on measures of iron nutriture in humans after hip fracture [17]. Various in vitro models of iron absorption are also discussed [18].
- Iodine: Databases of dietary supplements' composition are essential for improving the assessment of nutrient intakes and of the exposure to their ingredients in human populations. Some human studies and the process of database development for iodine in foods and dietary supplements are discussed [6].
- Non-Nutrient Bioactives: The topic of non-nutrient bioactives could fill several books because of the large number of ingredients they contain and the many scientific and regulatory challenges they pose. Only a few of the thousands of non-nutrient bioactives in supplements are discussed here, nonetheless the papers in this section provide an informative glimpse of the topic, including studies on the effects of carnitine [19], beetroot juice supplements [20], gingko biloba [21], creatine [22], various carotenoids [23], and other supplements [24]. The effects of xylitol, which is sometimes used as an ingredient in supplements, on altering an in vitro model of the microbiome are also described [25].
- Prevalence of Dietary Supplement Use: The prevalence of dietary supplement use in Australia is presented in depth in three comprehensive studies [26–28]. Two other contributions consider the prevalence of biomarkers in groups at high risk of micronutrient deficiency in the USA [29,30].
- Dietary Supplements and Micronutrient Deficiencies: Issues regarding dietary supplement use and

micronutrient deficiencies received attention in several papers [26–30].

- Sports and Athletic Performance: There is a very high interest among athletes in identifying ways to enhance their performance. This interest is reflected in six papers that describe regulatory issues and the effect of dietary supplements in sports and athletic performance [2,3,20–22,24].
- Databases of Dietary Supplements: Although the only contribution received on databases of dietary supplements was the paper on iodine [6], another collection of papers that describe such databases sponsored by NIH will be published in 2018 in the Journal of Nutrition.

Dietary supplements are products consumed widely by populations around the world, and consumers deserve the best possible information to perform the most advisable choices regarding their personal health. To that end, in the United States, the Congress established the ODS in 1994 to conduct and coordinate scientific research within the NIH relating to dietary supplements and the extent to which supplement use can limit or reduce the risk of diseases. The ODS serves as the principal advisor within the US Department of Health and Human Services on issues including the safety of dietary supplements, claims characterizing the relationship between the use of supplements and the prevention of disease or other health conditions and the maintenance of health, and scientific issues arising in connection with the labeling and composition of dietary supplements. Subsequent to the passage of the legislation establishing the office, Congressional mandates directed the ODS to: develop a botanical research center initiative (1999), conduct evidence-based reviews of the efficacy and safety of dietary supplements (2001), accelerate the validation of analytical methods and reference materials for dietary supplements (2001), and support the development of a dietary supplement label database (2004). Much progress has been made, but much remains to be done to fulfill these mandates.

It is gratifying that there is an increasing number of resources available to researchers, regulators, industry, and consumers. We hope that this book will add to the resources for researchers, regulators, and industry members and engage them in an exuberant and continued discussion of the opportunities–as well as the challenges–in the research on dietary supplements [1].

Johanna T. Dwyer and Paul M. Coates
Special Issue Editors

References

1. Dwyer, J.; Coates, P.; Smith, M. Dietary Supplements: Regulatory Challenges and Research Resources. *Nutrients* **2018**, *10*, 41, doi:10.3390/nu10010041.
2. Martínez-Sanz, J.; Sospedra, I.; Baladía, E.; Arranz, L.; Ortiz-Moncada, R.; Gil-Izquierdo, A. Current Status of Legislation on Dietary Products for Sportspeople in a European Framework. *Nutrients* **2017**, *9*, 1225, doi:10.3390/nu9111225.
3. Martínez-Sanz, J.; Sospedra, I.; Ortiz, C.; Baladía, E.; Gil-Izquierdo, A.; Ortiz-Moncada, R. Intended or Unintended Doping? A Review of the Presence of Doping Substances in Dietary Supplements Used in Sports. *Nutrients* **2017**, *9*, 1093, doi:10.3390/nu9101093.
4. Balk, E.; Lichtenstein, A. Omega-3 Fatty Acids and Cardiovascular Disease: Summary of the 2016 Agency of Healthcare Research and Quality Evidence Review. *Nutrients* **2017**, *9*, 865, doi:10.3390/nu9080865.
5. Taylor, C.; Sempos, C.; Davis, C.; Brannon, P. Vitamin D: Moving Forward to Address Emerging Science. *Nutrients* **2017**, *9*, 1308; doi:10.3390/nu9121308.
6. Ershow, A.; Skeaff, S.; Merkel, J.; Pehrsson, P. Development of Databases on Iodine in Foods and Dietary Supplements. *Nutrients* **2018**, *10*, 100; doi:10.3390/nu10010100.
7. Brannon, P.; Taylor, C. Iron Supplementation during Pregnancy and Infancy: Uncertainties and Implications for Research and Policy. *Nutrients* **2017**, *9*, 1327, doi:10.3390/nu9121327.

8. Devlin, A.; Chau, C.; Dyer, R.; Matheson, J.; McCarthy, D.; Yurko-Mauro, K.; Innis, S.; Grunau, R. Developmental Outcomes at 24 Months of Age in Toddlers Supplemented with Arachidonic Acid and Docosahexaenoic Acid: Results of a Double Blind Randomized, Controlled Trial. *Nutrients* **2017**, *9*, 975, doi:10.3390/nu9090975.

9. Lambert, C.; Cubedo, J.; Padró, T.; Sánchez-Hernández, J.; Antonijoan, R.; Perez, A.; Badimon, L. Phytosterols and Omega 3 Supplementation Exert Novel Regulatory Effects on Metabolic and Inflammatory Pathways: A Proteomic Study. *Nutrients* **2017**, *9*, 599, doi:10.3390/nu9060599.

10. Chilton, F.; Dutta, R.; Reynolds, L.; Sergeant, S.; Mathias, R.; Seeds, M. Precision Nutrition and Omega-3 Polyunsaturated Fatty Acids: A Case for Personalized Supplementation Approaches for the Prevention and Management of Human Diseases. *Nutrients* **2017**, *9*, 1165, doi:10.3390/nu9111165.

11. Rajaram, S.; Yip, E.; Reghunathan, R.; Mohan, S.; Sabaté, J. Effect of Altering Dietary n-6:n-3 Polyunsaturated Fatty Acid Ratio with Plant and Marine-Based Supplement on Biomarkers of Bone Turnover in Healthy Adults. *Nutrients* **2017**, *9*, 1162, doi:10.3390/nu9101162.

12. Tullberg, C.; Vegarud, G.; Undeland, I.; Scheers, N. Effects of Marine Oils, Digested with Human Fluids, on Cellular Viability and Stress Protein Expression in Human Intestinal Caco-2 Cells. *Nutrients* **2017**, *9*, 1213, doi:10.3390/nu9111213.

13. Halmenschlager, L.; Lehnen, A.; Marcadenti, A.; Markoski, M. Omega-3 Fatty Acids Supplementation Differentially Modulates the SDF-1/CXCR-4 Cell Homing Axis in Hypertensive and Normotensive Rats. *Nutrients* **2017**, *9*, 826, doi:10.3390/nu9080826.

14. Dix, C.; Bauer, J.; Martin, I.; Rochester, S.; Duarte Romero, B.; Prins, J.; Wright, O. Association of Sun Exposure, Skin Colour and Body Mass Index with Vitamin D Status in Individuals Who Are Morbidly Obese. *Nutrients* **2017**, *9*, 1094, doi:10.3390/nu9101094.

15. Chandler, P.; Tobias, D.; Wang, L.; Smith-Warner, S.; Chasman, D.; Rose, L.; Giovannucci, E.; Buring, J.; Ridker, P.; Cook, N.; Manson, J.; Sesso, H. Association between Vitamin D Genetic Risk Score and Cancer Risk in a Large Cohort of U.S. Women. *Nutrients* **2018**, *10*, 55, doi:10.3390/nu10010055.

16. Li, Y.; Jiang, H.; Huang, G. Protein Hydrolysates as Promoters of Non-Haem Iron Absorption. *Nutrients* **2017**, *9*, 609, doi:10.3390/nu9060609.

17. Aquilani, R.; Zuccarelli, G.; Condino, A.; Catani, M.; Rutili, C.; Del Vecchio, C.; Pisano, P.; Verri, M.; Iadarola, P.; Viglio, S.; Boschi, F. Despite Inflammation, Supplemented Essential Amino Acids May Improve Circulating Levels of Albumin and Haemoglobin in Patients after Hip Fractures. *Nutrients* **2017**, *9*, 637, doi:10.3390/nu9060637.

18. Uberti, F.; Morsanuto, V.; Ghirlanda, S.; Molinari, C. Iron Absorption from Three Commercially Available Supplements in Gastrointestinal Cell Lines. *Nutrients* **2017**, *9*, 1008, doi:10.3390/nu9091008.

19. Marx, W.; Teleni, L.; Opie, R.; Kelly, J.; Marshall, S.; Itsiopoulos, C.; Isenring, E. Efficacy and Effectiveness of Carnitine Supplementation for Cancer-Related Fatigue: A Systematic Literature Review and Meta-Analysis. *Nutrients* **2017**, *9*, 1224, doi:10.3390/nu9111224.

20. Nyakayiru, J.; Jonvik, K.; Trommelen, J.; Pinckaers, P.; Senden, J.; van Loon, L.; Verdijk, L. Beetroot Juice Supplementation Improves High-Intensity Intermittent Type Exercise Performance in Trained Soccer Players. *Nutrients* **2017**, *9*, 314, doi:10.3390/nu9030314.

21. Sadowska-Krepa, E.; Kłapcińska, B.; Pokora, I.; Domaszewski, P.; Kempa, K.; Podgórski, T. Effects of Six-Week Ginkgo biloba Supplementation on Aerobic Performance, Blood Pro/Antioxidant Balance, and Serum Brain-Derived Neurotrophic Factor in Physically Active Men. *Nutrients* **2017**, *9*, 803, doi:10.3390/nu9080803.

22. Wang, C.; Lin, S.; Hsu, S.; Yang, M.; Chan, K. Effects of Creatine Supplementation on Muscle Strength and Optimal Individual Post-Activation Potentiation Time of the Upper Body in Canoeists. *Nutrients* **2017**, *9*, 1169, doi:10.3390/nu9111169.

23. Phelan, D.; Prado-Cabrero, A.; Nolan, J. Stability of Commercially Available Macular Carotenoid Supplements in Oil and Powder Formulations. *Nutrients* **2017**, *9*, 1133, doi:10.3390/nu9101133.

24. Collins, P.; Earnest, C.; Dalton, R.; Sowinski, R.; Grubic, T.; Favot, C.; Coletta, A.; Rasmussen, C.; Greenwood, M.; Kreider, R. Short-Term Effects of a Ready-to-Drink Pre-Workout Beverage on Exercise Performance and Recovery. *Nutrients* **2017**, *9*, 823, doi:10.3390/nu9080823.

25. Uebanso, T.; Kano, S.; Yoshimoto, A.; Naito, C.; Shimohata, T.; Mawatari, K.; Takahashi, A. Effects of Consuming Xylitol on Gut Microbiota and Lipid Metabolism in Mice. *Nutrients* **2017**, *9*, 756, doi:10.3390/nu9070756.

26. McKenna, E.; Hure, A.; Perkins, A.; Gresham, E. Dietary Supplement Use during Preconception: The Australian Longitudinal Study on Women's Health. *Nutrients* **2017**, *9*, 1119, doi:10.3390/nu9101119.

27. O'Brien, S.; Malacova, E.; Sherriff, J.; Black, L. The Prevalence and Predictors of Dietary Supplement Use in the Australian Population. *Nutrients* **2017**, *9*, 1154, doi:10.3390/nu9101154.

28. Burnett, A.; Livingstone, K.; Woods, J.; McNaughton, S. Dietary Supplement Use among Australian Adults: Findings from the 2011–2012 National Nutrition and Physical Activity Survey. *Nutrients* **2017**, *9*, 1248, doi:10.3390/nu9111248.

29. Bird, J.; Murphy, R.; Ciappio, E.; McBurney, M. Risk of Deficiency in Multiple Concurrent Micronutrients in Children and Adults in the United States. *Nutrients* **2017**, *9*, 655, doi:10.3390/nu9070655.

30. Bruins, M.; Bird, J.; Aebischer, C.; Eggersdorfer, M. Considerations for Secondary Prevention of Nutritional Deficiencies in High-Risk Groups in High-Income Countries. *Nutrients* **2018**, *10*, 47, doi:10.3390/nu10010047.

nutrients

MDPI

Review

Dietary Supplements: Regulatory Challenges and Research Resources

Johanna T. Dwyer [1,*], Paul M. Coates [1] and Michael J. Smith [2,3]

1   Office of Dietary Supplements, National Institutes of Health, Bethesda, MD 20892-7517, USA;
    coatesp@od.nih.gov
2   National Center for Natural Products Research, University of Mississippi, MS 38677, USA;
    mjsmith073@olemiss.edu or m.j.smith@westernsydney.edu.au
3   National Institute of Complementary Medicine, Western Sydney University, Penrith, NSW 2751, Australia
*   Correspondence: dwyerj1@od.nih.gov; Tel.: +1-301-496-0048

Received: 9 November 2017; Accepted: 12 December 2017; Published: 4 January 2018

Abstract: Many of the scientific and regulatory challenges that exist in research on the safety, quality and efficacy of dietary supplements are common to all countries as the marketplace for them becomes increasingly global. This article summarizes some of the challenges in supplement science and provides a case study of research at the Office of Dietary Supplements at the National Institutes of Health, USA, along with some resources it has developed that are available to all scientists. It includes examples of some of the regulatory challenges faced and some resources for those who wish to learn more about them.

Keywords: dietary supplements; food supplements; supplement science; scientific challenges; regulatory challenges; natural health product; complementary medicine; traditional medicines; National Institutes of Health; Office of Dietary Supplements

1. Introduction

The fundamental challenge in any discussion about the regulation of dietary supplements is that there is no global consensus on how the category of products known variously as dietary supplements, natural health products (NHPs), complementary medicines or food supplements in different countries is defined. For example, a product considered to be a dietary supplement and regulated as a food in the USA, in another jurisdiction may be considered a food supplement or a therapeutic good (complementary medicine) or a therapeutic good (prescription medicine) or potentially even a controlled substance. The situation is even more complicated when countries like China or India that have an existing regulatory framework for traditional medicine or phytomedicine that includes crude botanicals are considered. To add further to the confusion, many regulatory frameworks are changing.

Another challenge is that while all regulatory scientists want to protect consumers from harm, ensure that consumers have the ability to make informed choices about the products they use, and do the right thing, the scientific challenges and regulatory systems that have arisen to deal with them vary greatly from country to country. Even in countries with similar cultures, legal systems, and levels of economic development, regulations applying to dietary supplements vary considerably. Some of these differences are explored below, using examples from Australia, Canada and the USA, all English-speaking countries with largely similar cultures and legal systems to illustrate this point. The discussion of other countries with similar legal systems such as the United Kingdom, New Zealand and South Africa or other nations in the Americas, Europe, Africa and Asia, often with different cultures, legal systems, and levels of economic development is left for others with greater expertise and experience.

A final challenge is that "dietary supplement" health products are often very emotive and polarizing topics, evoking a diverse range of opinions and viewpoints. While some observers may contend that these products should be considered in a similar fashion to conventional drugs and foods, others believe that a more tailored approach is necessary since there is often a traditional or historical evidence base and products often contain multiple ingredients. Increasingly, this situation has become even more complex because of the lucrative nature of the global dietary supplement sector, increased involvement of a growing industry sector producing them, and the introduction of many new and innovative products onto the market. A detailed discussion of the politics of the subject is outside the scope of this paper. However, it must be recognized that politics may play both a positive and negative role in shaping both regulatory frameworks and research agendas. Irrespective of the reader's point of view, this context is important in any discussion of dietary supplement products.

1.1. Importance of Research on Dietary Supplements

Until relatively recently, there was limited scientific research on dietary supplements and so little was known about them [1]. However, the prevalence of supplement use has increased dramatically over the past 20 years [2], and they have become a matter of consumer interest [3,4]. At the same time, the application of state-of-the art scientific methods to explore issues involving dietary supplements has advanced rapidly. The other invited articles in this special issue illustrate progress in our understanding of supplement science as it applies to several nutrients, including vitamin D, iron, omega-3 fatty acids, and iodine. Progress on botanicals and other non-nutrient ingredients (e.g., glucosamine, methylsulfonylmethane (MSM), coenzyme Q10) has been more challenging [5]. There is no global consensus in terminology for the category of products known variously as dietary supplements, NHPs, and food supplements in different countries and while we recognize this limitation, for the purpose of this article the term dietary supplement will be used to refer to such products as nutritional supplements, herbal medicines and traditional medicines. This article summarizes some of the scientific challenges in supplement research and some resources that may be useful in studying them. Most of the scientific challenges in supplement science are ubiquitous and global, so it is vital for scientists to collaborate across nations to help meet them without duplicating effort. A case study is provided by the work of the NIH Office of Dietary Supplements (ODS) which has been pursuing this goal since 2000. Some freely available resources and tools that ODS has developed for advancing health-related scientific knowledge on supplements are presented. The supplement marketplace is increasingly international, making collaboration between regulators essential since national decisions have international implications. Since products are consumed world-wide, calls for global quality standards are emerging. The remainder of the article focuses on regulatory challenges involving dietary supplements, and perspectives on how the regulatory systems in a number of different countries deal with them. Key resources for learning more about these approaches are provided.

1.2. Areas of Scientific Consensus about Supplement Science

Although there is broad consensus on the need for advances in science to make progress, opinions vary on the best paths to take and on priority areas for consideration.

1.2.1. Quality

The supply of ingredients used in supplements has outpaced the availability of methods and trained personnel to analyze them [6]. For example, in 1994, when the Dietary Supplement Health and Education Act (DSHEA) first became law in the USA, about 600 U.S. manufacturers of supplements were producing an estimated 4000 products. By 2000, more than 29,000 supplement products were on the US market but few documented analytical methods or reference materials (RM) were available for these products. This growth in the market has also been evident internationally. For example, there are anecdotal reports that over 100,000 product license applications have been approved in Canada since the Natural Health Products Regulations came into force in 2005. The need for improving quality continues today, since now there are estimated to be more than 85,000 supplement products in the US marketplace and concerns about ingredient misidentification, safety concerns, and quality assurance/control problems continue to be important for the industry and the public [7,8].

The first step in characterizing supplement products is generally identifying the ingredients [9]. Plant identification is a particular challenge. Even when easily identified whole plants or plant parts are used, unless the chain of custody is tight, and the exact manufacturing process is known and well characterized, the quality of extracts and blends such as those found in many botanical products is difficult to ascertain. Reliable analytical methods to characterize the bioactive components in supplements are helpful, but even for the nutrients in supplements, specific analytical chemistry methods must be often developed [10]. The bioactives in supplements differ from those in foods in their matrices in that the forms, combinations, and doses in which they are consumed, and the circumstances under which they are used are likely to differ. Analytical techniques for other bioactives in supplements are further complicated because the active compound(s) are often unknown, and even when they are known, validated analytical methods may not exist for determining their content. Reference materials are often unavailable to compare results between different laboratories for research purposes and to monitor data and supplement quality.

1.2.2. Safety

Manufacturers are prohibited from marketing supplement products that are unsafe or contain unsafe ingredients. This includes assuring that safe upper levels of intake for nutrients or maximum dosages for other constituents are not exceeded and ensuring that toxic contaminants are absent. Improved accuracy and precision of the nutrient measurements, bioactive marker compounds for other ingredients, natural toxins, toxic elements and/or pesticides in dietary supplement ingredients and finished products will be helpful to regulatory agencies.

1.2.3. Efficacy

Demonstration of efficacy typically depends on a number of research approaches ranging from basic in-vitro research on the mechanisms of action to animal and human studies. For example, in the past, large and expensive clinical trials using poorly characterized herbal supplement products for which the mechanisms of action were not understood were performed, leading to results that were inconclusive and irreproducible [11–13]. These experiences led publishers and funders to demand better product characterization and funders to demand more mechanistic evidence of bioactivity. Once mechanistic plausibility is established, animal and small phase 1 and phase 2 trials should precede the launch of large phase 3 studies of efficacy. More and better clinical studies of the safety and efficacy of dietary supplements on "hard" health outcomes are also sorely needed. Health outcomes such as changes in validated surrogate markers for performance, functions, morbidity, and mortality from diseases or conditions are required rather than changes in biochemical measures in blood with unvalidated surrogate markers. The question of the use of evidence from traditional forms of health and healing such as Traditional Chinese Medicine (TCM) makes the question of efficacy often more complex. This is briefly explored in the regulatory section below.

1.2.4. Translation of the Science

Widespread consensus exists on the need to translate the scientific evidence on supplements into appropriate recommendations, regulations, and policies that ensure the public health. Population-based prevalence estimates of supplement use are needed to estimate total exposures to nutrients or other bioactives that can be related to health outcomes [14]. Monitoring is especially important when supplementation is used as a public health strategy to fill nutrient gaps in deficient populations. It is also needed in other countries such as the USA where use of certain supplements is high, and where substantial proportions of total intakes of nutrients such as vitamin D and calcium come from supplements, especially among older adults [15].

2. Challenges and Resources: Regulatory Perspectives

As with other categories of regulated goods such as foods and drugs, the development of regulations is a balancing act where many different factors need to be taken into account. Notable among these are ensuring that products are of high quality and safe, that any claims made are truthful and not misleading, and that there is reasonable and appropriate access to the marketplace. All regulatory scientists want to both protect consumers from harm and support them in making informed choices about the products they include—or as importantly do not include—in their healthcare options. Appropriate regulatory oversight of this category is very challenging, and requires that scientists and regulators work together, as the former director general of the World Health Organization, Margaret Chan, MD urged [16]. This section provides a concise overview of how these regulations have been developed, and common themes as well as challenges faced in a global market.

2.1. Definition of "Dietary Supplements"

Although the definition of dietary supplement within a specific jurisdiction such as the USA is quite precise [17,18], a fundamental challenge to any discussion on regulation is that there is no global consensus on either what falls within this category or even what the category is called. Intuitively many equate a dietary supplement in the USA with a NHP in Canada or a traditional herbal medicine in the European Union or a complementary medicine in Australia, but this is not the case. For example, while melatonin is regulated in the USA as a dietary supplement and in Canada as a NHP, in Australia it is considered as a prescription medicine [19–21]. Dehydroepiandrosterone (DHEA) is readily available as a dietary supplement in the US, while in many other jurisdictions it is regulated as a controlled substance and is subject to significant regulatory oversight [22].

This situation is even more complicated when one considers that in addition to dietary supplements such as vitamins and minerals, many of these products come from traditional systems of health and healing such as TCM in China and Ayurvedic/Unani/Siddha medicine in India. For this reason, we must differentiate between the manner in which nations regulate the practice of medicine and the manner in which they regulate marketed products used in medical practice or as foods. In the U.S., the practice of medicine is regulated by the states, while marketed food and drug products in interstate commerce are regulated by the Federal government. Approaches and regulatory frameworks in many parts of the world, notably in Asia, reflect this fact with terminology and categories developed accordingly [23].

To assist in development of its Traditional Medicine Strategy 2014–2023, the World Health Organization refers to this category as Traditional and Complementary Medicines (T & CM) [16]. Although this classification does have significant limitations, it recognizes the fact that definitions for this category vary significantly globally. Descriptions of specific national/regional definitions and categories can be found through the list of resources in Table 1.

Table 1. Useful Global Resources on Dietary Supplement Regulatory Issues and Definitions.

Name	URL	Comments
USA		
FDA Food and Drug Administration Dietary Supplements	www.fda.gov/food/dietarysupplements/	Details on regulations, policies and guidelines dealing with dietary supplements
Australia		
Therapeutic Goods Administration (TGA)	www.tga.gov.au/complementary-medicines	Details of existing complementary medicine regulations, policies and guidelines
Food Standards Australia and New Zealand	www.foodstandards.gov.au/Pages/default.aspx	Details on food standards, policies and guidelines.

Table 1. *Cont.*

Name	URL	Comments
Canada		
Health Canada	www.canada.ca/en/health-canada/services/drugs-health-products/natural-non-prescription.html	Details on the existing NHP regulations, policies and guidelines as well as work underway with regards to a comprehensive approach to self care products
	www.canada.ca/en/health-canada/services/food-nutrition/legislation-guidelines/guidance-documents/category-specific-guidance-temporary-marketing-authorization-supplemented-food.html	Information on supplemented food category.
EU European Union		
EU Parliament and Council	ec.europa.eu/health/human-use/herbal-medicines_en	Details on the traditional herbal medicine directive re: member states.
European Food Safety Authority (EFSA)	www.efsa.europa.eu	Provides details and links to regulation of foods and food supplements.
China		
China Food and Drugs Administration (CFDA)	eng.sfda.gov.cn/WS03/CL0755/	Information on health food regulations including 'blue hat' process. (Note: English translation was not available).
China—Special Administrative Region of Hong Kong		
Health Ministry—Chinese Medicine Division	www.cmd.gov.hk/html/eng/important_info/regulation.html	Information on policies and regulation related to Chinese proprietary medicines.
Japan	www.mhlw.go.jp/english/topics/foodsafety/fhc/02.html	
Singapore		
Health Sciences Authority	www.hsa.gov.sg/content/hsa/en.html	Information on policies, regulation and guidelines related to health products and Chinese proprietary medicines. As a member state, resource to access work on regulatory harmonization of products within Association of South East Asian Nations (ASEAN).
New Zealand		
Medsafe	www.medsafe.govt.nz/regulatory/DietarySupplements/Regulation.asp	Provides information related to regulation, policies and guidelines dealing with dietary supplements.
India		
Food Safety and Standards Authority of India (FSSAI)	fssai.gov.in/home	Government direction, standards and regulation of health supplements and nutraceuticals. New regulations published in November 2016 take effect in January 2018. Health supplements are intended to supplement the diet of healthy individuals over 5 year, and levels of nutrients should not exceed RDA amounts.
Ministry of Ayurveda, Yoga, Unani, Siddha and Homeopathy (AYUSH)	ayush.gov.in	Policies, guidelines and regulations dealing with Indian traditional medicines.
WHO World Health Organization	who.int/medicines/areas/traditional/en/	Provides links to on-going work by the WHO including the Traditional Medicine Strategy 2014-2023, the International Regulation on the Cooperation of Herbal Medicines and various technical guidelines.
World Self Medication Industry	www.wsmi.org	Industry association website providing details on international approaches to over-the-counter medicines including dietary supplements.
International Alliance of Dietary/Food Supplement Associations (IADSA)	www.iadsa.org	Industry association website providing details on international approaches to dietary supplements.

While it would be easy just to consider that the substance itself is the defining factor in determining whether or not a product is a dietary supplement, this is not the case. Two other important factors considered are the claim that the product is making and how the product is supplied or recommended (intended use). In many jurisdictions such as the USA, Canada and Australia, dietary supplements are considered suitable for self-selection without the need for the intervention of a practitioner or prescription. Here the claims that can be made are limited to minor conditions and to the support of health and wellness depending on the jurisdiction [24,25]. In other jurisdictions, notably those where a traditional form of health and healing is recognized, traditional and complementary medicine products are often prescribed, and in some cases supply is limited only to trained practitioners.

2.2. Regulatory Models

As with the definition of the products themselves, there is no consistent global approach to regulation, with many different frameworks developed that largely reflecting national and regional priorities and needs. That being said, there are a number of common themes and approaches that have been taken internationally.

2.2.1. Where Does the Category Fall within Existing Legislation?

With a few exceptions, notably where traditional forms of health and healing exist, most countries do not regulate dietary supplements as a stand-alone category. Rather, they include them as a subset of existing legislation [17,18]. That is, they "hang from the hook" that is set in existing legislation. In the past, this was largely a question of whether these products should be considered a subset of drugs or foods; increasingly though, a third option is to capture them under existing regulations for biologics. It is important to note that overarching legislation is often one of the most important factors impacting the type of claim that can be made and what level of scrutiny and oversight will exist. For example, countries that regulate these products as a subset of drugs or therapeutic goods such as Australia, Canada and the European Union (EU) for traditional herbal medicines allow far more specific clinical claims to be made than in a jurisdiction such as the USA, where dietary supplements are captured in regulations under the existing food legislation, with their advertising regulated by trade regulations [20,25,26].

2.2.2. Should They Be Regulated as a Group?

As noted above in many jurisdictions dietary supplements are simply captured under the existing food or drug regulations and legislation with no specific consideration for these products, in some cases specific regulations have developed to reflect the category. In these cases, two different regulatory models have typically been adopted that reflect their domestic use, national priorities and public health needs. In many jurisdictions, the first model applies. Dietary supplements are simply captured under the existing food or drug regulations and legislation. In that model, a wide range of products (typically herbal medicines, traditional medicines and dietary or nutritional supplements) reside under an umbrella term such as dietary supplements in the USA, complementary medicines in Australia or NHP in Canada [20,24,25]. In the second model, specific regulations are developed to deal with these products. In this case, specific categories are developed with very structured regulatory frameworks for specific types of T&CMs. This is particularly the case in countries with a strong traditional form of health and healing such as Chinese proprietary medicines in China (TCM), Ayurvedic medicines in India and Kampo medicines in Japan [23].

Irrespective of the approach taken, it is rare that one set of regulations will encompass all products commonly considered to be dietary supplement-like. Typical examples of this are guidelines and legislation related to advertising that apply irrespective of whether or not a product is considered to be a dietary supplement.

2.2.3. Common Elements of Regulatory Frameworks

As with other forms of regulations, independent and irrespective of the approach taken, frameworks that deal with dietary supplements may contain a number of common elements, in this case often specifically developed to reflect the challenges and nature of the products. These common elements include: process for approval of a product to be sold; provisions related to manufacture and Good Manufacturing Practices (GMPs); reporting of adverse events; controls on labeling related to indications, contraindications and warnings; and, where claims are permitted, the type and quality of supporting evidence required. Again, the number and nature of these elements applied are determined by the specific regulations in place.

2.2.4. Risk-Based Approach

Operationally, the regulation of dietary supplements faces a number of issues and challenges not shared with conventional drugs or even food products. Notable amongst these are the sheer number of individual dietary supplements on the domestic markets, often numbering in the tens of thousands, and the fact that the sector contains many different types of products often posing very different risks that are grouped together often by the fact that they do not fit under any other regulatory regime. In particular, considerable challenges are posed especially by herbal and traditional medicine products that contain crude botanicals and a complex milieu of potentially active moieties, unlike conventional allopathic pharmaceuticals.

While a completely pre-market approach, where all products and manufacturing sites are 'approved' before the dietary supplement is marketed would be the optimal situation, given the challenges mentioned above, this is often impractical. This has led to the development of regulatory frameworks that increasingly blend elements looking at products and sites both before they come to market as well as once they are available to consumers, or post-market. This regulatory oversight is sometimes referred to as a "life-cycle" approach. Examples of post-market regulatory approaches (i.e., once the dietary supplement is on the market) include target audits where dietary supplements already on the market are analyzed for quality or manufacturers are requested to submit evidence they may hold that supports a specific claim. The determining factor on which approach is applied is largely determined by risk posed to the consumer. Since most dietary supplements when appropriately manufactured are considered to be inherently low risk, increasingly regulatory frameworks are increasingly focused more on post-market review than pre-market licensure.

Even in countries that are in many ways socially, economically and legally similar, different approaches to the definition and regulation of dietary supplement health products are evident although they contain some common elements. Illustrative examples of this are evident in the different regulatory frameworks in place in the United States, Australia and Canada.

In the United States, dietary supplements are regulated under the Dietary Supplements Health Education Act of 1994 (DSHEA) as a subset of foods and limited to those taken orally. This approach is primarily post-market in nature. However, it does contain pre-market elements. For example, manufacturers must hold evidence to support their claims and they cannot make specific disease treatment claims but only claims related to nutritional support (which includes physiological structure and function) [20]. All products must carry a disclaimer on the label stating that claims have not been reviewed by the US Food and Drug Administration (FDA). Provisions also include a post-market site audit process for manufacturing sites for Good Manufacturing Practice compliance and mandatory reporting of serious adverse effects by manufacturers. Companies must notify the Food and Drug Administration before marketing products with new dietary ingredients (NDI) [27]. There is at present no indication that DSHEA will be substantially changed or modified by Congress, in recent years the regulatory authority has given more attention to the notification and classification of NDIs as well as the importance of Good Manufacturing Practices (GMP) [20].

In Australia, although a small number of these products are captured by a food standard, most are regulated as therapeutic goods under the Australian Therapeutic Goods Act. Products are referred to as complementary medicines and are legally defined as being a listed therapeutic good or a registered therapeutic good. The legislation itself does not define these terms, but a comprehensive set of guidelines describes how they are considered. Most complementary medicines are listed medicines and are managed through an online portal called the Electronic Listing Facility (ELF). Permitted claims are limited to minor, self-limited considerations and those traditional forms of health and healing such as traditional Chinese medicine. Evidence for efficacy is assured through a random and targeted post-market audit system and new listable substances are evaluated pre-market. As with all registered therapeutic goods, registered complementary medicines are evaluated pre-market for safety, quality and efficacy. Manufacturers of either finished listed or registered complementary medicines must undergo an on-site audit to ensure GMP [28].

In 2014, complementary medicines were included within a comprehensive review of regulations for all therapeutic goods and medical devices to be conducted by an external expert panel [29]. The Commonwealth government accepted the majority of the recommendations from the panel and preliminary draft legislation was made public in September 2017. Although one of the recommendations was to keep complementary medicines as a distinct category, some significant changes are proposed, allowing mid-level claims through a new third regulatory route between the listed and registered therapeutic goods process as well as changes to how advertising is approved and compliance management [25,30].

In Canada, the majority of these dietary supplement products are referred to as natural health products (NHPs) and are considered a subset of drugs under a specific set of regulations—the Natural Health Products Regulations. Products must undergo a premarket assessment for safety, quality and efficacy. This is done in part through an online submission process with permissible claims supported by Health Canada monographs. Producers of NHPs who wish to make novel claims not supported through the monograph process must submit a full dossier of evidence for review. The products can make therapeutic claims, but their use is limited to self-care situations. While manufacturers are required to have a valid site license following approved GMP guidelines, no pre-market site audit is needed; the process being primarily paper based [24]. To address the growing number of NHPs sold in a food-like format, Health Canada has created a new category of food currently defined through regulatory policy called "supplemented foods". The category does allow for some health claims, but they are limited reflecting the nature of the products [31].

Unlike Australia, Canada is proposing to take different approach and rather than keeping NHPs as a distinct category, will include them in a self-care health product category together with non-prescription medicines and cosmetics. The intent of this initiative is to support informed consumer choice through a more consistent regulatory approach to these product categories that is based on risk. Key questions being explored deal with topics including evidence needed to support claims, provisions ensuring safety and quality and introduction of cost recovery framework [32].

The overviews above are brief and concise with more detailed information on these country specific approaches to be found through the list of resources in Table 1.

2.2.5. Competing Types of Evidence

While it is clear that high quality scientific evidence is always required to support the quality of a dietary supplement, from a regulatory perspective the same may not always be true with regard the type and nature of the evidence required to support a product claim. Given the nature of the dietary supplement sector and the fact that it often encompasses traditional medicines with a long history of use, the question faced by regulators is how to balance the need for robust scientific evidence with a respect for diverse forms of health and healing.

Globally, no consistent approach has been taken in answering this question. In some jurisdictions such as Canada and Australia, the approach has been to link the form of evidence, whether it be traditional or evidence based from scientific research, to the level and type of claim that can be made. In these cases, typically products based on traditional evidence making traditional health care claims are 'approved' according to pre-cleared and approved sources of information such as monographs or labeling standards. For products making higher level, clinical claims, in a way similar to that for conventional pharmaceuticals, companies must supply a full dossier with appropriate supporting evidence such as that from randomized controlled trials (RCTs) [24,28]. In many countries such as the United States with no pre-market approval framework system, claims that can be made are more limited [17,18]. In countries with long-established traditional forms of medicines such as in China,

India, and Japan, specific regulatory frameworks have been developed for these types of products with the type of claim that can be made and the evidence required to reflect this approach [23].

As the dietary supplement sector matures and develops and the market for raw ingredients becomes more global, establishing a balance between evidence generated by scientific research and that coming from traditional forms of health and healing is becoming increasingly demanding. This will be discussed later.

2.3. Evolving Regulatory Landscape—Challenging Issues

International regulatory frameworks are still considered by many to be a new and novel sector, although many of them are now more than two decades old. They were developed to reflect a time when the sector and nature of the market, not to mention the needs and demands of the consumer, were very different. This has meant that some decisions made in the past around policies and regulatory decisions may need to be revisited. These include the need to evaluate evidence of the "grandfathering" of dietary supplements already on the market when new regulations were implemented, the need to ensure that approaches are sustainable through cost-recovery mechanisms and the more global nature of the market place. Table 1 provides links to some of the regulatory frameworks of different countries that provide insights into the ways issues are dealt with in them.

Some of the key issues that commonly arise are:

2.3.1. Evaluating Evidence for Product Claims

As the market for dietary supplements has increased, so has the amount and diversity of scientific evidence and research to support, or not support, their use. This market is made more complex when there are conflicting evidence bases and conflicting ways for evaluating them. For example, how, or should, traditional evidence be evaluated within the framework of traditional healing theories or those of allopathic evidence based medicine; what should be done when evidence from traditional forms of health and healing are not supported by more conventional evaluation mechanisms such as randomized clinical trials; and how can consumers, often wanting to explore both conventional and traditional medicine, be supported in making informed choices about including, or not including, these products in their health care options.

The original concept of Evidence Based Medicine is based on three basic premises—individual clinical expertise, the best external evidence and patients' values and expectations [33]. The challenge faced by the regulator is to ensure that these are in play and to support consumers in making informed choices that are often made in a self-care setting.

2.3.2. Questions at the Regulatory Interface

It has never been easy to distinguish between a dietary supplement and other categories such as conventional foods, drugs and biologics. As all these sectors have evolved, this question of product classification has become even more complex. Two of the main questions at the regulatory interface are: what are the boundaries are between dietary supplements and conventional foods and between dietary supplements and over-the-counter drugs?.

As the popularity of dietary supplements available in a food-like format such as a pre-prepared drink or bar has increased, the line between what a consumer would understand to be a food as compared to a dietary supplement has become increasingly blurred. In essence, how does the regulator provide for appropriate regulatory oversight? This has been particularly challenging for those jurisdictions that consider these products as a sub-set of drugs with regulation and often legislation governing them that is very different from that for foods. In these cases, the regulatory frameworks are more specific to such dosage forms as capsules, tablets and tinctures. The challenge is one primarily of balance in providing a regulatory approach that is appropriate and not unnecessarily restrictive with the need to ensure that consumers are aware that these food-like dietary supplements that they are considering are not typical foods. This lack of clarity is also challenging for the private sector in determining what regulatory framework applies to a product, either food or drug, that they wish to develop and bring to market. In Canada, this concern required the government to create a new category called "supplemented foods" distinct from NHPs where products in a food like format are considered as a subset of foods and not as natural health products [31]. In other jurisdictions such as Australia, authority has been given to the respective regulators to deem something to be either a therapeutic good or a food based a specific set of criteria [34].

The challenge at the over-the-counter (OTC)/dietary supplement interface is even more pronounced. A number of herbal medicines with a long history of use within the conventional health care model, such as senna and cascara, are regulated in most countries as OTC drugs rather than dietary supplements. As described above, Health Canada is proposing to address this issue in part by considering both NHPs and OTC drugs within a single regulatory approach for self-care products [32].

2.3.3. Working on the Global Stage

Although science and research may be global, regulations are still made primarily to reflect domestic needs and pressures. This poses a challenge regarding dietary supplements and dietary supplement ingredients that are now often sourced and/or manufactured outside of the country where they are sold. In spite of calls for regulatory harmonization, examples of true harmonization are limited to regions such as countries in the Association of South East Asian Nations (ASEAN) with the lack of a coherent and consistent regulatory approach prohibiting this globally [35]. Even if regulatory harmonization is not possible, regulatory cooperation is often a viable option, taking into account inputs from stakeholder groups such as industry and not just governments. For example, to support cooperation between regulators, in 2005 in Ottawa, the World Health Organization supported the creation of the International Cooperation on Herbal Medicine (IRCH). IRCH now has over twenty members and provides a forum and mechanism for regulators to share information on safety issues and common challenges they all face [36]. Increasingly governments are working together as well as with other stakeholders such as industry and consumers to address common problems and in some cases to provide regulatory decisions in one jurisdiction that can be used as a basis for action in another.

2.3.4. Strengthening Product Quality

As the dietary supplement market has become more global and lucrative, so have the importance of ensuring product quality and the challenges in doing so. There are increasing numbers of cases of adverse reactions and some fatalities due to contaminants or adulterants in the product rather than in the dietary supplement ingredients themselves. In some cases this has been due to intentional fraud by producers of these poor quality products who have developed sophisticated methods for overcoming existing regulations and oversight. This situation is explored in greater depth elsewhere in this paper.

2.4. Need for Continued Science in Support of Regulation

Irrespective of whether the goal is to support production of high quality products or to develop, apply or modify methods for evaluation of evidence in support of claims, the need for robust and relevant science and research on dietary supplements has never been more necessary. As regulatory frameworks evolve, many of the questions posed above will need to be addressed, balancing the need for robust science with a respect for traditional forms of health and healing.

3. Challenges: Scientific Perspectives

3.1. Issues Involving Human Requirements

Scientists often disagree about definitions of human requirements for bioactives and the implications for supplements. They differ on whether some non-nutrient bioactives are required for certain population subgroups and also on the health effects associated with the use of non-nutrient bioactives. It has been known for over 100 years that inborn errors of nutrient metabolism exist that can be remediated by supplying the lacking nutrient that has become conditionally essential. However, it is not clear that such a model based on single gene defects is useful for the amelioration of multigenic complex diseases. It is unclear that there are large numbers of individuals with common diseases and conditions such as type 2 diabetes or depression whose unique genetic characteristics cause them to have special nutritional requirements requiring supplements or medical foods [37].

Discoveries of genetic polymorphisms and the advent of inexpensive genetic tests that are widely available to consumers have nutritional implications. They have led to the rise of personalized or "precision nutrition" [38] and to the proliferation of boutique "personalized" eating plans and "precision" dietary supplements supposedly tailored to an individual's genetic profile. The extent to which such supplements are efficacious in reducing chronic degenerative disease remains to be determined.

3.2. Supplement Quality, Safety and Efficacy

Challenges remain on the appropriate means for assuring supplement quality, safety and efficacy.

3.2.1. Quality

Regulators, health professionals and manufacturers often disagree on how much quality testing is necessary for supplements. This is echoed by the World Health Organization's Strategy on Traditional Medicines 2014–2023 [39] where quality is seen as a cornerstone of the sector. Botanical extracts and blends present particular challenges for detecting misidentification and contamination. The presence of adulterants and contaminants of both a biological and chemical nature in supplements is also challenging. Certain categories of supplements, such as athletic performance, sexual performance, and weight loss products, are particularly prone to the deliberate "spiking" with unlabeled extraneous or synthetic substances to confuse analytical techniques and even occasionally the addition of active synthetic drugs. Purity is a special problem for individuals with inborn errors of metabolism for specific nutrients such as vitamin B-6 or choline who require reliable, high quality sources of the nutrient. In countries that do not require that added nutrients be pharmaceutical grade or provide nutrients free to such patients, afflicted individuals must buy products that vary greatly in their quality on the open market.

The scientific challenges involved in all of the problems cited above depend in part on the adequacy and application of analytical methods. Analytical methods and reference standards are lacking for many of the thousands of different bioactive ingredients in dietary supplements. There is still disagreement about whether only a single officially endorsed method of analysis is acceptable. Any analytical method that is appropriately calibrated to a recognized reference standard should suffice but the onus is on the user of the method to demonstrate that affirmative requirements are met and that the method is suitable for its intended use and yields results that are accurate and precise. Methods that are suitable for foods may not be so for dietary supplements. Opinions also differ on whether government or the private sector is responsible for developing reference standards and analytical methods, and, if the private sector develops them, how they can be both kept independent and objective and made publicly available to avoid duplication of effort while preserving the marketing advantage of the developer. Tension also exists between researchers who desire ever more precise analytical methods for ingredients in dietary supplements and manufacturers who are concerned about the expertise and monetary costs required to apply some of the methods. A balance needs to be struck between the two.

3.2.2. Safety

Apart from concerns related to product quality, the safety of dietary supplements depends largely on dose. High doses of some nutrients are more likely to pose problems than others, although there is disagreement about the levels at which problems arise. For example, some dialysis patients who are receiving very large doses of calcium and the active form of vitamin D on a chronic basis may exceed the Tolerable Upper Level (UL) and incur adverse effects on health, including calcification of the soft tissues [40]. Very high doses of vitamin D may also cause adverse effects in people with normal kidney function [41]. There is little evidence that usual doses and forms of these nutrients give rise to health problems [42]. The possibilities of excessive intakes of nutrients from dietary supplements are greater in countries with programs to fortify their food supplies than in others, and therefore they must also be evaluated [43–46].

Dose-response data for establishing safe levels of intakes of non-nutrient bioactives in supplements is frequently lacking [47,48]. Some dietary supplements containing non-target herbs added intentionally (like germander as an adulterant for skullcap), or others such as black cohosh, kava extract, green tea and others have been associated with liver injures of various types even after taking into account concomitant use with acetaminophen and alcohol and consumption while fasting [49]. Extracts that are used in bodybuilding and weight loss have also been linked to liver injury. This has led to studies of the composition of different supplements [50,51]. Causes of liver toxicity from supplements appear to be due to insufficient regulatory authority, inaccurate product labeling, adulterants and inconsistent sourcing of ingredients [52]. There is controversy about whether evidence of causality is sufficient for regulators to take action against supplements that seem to pose a hepatotoxic risk [53]. Some possible actions include requirements for warning labels with usage instructions as is done for drugs, or/and removal of products from the market. Adulterated or fraudulent tainted products sold as dietary supplements are already illegal and subject to recall [54].

Interactions of some ingredients in supplements with other dietary supplements, nutrients, prescription or over-the-counter drugs are well documented. Of particular concern are adverse reactions occurring with commonly used medications, such as anti-hypertensive and cardiovascular preparations [55]. In addition, much interest focuses around concomitant use of herbal medicines such as St. John's Wort which has been shown to alter drug metabolism of a number of drugs notably those used in the treatment of HIV/AIDS, warfarin, insulin, aspirin and digoxin [56].

3.2.3. Efficacy

Among the most hotly debated issues in supplement research is the type and amount of evidence needed to demonstrate the efficacy of dietary supplements. Many of the issues involving efficacy include those common in testing of all medications such as study designs, significance testing, appropriate outcomes, effect sizes, acceptable biomarkers of effect, and the differences between statistical and clinical significance. In order to be efficacious, dietary supplements must be bioavailable, and yet in some countries regulations do not require testing of supplements for disintegration and dissolution and some products on the market fail such tests. This is a matter of concern both to researchers and regulators since such results have a negative impact on studies of dietary supplement efficacy. In-vitro methods are available for testing disintegration and dissolution of drugs, and these are adaptable for use with dietary supplement products. Regulators in some countries insist on changes in health outcomes or in validated surrogate biochemical markers of effect on the causal pathway to a health or performance outcome. Others accept changes in intermediary biochemical markers that may or may not be surrogates of health outcomes. These considerations have come to the fore because supplements on the market in some countries apparently have little or no demonstrated efficacy. For example, one recent review of 63 randomized, placebo-controlled clinical trials of dietary supplements in Western adults found that in 45 of them no benefits were found, 10 showed a trend toward harm and 2 showed a trend toward benefit, while 4 reported actual harm, and 2 both harms and benefits; only vitamin D and omega 3 fatty acids had strong enough benefits and lack of harm to suggest possible efficacy [3]. This is an area of controversy that is highly polarized with questions being raised that depend on the type of dietary supplement being used, notably herbal medicines, the quality of the studies included in the review, and additional factors such as product quality of the supplement being evaluated that need to be taken into account [57].

3.2.4. Standards of Efficacy for Traditional Natural Products

The traditional use of Chinese medicines, Ayurvedic medicines and other remedies is embedded in larger healing systems and cultural or metaphysical beliefs that are part of users' larger and more holistic world views. Should usual standards for efficacy should apply to them when they are used in the traditional manner? Clearly such uses are quite different than the use of a single product or ingredient at much higher traditional doses and without such a cultural context.

3.3. Policy

Although policy issues arise with all types of dietary supplements, the examples below will focus on nutrient-containing dietary supplements since these are particularly germane to discussions of nutritional status.

3.3.1. Nutrient Supplements Are Only One of Many Strategies for Improving Nutrient Intakes

There are many strategies for filling nutrient gaps in dietary intakes. They include nutrition education on appropriate food choices, fortification and enrichment that add nutrients to staple foods, genetic engineering that increases the nutrient content of a commodity itself either by genetic engineering/biotechnology, biofortification involving conventional breeding, and the use of nutrient containing dietary supplements. Dietary supplements provide concentrated sources of bioactives that are low or lacking in some individuals' ordinary dietary intakes. The supplements can be used selectively by those whose diets have gaps in them. However, supplements have disadvantages. Their use depends upon individual motivations. Because they provide concentrated sources of bioactives at relatively high levels, they may increase the risks that some individuals will ingest excessive quantities and suffer health risks. Moreover, since dietary supplements can contain ingredients that lack a history of safe use, their long-term health effects may be unknown. The advantages and disadvantages of dietary supplements as a strategy to improve dietary intakes therefore must be carefully considered.

3.3.2. Supplementation as a Strategy to Achieve Nutritional Adequacy

The cost-effectiveness of using supplements to fill gaps in nutrient intakes as opposed to other means such as fortification or nutrition education varies from one nutrient to another and by country, and so each situation is unique and must be evaluated independently. There are also questions about what the supplement should be, if supplementation is chosen. In countries where nutrient containing dietary supplements are common, the use of multivitamin-multi-mineral (MVM) supplements is often associated with a greater proportion of the population reaching the estimated average requirement (EAR) for nutrients [58]. However, for some of these nutrients, intakes are already adequate, so that the increased intakes may do little good, and in some cases supplements may increase the risk of exceeding the upper safe level (UL) of intakes.

3.3.3. Monitoring of Supplement Use

Monitoring of supplement use is particularly important in countries where premarket approval is not required to detect potential adverse reactions. Dietary indicators are known to be imprecise and estimates of usual intake are lacking for many nutrients [59]. Biochemical indicators of deficiency are often not well linked with adverse health outcomes, underscoring the need for more attention to be paid to the development of agreed on measures of deficiency and excess [60]. Recent work on key nutrient biomarkers is now available, facilitating the monitoring of high risk groups, such as pregnant women for folate status [61,62].

3.3.4. Authoritative Recommendations for Dietary Supplements

Health and nutrition experts differ on whether it is appropriate to include recommendations for nutrient containing dietary supplements in national health promotion and disease prevention recommendations. Many countries opt to recommend that adequate nutrient intake for the general public be achieved solely from foods, and reserve recommendations of specific nutrient supplements for specific subgroups in the population. Others recommend only food alone with no recommendations for special populations.

3.3.5. Inclusion of Dietary Supplements in Food Programs to Reduce Malnutrition

There is pressure by industry to include MVM or other dietary supplements in food programs. However, there is little evidence that the target groups are deficient in the ingredients in the supplements, nor has it been demonstrated that provision of a supplement leads to better health outcomes.

3.3.6. Stimulating Innovation

The development of new and more highly bioavailable forms of the nutrients, timed release, dosage forms, novel bioactive constituents and the appropriate application of new technologies such as nanotechnology are all important, but some pose new scientific and regulatory challenges.

4. Case Study: Office of Dietary Supplements (ODS), National Institutes of Health (NIH), USA

This case study highlights some examples of dietary supplement research supported by or conducted at the ODS, and provides some research tools it has developed that may be useful resources for scientists both there and abroad.

4.1. Background

Since its establishment in 1995 as part of the implementation of the Dietary Supplement and Health Education Act [17,18] of 1994, the ODS is the lead federal agency devoted to the scientific exploration of dietary supplements. Its mission is to support, conduct and coordinate scientific research and provide intellectual leadership to strengthen the knowledge and understanding of dietary supplements in order to enhance the US population's health and quality of life. ODS's four goals are to: expand the scientific knowledge base on dietary supplements by stimulating and supporting a full range of biomedical research and by developing and contributing to collaborative initiatives, workshops, meetings and conferences; enhance the dietary supplement research workforce through training and career development; foster development and dissemination of research resources and tools to enhance the quality of dietary supplement research; and translate dietary supplement research findings into useful information for consumers, health professionals, researchers, and policymakers.

Several of its major initiatives that have expanded the scientific knowledge base on dietary supplements are described elsewhere in this special issue of NUTRIENTS. They include studies to clarify the implications for public health of omega-3 fatty acids [63], iodine [64], vitamin D [65], and iron [66].

4.2. Research Resources and Tools

This section provides the details on freely available research resources developed by ODS that are available for scientists to use to enhance the quality of dietary supplement research and meet public health priorities, with a focus on those that may be useful to scientists in other countries.

4.3. Analytical Methods for Dietary Supplements

The rigorous assessment of dietary supplement ingredients requires accurate, precise and reliable analytical methods and matching reference materials. The ODS Analytical Methods and Reference Materials program accelerates the creation and dissemination of validated methods and reference materials. It provides resources for characterization and verification of supplement product content that enhance the reliability and reproducibility of research using these products and supports product quality [67].

The genesis of the program was the paucity of publicly available methods for the analysis of supplement ingredients [68,69]. In 2000, the US dietary supplement community tended to use proprietary or compendial methods for quality control operations, and scientists and laboratories often kept their proprietary methods to themselves. Negative publicity about discrepancies between label claims and the results of product testing performed by third parties led to some unsuccessful efforts on the part of the industry to pay a laboratory to develop and validate methods through the Association of Official Analytical Chemists International (AOACI). The program was not successful for several reasons, including lack of expert technical guidance and conflicting sponsor priorities. However, this early effort led to a collaboration between trade associations, ODS, the AOACI, the United States Pharmacopoeia (USP), NSF International, and others in an attempt to establish standard methods for dietary supplement analysis. The ODS became involved because explicit wording in DSHEA required the Government to use "publicly available" analytical methods for enforcement actions involving dietary supplements. In response to the need for such publicly available methods and to support efforts to validate methods used in biomedical research on dietary supplement ingredients, ODS established the Analytical Methods and Reference Materials (AMRM) program in 2002.

ODS has been involved in sponsoring the creation of AOAC Official Methods of Analysis for dietary supplements and in the development and dissemination of numerous analytical methods and reference materials for 15 ingredients in dietary supplements in the USA, 32 botanical identification and documentation projects, and 45 studies determining contamination and adulterants. It has also helped to develop guidance on the validation of identity methods for botanical ingredients [70] and the conduct of single-laboratory validation studies for dietary supplements, Appendix K, AOAC Official Methods of Analysis, and provided guidance to evaluation of the literature on botanical supplements [71,72]. The portion of the ODS website includes a searchable database of analytical methods; these can be accessed at: https://ods.od.nih.gov/Research/AMRMProgramWebsite.aspx.

ODS also supports the Dietary Supplement Laboratory Quality Assurance Program in which participants measure concentrations of active and/or marker compounds and nutritional and toxic elements in practice and test materials. Exercises have included water and fat-soluble vitamins, nutritional and toxic elements, fatty acids, contaminants (e.g., aflatoxins, polyaromatic hydrocarbons (PAH's)) and botanical markers (e.g., phytosterols and flavonoids).

4.4. Reference Materials

ODS supports the development of certified reference materials for dietary supplement ingredients with assigned values for concentrations of active and/or marker compounds, pesticides, and toxic metals to assist in the verification of product label claims and in quality control during the manufacturing process. A reference material is a material that is sufficiently homogeneous and stable with respect to one or more specified properties, which have been established to be fit for its intended use in a measurement process. A certified reference material (CRM) is a reference material characterized by a metrologically valid procedure for one or more specified properties, accompanied by a certificate that provides the value of the specified property, its associated uncertainty, and a statement of metrological traceability. Certified reference materials can be used for laboratory proficiency studies, methods development, method verification, and method validation studies. Calibration standards are the single chemical entities necessary for construction of calibration curves for quantitative analysis and for confirming analyte identity. Several processes are used to produce calibration standards. ODS provided funding to the U.S. Department of Commerce's National Institute of Standards and Technology (NIST) for the development and distribution of calibration standard solutions and matrix standard reference materials (SRM®; a NIST-trademarked type of CRM). The materials fall into one of the following categories: (1) pure chemical entities or their mixtures, including many nutrients and other ingredients in dietary supplements for use in establishing analyte identity and for calibrating instruments; (2) natural matrix materials that represent the supply chain of a particular dietary supplement, e.g., biomass (ginkgo leaves and powder), processed botanical ingredient (ginkgo extract), finished product; (3) natural matrix materials that cover a range of analytes including nutritional compounds, botanical marker compounds, and compounds with known health concerns (heavy metals, pesticides, plant toxins); and (4) Clinical materials that can be used to assist clinical laboratories assess nutrient status or exposure, such as the measure of measure of vitamin D status commonly used around the world, serum 25-hydroxyvitamin D [73–75]. ODS is now expanding efforts to develop biomarkers of nutrient exposure and status in blood and other biological specimens in relation to chronic disease risk in individuals and populations. ODS has worked with NIST to produce and make available reference materials for calibration of various laboratory methods. Supplementary Table S1 shows NIST Standard Reference Materials (SRM®) now available. Supplementary Table S2 shows dietary supplement and nutritional assessment SRMs that are currently in progress.

4.5. Dietary Supplement Databases

Two databases have been developed by ODS that are described elsewhere in detail [76–80]. The goal of the Dietary Supplement Label Database (DSLD) is to include labels for virtually all dietary supplements sold in the USA. This provides all the information on the product label including composition, claims, and manufacturer contact information. It now contains over 72,000 dietary supplement labels, with new labels added at the rate of 1000 per month. Used together with food composition databases it is possible to estimate total daily intakes of nutrients and other bioactive ingredients from both foods and dietary supplements. A mobile version of DSLD is now available for use on smartphones to enhance consumer access to it [78,80]. It is primarily aimed at researchers and so contains information about products that are currently on the market, as well as those that have been removed from the market.

The Dietary Supplement Ingredient Database (DSID) provides analytically derived information on the amount of labeled ingredients of a representative sample of commonly used categories of supplement products sold in the USA, including adult, child and prenatal MVM supplements and omega-3 fatty acids. DSID is now being expanded to examine botanicals and other ingredients in supplements that are of public health interest, such as green tea products. Calculators included with the DSID permit a consumer to examine how closely the labeled contents of a nutrient in a product compare to chemical analyses of all products in the category [79].

4.6. Nutrition Research Methods and Review Methodology

Systematic reviews of dietary supplements require special techniques. ODS has sponsored a series of technical reports on the application of review methodology to the field of nutrition and dietary supplements [81–86]. Staff have also collaborated in performing systematic reviews with other groups [87,88].

4.7. Population-Based Monitoring of Dietary Supplement Use

In collaboration with the National Health and Nutrition Examination Survey (NHANES) of the National Center for Health Statistics, ODS investigates patterns of dietary supplement use using national and other large cohorts, and assesses supplements' effects on total nutrient intakes. Several studies have focused on adults [89], children [90,91], and others in the population and their supplement use. Other studies have focused on the contributions to total intakes of nutrients made by dietary supplements. Investigators at ODS have been active in funding monitoring efforts on the links between intakes of folic acid and health [92]. They have devoted particular attention to blood levels of folic acid and dietary intake patterns that are associated with very low and very high intakes of the nutrient [93–95]. The survey methods used are well documented and they may be useful for those in other countries planning similar population-based surveys to consult [96].

The motivations for use of dietary supplements are also documented; they often differ from those specified in regulations. NHANES contains several items that are consumer tested and available for use in other surveys on motivations. Knowledge of motivations can improve understanding of how people use these products and may provide clues for encouraging appropriate supplement use.

4.8. Translation of Supplement Science for Health Professionals and the Public

ODS has produced and periodically updates a library of more than two dozen fact sheets on the ingredients in supplements such as vitamin D, magnesium, and special products such as MVM supplements and products marketed for weight loss. There is a detailed version for professionals that is complete with detailed references, as well as easy-to-read versions for consumers in both English and Spanish. ODS also works with the National Library of Medicine (NLM) to produce and update a Dietary Supplement Subset of NLM's PubMed. The National Center for Complementary and Integrative Health (NCCIH) at NIH produces a series of fact sheets on many botanicals and other non-nutrient bioactives in supplements that are also useful. They can be accessed at https://www.nccih.nih.gov. ODS also hosts an intensive, free 3-day course on issues in dietary supplement research annually for researchers. Further information about these and other projects is accessible at: https://www.ods.od.nih.gov.

4.9. Other Resources

In order to foster the development of appropriate study methods for dietary supplement research, ODS sponsors workshops on the latest knowledge and emerging approaches to the study of dietary supplements. It also supports the development of cutting–edge approaches to elucidate the mechanisms of action of complex botanical dietary supplements. It co-funds the Centers for Advancing Research on Natural Products (CARBON) with the NCCIM, including its program to develop high content high throughput methods to rapidly generate hypotheses on active compounds and the cellular targets. These and other resources are announced as they become available on the ODS website.

4.10. Fostering Use of Systematic Evidence Reviews in Policy Making and Clinical Practice

ODS has strengthened the scientific framework for developing dietary recommendations by encouraging the incorporation of systematic reviews into the development of the DRI. It has sponsored 18 systematic reviews on topics related to dietary supplements. These include ephedra, B vitamins, MVM supplements, omega-3 fatty acids, soy, probiotics, and vitamin D. The ephedra systematic review was helpful to the US government in banning ephedra products from the US market. The systematic reviews of omega-3 fatty acids funded over a decade ago and more recent updates on their associations with cardiovascular disease and infant health outcomes have been useful for planning intervention programs as well as for regulatory purposes. Current AHRQ reviews are available on the AHRQ website (https://www.ahrq.gov).

5. Future Needs

Attitudes toward safety, efficacy, and values about what is important in food and life will be important in determining future needs involving supplement science in the countries we have discussed and perhaps elsewhere in the world. Safety is critical, and requires better chains of custody and product characterization that exists at present for these products, particularly those involving global markets. Efficacy, that is that the health promotion claims for the product are true and not misleading is also critical. Demonstrating efficacy requires clinical studies with well defined products and rigorous experimental designs, and the studies must be replicable. To that end, many publishers now require that submitted manuscripts comply with established guidelines for the reporting of clinical trial results (e.g., CONSORT guidelines), while funders require demonstration of product integrity by applicants [97,98]. Finally there are issues of personal choice and values, sometimes involving the efficacy of supplements as complementary and alternative therapies that are part of a larger philosophical or religious world views and systems. These must be accommodated without abandoning safety.

Both basic and more applied challenges will continue well into the future. Much remains to be learned about the effects of bioactive constituents such as flavonoids in foods and dietary supplements on health outcomes, as many recent papers in Nutrients and elsewhere indicate [99–101]. More and better biomarkers need to be developed and their associations with health outcomes clarified [102]. Supplements intended to enhance sports performance [103] botanicals used for disease treatment [104] and those ingredients thought to slow aging [105] all require identification of valid biomarkers of efficacy as well as of exposure. The role of supplements and the gut microbiome also must be explored for its associations with common diseases and conditions [106]. The associations between supplement ingredients and health outcomes in chronic degenerative disease must be clarified [47,105,107–109]. High risk groups need more attention Certain subgroups within the population such as athletes consume very high amounts of some supplements and it is important to monitor them to prevent adverse outcomes and study the effects, if any, on athletic performance [110]. Others use supplements in the hope that they will improve cognitive performance [103]. Those who practice polypharmacy with prescription, non-prescription drugs and dietary supplements represent another high-risk group, and interventions to limit the potential for adverse events are needed [111,112]. Collaborations among scientists in many countries are needed to drive supplement science forward.

Irrespective of the type of health product, high quality science is fundamental to the success of any regulatory framework. Assessments of the safety, quality and efficacy of nutrients and other bioactives are needed to provide the scientific information that regulators need [113]. As mentioned earlier, the nature and diversity of the sector means that regulators face a number of very specific challenges for these low risk products. These include evaluating traditional evidence, dealing with products that contain multiple bio-actives and addressing the growing challenges of ensuring product quality. It is critical that scientists and regulators work together and learn from each other in both identifying issues and developing ways in which they can be addressed. Although regulatory challenges must be met at the national level, there must be due regard paid to the fact that national regulatory decisions about supplements have global implications.

6. Conclusions

Science is vital in regulatory settings, and there is no reason that science and regulation should be incompatible [114]. The challenges in supplement science and its regulation provide new opportunities for scientists and regulators to work together both nationally and internationally, to learn from each other, and to cooperate and when appropriate harmonize approaches to improve the public health.

Supplementary Materials: The following are available online at www.mdpi.com/2072-6643/10/1/41/s1, Tables S1 and S2 Table S1 Standard Reference Materials (SRM®) available from the National Institute of Science and Technology, US Department of Commerce. Table S2 Dietary supplement and nutritional assessment Standard Reference Materials (SRM®) currently under development at the National Institute of Science and Technology, US Department of Commerce (as of December 2016).

Acknowledgments: Funded by the National Institutes of Health, Bethesda, MD, USA. We thank Joseph M. Betz, Leila Saldanha, Cara Welsh, for their thoughtful and critical reviews of the manuscript, and Joyce Merkel, for technical editing and support.

Author Contributions: J.T.D. and P.M.C. developed the concept for the manuscript. J.T.D., P.M.C. and M.J.S. wrote the manuscript.

Conflicts of Interest: Johanna T. Dwyer holds stock in several food and drug companies, and serves on the scientific advisory boards of Conagra Foods, McCormick Spices, and as a consultant for Gerber/Nestle. She accepted partial travel and per diem expenses to speak at a symposium on dietary supplements sponsored by the International Association of Dietary/Food Supplement Associations at the International Congress of Nutrition in Buenos Aires, Argentina in October 2017. Michael J. Smith holds stock in several food and drug companies as well as acting as a consultant with clients in both the private and public sector including companies in dietary supplement and natural health products sector. He sits on the scientific advisory board of ISURA and the advisory board of the American Botanical Council. Paul M. Coates reports no conflicts of interest.

References

1.   White, A. Growth-inhibition produced in rats by the oral administration of sodium benzoate: Effects of various dietary supplements. *Yale J. Biol. Med.* **1941**, *13*, 759–768. [PubMed]

2. Kantor, E.D.; Rehm, C.D.; Du, M.; White, E.; Giovannucci, E.L. Trends in dietary supplement use among US adults from 1999–2012. *JAMA Intern. Med.* **2016**, *316*, 1464–1474. [CrossRef] [PubMed]
3. Marik, P.E.; Flemmer, M. Do dietary supplements have beneficial health effects in industrialized nations: What is the evidence? *JPEN J. Parenter. Enter. Nutr.* **2012**, *36*, 159–168. [CrossRef] [PubMed]
4. Manson, J.E.; Brannon, P.M.; Rosen, C.J.; Taylor, C.L. Vitamin D deficiency—Is there really a pandemic? *N. Engl. J. Med.* **2016**, *375*, 1817–1820. [CrossRef] [PubMed]
5. Balentine, D.A.; Dwyer, J.T.; Erdman, J.W., Jr.; Ferruzzi, M.G.; Gaine, P.C.; Harnly, J.M.; Kwik-Uribe, C.L. Recommendations on reporting requirements for flavonoids in research. *Am. J. Clin. Nutr.* **2015**, *101*, 1113–1125. [CrossRef] [PubMed]
6. Betz, J.M.; (NIH Office of Dietary Supplements, Bethesda, MD, USA). Personal communication, 2017.
7. Mudge, E.M.; Betz, J.M.; Brown, P.N. The importance of method selection in determining product integrity for nutrition research. *Adv. Nutr.* **2016**, *7*, 390–398. [CrossRef] [PubMed]
8. Orhan, I.E.; Senol, F.S.; Skalicka-Wozniak, K.; Georgiev, M.; Sener, B. Adulteration and safety issues in nutraceuticals and dietary supplements: Innocent or risky? In *Nutraceuticals, Nanotechnology in the Agri-Food Industry*; Grumezescu, A.M., Ed.; Academic Press: Amsterdam, The Netherlands, 2016; Volume 4, pp. 153–182.
9. AOAC International. AOAC International guidelines for validation of botanical identification methods. *J. AOAC Int.* **2012**, *95*, 268–272.
10. Dwyer, J.T.; Holden, J.; Andrews, K.; Roseland, J.; Zhao, C.; Schweitzer, A.; Perry, C.R.; Harnly, J.; Wolf, W.R.; Picciano, M.F.; et al. Measuring vitamins and minerals in dietary supplements for nutrition studies in the USA. *Anal. Bioanal. Chem.* **2007**, *389*, 37–46. [CrossRef] [PubMed]
11. Swanson, C.A. Suggested guidelines for articles about botanical dietary supplements. *Am. J. Clin. Nutr.* **2002**, *75*, 8–10. [PubMed]
12. Wolsko, P.M.; Solondz, D.K.; Phillips, R.S.; Schachter, S.C.; Eisenberg, D.M. Lack of herbal supplement characterization in published randomized controlled trials. *Am. J. Med.* **2005**, *118*, 1087–1093. [CrossRef] [PubMed]
13. Gagnier, J.J.; DeMelo, J.; Boon, H.; Rochon, P.; Bombardier, C. Quality of reporting of randomized controlled trials of herbal medicine interventions. *Am. J. Med.* **2006**, *119*, 800.e1–800.e11. [CrossRef] [PubMed]
14. Dwyer, J.; Costello, R.B.; Merkel, J. Assessment of dietary supplements. In *Nutrition in the Prevention and Treatment of Disease*, 4th ed.; Coulston, A.M., Boushey, C.J., Rerruzai, M.G., Delahaty, L.M., Eds.; Academic Press: London, UK, 2017; pp. 49–70.
15. Ahluwalia, N.; Dwyer, J.; Terry, A.; Moshfegh, A.; Johnson, C. Update on NHANES dietary data: Focus on collection, release, analytical considerations, and uses to inform public policy. *Adv. Nutr.* **2016**, *7*, 121–134. [CrossRef] [PubMed]
16. Chan, M. Forward. In *WHO Traditional Medicine Strategy: 2014–2023*; WHO: Hong Kong, China, 2013; pp. 7–8.
17. Dickinson, A. History and overview of DSHEA. *Fitoterapia* **2011**, *82*, 5–10. [CrossRef] [PubMed]
18. Taylor, C.L. Regulatory frameworks for functional foods and dietary supplements. *Nutr. Rev.* **2004**, *62*, 55–59. [CrossRef] [PubMed]
19. Australian Government Department of Health Therapeutic Goods Administration. The Poisons Standard (the SUSMP). Available online: https://www.tga.gov.au/publication/poisons-standard-susmp (accessed on 17 September 2017).
20. U.S. Food and Drug Administration. Dietary Supplements. Available online: https://www.fda.gov/food/dietarysupplements/ (accessed on 17 September 2017).
21. Health Canada. Monograph: Melatonin—Oral. Available online: http://webprod.hc-sc.gc.ca/nhpid-bdipsn/monoReq.do?id=136 (accessed on 17 September 2017).
22. Ventola, C.L. Current issues regarding complementary and alternative medicine (CAM) in the United States: Part 2: Regulatory and safety concerns and proposed governmental policy changes with respect to dietary supplements. *P T* **2010**, *35*, 514–522. [PubMed]
23. World Health Organization. National Policy on Traditional Medicine and Regulation of Herbal Medicines—Report of a WHO Global Survey. Available online: http://apps.who.int/medicinedocs/en/d/Js7916e/ (accessed on 6 November 2017).

24. Health Canada Natural and Non-prescription Health Products Directorate (NNHPD) About Natural Health Product Regulation in Canada. Available online: https://www.canada.ca/en/health-canada/services/drugs-health-products/natural-non-prescription/regulation.html (accessed on 5 September 2017).
25. Australian Government Department of Health Therapeutic Goods Administration. Exposure Drafts: Therapeutic Goods Amendment (2017 Measures No. 1) Bill 2017 and Therapeutic Goods (Charges) Amendment Bill 2017. Available online: https://www.tga.gov.au/consultation/consultation-exposure-drafts-2017 (accessed on 17 September 2017).
26. European Commission Directorate-General for Health and Food Safety. Herbal Medicinal Products. Available online: https://ec.europa.eu/health/human-use/herbal-medicines_en (accessed on 17 September 2017).
27. U.S. Food and Drug Administration. New Dietary Ingredients (NDI) Notification Process. Available online: https://www.fda.gov/food/dietarysupplements/newdietaryingredientsnotificationprocess/default.htm (accessed on 17 September 2017).
28. Australian Government Department of Health Therapeutic Goods Administration. Australian Regulatory Guidelines for Complementary Medicines (ARGCM). Available online: https://www.tga.gov.au/publication/australian-regulatory-guidelines-complementary-medicines-argcm (accessed on 17 September 2017).
29. Australian Government Department of Health Therapeutic Goods Administration. Medicines and Medical Devices Regulation Review. Available online: https://www.tga.gov.au/mmdr (accessed on 17 September 2017).
30. Australian Government Department of Health Therapeutic Goods Administration. Australian Government Response to the Review of Medicines and Medical Devices Regulation. Available online: https://www.tga.gov.au/australian-government-response-review-medicines-and-medical-devices-regulation (accessed on 17 September 2017).
31. Government of Canada. Category Specific Guidance for Temporary Marketing Authorization: Supplemented Food. Available online: https://www.canada.ca/en/health-canada/services/food-nutrition/legislation-guidelines/guidance-documents/category-specific-guidance-temporary-marketing-authorization-supplemented-food.html (accessed on 17 September 2017).
32. Government of Canada Health Canada. Consulting Canadians on the Regulation of Self-Care Products in Canada. Available online: https://www.canada.ca/en/health-canada/programs/consultation-regulation-self-care-products/consulting-canadians-regulation-self-care-products-canada.html (accessed on 17 September 2017).
33. Physiopedia. Evidence Based Practice (EBP). Available online: https://www.physio-pedia.com/Evidence_Based_Practice_(EBP) (accessed on 17 September 2017).
34. Australian Government Department of Health Therapeutic Goods Administration. Complementary Medicine Interface Issues. Available online: https://www.tga.gov.au/complementary-medicine-interface-issues (accessed on 17 September 2017).
35. Singapore Government Health Science Authority. ASEAN Harmonization of Traditional Medicines and Health Supplements. Available online: http://www.hsa.gov.sg/content/hsa/en/Health_Products_Regulation/Complementary_Health_Products/Overview/ASEAN_Harmonization_of_Traditional_Medicines_and_Health_Supplements.html (accessed on 17 September 2017).
36. World Health Organization. International Regulatory Cooperation for Herbal Medicines (IRCH). Available online: http://www.who.int/medicines/areas/traditional/irch/en/ (accessed on 17 September 2017).
37. Gorman, U.; Mathers, J.C.; Grimaldi, K.A.; Ahlgren, J.; Nordstrom, K. Do we know enough? A scientific and ethical analysis of the basis for genetic-based personalized nutrition. *Genes Nutr.* **2013**, *8*, 373–381. [CrossRef] [PubMed]
38. De Toro-Martin, J.; Arsenault, B.J.; Despres, J.P.; Vohl, M.C. Precision nutrition: A review of personalized nutritional approaches for the prevention and management of metabolic syndrome. *Nutrients* **2017**, *9*, 913. [CrossRef] [PubMed]
39. World Health Organization. WHO Traditional Medicine Strategy: 2014–2023. Available online: http://www.who.int/medicines/publications/traditional/trm_strategy14_23/en/ (accessed on 17 September 2017).
40. Drueke, T.B.; Massy, Z.A. Role of vitamin D in vascular calcification: Bad guy or good guy? *Nephrol. Dial. Transplant.* **2012**, *27*, 1704–1707. [CrossRef] [PubMed]
41. Rooney, M.R.; Harnack, L.; Michos, E.D.; Ogilvie, R.P.; Sempos, C.T.; Lutsey, P.L. Trends in use of high-dose vitamin D supplements exceeding 1000 or 4000 international units daily, 1999–2014. *JAMA Intern. Med.* **2017**, *317*, 2448–2450. [CrossRef] [PubMed]

42. Prentice, R.L.; Pettinger, M.B.; Jackson, R.D.; Wactawski-Wende, J.; Lacroix, A.Z.; Anderson, G.L.; Chlebowski, R.T.; Manson, J.E.; Van Horn, L.; Vitolins, M.Z.; et al. Health risks and benefits from calcium and vitamin D supplementation: Women's Health Initiative clinical trial and cohort study. *Osteoporos. Int.* **2013**, *24*, 567–580. [CrossRef] [PubMed]
43. Fulgoni, V.L., 3rd; Keast, D.R.; Bailey, R.L.; Dwyer, J. Foods, fortificants, and supplements: Where do Americans get their nutrients? *J. Nutr.* **2011**, *141*, 1847–1854. [CrossRef] [PubMed]
44. Boyles, A.L.; Yetley, E.A.; Thayer, K.A.; Coates, P.M. Safe use of high intakes of folic acid: Research challenges and paths forward. *Nutr. Rev.* **2016**, *74*, 469–474. [CrossRef] [PubMed]
45. Dwyer, J.T.; Wiemer, K.L.; Dary, O.; Keen, C.L.; King, J.C.; Miller, K.B.; Philbert, M.A.; Tarasuk, V.; Taylor, C.L.; Gaine, P.C.; et al. Fortification and health: Challenges and opportunities. *Adv. Nutr.* **2015**, *6*, 124–131. [CrossRef] [PubMed]
46. Dwyer, J.T.; Woteki, C.; Bailey, R.; Britten, P.; Carriquiry, A.; Gaine, P.C.; Miller, D.; Moshfegh, A.; Murphy, M.M.; Smith Edge, M. Fortification: New findings and implications. *Nutr. Rev.* **2014**, *72*, 127–141. [CrossRef] [PubMed]
47. Yetley, E.A.; MacFarlane, A.J.; Greene-Finestone, L.S.; Garza, C.; Ard, J.D.; Atkinson, S.A.; Bier, D.M.; Carriquiry, A.L.; Harlan, W.R.; Hattis, D.; et al. Options for basing Dietary Reference Intakes (DRIs) on chronic disease endpoints: Report from a joint US-/Canadian-sponsored working group. *Am. J. Clin. Nutr.* **2017**, *105*, 249s–285s. [CrossRef] [PubMed]
48. Gaine, P.C.; Balentine, D.A.; Erdman, J.W., Jr.; Dwyer, J.T.; Ellwood, K.C.; Hu, F.B.; Russell, R.M. Are dietary bioactives ready for recommended intakes? *Adv. Nutr.* **2013**, *4*, 539–541. [CrossRef] [PubMed]
49. Brown, A.C. Liver toxicity related to herbs and dietary supplements: Online table of case reports. Part 2 of 5 series. *Food Chem. Toxicol.* **2017**, *107*, 472–501. [CrossRef] [PubMed]
50. Saldanha, L.; Dwyer, J.; Andrews, K.; Betz, J.; Harnly, J.; Pehrsson, P.; Rimmer, C.; Savarala, S. Feasibility of including green tea products for an analytically verified dietary supplement database. *J. Food Sci.* **2015**, *80*, H883–H888. [CrossRef] [PubMed]
51. Sander, L.C.; Bedner, M.; Tims, M.C.; Yen, J.H.; Duewer, D.L.; Porter, B.; Christopher, S.J.; Day, R.D.; Long, S.E.; Molloy, J.L.; et al. Development and certification of green tea-containing standard reference materials. *Anal. Bioanal. Chem.* **2012**, *402*, 473–487. [CrossRef] [PubMed]
52. De Boer, Y.S.; Sherker, A.H. Herbal and dietary supplement-induced liver injury. *Clin. Liver Dis.* **2017**, *21*, 135–149. [CrossRef] [PubMed]
53. Avigan, M.I.; Mozersky, R.P.; Seeff, L.B. Scientific and regulatory perspectives in herbal and dietary supplement associated hepatotoxicity in the United States. *Int. J. Mol. Sci.* **2016**, *17*, 331. [CrossRef] [PubMed]
54. Brown, A.C. An overview of herb and dietary supplement efficacy, safety and government regulations in the United States with suggested improvements. Part 1 of 5 series. *Food Chem. Toxicol.* **2017**, *107*, 449–471. [CrossRef] [PubMed]
55. Gardiner, P.; Phillips, R.; Shaughnessy, A.F. Herbal and dietary supplement-drug interactions in patients with chronic illnesses. *Am. Fam. Physician* **2008**, *77*, 73–78. [PubMed]
56. Tsai, H.H.; Lin, H.W.; Simon Pickard, A.; Tsai, H.Y.; Mahady, G.B. Evaluation of documented drug interactions and contraindications associated with herbs and dietary supplements: A systematic literature review. *Int. J. Clin. Pract.* **2012**, *66*, 1056–1078. [CrossRef] [PubMed]
57. Gagnier, J.J.; Boon, H.; Rochon, P.; Moher, D.; Barnes, J.; Bombardier, C.; Group, C. Reporting randomized, controlled trials of herbal interventions: An elaborated CONSORT statement. *Ann. Intern. Med.* **2006**, *144*, 364–367. [CrossRef] [PubMed]
58. Blumberg, J.B.; Frei, B.B.; Fulgoni, V.L.; Weaver, C.M.; Zeisel, S.H. Impact of frequency of multi-vitamin/multi-mineral supplement intake on nutritional adequacy and nutrient deficiencies in U.S. adults. *Nutrients* **2017**, *9*, 849. [CrossRef] [PubMed]
59. Raghavan, R.; Ashour, F.S.; Bailey, R. A review of cutoffs for nutritional biomarkers. *Adv. Nutr.* **2016**, *7*, 112–120. [CrossRef] [PubMed]
60. Centers for Disease Control and Prevention National Center for Environmental Health Division of Laboratory Sciences. *Second National Report on Biochemical Indicators of Diet and Nutrition in the U.S. Population*; Centers for Disease Control and Prevention: Atlanta, GA, USA, 2012.
61. Bailey, L.B.; Stover, P.J.; McNulty, H.; Fenech, M.F.; Gregory, J.F., 3rd; Mills, J.L.; Pfeiffer, C.M.; Fazili, Z.; Zhang, M.; Ueland, P.M.; et al. Biomarkers of nutrition for development-folate review. *J. Nutr.* **2015**, *115*, 1636s–1680s. [CrossRef] [PubMed]

62. Branum, A.M.; Bailey, R.; Singer, B.J. Dietary supplement use and folate status during pregnancy in the United States. *J. Nutr.* **2013**, *143*, 486–492. [CrossRef] [PubMed]
63. Balk, E.M.; Lichtenstein, A.H. Omega-3 fatty acids and cardiovascular disease: Summary of the 2016 Agency of Healthcare Research and Quality evidence review. *Nutrients* **2017**, *9*, 865. [CrossRef] [PubMed]
64. Ershow, A.G.; Skaeff, S.; Merkel, J.; Pehrsson, P. Development of databases on iodine in foods and dietary supplements. *Nutrients* **2018**, in press.
65. Taylor, C.L.; Sempos, C.T.; Davis, C.D.; Brannon, P.M. Vitamin D: Moving forward to address emerging science. *Nutrients* **2017**, *9*, 1308. [CrossRef] [PubMed]
66. Brannon, P.M.; Taylor, C.L. Iron supplementation during pregnancy and infancy: Uncertainties and implications for research and policy. *Nutrients* **2017**, *9*, 1327. [CrossRef] [PubMed]
67. Kuszak, A.J.; Hopp, D.C.; Williamson, J.S.; Betz, J.M.; Sorkin, B.C. Approaches by the U.S. National Institutes of Health to support rigorous scientific research on dietary supplements and natural products. *Drug Test. Anal.* **2016**, *8*, 413–417. [CrossRef] [PubMed]
68. Betz, J.M.; Fisher, K.D.; Saldanha, L.G.; Coates, P.M. The NIH analytical methods and reference materials program for dietary supplements. *Anal. Bioanal. Chem.* **2007**, *389*, 19–25. [CrossRef] [PubMed]
69. Betz, J.M.; Brown, P.N.; Roman, M.C. Accuracy, precision, and reliability of chemical measurements in natural products research. *Fitoterapia* **2011**, *82*, 44–52. [CrossRef] [PubMed]
70. LaBudde, R.A.; Harnly, J.M. Probability of identification: A statistical model for the validation of qualitative botanical identification methods. *J. AOAC Int.* **2012**, *95*, 273–285. [CrossRef] [PubMed]
71. Betz, J.M.; Hardy, M.L. Evaluating the botanic dietary supplement literature. In *The HERBAL Guide: Dietary Supplement Resources for the Clinician*; Bonakdar, R.A., Ed.; Lippincott Williams and Wilkins: Philadelphia, PA, USA, 2010; pp. 175–184.
72. Betz, J.M.; Hardy, M.L. Evaluating the botanical dietary supplement literature: How healthcare providers can better understand the scientific and clinical literature on herbs and phytomedicines. *HerbalGram* **2014**, *101*, 58–67.
73. Brooks, S.P.J.; Sempos, C.T. The importance of 25-hydroxyvitamin D assay standardization and the Vitamin D Standardization Program. *J. AOAC Int.* **2017**, *100*, 1223–1224. [CrossRef] [PubMed]
74. Phinney, K.W.; Tai, S.S.; Bedner, M.; Camara, J.E.; Chia, R.R.C.; Sander, L.C.; Sharpless, K.E.; Wise, S.A.; Yen, J.H.; Schleicher, R.L.; et al. Development of an improved standard reference material for vitamin D metabolites in human serum. *Anal. Chem.* **2017**, *89*, 4907–4913. [CrossRef] [PubMed]
75. Phinney, K.W.; Bedner, M.; Tai, S.S.; Vamathevan, V.V.; Sander, L.C.; Sharpless, K.E.; Wise, S.A.; Yen, J.H.; Schleicher, R.L.; Chaudhary-Webb, M.; et al. Development and certification of a standard reference material for vitamin D metabolites in human serum. *Anal. Chem.* **2012**, *84*, 956–962. [CrossRef] [PubMed]
76. Dwyer, J.T.; Picciano, M.F.; Betz, J.M.; Fisher, K.D.; Saldanha, L.G.; Yetley, E.A.; Coates, P.M.; Milner, J.A.; Whitted, J.; Burt, V.; et al. Progress in developing analytical and label-based dietary supplement databases at the NIH Office of Dietary Supplements. *J. Food Compost. Anal.* **2008**, *21*, S83–S93. [CrossRef] [PubMed]
77. Dwyer, J.T.; Saldanha, L.G.; Bailen, R.A.; Bailey, R.L.; Costello, R.B.; Betz, J.M.; Chang, F.F.; Goshorn, J.; Andrews, K.W.; Pehrsson, P.R.; et al. A free new dietary supplement label database for registered dietitian nutritionists. *J. Acad. Nutr. Diet.* **2014**, *114*, 1512–1517. [CrossRef] [PubMed]
78. Dwyer, J.T.; (NIH Office of Dietary Supplements, Bethesda, MD, USA). Personal communication, 2017.
79. Andrews, K.W.; (USDA-ARS Beltsville Human Nutrition Research Center, Beltsville, MD, USA). Personal communication, 2017.
80. Saldanha, L.G.; (NIH Office of Dietary Supplements, Bethesda, MD, USA). Personal communication, 2017.
81. Lichtenstein, A.H.; Yetley, E.A.; Lau, J. *Application of Systematic Review Methodology to the Field of Nutrition: Nutritional Research Series*; Agency for Healthcare Research and Quality: Rockville, MD, USA, 2009; Volume 1.
82. Helfand, M.; Balshem, H. AHRQ series paper 2: Principles for developing guidance: AHRQ and the effective health-care program. *J. Clin. Epidemiol.* **2010**, *63*, 484–490. [CrossRef] [PubMed]
83. Trikalinos, T.A.; Lee, J.; Moorthy, D.; Yu, W.W.; Lau, J.; Lichtenstein, A.H.; Chung, M. *Effects of Eicosapentanoic Acid and Docosahexanoic Acid on Mortality across Diverse Settings: Systematic Review and Meta-Analysis of Randomized Trials and Prospective Cohorts: Nutritional Research Series*; Agency for Healthcare Research and Quality: Rockville, MD, USA, 2012; Volume 4.

84. Trikalinos, T.A.; Moorthy, D.; Chung, M.; Yu, W.W.; Lee, J.H.; Lichtenstein, A.H.; Lau, J. *Comparison of Translational Patterns in Two Nutrient-Disease Associations*; Agency for Healthcare Research and Quality: Rockville, MD, USA, 2011.

85. Moorthy, D.; Chung, M.; Lee, J.; Yu, W.W.; Lau, J.; Trikalinos, T.A. *Concordance between the Findings of Epidemiological Studies and Randomized Trials in Nutrition: An Empirical Evaluation and Citation Analysis*; Agency for Healthcare Research and Quality: Rockville, MD, USA, 2013.

86. Brannon, P.M.; Taylor, C.L.; Coates, P.M. Use and applications of systematic reviews in public health nutrition. *Annu. Rev. Nutr.* **2014**, *34*, 401–419. [CrossRef] [PubMed]

87. Ko, R.; Low Dog, T.; Gorecki, D.K.; Cantilena, L.R.; Costello, R.B.; Evans, W.J.; Hardy, M.L.; Jordan, S.A.; Maughan, R.J.; Rankin, J.W.; et al. Evidence-based evaluation of potential benefits and safety of beta-alanine supplementation for military personnel. *Nutr. Rev.* **2014**, *72*, 217–225. [CrossRef] [PubMed]

88. Brooks, J.R.; Oketch-Rabah, H.; Low Dog, T.; Gorecki, D.K.; Barrett, M.L.; Cantilena, L.; Chung, M.; Costello, R.B.; Dwyer, J.; Hardy, M.L.; et al. Safety and performance benefits of arginine supplements for military personnel: A systematic review. *Nutr. Rev.* **2016**, *74*, 708–721. [CrossRef] [PubMed]

89. Bailey, R.L.; Gahche, J.J.; Miller, P.E.; Thomas, P.R.; Dwyer, J.T. Why US adults use dietary supplements. *JAMA Intern. Med.* **2013**, *173*, 355–361. [CrossRef] [PubMed]

90. Bailey, R.L.; Gahche, J.J.; Thomas, P.R.; Dwyer, J.T. Why US children use dietary supplements. *Pediatr. Res.* **2013**, *74*, 737–741. [CrossRef] [PubMed]

91. Berner, L.A.; Keast, D.R.; Bailey, R.L.; Dwyer, J.T. Fortified foods are major contributors to nutrient intakes in diets of US children and adolescents. *J. Acad. Nutr. Diet.* **2014**, *114*, 1009–1022.e8. [CrossRef] [PubMed]

92. Taylor, C.L.; Bailey, R.L.; Carriquiry, A.L. Use of folate-based and other fortification scenarios illustrates different shifts for tails of the distribution of serum 25-hydroxyvitamin D concentrations. *J. Nutr.* **2015**, *145*, 1623–1629. [CrossRef] [PubMed]

93. Pfeiffer, C.M.; Hughes, J.P.; Lacher, D.A.; Bailey, R.L.; Berry, R.J.; Zhang, M.; Yetley, E.A.; Rader, J.I.; Sempos, C.T.; Johnson, C.L. Estimation of trends in serum and RBC folate in the U.S. population from pre- to postfortification using assay-adjusted data from the NHANES 1988–2010. *J. Nutr.* **2012**, *142*, 886–893. [CrossRef] [PubMed]

94. Pfeiffer, C.M.; Sternberg, M.R.; Hamner, H.C.; Crider, K.S.; Lacher, D.A.; Rogers, L.M.; Bailey, R.L.; Yetley, E.A. Applying inappropriate cutoffs leads to misinterpretation of folate status in the US population. *Am. J. Clin. Nutr.* **2016**, *104*, 1607–1615. [CrossRef] [PubMed]

95. Pfeiffer, C.M.; Lacher, D.A.; Schleicher, R.L.; Johnson, C.L.; Yetley, E.A. Challenges and lessons learned in generating and interpreting NHANES nutritional biomarker data. *Adv. Nutr.* **2017**, *8*, 290–307. [CrossRef] [PubMed]

96. Gahche, J.J.; (NIH Office of Dietary Supplements, Bethesda, MD, USA). Personal communication, 2017.

97. NIH National Center for Complementary and Integrative Health. NCCIH Policy: Natural Product Integrity. Available online: https://nccih.nih.gov/research/policies/naturalproduct.htm (accessed on 7 November 2017).

98. NIH Office of Extramural Research. Grants & Funcing—Rigor and Reproducibility. Available online: https://grants.nih.gov/reproducibility/index.htm#guidance (accessed on 7 November 2017).

99. Sebastian, R.S.; Wilkinson Enns, C.; Goldman, J.D.; Moshfegh, A.J. Dietary flavonoid intake is inversely associated with cardiovascular disease risk as assessed by body mass index and waist circumference among adults in the United States. *Nutrients* **2017**, *9*, 827. [CrossRef] [PubMed]

100. Dwyer, J.T.; Peterson, J. Tea and flavonoids: Where we are, where to go next. *Am. J. Clin. Nutr.* **2013**, *98*, 1611s–1618s. [CrossRef] [PubMed]

101. González-Sarrías, A.; Combet, E.; Pinto, P.; Mena, P.; Dall'Asta, M.; Garcia-Aloy, M.; Rodríguez-Mateos, A.; Gibney, E.R.; Dumont, J.; Massaro, M.; et al. A systematic review and meta-analysis of the effects of flavanol-containing tea, cocoa and apple products on body composition and blood lipids: Exploring the factors responsible for variability in their efficacy. *Nutrients* **2017**, *9*, 746. [CrossRef]

102. Kim, K.; Vance, T.; Chun, O. Greater total antioxidant capacity from diet and supplements is associated with a less atherogenic blood profile in U.S. adults. *Nutrients* **2016**, *8*, 15. [CrossRef] [PubMed]

103. Kuhman, D.J.; Joyner, K.J.; Bloomer, R.J. Cognitive performance and mood following ingestion of a theacrine-containing dietary supplement, caffeine, or placebo by young men and women. *Nutrients* **2015**, *7*, 9618–9632. [CrossRef] [PubMed]

104. Costello, R.B.; Dwyer, J.T.; Bailey, R.L. Chromium supplements for glycemic control in type 2 diabetes: Limited evidence of effectiveness. *Nutr. Rev.* **2016**, *74*, 455–468. [CrossRef] [PubMed]
105. Delmas, D. Nutrients Journal Selected Papers from Resveratrol Regional Meeting 2015—Special Issue. Available online: http://www.mdpi.com/journal/nutrients/special_issues/resveratrol_regional_meeting_2015 (accessed on 30 August 2017).
106. Davis, C.D. The gut microbiome and its role in obesity. *Nutr. Today* **2016**, *51*, 167–174. [CrossRef] [PubMed]
107. Perez-Cano, F.J.; Castell, M. Flavonoids, inflammation and immune system. *Nutrients* **2016**, *8*, 659. [CrossRef] [PubMed]
108. Chamcheu, J.C.; Syed, D.N. Nutrients Journal Special Issue "Nutraceuticals and the Skin: Roles in Health and Disease". Available online: http://www.mdpi.com/journal/nutrients/special_issues/nutraceuticals_skin (accessed on 17 September 2017).
109. Castell, M.; Perez Cano, F.J. Nutrients Journal Special Issue "Flavonoids, Inflammation and Immune System". Available online: http://www.mdpi.com/journal/nutrients/special_issues/flavonoids-inflammation-immune-system (accessed on 1 November 2017).
110. Wardenaar, F.; Brinkmans, N.; Ceelen, I.; Van Rooij, B.; Mensink, M.; Witkamp, R.; De Vries, J. Micronutrient intakes in 553 Dutch elite and sub-elite athletes: Prevalence of low and high intakes in users and non-users of nutritional supplements. *Nutrients* **2017**, *9*, 142. [CrossRef] [PubMed]
111. Chiba, T.; Sato, Y.; Suzuki, S.; Umegaki, K. Concomitant use of dietary supplements and medicines in patients due to miscommunication with physicians in Japan. *Nutrients* **2015**, *7*, 2947–2960. [CrossRef] [PubMed]
112. Chiba, T.; Sato, Y.; Nakanishi, T.; Yokotani, K.; Suzuki, S.; Umegaki, K. Inappropriate usage of dietary supplements in patients by miscommunication with physicians in Japan. *Nutrients* **2014**, *6*, 5392–5404. [CrossRef] [PubMed]
113. Taylor, C.L.; Yetley, E.A. Nutrient risk assessment as a tool for providing scientific assessments to regulators. *J. Nutr.* **2008**, *138*, 1987s–1991s. [PubMed]
114. Yetley, E.A. Science in the regulatory setting: A challenging but incompatible mix? *Novartis Found. Symp.* **2007**, *282*, 59–68; discussion 69–76, 212–218. [PubMed]

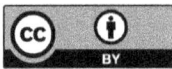

nutrients

MDPI

Review

Current Status of Legislation on Dietary Products for Sportspeople in a European Framework

José Miguel Martínez-Sanz [1,2,*], Isabel Sospedra [1,2], Eduard Baladía [2,3] , Laura Arranz [4], Rocío Ortiz-Moncada [2,5] and Angel Gil-Izquierdo [2,6]

[1]   Nursing Department, Faculty of Health Sciences, University of Alicante, 03690 Alicante, Spain; isospedra@ua.es

[2]   Research Group on Food and Nutrition (ALINUT), University of Alicante, 03690 Alicante, Spain; e.baladia@academianutricion.org (E.B.); rocio.ortiz@ua.es (R.O.-M.); angelgil@cebas.csic.es (A.G.-I.)

[3]   Evidence-Based Nutrition Network (RED-NuBE), Spanish Academy of Nutrition and Dietetics (AEND), 31006 Navarra, Spain

[4]   Department of Nutrition and Food Science, Faculty of Pharmacy, University of Barcelona, 08007 Barcelona, Spain; gana_bcn@yahoo.es

[5]   Department of Community Nursing, Preventive Medicine and Public Health and History of Science Health, University of Alicante, 03690 Alicante, Spain

[6]   Quality, Safety, and Bioactivity of Plant Foods Group, Department of Food Science and Technology, CEBAS-CSIC, University of Murcia, 30100 Murcia, Spain

*   Correspondence: josemiguel.ms@ua.es; Tel.: +34-965909408

Received: 14 September 2017; Accepted: 5 November 2017; Published: 8 November 2017

Abstract: The consumption of nutritional ergogenic aids is conditioned by laws/regulations, but standards/regulations vary between countries. The aim of this review is to explore legislative documents that regulate the use of nutritional ergogenic aids intended for sportspeople in a Spanish/European framework. A narrative review has been developed from official websites of Spanish (Spanish Agency of the Consumer, Food Safety, and Nutrition) and European (European Commission and European Food Safety Authority) bodies. A descriptive analysis of documents was performed. Eighteen legislative documents have been compiled in three sections: (1) Advertising of any type of food and/or product; (2) Composition, labeling, and advertising of foods; (3) Nutritional ergogenic aids. In spite of the existence of these legal documents, the regulation lacks guidance on the use/application of nutritional ergogenic aids for sportspeople. It is essential to prevent the introduction or dissemination of false, ambiguous, or inexact information and contents that induce an error in the receivers of the information. In this field, it is worth highlighting the roles of the European Food Safety Authority and the World Anti-Doping Agency, which provide information about consumer guidelines, prescribing practices, and recommendations for the prudent use of nutritional ergogenic aids.

Keywords: food legislation; health claims; nutritional ergogenic aids

1. Introduction

Ergogenic aids have been defined as substances or methods used to improve endurance, total fitness level, and sports performance; they could be anything that gives a mental or physical edge while exercising or competing. These aids are classified as nutritional, pharmacologic, physiologic, or psychological [1,2]. In the field of nutrition, foods and food components that can improve the capacity of an individual to perform an exercise task have also been described as ergogenic aids [3].

In the context of sport, nutritional ergogenic aids are commonly known as dietary or sport supplements, sports food, or food aids, and have been used for different purposes: in particular, to increase energy, maintain strength, health and the immune system, enhance performance, and prevent nutritional deficiencies [4–7]. However, the use of sports food involves both benefits and risks. Its inadequate consumption can cause adverse effects on the athlete's health [6,8]. An example of these undesirable effects are unintentional doping situations, caused by the intake of nutritional ergogenic aids containing substances prohibited by the World Anti-Doping Agency (WADA) [9].

The consumption of nutritional ergogenic aids by athletes is conditioned by specific laws, regulations, or instructions. Such legislation should provide advice or recommendations regarding the usage, dose, security, and any precautions and warnings for these substances. It should also provide information about their market access and availability, as well as their efficiency with respect to enhancing sport performance.

These are general principles of action on public health to ensure that the population can achieve or maintain the highest standard of health [10]. However, some popular products are marketed as ergogenic aids despite a lack of objective evidence to support claims of an ergogenic effect [11].

Standards and regulations on nutritional ergogenic aids vary between countries and also between different types of products. In the European Union and its member states, several provisions on sport foods can be found. All of them include labeling (health or performance claims in labels), safety, and marketing aspects and the contents of vitamins, minerals, and other substances [12,13]. However, currently there is no specific legislation on nutritional ergogenic aids.

Misleading advertising as well as an incomplete labeling may also have consequences for the health of the consumers due to a chemical risk linked to doping substances, if non-approved ingredients are used or contamination occurs [14,15].

Beyond European borders, similar situations can be found. In the United States, the Food and Drug Administration (FDA), broadly speaking, regulates quality and the Federal Trade Commission supervises the marketing and advertising of dietary supplements [16]. According to the Dietary Supplement Health and Education Act (DSHEA) [17], dietary supplements, including nutritional ergogenic aids, that are not intended to diagnose, treat, cure, or prevent any disease currently do not need to be evaluated by the FDA prior to their commercialization. The manufacturers are responsible for the determination of the purity, benefits, efficacy, safety, and compositional specifications that the supplement is required to meet [18].

On the basis of the level of scientific evidence and its practical applications, the American Dietetic Association and the Australian Institute of Sport proposed a provisional classification of nutritional ergogenic aids: (1) Supported for use in specific situations in sport using evidence-based protocols; (2) Deserving of further research and could be considered for provision to athletes under a research protocol or case-managed monitoring situation; (3) Having little meaningful proof of beneficial effects; (4) Banned or at high risk of contamination with substances that could lead to a positive drug test [19].

The absence of supporting legislation in Europe contributes to the misleading advertising. As a result of this lack of legislation on nutritional ergogenic aids, the companies can make unsubstantiated claims about the efficacy of the products. Advertisements and health/performance claims in labels with references to improved athletic performance without any scientific evidence can be found on the market.

Thus, since there is no specific legislation on nutritional ergogenic aids, the aim of the present study is to explore legislative documents that regulate the use of nutritional ergogenic aids intended for sportspeople in the Spanish and European frameworks.

2. Materials and Methods

The methodology was developed by different strategies, as follows:

(1) A narrative review of legislative documents related to nutritional ergogenic aids, especially for sportspeople, has been developed. The information was extracted from the official websites of Spanish and European bodies. A legislative document is considered to be the laws, regulations, and/or standards laid down by the competent authority in the national or European field.

The search for Spanish documents was carried out on the website of the Spanish Agency for the Consumer, Food Safety, and Nutrition (AECOSAN) of the Spanish Ministry of Health, Social Policy, and Equality and, in particular, on the "legislation" section (http://aesan.msssi.gob.es/AESAN/web/legislacion/seccion/especifica_ambito_alimentario.shtml). The "General" category was consulted to obtain information about "Labeling and advertising of foods" and the "By Sectors" category was explored to compile information about "Food products for special groups".

In the search for European legislation, the section "Dietetic Foods/Foods for specific groups" on the European Commission website was consulted: http://ec.europa.eu/food/safety/labelling_nutrition/special_groups_food/sportspeople/index_en.htm. Also consulted was the section "The Panel on Dietetic Products, Nutrition and Allergies (NDA)" from the European Food Safety Authority (EFSA) (http://www.efsa.europa.eu/en/panels/nda).

(2) The selection process was performed by two independent reviewers, reaching a consensus and finally approving its inclusion or exclusion.

(3) The selection of the compiled documents was carried out using classification criteria according to the information contained in the publication. Three sections were established:

- Section 1: legislative documents on advertising (for every type of products including foods).
- Section 2: legislative documents on the composition, labeling, and advertising of foods (only for foods).
- Section 3: specific legislative documents on nutritional ergogenic aids (only nutritional/dietary supplements).

3. Results

A total of 18 relevant legislative documents have been compiled. All of them deal with nutritional ergogenic aids in a general or specific way and in the Spanish or European framework. For the sake of clarity, the documents are grouped in sections as follows:

Section 1, documents that refer to the advertising for any type of food and/or product. Six documents applicable in Spain were found; the results are shown in Table 1.

Table 1. Legislative documents on advertising.

Legislative Documents	Information Related to Nutritional Ergogenic Aids
Law 34/1988, of 11 November of General Advertising. Official State Bulletin No. 274. [20]	Applicable law in Spain about advertising. It establishes the requirement about legal and illegal advertising (misleading, unfair, subliminal) in product labeling. Article 8 speaks about the need to declare derived risks arising out of their normal use.
Law 3/1991, of 10 January of Unfair Competition, Official State Bulletin No. 10. [21]	Unfair Commercial Practices Spanish Directive. This Directive states the laws on unfair commercial practices, including unfair advertising, which directly harm the consumers' economic interests and thereby indirectly harm the economic interests of legitimate competitors. The law describes the situations that can be considered unfair competition and the actions deriving from it.
Ministry of Health and Consumer Affairs and the Spanish Federation of Food and Drink Industries. Interpretative agreement on the advertising of the properties of food in relation to health. 1998. [22]	Voluntary agreement applicable in Spain on health claims in advertising of food. This labeling legislation prohibits the attribution to any foodstuff of the property of preventing, treating, or curing a human disease or referring to such properties. -Each health claim should be adequately and sufficiently demonstrated, based on and substantiated by generally accepted scientific evidence. -In order to ensure that the claims made are truthful, it is necessary that the substance that is the subject of the claim is present in the final product in quantities that are sufficient, or that the substance is absent or present in suitably quantities, to produce the nutritional or physiological effect claimed. -Health claims in labeling and advertising should be accompanied by a declaration on the importance of a varied and balanced diet to address feeding requirements. -A particular brand should not be suggested if similar products can produce the same health effects.

Table 1. *Cont.*

Legislative Documents	Information Related to Nutritional Ergogenic Aids
Royal Legislative Decree 1/2007 of 16 November, approving the revised text of the General Law for the Protection of Consumers and Users and other complementary laws. Official State Bulletin No. 287. [23]	Law applicable in Spain about relations between users or consumers and businesspeople. The law establishes the basic rights of consumers and the protection against risks that may affect their health or safety.
Law 7/2010, of 31 March, General Audiovisual Communication. Official State Bulletin No. 79. [24]	Law regulating the audio-visual communication of state coverage. It establishes the basic rules in the audiovisual field. Article 18 talks about commercial practices that are prohibited, such as "Any commercial practice that encourages behavior prejudicial to health or safety is prohibited".
Royal Decree 1907/1996, of 2 August, on advertising and sales promotion products, activities or services intended for health purposes. Official State Bulletin No. 189. [25]	Article 4. Prohibitions and Limitations of advertising intended for health purposes. Any advertising, direct or indirect, massive or individualized promotion of products or substances that suggest/indicate their use/consumption improves physical, mental, or sexual performance sports is prohibited.

Section 2, laws and legislative records related to the composition, labeling, and advertising that affect all food and products. Six documents, mostly applicable in Europe, were compiled (Table 2).

Table 2. Legislative documents on composition, labeling, and advertising of foods.

Legislative Documents	Information Related to Nutritional Ergogenic Aids
Commission of the European Communities. White Paper on food safety of 12/1/2000. [26]	The establishment of an independent European Food Authority is considered by the Commission to be the most appropriate response to the need to guarantee a high level of food safety. To outline a comprehensive range of actions needed to complement and modernize existing EU food legislation, to make it more coherent, understandable and flexible, to promote better enforcement of that legislation, and to provide greater transparency to consumers; in addition, to guarantee a high level of food safety.
Regulation (EC) No. 178/2002 of the European Parliament and of the Council of 28 January 2002 laying down the general principles and requirements of food law, establishing the European Food Safety Authority and laying down procedures in matters of food safety. [27]	Establishing the European Food Safety Authority and laying down procedures in matters of food safety. This Regulation provides the basis for the assurance of a high level of protection of human health and consumers' interest in relation to food, taking into account in particular the diversity in the supply of food including traditional products, whilst ensuring the effective functioning of the internal market. Note the creation of a Scientific Committee and Scientific Panels as the Panel on dietetic products, nutrition and allergies (Section 2).
Regulation (EC) No. 1924/2006 of the European Parliament and of the Council of 20 December 2006 on nutrition and health claims made on foods. [28]	This Regulation harmonizes the provisions laid down by law, regulation or administrative action in Member States that relate to nutrition and health claims in order to ensure the effective functioning of the internal market whilst providing a high level of consumer protection. Also apply to nutrition and health claims made in commercial communications, whether in the labeling, presentation or advertising of foods to be delivered as such to the final consumer, including foods that are placed on the market unpacked or supplied in bulk.
Commission Regulation (EC) No. 353/2008 of 18 April 2008 establishing implementing rules for applications for authorization of health claims as provided for in Article 15 of Regulation (EC) No. 1924/2006 of the European Parliament and of the Council. [29]	This Regulation establishes implementing rules for the following: 1. Applications for authorization, submitted in accordance with Article 15 of Regulation (EC) No. 1924/2006; and 2. Applications for the inclusion of a claim in the list provided for in Article 13(3) submitted in accordance with Article 18 of Regulation (EC) No. 1924/2006.

Table 2. *Cont.*

Legislative Documents	Information Related to Nutritional Ergogenic Aids
Regulation (EU) No. 1169/2011 of the European Parliament and of the Council of 25 October 2011 on the provision of food information to consumers, amending Regulations (EC) No. 1924/2006 and (EC) No. 1925/2006 of the European Parliament and of the Council, and repealing Commission Directive 87/250/EEC, Council Directive 90/496/EEC, Commission Directive 1999/10/EC, Directive 2000/13/EC of the European Parliament and of the Council, Commission Directives 2002/67/EC and 2008/5/EC and Commission Regulation (EC) No. 608/2004. [30]	This Regulation provides the basis for the assurance of a high level of consumer protection in relation to food information, taking into account the differences in the perception of consumers and their information needs. Establishes the general principles, requirements and responsibilities governing food information, and in particular food labeling. It lays down the means to guarantee the right of consumers to information and procedures for the provision of food information, taking into account the need to provide sufficient flexibility to respond to future developments and new information requirements (Chapter IV, Sections 1, 2 and Chapter VII).
EU Register on nutrition and health claims. [31]	European Union Register of nutrition and health claims made on foods, showing: 1. Permitted nutrition claims and their conditions of use; 2. Authorized health claims, their conditions of use and applicable restrictions, if any; 3. Non-authorized health claims and the reasons for their non-authorization; 4. EU legal acts for the specific health claims; and 5. National measures mentioned in Art. 23(3) of Regulation EC 1924/2006. URL: http://ec.europa.eu/nuhclaims/

Section 3, this section contains the main specific legislative documents about foodstuffs intended for particular nutritional uses. Among them are the foods intended to satisfy the expenditure of intense muscular effort, especially for sportspeople. This section also includes reports issued by the EFSA on the health claims made for nutritional ergogenic aids. Table 3 shows the information about the six documents found.

Table 3. Specific legislative documents on nutritional ergogenic aids.

Legislative Documents	Information Related to Nutritional Ergogenic Aids
Royal Decree 2685/1976 Technical health regulations on foodstuffs intended for particular nutritional uses. Official State Bulletin No. 284. [32]	This Regulation defines food prepared for dietary regimens and/or special uses and establishes the legal regulation of such products.
Directive 2009/39/EC of the European Parliament and of the Council of 6 May 2009 on foodstuffs intended for particular nutritional uses. [33]	The Directive defines foodstuffs for particular nutritional uses are foodstuffs. Annex 1. Groups of foodstuffs for particular nutritional uses for which specific provisions will be laid down by specific Directives: Group 5 "foods intended to meet the expenditure of intense muscular effort, especially for sportsmen".
Commission Regulation (EC) No. 953/2009 of 13 October 2009 on substances that may be added for specific nutritional purposes in foods for particular nutritional uses. [34]	Article 1. Regulation shall apply to foods for particular nutritional uses, excluding those covered by Directive 2006/125/EC and Directive 2006/141/EC. Article 2. Among the substances belonging to the categories appearing in Annex to this Regulation, only those listed in that Annex, complying with the relevant specifications as necessary may be added for specific nutritional purposes in the manufacture of foodstuffs for particular nutritional uses covered by Directive 2009/39/EC. Without prejudice to Regulation (EC) No. 258/97 of the European Parliament and of the Council (6), also substances not belonging to the categories appearing in the Annex to this Regulation may be added for specific nutritional purposes in the manufacture of foods for particular nutritional uses.

Table 3. *Cont.*

Legislative Documents	Information Related to Nutritional Ergogenic Aids
Regulation (EU) No. 609/2013 of the European Parliament and of the Council of 12 June 2013 on food intended for infants and young children, food for special medical purposes, and total diet replacement for weight control and repealing Council Directive 92/52/EEC, Commission Directives 96/8/EC, 1999/21/EC, 2006/125/EC and 2006/141/EC, Directive 2009/39/EC of the European Parliament and of the Council and Commission Regulations (EC) No. 41/2009 and (EC) No. 953/2009. [35]	This regulation excludes products for athletes from the category of "dietetics". Applicable from 20 July 2016. With regard to food intended to meet the expenditure of intense muscular effort, especially for sportsmen, no successful conclusion could be reached as regards the development of specific provisions due to widely diverging views among the Member States and stakeholders concerning the scope of specific legislation, the number of subcategories of food to be included, the criteria for establishing compositional requirements and the potential impact on innovation in product development. Therefore, specific provisions should not be developed at this stage. Meanwhile, on the basis of requests submitted by food business operators, relevant claims have been considered for authorization in accordance with Regulation (EC) No. 1924/2006. Different views exist as to whether additional rules are needed to ensure an adequate protection of consumers of food intended for sportsmen, also called food intended to meet the expenditure of intense muscular effort. The Commission should, therefore, be invited, after consulting the Authority, to submit to the European Parliament and to the Council a report on the necessity, if any, of provisions concerning food intended for sportsmen. The consultation of the Authority should take into account the report of 28 February 2001 of the Scientific Committee on Food on composition and specification of food intended to meet the expenditure of intense muscular effort, especially for sportsmen. In its report, the Commission should, in particular, evaluate whether provisions are necessary to ensure the protection of consumers. Taking into account the existing situation on the market and Directives 2006/125/EC and 2006/141/EC, and Regulation (EC) No. 953/2009, it is appropriate to establish and include in the Annex to this Regulation a Union list of substances belonging to the following categories of substances: vitamins, minerals, amino acids, carnitine and taurine, nucleotides, choline and inositol. Article 13. Food intended for sportspeople. By 20 July 2015, the Commission shall, after consulting the Authority, present to the European Parliament and to the Council a report on the necessity, if any, of provisions for food intended for sportspeople. Such a report may, if necessary, be accompanied by an appropriate legislative proposal.
EFSA Panel on Dietetic Products, Nutrition and Allergies (NDA). Guidance on the scientific requirements for health claims related to physical performance. EFSA Journal 2012;10(7):2817. [36]	Document prepared by The Panel on Dietetic Products, Nutrition and Allergies (NDA) of the EFSA about scientific requirements for health claims related to physical performance.
Scientific and technical assistance on food intended for sportspeople. Question Number: EFSA-Q-2015-00403. [37]	Technical report of the EFSA to compile existing scientific advice in the area of nutrition and health claims and Dietary Reference Values for adults that is relevant to sportspeople and to inform the Commission on how such scientific advice relates to the different conclusions and specifications of the report of the Scientific Committee on Food (SCF) of 2001 on the composition and specification of food intended to meet the expenditure of intense muscular effort, especially for sportspeople.

4. Discussion

In the present work the importance of the creation of the EFSA in 2002 is emphasized. This agency is an essential asset for Europe's food security in the context of public health.

In the European framework, and according to Action plan No. 55 of the European Commission, there are several legislative documents for food destined to alleviate intense muscle loss, particularly in athletes. Nevertheless, despite the existence of the EFSA, the analyses of legislative documents uncovered ambiguity in the regulations.

The documents related to laws and resolutions in Spain and Europe are orientated towards the general regulation of advertising and food marketing. However, specific documents referring to nutritional ergogenic aids show more ambiguity or are inconsistent or are inexistent.

Action plan No. 56 of the European Commission (2001) has been reflected in Directive 2009/39/C [33] and in Regulation (EC) No. 953/2009 [34]. Both documents highlight the need to create a more specific legislation for ergonutritional aids. However, in both of them, ergonutritional aids and sport foods are considered together as the group of "foods intended to meet the expenditure of intense muscular effort, especially for sportsmen".

The guidance of the EFSA on the scientific requirements for health claims related to physical performance [36] represents the views of the NDA panel based on its experience with the evaluation of health claims for physical performance, endurance capacity, muscle function, and physiological effects. This is a compilation about scientific opinions from NDA panel that have been approved by the European Commission to be applied on the European Union countries.

4.1. Legislative Documents in Spain

This guide is based on Regulation (EC) No. 1924/2006 [28] and its subsequent amendments, concerning nutrition and health claims made for foods, and also on Regulation (EU) No. 1169/2011 [30], concerning the provision of food information to consumers.

Domestically, in Spain, several regulations on the advertising of any food and/or product exist. These establish common considerations related to unfair competition and illicit advertising on labeling [20,21,23,24].

In this context, it is worth noting the agreement signed in 1998 between the Ministry of Health and Consumer Affairs and the Spanish Federation of Food and Drink Industries (FIAB). This provides criteria for assessing the conformity of a product with the general safety requirements and the right of consumers to obtain accurate, truthful, and reliable information. These criteria have subsequently been reinforced by Law 17/2011, of 5 July 2011, on food safety and nutrition [38] and more especially by the Co-regulation Codex on food and beverages advertising targeted at minors, obesity prevention, and health (PAOS Codex) [39].

In Spain, sports food has been regulated for 40 years through the Royal Decree 2685/1976 "Healthcare Regulation on Formula Foods for Use in Weight Control Diets and/or in Special Situations" [32]. This Royal Decree defined the "food destined to those people who make extraordinary efforts or live in special environmental conditions" as "food that provides complementary nutrients" in Section 3.1.2.2 and this is also included in Section 3.1.2 as "complementary food for situations of great physical exertion". Even so, the Annex constitutes an indication of the need to create specific regulations for sports food.

4.2. Legislative Documents in Europe

In February 2001, the Health & Consumer Protection Directorate-General of the European Commission ordered the Scientific Committee on Food (SCF) (European Commission. Health and Consumer Protection, 2001) to write a report on the food composition and specification of food intended to meet the expenditure of intense muscular effort, especially for sportsmen [40]. The document concluded that a well-balanced diet is the basic nutritional requirement for athletes. Nevertheless, taking into consideration the distinct aspects of intense muscular exercise—such as intensity, duration, and frequency as well as specific constraints like time and convenience—individuals can benefit from particular foods or food ingredients. Specially adapted nutritious foods or fluids may help to solve specific problems so that an optimal nutritional balance can be reached. On the basis of such considerations, four food categories, for which essential requirements were formulated, were identified: (1) Carbohydrate-rich energy food products; (2) Carbohydrate–electrolyte solutions; (3) Protein and protein components; (4) Supplements and other food components.

This report was the first step in the categorization and legislation of sport foods, as indicated in the Action plan No. 55 of the White Paper on Food Safety [26].

Directive 2009/39/EC states the conditions that foodstuffs must comply with in order to bear the words dietetic or dietary. Foodstuffs for particular nutritional uses are defined as "foodstuffs which, owing to their special composition or manufacturing process, are clearly distinguishable from foodstuffs for normal consumption, which are suitable for their claimed nutritional purposes and which are marketed in such a way as to indicate such suitability". This Directive also establishes that "A particular nutritional use shall fulfil the particular nutritional requirements of certain categories of persons who are in a special physiological condition and who are therefore able to obtain special benefit from controlled consumption of certain substances in foodstuffs". Among the products destined for a special diet, adapted food for intense muscle wastage is found, especially for athletes [33]. Consequently, from the evaluation of new substances by the EFSA, the necessity to update and complete lists of substances that can be added to dietetic products through Regulation (EC) No. 953/2009 arises [34]. Substances like vitamins, minerals, amino acids, L-carnitine, taurine, nucleotides, choline, and inositol are on this list. These compounds are frequently used for the preparation of dietetic products and sport foods, but their use to improve sport performance has questionable benefits [41,42].

In addition to the lack of scientific evidence about sport performance benefits, important inaccuracies and legal loopholes can be found in this Regulation. Two examples are the sentence "the inclusion of substances in the list of those that may be used in the manufacture of foodstuffs for particular nutritional uses does not mean that their addition to those foodstuffs is necessary or desirable" and point 2 of Article 2: "also substances not belonging to the categories appearing in the Annex to this Regulation may be added for specific nutritional purposes in the manufacture of foods for particular nutritional uses".

Directive 2009/39/CE foresees a specific legislation of foods intended to meet the expenditure of intense muscular effort, especially for sportsmen [33].

Due to these legal loopholes, the European Commission has elaborated recently the Regulation (EU) No. 609/2013 on food intended for infants and young children, food for special medical purposes, and total diet replacement for weight control and has repealed Council Directive 92/52/EEC [35]. This suppose a clear fault on food safety and consequently, inefficient control of these nutritional/dietary supplements. This new Regulation will replace Directive 2009/39/CE [19] and specifies that "food intended to meet the expenditure of intense muscular effort, especially for sportsmen, no successful conclusion could be reached as regards the development of specific provisions due to widely diverging views among the Member States and stakeholders concerning the scope of specific legislation, the number of subcategories of food to be included, the criteria for establishing compositional requirements and the potential impact on innovation in product development. Therefore, specific provisions should not be developed at this stage". Section 13 of this Regulation discusses food intended for sportspeople and mentions that "By 20 July 2015, the Commission shall, after consulting the Authority, present to the European Parliament and to the Council a report on the necessity, if any, of provisions for food intended for sportspeople. Such a report may, if necessary, be accompanied by an appropriate legislative proposal". Considerations previous to this Regulation indicate that the report of 28 February 2001 of the SCF should be taken into account [40]. Today, there is no law/rule on these products and this type of food will be exclusively governed by horizontal rules of food law.

4.3. Specific Legislation on Nutritional Ergogenic Aids or Sports Food

Until now, the European Commission has not proposed any specific legislation concerning this field, but the Directorate General for Health and Food Safety ordered that a report be drawn up on food for sportspeople [35]. This report indicates that there is no universally accepted definition of what constitutes "sports food". The scope of the report is not limited only to foods available on the market under Directive 2009/39/EC, but considers all products specifically targeting sportspeople regardless of their method of market placement.

Its objective is to provide the information missing in current legislation and aims to provide: (1) A description and analysis of the market of foods intended for sportspeople; (2) A description and analysis of the different marketing techniques and practices used for foods intended for sportspeople, with particular attention to the use of nutrition and health claims; (3) A description and analysis of the consumers of foods intended for sportspeople, with particular focus on their behavior, interest, and understanding; (4) A description of the national legislation in the 28 Member States related to foods intended for sportspeople, when this exists, and an analysis of how this is performing; and (5) A description and analysis of the legislations in the main trading partner countries related to foods intended for sportspeople.

The study will help the development of a legislative proposal, in which Regulation No. 609/2013 [35] will be applied, repealing Directive 2009/39/E [33]. Foodstuffs currently considered as "dietary products", but not included in Regulation 609/2013, will be regulated by legal acts applicable to all foods so long as they do not contradict the horizontal rules of EU food law after 20 July 2016 [37,38]: (a) Regulation (EC) No. 1924/2006 on nutrition and health claims made on foods [28]; (b) Regulation (EC) No. 353/2008, establishing the implementation of rules for applications for authorization of health claims as provided for in Article 15 of Regulation (EC) No. 1924/2006 of the European Parliament and of the Council [29]; (c) Regulation (EC) No. 1925/2006 on the addition of vitamins and minerals and certain other substances to foods [43]; (d) Regulation (EU) No. 1169/2011 on the provision of food information to consumers [30]; (e) Directive 2002/46/EC on the approximation of the laws of the Member States relating to food supplements [44]; and (f) Regulation (EC) No. 258/97 on novel foods and novel food ingredients [45] (this Regulation will be replaced, as of 1 January 2018, by Regulation (EU) 2015/2283 on novel food [46]). Compared to the legislative framework of Directive 2009/39/EC, there are differences regarding how and which information can be provided to the consumer and regarding the composition of the product concerned.

Regulation (EC) No. 1924/2006 provides the legal framework and the rules for these statements. It would facilitate the consumer's choice, while avoiding ambiguous, illegal, misleading, or false advertising [47]. While nutritional declarations are strictly, explicitly, and clearly defined in the regulation, declarations of healthy properties must be requested, examined based on generally accepted scientific tests, and be finally accepted by the European Union in positive lists [48].

General documental requirements are established for the use of health claims [49] and also there are more specific requirements for nutritional ergogenic aids [36]. Health claims should adequately and sufficiently demonstrate that they are based on and substantiated by generally accepted scientific evidence, by taking into account the totality of the available scientific data and by weighing the evidence. Health claims must satisfy the following principles [47]: (a) a comprehensive and systematic review of data from human subjects should be conducted; (b) published and unpublished data must be included; (c) positive and negative data must be evaluated; (d) priority must be given (in this order) to intervention studies, observational studies, human studies, animal model studies, and studies with cell models, and (e) the methodological quality of intervention studies, observational studies, and meta-analysis must be evaluated.

These requirements, that would demonstrate a clear cause–effect relationship between nutritional ergogenic aids and the declared effect, could be the cause of the scarce approval of the declarations of healthy properties related to sports performance. While more than 2200 general declarations have been presented, just a few of them have been approved [31]. Some examples of claims for substances approved by the EFSA are creatine (increases physical performance in successive bursts of short-term, high-intensity exercise) [50], carbohydrates (contribute to the recovery of normal muscle function after highly intensive and/or long-lasting physical exercise leading to muscle fatigue and the depletion of glycogen stores in skeletal muscle) [51], carbohydrate–electrolyte solutions (contribute to the maintenance of endurance performance during prolonged endurance exercise or enhance the absorption of water during physical exercise) [52], and vitamin C (contributes to maintaining the normal function of the immune system during and after intense physical exercise) [53]. These approvals are based on scientific opinions issued by the American Academy of Nutrition and Dietetics [41] and the Australian Sport Commission and these substances have a relationship with sportspeople's health and performance [19]. For example, the health effect of carbohydrate–electrolyte solutions is maintenance of endurance performance, while that of Vitamin C is to maintain the function of the immune system during and after extreme physical exercise. It should be noted that caffeine is an exceptional case. Although it has a positive evaluation by the EFSA [54], it was not authorized by the European Commission. The latest scientific opinion, after public consultation, informed that a dosage of 3 mg/kg (200 mg approx.) consumed within 2 h before intense physical exercise in normal environmental conditions does not show any problem [55].

Nutrition claims and the health claims made for proteins, vitamins, and minerals based on Regulation (EC) No. 1924/2006 are, by and large, general in nature but are also applicable to nutritional ergogenic aids [28,31].

According to Directive 2002/46/EC, a food supplement "means foodstuffs the purpose of which is to supplement the normal diet and which are concentrated sources of nutrients or other substances with a nutritional or physiological effect, alone or in combination, marketed in dose form, namely forms such as capsules, pastilles, tablets, pills and other similar forms, sachets of powder, ampoules of liquids, drop dispensing bottles, and other similar forms of liquids and powders designed to be taken in measured small unit quantities" [44]. These represent the most common forms of presentation for companies commercializing nutritional ergogenic aids. The labeling of nutritional ergogenic aids is regulated by Regulation No. 1169/2011 on the provision of food information to consumers [30].

With the entry into force of Regulation No. 1169/2011, nutritional labeling became compulsory. In addition to the declaration of particular elements of the qualitative and quantitative compositions, the declaration of allergens and nano-nutrients has become mandatory, as well as an increase in the size of the letters. Regulation No. 1169/2011 amends rule 7 of Regulation (CE) No. 1924/2006: "Nutrition labeling of products on which a nutrition and/or health claim is made shall be mandatory, with the exception of generic advertising. The information to be provided shall consist of that specified in Article 30(1) of Regulation (EU) No. 1169/2011 of the European Parliament and of the Council of 25 October 2011 on the provision of food information to consumers (*). Where a nutrition and/or health claim is made for a nutrient referred to in Article 30(2) of Regulation (EU) No. 1169/2011 the amount of that nutrient shall be declared in accordance with Articles 31 to 34 of that Regulation" and "The amount(s) of the substance(s) to which a nutrition or health claim relates that does not appear in the nutrition labeling shall be stated in the same field of vision as the nutrition labeling and be expressed in accordance with Articles 31, 32 and 33 of Regulation (EU) No. 1169/2011. The units of measurement used to express the amount of the substance shall be appropriate for the individual substances concerned".

On 24 September 2015, the EFSA issued a technical report called "Scientific and technical assistance on food intended for sportspeople" based on the SCF report of 2001 [37,40] and on EFSA scientific opinions about sports. The report does not take into account new scientific reports about nutritional ergogenic aids published in recent years, after the issue of its scientific views. Because of this, the report could be outdated and out of context [41,56,57]. On the other hand and according to the Directorate General for Health and Food Safety, the report should contribute to the development of a legislative proposal. However, none of the points it mentions have been accomplished.

The majority of national competent authorities believe that the existing horizontal rules of food law are either quite suitable or very suitable for the regulation of sports food. Six national competent authorities have recognized the need for specific rules for sports food [58].

4.4. Considerations of the World Anti-Doping Agency

Finally, the list of forbidden substances issued by the WADA [59] and its World Anti-Doping Code [60] must be heeded. Although this information is important because prohibited substances could be a health risk for athletes and their sporting careers [61], the WADA reports are not taken into account in the current legislation on control measures, product supervision, and food complements that contain substances prohibited in sports activities. The WADA warns that dietetic products and herbal products, especially those destined for sport, can contain non-declared substances that could give positive results in anti-doping controls (ephedrine and anabolic substances). The agency also points out that control policies regarding dietetic products are usually quiet lax [62].

The scientific literature contains studies that prove the presence of doping substances in supplements like growth hormones [41], androgen receptor modulators, anabolic hormones [63–65], and stimulants [66]. Many supplements contain hazardous substances, such as illegal anabolic steroids, that have serious known side effects. In more than 15% of the supplements analyzed, substances were identified at concentrations that are potential positives in "anti-doping" tests and with potential secondary effects for consumers [67–69]. The main causes were cross-contamination during manufacturing, processing, or packaging, poor quality control, or bad labeling [14,70,71]. Studies related to the WADA considerations recommend the establishment of better and more effective controls in the elaboration and commercialization of dietetic products. Hence, the WADA has approved programs that guarantee the quality of nutritional ergogenic aids. The quality of the products, suppliers, factory installations, and anti-doping laboratories is certified with a logo that guarantees that these products do not contain prohibited substances.

5. Conclusions

Currently, legislation related to the regulation and application of nutritional ergogenic aids or sports food products can be found in the following documents: Regulation (EU) No. 1169/2011, Regulation (EC) No. 353/2008, Regulation (EC) No. 1924/2006, Regulation (EC) No. 1925/2006, Directive 2002/46/EC, and Regulation (EC) No. 258/97. Regulation (EU) No. 609/2013, proposed by the European Commission, came into force on 20 July 2016. In spite of the existence of this legal framework, the regulation lacks a normative sector regarding the use and application of nutritional ergogenic aids by sports food consumers. These legislative documents should also take into account the WADA considerations on the quality control programs of these substances.

The direct marketing and free sale of sports food could be a health risk in the case of indiscriminate consumption by athletes. So, Regulation (EC) No. 1924/2006, Regulation (EU) No. 1169/2011, and the guidance on the scientific requirements for health claims related to physical performance are essential for the commercialization and advertising of sports food. It is essential to prevent the introduction or dissemination of false, ambiguous, or inexact information and contents that induce an error in the receivers of the information.

We wish to highlight the importance of the steps taken by the authorities and institutions regarding legislative measures for sports food products. Among them stand out the institutionalization of the EFSA as a European body and the work developed by international scientific societies/companies such as the WADA. All of them have contributed information about consumer guidelines, prescribing practices, prudent use recommendations, and the advantages and limitations of nutritional ergogenic aids.

However, the results obtained show the absence in the European legislation of a normative sector applied directly to nutritional ergogenic aids for sportspeople. To establish a policy recommendation and to move this process forward, an appropriate institutional setting is needed. Consumer protection provisions should promote greater levels of policy development, regulatory enforcement, and consumer education. Public health measures must be based on the principles of precaution, evaluation, transparency, and the safety of nutritional ergogenic supplements.

Acknowledgments: This work has been partially funded by the "Fundación Séneca de la Región de Murcia" Grupo de Excelencia 19900/GERM/15. We are grateful to David Walker (native English speaker) and for their reviews of the English grammar and style of the current report.

Author Contributions: All authors participated in the work and the contribution of each author is detailed below: Study design: José Miguel Martínez Sanz, Laura Arranz, Eduard Baladia, and Rocio Ortiz Moncada; Data acquisition: José Miguel Martínez Sanz, Laura Arranz, and Isabel Sospedra; Analysis and interpretation of data: José Miguel Martínez Sanz, Laura Arran, Isabel Sospedra, and Angel Gil Izquierdo; Drafting of manuscript: José Miguel Martínez Sanz, Laura Arranz, Eduard Baladia, Isabel Sospedra, Angel Gil Izquierdo, and Rocio Ortiz Moncada; Critical review: Laura Arranz, Eduard Baladia, Isabel Sospedra, Angel Gil Izquierdo, and Rocio Ortiz Moncada.

Conflicts of Interest: The authors declare no conflict of interest.

References

1. Thein, L.A.; Thein, J.M.; Landry, G.L. Ergogenic aids. *Phys. Ther.* **1995**, *75*, 426–439.
2. Prada Pérez, A. Ayudas Ergogénicas en el Deporte. Ministerio de Educación: Edusport. Available online: http://recursos.cnice.mec.es/edfisica/publico/articulos/articulo13/articulo_13.php (accessed on 14 May 2016).
3. Williams, M.H. *Ergogenic Aids in Sport*; Human Kinetics Publishers: Champaign, IL, USA, 1983; 404p.
4. Buck, C.L.; Wallman, K.E.; Dawson, B.; Guelfi, K.J. Sodium phosphate as an ergogenic aid. *Sports Med.* **2013**, *43*, 425–435.
5. Maughan, R.J. Nutritional ergogenic aids and exercise performance. *Nutr. Res. Rev.* **1999**, *12*, 255–280.
6. Maughan, R.J.; Greenhaff, P.L.; Hespel, P. Dietary supplements for athletes: Emerging trends and recurring themes. *J. Sports Sci.* **2011**, *29* (Suppl. 1), S57–S66.
7. Heikkinen, A.; Alaranta, A.; Helenius, I.; Vasankari, T. Use of dietary supplements in Olympic athletes is decreasing: A follow-up study between 2002 and 2009. *J. Int. Soc. Sports Nutr.* **2011**, *8*, 1. [CrossRef]
8. Australian Sports Commission. Australia. Sports Nutrition. Nutrition. Available online: http://www.ausport.gov.au/ais/nutrition (accessed on 12 December 2015).
9. Martínez-Sanz, J.M.; Sospedra, I.; Ortiz, C.M.; Baladía, E.; Gil-Izquierdo, A.; Ortiz-Moncada, R. Intended or Unintended Doping? A Review of the Presence of Doping Substances in Dietary Supplements Used in Sports. *Nutrients* **2017**, *9*. [CrossRef]
10. Ley 33/2011, de 4 de Octubre, General de Salud Pública. *Boletín Oficial del Estado*, 5 October 2011, No. 240, pp. 104593–104626.
11. Juhn, M. Popular sports supplements and ergogenic aids. *Sports Med.* **2003**, *33*, 921–939.
12. Petrenko, A.S.; Ponomareva, M.N.; Sukhanov, B.P. Regulation of food supplements in the European Union and its member states. Part I. *Vopr. Pitan.* **2014**, *83*, 32–40.
13. Petrenko, A.S.; Ponomareva, M.N.; Sukhanov, B.P. Regulation of food supplements in the European Union and its member states. Part 2. *Vopr. Pitan.* **2014**, *83*, 52–57.
14. Gabriels, G.; Lambert, M. Nutritional supplement products: Does the label information influence purchasing decisions for the physically active? *Nutr. J.* **2013**, *12*, 133.
15. Heneghan, C.; Howick, J.; O'Neill, B.; Gill, P.J.; Lasserson, D.S.; Cohen, D.; Davis, R.; Ward, A.; Smith, A.; Jones, G.; et al. The evidence underpinning sports performance products: A systematic assessment. *Br. Med. J. Open.* **2012**, *2*, e001702.
16. Starr, R.R. Too little, too late: Ineffective regulation of dietary supplements in the United States. *Am. J. Public Health* **2015**, *105*, 478–485.
17. Dietary Supplement Health and Education (DSHEA) Act of 1994. Available online: https://ods.od.nih.gov/About/DSHEA_Wording.aspx (accessed on 16 May 2016).
18. Food and Drug Administration (FDA). New Dietary Ingredients in Dietary Supplements—Background for Industry. Available online: http://www.fda.gov/Food/DietarySupplements/NewDietaryIngredientsNotificationProcess/ucm109764.htm (accessed on 14 July 2016).
19. Australian Institute of Sport (AIS). Australian Sport Commission. Classification. Available online: http://www.ausport.gov.au/ais/nutrition/supplements/classification (accessed on 9 May 2015).
20. Ley 34/1988, de 11 de noviembre, General de Publicidad. *Boletín Oficial del Estado*, 15 November 1988, No. 274, pp. 32464–32467.
21. Ley 3/1991, de 10 de enero, de Competencia desleal. *Boletín Oficial del Estado*, 1 November 1991, No. 10, pp. 959–962.
22. Ministerio de Sanidad y Consumo (MSC), Federación Española de Industrias de la Alimentación y Bebidas (FIAB). Acuerdo Interpretativo Sobre la Publicidad de las Propiedades de los Alimentos en Relación con la Salud. Madrid: MSC–FIAB; 1998. Available online: http://www.autocontrol.es/pdfs/pdfs_codigos/cod0012.pdf (accessed on 15 May 2016).

23. Real Decreto Legislativo 1/2007, de 16 de noviembre, por el que se aprueba el texto refundido de la Ley General para la Defensa de los Consumidores y Usuarios y otras leyes complementarias. *Boletín Oficial del Estado*, 30 November 2007, No. 287, pp. 49181–49215. Available online: https://www.boe.es/buscar/act.php?id=BOE-A-2007-20555 (accessed on 15 May 2016).

24. Ley 7/2010, de 31 de marzo, General de la Comunicación Audiovisual. *Boletín Oficial del Estado*, 1 April 2010, No. 79, pp. 30157–30209. Available online: https://www.boe.es/buscar/pdf/2010/BOE-A-2010-5292-consolidado.pdf (accessed on 9 May 2016).

25. Real decreto 1907/1996, de 2 de agosto, sobre publicidad y promoción comercial de productos, actividades 0 servicios con pretendida finalidad sanitaria. *Boletín Oficial del Estado*, 6 August 1996, No. 189, pp. 24322–24325.

26. White Paper on Food Safety. Commission of the European Communities: Brussels, Belgium, 12 January 2000. Available online: http://ec.europa.eu/dgs/health_food-safety/library/pub/pub06_en.pdf (accessed on 1 December 2016).

27. Regulation (EC) No. 178/2002 of the European Parliament and of the Council of 28 January 2002 laying down the general principles and requirements of food law, establishing the European Food Safety Authority and laying down procedures in matters of food safety. *Official Journal of the European Union*, 1 February 2002, No. 31, pp. 1–24.

28. Regulation (EC) No. 1924/2006 of the European Parliament and of the Council of 20 December 2006 on nutrition and health claims made on foods. *Official Journal of the European Union*, 20 December 2006, No. 404, pp. 9–25. Available online: https://www.fsai.ie/uploadedFiles/Cor_Reg1924_2006.pdf (accessed on 11 December 2016).

29. Commission Regulation (EC) No. 353/2008 of 18 April 2008 establishing implementing rules for applications for authorisation of health claims as provided for in Article 15 of Regulation (EC) No. 1924/2006 of the European Parliament and of the Council. *Official Journal of the European Union*, 18 April 2008, No. 109, pp. 11–16.

30. Regulation (EU) No. 1169/2011 of the European Parliament and of the Council of 25 October 2011 on the provision of food information to consumers, amending Regulations (EC) No. 1924/2006 and (EC) No. 1925/2006 of the European Parliament and of the Council, and repealing Commission Directive 87/250/EEC, Council Directive 90/496/EEC, Commission Directive 1999/10/EC, Directive 2000/13/EC of the European Parliament and of the Council, Commission Directives 2002/67/EC and 2008/5/EC and Commission Regulation (EC) No. 608/2004. *Official Journal of the European Union*, 25 October 2011, No. 304, pp. 18–63. Available online: http://eur-lex.europa.eu/legal-content/EN/ALL/?uri=CELEX%3A32011R1169 (accessed on 1 December 2016).

31. EU Register of Nutrition and Health Claims Made on Foods. European Commission—Health and Consumers. Available online: http://ec.europa.eu/nuhclaims/ (accessed on 15 May 2016).

32. Real Decreto 2685/1976, de 16 de octubre, por el que se aprueba la Reglamentación Técnico-Sanitaria para la Elaboración, Circulación y Comercio de Preparados Alimenticios para Regímenes Dietéticos y/o Especiales. *Boletín Oficial del Estado*, 26 November 1976, No. 284, pp. 23543–23549.

33. Directive 2009/39/EC of the European Parliament and of the Council of 6 May 2009 on foodstuffs intended for particular nutritional uses. *Official Journal of the European Union*, 6 May 2009, No. 124, pp. 21–29. Available online: http://eur-lex.europa.eu/legal-content/EN/ALL/?uri=CELEX%3A32009L0039 (accessed on 7 May 2016).

34. Commission Regulation (EC) No. 953/2009 of 13 October 2009 on substances that may be added for specific nutritional purposes in foods for particular nutritional uses. *Official Journal of the European Union*, 13 October 2009, No. 269, pp. 9–19. Available online: https://www.fsai.ie/uploadedFiles/Reg953_2009.pdf (accessed on 1 June 2016).

35. Regulation (EU) No. 609/2013 of the European Parliament and of the Council of 12 June 2013 on food intended for infants and young children, food for special medical purposes, and total diet replacement for weight control and repealing Council Directive 92/52/EEC, Commission Directives 96/8/EC, 1999/21/EC, 2006/125/EC and 2006/141/EC, Directive 2009/39/EC of the European Parliament and of the Council and Commission Regulations (EC) No. 41/2009 and (EC) No. 953/2009. *Official Journal of the European Union*, 12 June 2013, No. 181, pp. 35–56. Available online: http://eur-lex.europa.eu/legal-content/EN/ALL/?uri=celex%3A32013R0609 (accessed on 1 December 2016).

36. EFSA Panel on Dietetic Products, Nutrition and Allergies (NDA). Guidance on the scientific requirements for health claims related to physical performance. *Eur. Food Saf. Auth. J.* **2012**, *10*, 2817.

37. European Food Safety Authority (EFSA). Scientific and Technical Assistance on Food Intended for Sportspeople. Available from: http://www.efsa.europa.eu/en/supporting/pub/871e (accessed on 15 May 2016).

38. Ley 17/2011, de 5 de julio, de seguridad alimentaria y nutrición. *Boletín Oficial del Estado*, 5 July 2011, No. 160, pp. 71283–71319. Available online: http://www.pap.es/FrontOffice/PAP/front/Articulos/Articulo/_IXus5l_LjPrOfNrft0uEHcQuKtNbft-T (accessed on 14 December 2016).

39. Código Corregulación de la Publicidad de Alimentos y Bebidas Dirigida a Menores, Prevención de la Obesidad y Salud (CODIGO PAOS); Modificado en 2013. FIAB-Ministerio Sanidad, Política Social e Igualdad, 2005. Available online: http://www.aecosan.msssi.gob.es/AECOSAN/docs/documentos/nutricion/Nuevo_Codigo_PAOS_2012_espanol.pdf (accessed on 1 May 2016).

40. European Commission. Health and Consumer Protection. Report of the Scientific Committee on Food Composition and Specification of Food Intended to Meet the Expenditure of Intense Muscular Effort, Especially for Sportsmen; Adopted by tche SCF on 22/6/2000, Corrected by the SCF on 28/2/2001; Brussels, Belgium, 28 February 2001. Available online: https://ec.europa.eu/food/sites/food/files/safety/docs/sci-com_scf_out64_en.pdf (accessed on 7 November 2017).

41. Thomas, D.T.; Erdman, K.A.; Burke, L.M. Position of the Academy of Nutrition and Dietetics, Dietitians of Canada, and the American College of Sports Medicine: Nutrition and Athletic Performance. *J. Acad. Nutr. Diet.* **2016**, *116*, 501–528.

42. Australian Sports Commission. Australia. Sports Nutrition. Supplements. Available online: http://www.ausport.gov.au/ais/nutrition/supplements (accessed on 9 March 2015).

43. Regulation (EC) No. 1925/2006 of the European Parliament and of the Council of 20 December 2006 on the addition of vitamins and minerals and of certain other substances to foods. *Official Journal of the European Union.* 20 December 2006, No. 404, pp. 26–38. Available online: https://www.fsai.ie/uploadedFiles/Consol_Reg1925_2006.pdf (accessed on 17 May 2016).

44. Directive 2002/46/EC of the European Parliament and of the Council of 10 June 2002 on the approximation of the laws of the Member States relating to food supplements. *Official Journal of the European Communities.* 10 June 2002, No. 183, pp. 51–57. Available online: http://www.fao.org/faolex/results/details/en/c/LEX-FAOC037787/ (accessed on 14 May 2017).

45. Regulation, H.A.T. Regulation (EC) No. 258/97 of the European Parliament and of the Council of 27 January 1997 concerning novel foods and novel food ingredients. *Off. J. Eur. Communities* **1997**, *40*, 1–7.

46. Regulation (EU) No. 2015/2283 of the European Parliament and of the Council of 25 November 2015 on novel foods. *Open J. Leadersh.* **2015**, *327*, 1–22.

47. Perales-Albert, A.; Bernácer-Martínez, R.; García-Gómez, J.; Álvarez-Dardet, C.; Ortiz-Moncada, R. Actualizaciones sobre declaraciones nutricionales y de propiedades saludables. *Rev. Española Nutr. Humana Diet.* **2013**, *17*, 179–186.

48. Buttriss, J.L.; Benelam, B. Nutrition and health claims: The role of food composition data. *Eur. J. Clin. Nutr.* **2010**, *64* (Suppl. 3), S8–S13.

49. AECOSAN. Dietéticos Sin Legislación Específica—Agencia Española de Consumo, Seguridad Alimentaria y Nutrición. Available online: http://www.aecosan.msssi.gob.es/AECOSAN/web/seguridad_alimentaria/subdetalle/dieteticos_sin_legislacion.shtml (accessed on 14 May 2016).

50. EFSA Panel on Dietetic Products, Nutrition and Allergies (NDA). Scientific Opinion on the substantiation of health claims related to creatine and increase in physical performance during short-term, high intensity, repeated exercise bouts (ID 739, 1520, 1521, 1522, 1523, 1525, 1526, 1531, 1532, 1533, 1534, 1922, 1923, 1924), increase in endurance capacity (ID 1527, 1535), and increase in endurance performance (ID 1521, 1963) pursuant to Article 13(1) of Regulation (EC) No. 1924/2006. *Eur. Food Saf. Auth. J.* **2011**, *9*, 2303.

51. EFSA Panel on Dietetic Products, Nutrition and Allergies (NDA). Scientific Opinion on the substantiation of a health claim related to glycaemic carbohydrates and recovery of normal muscle function (contraction) after strenuous exercise pursuant to Article 13(5) of Regulation (EC) No. 1924/2006. *Eur. Food Saf. Auth. J.* **2013**, *11*, 3409.

52. EFSA Panel on Dietetic Products, Nutrition and Allergies (NDA). Scientific Opinion on the substantiation of health claims related to carbohydrate-electrolyte solutions and reduction in rated perceived exertion/effort during exercise (ID 460, 466, 467, 468), enhancement of water absorption during exercise (ID 314, 315, 316, 317, 319, 322, 325, 332, 408, 465, 473, 1168, 1574, 1593, 1618, 4302, 4309), and maintenance of endurance performance (ID 466, 469) pursuant to Article 13(1) of Regulation (EC) No. 1924/2006. *Eur. Food Saf. Auth. J.* **2011**, *9*, 2211.

53. EFSA Panel on Dietetic Products, Nutrition and Allergies (NDA). Scientific Opinion on the substantiation of health claims related to vitamin C and protection of DNA, proteins and lipids from oxidative damage (ID 129, 138, 143, 148), antioxidant function of lutein (ID 146), maintenance of vision (ID 141, 142), collagen formation (ID 130, 131, 136, 137, 149), function of the nervous system (ID 133), function of the immune system (ID 134), function of the immune system during and after extreme physical exercise (ID 144), non-haem iron absorption (ID 132, 147), energy-yielding metabolism (ID 135), and relief in case of irritation in the upper respiratory tract (ID 1714, 1715) pursuant to Article 13(1) of Regulation (EC) No. 1924/2006. *Eur. Food Saf. Auth. J.* **2009**, *7*, 1226.

54. European Food Safety Authority (EFSA). Scientific Opinion on the substantiation of health claims related to caffeine and increase in physical performance during short-term high-intensity exercise (ID 737, 1486, 1489), increase in endurance performance (ID 737, 1486), increase in endurance capacity (ID 1488) and reduction in the rated perceived exertion/effort during exercise (ID 1488, 1490) pursuant to Article 13(1) of Regulation (EC) No. 1924/2006. *Eur. Food Saf. Auth. J.* **2011**, *9*, 2053.

55. EFSA Panel on Dietetic Products, Nutrition and Allergies (NDA). Scientific Opinion on the Safety of Caffeine. *Eur. Food Saf. Auth. J.* **2015**, *13*, 4102.

56. Trexler, E.T.; Smith-Ryan, A.E.; Stout, J.R.; Hoffman, J.R.; Wilborn, C.D.; Sale, C.; Kreider, R.B.; Jäger, R.; Earnest, C.P.; Bannock, L.; et al. International society of sports nutrition position stand: Beta-Alanine. *J. Int. Soc. Sports Nutr.* **2015**, *12*, 30.

57. Wilson, J.M.; Fitschen, P.J.; Campbell, B.; Wilson, G.J.; Zanchi, N.; Taylor, L.; Wilborn, C.; Kalman, D.S.; Stout, J.R.; Hoffman, J.R. International Society of Sports Nutrition Position Stand: Beta-hydroxy-beta-methylbutyrate (HMB). *J. Int. Soc. Sports Nutr.* **2013**, *10*. [CrossRef]

58. European Commission. *Directorate General for Health and Food Safety. Study on Food Intended for Sportspeople*; Final Report; European Commission: Brussels, Belgium, June 2015. Available online: https://ec.europa.eu/food/sites/food/files/safety/docs/fs_labelling-nutrition_special_study.pdf (accessed on 14 January 2017).

59. World Anti-Doping Agency (WADA). Sustancias Prohibidas | Lista de Sustancias y Métodos Prohibidos. Español. Available online: http://list.wada-ama.org/es/prohibited-all-times/prohibited-substances/ (accessed on 17 May 2016).

60. World Anti-Doping Agency (WADA). *World Anti-Doping Code*; World Anti-Doping Agency: Montreal, QC, Canada, 2013. Available online: https://www.wada-ama.org/en/what-we-do/the-code (accessed on 15 May 2016).

61. Judkins, C.; Prock, P. Supplements and inadvertent doping—How big is the risk to athletes. *Med. Sport Sci.* **2012**, *59*, 143–152.

62. World Anti-Doping Agency (WADA). *Dietary and Nutritional Supplements*; World Anti-Doping Agency: Montreal, QC, Canada, 2014. Available online: https://www.wada-ama.org/en/questions-answers/dietary-and-nutritional-supplements (accessed on 15 June 2016).

63. Kohler, M.; Thomas, A.; Geyer, H.; Petrou, M.; Schänzer, W.; Thevis, M. Confiscated black market products and nutritional supplements with non-approved ingredients analyzed in the Cologne Doping Control Laboratory 2009. *Drug Test. Anal.* **2010**, *2*, 533–537.

64. Geyer, H.; Parr, M.K.; Koehler, K.; Mareck, U.; Schänzer, W.; Thevis, M. Nutritional supplements cross-contaminated and faked with doping substances. *J. Mass Spectrom.* **2008**, *43*, 892–902.

65. Parr, M.K.; Fußhöller, G.; Schlörer, N.; Opfermann, G.; Geyer, H.; Rodchenkov, G.; Schänzer, W. Detection of Δ6-methyltestosterone in a "dietary supplement" and GC-MS/MS investigations on its urinary metabolism. *Toxicol. Lett.* **2011**, *201*, 101–104.

66. Maughan, R.J. Contamination of dietary supplements and positive drug tests in sport. *J. Sports Sci.* **2005**, *23*, 883–889.

67. Geyer, H.; Parr, M.K.; Mareck, U.; Reinhart, U.; Schrader, Y.; Schänzer, W. Analysis of non-hormonal nutritional supplements for anabolic-androgenic steroids—Results of an international study. *Int. J. Sports Med.* **2004**, *25*, 124–129.

68. Green, G.A.; Catlin, D.H.; Starcevic, B. Analysis of over-the-counter dietary supplements. *Clin. J. Sport Med.* **2001**, *11*, 254–259.

69. Kamber, M.; Baume, N.; Saugy, M.; Rivier, L. Nutritional supplements as a source for positive doping cases? *Int. J. Sport Nutr. Exerc. Metab.* **2001**, *11*, 258–263.

70. Pipe, A.; Ayotte, C. Nutritional supplements and doping. *Clin. J. Sport Med.* **2002**, *12*, 245–249.

71. Ayotte, C. Significance of 19-norandrosterone in athletes' urine samples. *Br. J. Sports Med.* **2006**, *40* (Suppl. 1), 25–29.

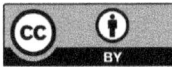

nutrients

MDPI

Review

Intended or Unintended Doping? A Review of the Presence of Doping Substances in Dietary Supplements Used in Sports

José Miguel Martínez-Sanz [1,2,*], Isabel Sospedra [1,2], Christian Mañas Ortiz [3], Eduard Baladía [2,4], Angel Gil-Izquierdo [2,5] and Rocio Ortiz-Moncada [2,6]

[1] Nursing Department, Faculty of Health Sciences, University of Alicante, 03690 Alicante, Spain; isospedra@ua.es

[2] Research Group on Food and Nutrition (ALINUT), University of Alicante, 03690 Alicante, Spain; e.baladia@academianutricion.org (E.B.); angelgil@cebas.csic.es (A.G.-I.); rocio.ortiz@ua.es (R.O.-M.)

[3] Pharmacy faculty, University of Valencia, 46100 Valencia, Spain; christianmanas@hotmail.es

[4] Evidence-Based Nutrition Network (RED-NuBE), Spanish Academy of Nutrition and Dietetics (AEND), 31006 Navarra, Spain

[5] Quality, Safety, and Bioactivity of Plant Foods Group, Department of Food Science and Technology, CEBAS-CSIC, University of Murcia, 30100 Murcia, Spain

[6] Department of Community Nursing, Preventive Medicine and Public Health and History of Science Health, University of Alicante, 03690 Alicante, Spain

* Correspondence: josemiguel.ms@ua.es

Received: 29 August 2017; Accepted: 29 September 2017; Published: 4 October 2017

Abstract: Introduction: The use of dietary supplements is increasing among athletes, year after year. Related to the high rates of use, unintentional doping occurs. Unintentional doping refers to positive anti-doping tests due to the use of any supplement containing unlisted substances banned by anti-doping regulations and organizations, such as the World Anti-Doping Agency (WADA). The objective of this review is to summarize the presence of unlabeled doping substances in dietary supplements that are used in sports. Methodology: A review of substances/metabolites/markers banned by WADA in ergonutritional supplements was completed using PubMed. The inclusion criteria were studies published up until September 2017, which analyzed the content of substances, metabolites and markers banned by WADA. Results: 446 studies were identified, 23 of which fulfilled all the inclusion criteria. In most of the studies, the purpose was to identify doping substances in dietary supplements. Discussion: Substances prohibited by WADA were found in most of the supplements analyzed in this review. Some of them were prohormones and/or stimulants. With rates of contamination between 12 and 58%, non-intentional doping is a point to take into account before establishing a supplementation program. Athletes and coaches must be aware of the problems related to the use of any contaminated supplement and should pay special attention before choosing a supplement, informing themselves fully and confirming the guarantees offered by the supplement.

Keywords: dietary supplements; doping; ergonutritional aids; WADA

1. Introduction

According to European Parliament Directive (2002/46/EC), a food supplement is defined as a product intended to supplement the normal diet, consisting of a concentrated source of a nutrient or of other substances that have a nutritional or physiological effect, in a simple or combined form, commercialized in dosed formulas, capsules, tablets, pills and other similar forms, bags of powder, vials of liquid, dropper bottles and other similar forms of liquids and powders, which is taken in small, quantified amounts [1]. In sport—understood as a set of motor situations codified in the form of competition, and institutionalized—athletes use ergogenic aids (any nutritional, physical, mechanical, psychological, or pharmacological maneuver or method) in order to increase their ability to perform physical work and improve performance [2]. In sport, dietary supplements (also known as ergonutritional aids) have been used since the first Olympic Games, although recently there has been a notable increase in their consumption by certain population groups [3–5]. Athletes consume a wide variety of dietary supplements and are the main target of the industry that produces them [6]. The "Sports Nutrition and Weight Loss Report", published by the Nutrition Business Journal, showed that sales of sports nutrition and weight loss products have increased year-on-year in the North American market, with nutritional supplements being in second place in the sales ranking [7].

This indicates that the sale and consumption of supplements have increased both in the general population and in the sports population. In a study of 3168 British Royal Army soldiers, a rate of supplement use of 38% at the time of the study was reported, reaching 54% when the use of supplements referred to the 12 months prior to the study [8]. In order of prevalence, the most used supplements were: protein powders/bars (66%), isotonic sports drinks (49%), creatine (38%), recovery drinks (35%), multivitamins (31%), and Vitamin C (25%). The work of Tscholl et al. was performed on 3887 athletes, and found a total consumption of 6523 supplements (1.7 per athlete) [9].

Some athletes have been reported to have tested positive for doping due to the intake of dietary supplements, which had either poor labeling or product contamination [5,10]. This poses a threat to the athlete's career or also to his or her health depending on the dose, as the World Anti-Doping Agency (WADA) states that it is the athlete's responsibility to ensure no prohibited substance or its metabolite or marker are in the samples [11]. An example of the presence of doping substances in supplements can be seen in the study published in 2003 by Geyer et al., where 94 of the 634 supplements analyzed (14.8%) had prohormones that were not mentioned on the label [12]. More current is the study by Judkins et al. in which, of the 58 supplements analyzed, 25% contained low levels of contaminating steroids and 11% were contaminated with stimulants [13]. These data have led to the investigation of contamination in different food supplements; in most of them, small quantities of banned substances have been found, due to cross-contamination during manufacturing, processing, or packaging [14–17]. In some cases, this contamination was not intentional and was due to poor quality control, but in others the adulteration of the substance was intentional [10]. In the United States (US), the Food and Drug Administration (FDA), broadly speaking, regulates quality, and the Federal Trade Commission supervises the marketing and advertising of dietary supplements [18]. However, according to the Dietary Supplement Health and Education Act (DSHEA), dietary supplements, including nutritional ergogenic aids, that are not intended to diagnose, treat, cure, or prevent any disease, currently do not need to be evaluated by the FDA prior to their commercialization [19].

Despite the proposed legislation and the pressure exerted by governments [20,21] and various organizations, such as the WADA, through the list of prohibited substances and methods, or the International Olympic Committee (IOC), with the acceptance of the World Anti-Doping Code [22,23], positive tests continue to occur in anti-doping checks due to products containing prohibited substances that are not listed in their labeling. One example is 19-norandrosterone, a substance found alongside stimulants, such as caffeine and epinephrine, in certain dietary supplements [24]. In 2003, after observing a series of repeated cases, a study was performed to determine the extent of the problem of unidentified prohormones in dietary supplements, giving positive results for 19-norandrosterone with the intake of only one capsule of product, while the proposed dose is four capsules, three times a day [25]. More recently, in a review of 24 different types of protein supplement, carried out in 2010 by ConsumerLab, 31% of products did not pass the proposed safety test, leaving in question the supposed safety that these products offer the consumer [26].

Therefore, the objective of the present work is to describe the presence of doping substances prohibited by the WADA in dietary supplements, used in the context of sport and published in research articles, thereby highlighting the problem of plausible positive tests in anti-doping checks and the health problems that could be generated by their unintended consumption.

2. Materials and Methods

This is a descriptive study, consisting of a bibliographic review of the presence of substances/metabolites/markers prohibited by the WADA in dietary supplements used in the sporting context. Contamination is understood as introduction into a medium of substances that cause it to be unsafe or unfit for use; in our case, the incorporation and non-declaration in the labeling of substances/metabolites/markers prohibited by WADA into ergonutritional supplements used by athletes. A data collection protocol was established for the research that met the inclusion criteria. The screening of the articles was performed by two researchers, independently.

A structured restrictive search was performed in the PubMed, Tripdatabase, and Epistemonikos databases using controlled and natural vocabulary descriptors related to "doping agents" and "Dietary supplements" concepts. The full electronic search strategy for PubMed was: ("prohibited substance" [tiab (title/abstract)] or "banned substance" [tiab] or "banned substances" [tiab] or "Doping in Sports" [Mesh] or "Doping in Sports" [tiab] or Doping [tiab] or "doping agent" [tiab] or "doping agents" [tiab]) AND ("Dietary Supplements" [Mesh] or "Dietary Supplements" [tiab] or "Dietary Supplement" [tiab] or Nutraceuticals [tiab] or Nutraceutical [tiab] or Nutriceutical [tiab] or Nutriceuticals [tiab] or Neutraceutical [tiab] or Neutraceuticals [tiab] or "Food Supplementations" [tiab] or "Food Supplementation" [tiab] or "Ergogenic aids" [tiab] or "Ergogenic aid" [tiab] or "dietary supplement, SPORT" [Supplementary Concept] or "nutritional supplement" [tiab] or "nutritional supplements" [tiab]). Also, relevant references related to the topic of the selected articles were searched for manually, using a snow-ball method. No additional filters were applied, and the last search was performed on 17 September 2017.

The eligibility criteria to select articles was:

- Evaluation of marketed dietary supplements for intended use in sports
- Evaluation of any type of prohibited substance, as defined by WADA (World Anti-Doping Agency. 2017 List of prohibited substances and methods. 2017 [22].)
- Only primary research was allowed, but secondary research was screened (by bibliography)
- No limits were set according language, years considered, or publication status or availability.

Two independent researchers screened titles and abstracts to pre-select studies from the list of articles retrieved by the search strategy. One researcher screened the pre-selected articles, by full-text reading, to apply eligibility criteria and a second researcher reviewed the selections, to ensure that all studies should be included. One researcher performed the data extraction without piloted forms, but a second researcher reviewed the extracted data to avoid extraction mistakes or missing information.

From selected studies, the extracted data set was composed of the following variables:

- Author/year: authors and year of publication.
- Country: geographical area from which the results obtained in the study come.
- Aim of the study: results that were intended to be achieved with the study.
- Sample: number and type of supplements analyzed.
- Methodology for the analysis of banned substances/metabolites/markers.
- Selected markers: tested substances/metabolites/markers that give positive results in anti-doping controls.
- Main results: final outcomes of the study, in which it is shown whether the proposed objectives have been achieved, and the main results obtained are listed.
- Conclusions: arguments and statements concerning the data obtained in the studies.

No risk of bias analysis in the included studies was performed and data was summarized through table summaries. No additional analysis was performed.

3. Results

The search strategy retrieved 446 articles (PubMed $n = 378$; Tripdatabase $n = 67$; Epistemonikos $n = 0$; 1 added manually from a review screening), which resulted in 423 unique articles after duplicate removal. After title and abstract screening, 54 titles were pre-selected, from which 23 were finally included, after full-text reading and eligibility criteria was applied.

Table 1 shows the study variables of the bibliographic review. The articles that met the inclusion requirements were published between 2000 and 2017. In regard to the countries of origin, six articles came from Germany, three from the USA, two from Switzerland, United Kingdom and Poland, while Belgium, Canada, Italy, Australia, Serbia, Czech Republic and South Africa contributed one article each (column 1 of Table 1). Column 2 shows that the goal of most of the studies was to identify doping substances (substances/metabolites/markers) in dietary supplements. Six studies determined whether the intake of contaminated dietary supplements could result in a positive test in anti-doping controls. The characteristics of the sample of supplements or study subjects are shown in column 3. Column 4 identifies the tested substances/metabolites/markers that give positive results in anti-doping controls. Column 5 refers to the main results, and column 6 to the conclusions of the studies included in the review.

Regarding the number of samples selected, more than 100 supplements were analyzed, when considering all the articles incorporated in this review. In five of the studies included, it was the subjects who had taken the substances of interest that were analyzed. In 13 of the 23 articles, more than two contaminating substances were studied, while in three articles, two contaminants were studied and in seven articles there was only a single substance under study. The contamination rate found in studies where more than two ergonutritional supplements were analyzed, ranged from 12% to 58%. While nine of the 10 studies that analyzed one or two supplements had rates of contamination of 100%, in the study by Goel et al. [27], where a single supplement was analyzed, the results obtained showed no contamination. In one of the 23 studies, the metabolic effects, produced two hours after the ingestion of an ergonomic supplement, contaminated by 19-nor-4-androstenedione and 4-androsten-3,17-dione, were identified after the collection of urine samples, for a total of five individuals. In five of the 23 studies, banned substances were sought in three specific supplements, by analyzing urine samples.

The most commonly used methodology for the detection of any unidentified substance or one prohibited in ergonomic supplementation by any of the official bodies was gas chromatography coupled to mass spectrometry (GC-MS) ($n = 10$), followed by liquid chromatography coupled to mass spectrometry (LC-MS) ($n = 3$), combined GC-MS + LC-MS ($n = 2$), nuclear magnetic resonance (NMR) ($n = 2$), HPLC-DAD ($n = 1$), UHPL-MS/MS ($n = 1$) and the modified Geyer method ($n = 1$).

Table 1. Information on studies analyzing contamination with substances/metabolites/markers prohibited by the World Anti-Doping Agency (WADA) in ergonutritional supplements.

Author/Year/Country	Aim	Sample	Selected Markers	Main Results	Conclusions
Van Thuyne, et al., 2006 [5] South Africa	Determine whether the intake of contaminated dietary supplements can make an athlete positive in an anti-doping test.	5 male volunteers (24–55 years old) (11–99.4 kg)	19-nor-4-androstenediona y 4-androsten-3,17-diona	All exceeded the minimum amount established by WADA 2 h post-intake. Two exceeded the minimum amount 36 h post-intake. The maximum value was 54.6 ng/mL (8 h post)	The intake of only micrograms of contaminated substance can provoke a positive in an antidoping test.
Geyer, H., et al., 2004 [12] Germany	Analysis of 634 non-hormonal supplements to identify possible contamination of undeclared prohormones.	634 supplements	Testosterone and its prohormones, nandrolone and its prohormones and baldonone	Of the 634 supplements analyzed, 94 presented unidentified contaminants on their labeling	Despite offering guarantees in terms of pollutants, the population must be cautious about using ergonutricional substances, since not all these products are free of doping substances.
Green, H., et al., 2001 [16] EEUU	Determine if steroids in supplements meet the Dietary Supplement Health and Education Act (DSHEA) labeling laws.	12 prohormones from 12 different brands, purchased from local stores.	5-androstenediol, 5-androstene-3,17-dione, 5-androstene-3b, 17b-diol, 4-androstene-3,17-dione, 5-androstene-3,17-diol, 19-Androstene-3b, 17b-diol, 4-androstene-3,17-diol, 19-nor-4-androstene-3,17-dione, 19-norandrostenedione, androstenedione, 19-nor-5-androstene-3,17-diol, Tribulus terrestris	Authors found that 11 of 12 brands tested did not meet the labeling requirements set out in the 1994 Dietary Supplement Health and Education Act. One brand contained 10 mg of testosterone, a controlled steroid, another contained 77% more than the label stated, and 11 of 12 contained less than the amount stated on the label.	The current study validates the concerns of physicians and sporting organizations that the labeling of some sports nutritional supplements does not accurately reflect what is contained in the product. This information may be helpful in deterring athletes from using substances that have unsubstantiated efficacy and unknown adverse effects.
Kamber, M., et al., 2001 [17] Switzerland	Determine whether the products tested contain anabolic steroids or stimulants not indicated or poorly described on the label.	75 products	Anabolic steroids or stimulants not listed or poorly described on labeling	In 7 out of 17 prohormones, different substances than indicated on the labels were found. This corresponds to 41% of the products in this class of supplements and 9% of all analyzed supplements. In two other products ("mental enhancers"), caffeine and ephedrine were found. Both compounds were either not, or not clearly declared, on the labels (e.g., declaration of the plant Ma Huang that contains ephedrine). The concentration of ephedrine in product 56 was so high that an athlete would test positive for doping if only one capsule was consumed just before competition.	It is recommended that athletes use only supplements that are registered in Switzerland (and even these supplements may not be entirely free of contaminates). In light of the easy availability of medicines and nutritional supplements through the Internet, we should strive to inform and educate users (especially adolescents) about nutritional supplements, and support international standards for accurate product labeling.

Table 1. *Cont.*

Author/Year/Country	Aim	Sample	Selected Markers	Main Results	Conclusions
Goel, D.P., et al., 2004 [27] Canada	Address and determine the feasibility of conducting clinical tests on a dietary supplement (Cold-FX®) under strict International Olympics Committee (IOC) doping-control procedures and to determine whether ingesting this ginseng extract would result in any doping-control infractions among athletes.	20 men and 20 women	Ginseng Extract (Cold-FX)	No positives were found for prohibited substances in any of the subjects' urine samples.	Cold-FX® substance is safe. This work could encourage companies to test dietary supplements so that athletes and athletic regulatory bodies have access to competent, comprehensive, credible, and unbiased information on the capacity for nutraceuticals and dietary supplements to induce positive urinalysis tests.
Baume, N., et al., 2006 [28] Switzerland	To screen the supplements for con-taminations with major anabolic steroid parent compounds, stimulants and traces of testosterone, nandrolone and their precursors	103 supplements, divided into creatine, prohormones, mental enhancers and branched amino acids, all purchased online.	4-Androstenediol, 4-Norandrostenediol, 5-Androstenedione, 5-Norandrostenediol, 19-Noranrostenedione, Androstenediol, Androstenedione, Bolasterone, Boldenone, Clostebol, Dehydroepiandrosterone (DHEA), Dihydrotestosterone (DHT), Drostanolone, Fluoxymesterone, Mesterolone, Metandienone, Metenolone, Methyltestosterone, Norethandrolone, Oxandrolone, Oxymesterone, Stanozol, Oxymetholone, Nandrolone, Testosterone, Testosterone Propionate, Turinabol, 5-Norandrostenedione.	Methandienone was found in 3 of the 103 products. 18% of the products had errors in the labeling, while 18 products were found to contain metabolites of testosterone or nandrolone. The most commonly used contaminant was testosterone and the most contaminated product was prohormonesl.	More studies are needed to analyze contamination in products or poorly labeling, in order to prevent and improve the quality of dietary supplements available in the market.

Table 1. *Cont.*

Author/Year/Country	Aim	Sample	Selected Markers	Main Results	Conclusions
Martello, S., et al., 2007 [29] Italy	Validation of a qualitative LC-MS/MS method for the determination of eight doping substances.	64 supplements obtained from stores and court proceedings.	4-androsten-3,17-dione, 4-oestrene-3,17-dione, 5α-androsten-17β-ol-3-one, Boldenone, Nandrolone, Nandrolone Decanolate, Testosterone, Testosterone Decanolate, Ephedrine	This LCMS/MS method was applied to 64 nutritional supplements and 12.5% of tested substances contained prohibited substances (anabolic steroids and ephedrine) not stated on the labeling.	The method reported is sufficiently sensitive, specific and selective for the detection and confirmation of prohibited substances in nutritional supplements. The low levels of the compounds found in the samples may indicate accidental contamination and not intentional admixture. However, athletes should consider only purchasing from companies that perform quality tests on prohormones, and which test for possible contamination during production.
Parr, M. K., et al., 2008 [30] Germany	Detection of clenbuterol in a sample of a fat burner	Sample of urine, 3 h post ingestion of a supplement tablet	Clenbuterol	After ingesting one tablet the participant reported tremor and delivered a urine sample. This urine was found to contain 2 ng/mL of clenbuterol utilizing LC-MS/MS analysis. Additionally the product itself was analyzed with gas chromatography coupled to mass spectrometry (GC-MS) for clenbuterol, yielding a content of about 30 µg per tablet.	The beta-2 agonist clenbuterol is only legally available on prescription and is classified as a prohibited doping substance in sports. The present case, for the first time, confirms the presence of clenbuterol in a dietary supplement. It again demonstrates the common problem with products on the supplement market, where non-licensed pharmaceuticals and doping substances are easily available. The ingestion of these products, containing additions of therapeutic drugs, can lead to side effects and/or interactions with conventional medicines.

Table 1. *Cont.*

Author/Year/Country	Aim	Sample	Selected Markers	Main Results	Conclusions
Van Poucke, C., et al., 2007 [31]	Belgium Determination of anabolic steroids in dietary supplements.	19 dietary supplements obtained via the internet from 12 different companies.	A and β Boldenone, α and β Nortestosterone, 17α-Hydroxyprogesterone, Algeston acetophenide, Chloromadinon Acetate, Clostebol Acetate, Delmadinone Acetate, Fluoximesterone, Formeblone, Megestrol Acetate, Melengestrol Acetate, Methylboldenone, Methyltestosterone, Norethandrolone, Noretistosterone, Norgestrel, Oxymetolone, Progesterone, Stanozol, Trenbolone, α and β Zeranol, D-equilenin, Dienestrol, Diethylstolbestrol, Ethinyl estradiol, Estradiol, Hexestrol, Testosterone, 16-dehydropnogesterone, 17α-acetoxyprogesterone, tenbolon 17β-acetate, 20β-hydroxyprogesterone, 3α and B-hydroxy-5β-estrane-17-one, α-testosterone, ethylstiltranediol, Flugestonacetate, Medroxyprogesterone acetate, Mestranol, Metandriol, Metenolone, Methenolone acetate, Methylandrantranediol, Norethystostosterone acetate, Noretilnodrel, Vinylstestone.	According to the labeling, 15 of the 19 products contained 1–5 prohormones. Eleven products contained at least one anabolic component, all of these products claimed to contain prohormones.	The analysis of the 19 dietary supplements, indicates that the supplements named are not suitable for athletes. In addition to having prohormones that can be activated in the body, anabolic steroids were found in their active form.

Table 1. *Cont.*

Author/Year/Country		Aim	Sample	Selected Markers	Main Results	Conclusions
Parr, M.K., et al., 2011 [32]	Germany	Identification of Δ6-methyltestosterone in a product named "Jungle Warfare", which was obtained from a web-based supplement store	1 subject (52 years, 77 kg, 1.70 m)	(Epi-) methyltestosterone	The presence of the study metabolite was confirmed both in the analysis of the supplement and in the urine sample of the study subject.	The Jungle Warfare supplement represents another product labeled as a dietary supplement that contains steroids not approved for medical use.
Watson, P., et al., 2009 [33]	UK	To detect urinary excretion of nandrolone metabolites after ingestion of a precursor of nandrolone.	20 subjects (11 men and 9 women) recreational athletes	19-norandrostenedione (nandrolone)	With the intake of a supplement contaminated with 1 μg, no athlete would give a positive result in a doping control. In the case of 2.5 μg, 5 subjects would give a positive result and 15 subjects, would pass the minimum level (2 ng/mL) allowed, giving a positive result in the test of 5 μg of nandrolone.	Ingestion of trace amounts of 19-norandrostenedione can result in transient elevations of urinary 19-NA and 19-NE concentrations. The addition of as little as 2.5 kg of 19-norandrostenedione to a supplement (0.00005% contamination) appears sufficient to result in a doping violation in some individuals.
Parr, M.K., et al., 2007 [34]	Germany	Check the lack of safety in the production of supplements and obtaining supplements.	2 dietary supplements were analyzed (Stanozol-S and Parabolon-S) obtained by telephone.	Methandienone, norandrostenedione, stanozolol, testosterone, 5α-dihydrotestosterone, boldenone and estrone.	In Parabolon-S, metandienone was found. In addition, Stanozolol-S, stanozol, testosterone, 5α-dihydrotestosterone and boldenone were found.	There is insufficient surveillance of the production and trade of dietary supplements. Consumers should be aware of the enormous health and doping risks connected with the use of such products. New regulations for trade, production and labeling should be adopted. The first step should be a public warning to consumers and the withdrawal of dietary supplements containing prescription drugs.

Table 1. *Cont.*

Author/Year/Country	Aim	Sample	Selected Markers	Main Results	Conclusions
Thevis, M., et al., 2013 [35]	Study the ability to detect the origin of clenbuterol (therapeutic use or food intake) depending on the presence of racemic mixtures (enantiomers).	6 urine samples, collected from 2 male subjects	Stereoisomers + and − of Clenbuterol		The determination of relative abundances of clenbuterol enantiomers can indicate the ingestion of clenbuterol via contaminated food; however, depletion of (−)-clenbuterol in edible animal tissue is time-dependent and thus results can still be inconclusive as to the inadvertent ingestion of clenbutero, 1 when clenbuterol administration to animals was conducted until slaughter.
Monakhova, Y.B., et al., 2014 [36]	Test an magnetic resonance (NMR)-based method with minimal sample preparation for determination of 1,3–dimethylamylamine (DMAA) in sports nutrition and dietary supplements.	16 sports nutrition products and dietary supplements	1,3–dimethylamylamine	9 of the 16 substances were contaminated with DMAA.	Routine application of NMR is an alternative to time-consuming chromatographic methods for DMAA quantification in various kinds of products. 1H NMR spectroscopy has proven to be a robust analytical tool, yielding highly reliable quantitative results regarding DMAA, in a very short time. The approach is advantageous as it minimizes sample preparation and allows for the analysis of a large number of samples without human intervention (120 samples in a batch). The developed NMR method is recommended for use in food testing, customs and doping control laboratories, for the routine control of DMAA.

Table 1. *Cont.*

Author/Year/Country	Aim	Sample	Selected Markers	Main Results	Conclusions
Abbate V., et al., 2014 [37]	United Kingdom	Determine any steroid present in the supplements, using full scan gas chromatography-mass spectrometry (GC-MS), accurate mass liquid chromatography-mass spectrometry (LC-MS), high pressure liquid chromatography with diode array detection (HPLC-DAD), UV-Vis, and nuclear magnetic resonance (NMR)	A total of 24 products were purchased from two fitness equipment shops—one in Merseyside and one in Cheshire—and three online shops.	Anabolic steroids	Of the 24 products tested, 23 contained steroids, including known anabolic agents; sixteen of these contained steroids that were different to those indicated on the packaging and one product contained no steroids at all. Overall, 13 different steroids were identified; 12 of these are controlled in the UK under the Misuse of Drugs Act 1971. Several of the products contained steroids that may be considered to have considerable pharmacological activity, based on their chemical structures and the amounts present. This could unwittingly expose users to a significant risk to their health, which is of particular concern for naive users.	The analytical methods used can play an essential role in the public health response to these drugs by providing methodologies to identify and quantify the active substance(s) present. This helps develop our understanding of this market, as well as allowing us to monitor the composition of supplements sold and the hazards that they may pose. When considered with other data, such as prevalence of use, these types of study play a central role in assessing and quantifying the risks to individual and public health.
Cooper E.R., et al. 2017 [38]	Australia	Characterize the androgenic bioactivity of sports supplements available from the Australian market, using yeast and mammalian cell androgen bioassays.	112 sports supplements available from the Australian market, either over the counter or via the Internet.	Androgens (Androgen bioactivity)	All 112 products did not declare an androgen on the label as an included ingredient. Our findings show that 6/112 supplements had strong androgenic bioactivity in the yeast cell bioassay, indicating products spiked or contaminated with androgens. The mammalian cell bioassay confirmed the strong androgenic bioactivity of 5/6 positive supplements. Supplement 6 was metabolized to weaker androgenic bioactivity in the mammalian cells. Further to this, supplement 6 showed a positive result in a yeast cell progestin bioassay.	These findings highlight that nutritional supplements, taken without medical supervision, could expose or predispose users to the adverse consequences of androgen abuse. The findings reinforce the need to increase the awareness of the dangers of nutritional supplements and highlight the challenges that clinicians face in the fast-growing market of nutritional supplements.

Table 1. *Cont.*

Author/Year/Country	Aim	Sample	Selected Markers	Main Results	Conclusions
Cohen E.A., et al., 2013 [39]	USA	Detect the presence and concentration of N-alpha-Diethylphenylethylamine (N,α-DEPEA) in supplement Craze (Driven Sports, Inc.)	Three samples from different lot numbers of Craze	N,α-DEPEA	The identity of N,α-DEPEA was confirmed using nuclear magnetic resonance and reference standards. Manufacturer recommended servings were estimated to provide 21 to 35 mg of N,α-DEPEA. N,α-DEPEA has never been studied in humans. N,α-DEPEA is a methamphetamine analog; however, its stimulant, addictive and other adverse effects in humans are entirely unknown.	If the findings are confirmed by regulatory authorities, the Food and Drug Administration (FDA) should take immediate action to warn consumers and remove all N,α-DEPEA-containing supplements from the marketplace.
Stepan R., et al., 2008 [40]	Czech Republic	Analytical approach employing ethyl acetate extraction, dispersive solid-phase extraction (SPE) clean-up using PSA followed by an analysis of underivatized compounds, using comprehensive two-dimensional gas chromatography with time-of-flight mass spectrometric detection (GC×GC–TOF MS) is presented.	Two types of commercially available solid nutritional supplements: protein concentrate and creatine monohydrate	Anabolic steroids	Results from this monitoring programme showed a total 6.3% (i.e., three) positive samples. Nandrolone (0.022 mg kg^{-1}), testosterone (0.070 mg kg^{-1}) and DHEA (0.063 mg kg^{-1}) were found in a whey protein gainer, 5-androstan-3,17-dione (0.398 mg kg^{-1}) and 19-norandrostendione (0.304 mg kg^{-1}) in creatine pyruvate, and one sample of synephrine-based 'fat burner' contained progesterone (0.102 mg kg^{-1}).	This analytical method, based on the comprehensive two-dimensional gas chromatography with time-of-flight mass spectrometric detection, provides an advantageous strategy for the determination of anabolic androgenic steroids and related compounds in nutritional supplements. The use of dispersive solid-phase extraction (SPE) with primary secondary amine (PSA) for the clean-up of crude extracts prepared from other matrices could likely be an efficient process for removing interferences and should be considered individually, according to the type of co-extracted matrix components.

Table 1. *Cont.*

Author/Year/Country	Aim	Sample	Selected Markers	Main Results	Conclusions
Parr M.K., et al., 2011 [41]	Warn about the presence of designer steroids in some dietary or nutritional supplements.	Reports a few doping cases caused by the use of supplements with doping substances by athletes, noted by two World Anti-Doping Agency (WADA) accredited laboratories (Cologne and Warsaw)	Steroids	Steroids that may be interpreted as metabolites of Δ6-methyltestosterone, were detected. The availability of the athletes' supplements allowed for confirmation of this interpretation, as one of the products indeed contained Δ6-methyltestosterone. These findings confirmed the presumption that such products are used by athletes and that their consumption may lead to positive results in doping controls.	Top level athletes use "dietary supplements" that contain so-called designer steroids. The statistics of the World Anti-Doping Agency in recent years has reported some more cases with steroids that are only available in dubious products and not as approved pharmaceuticals. However, people outside of elite sport were also found to have used such designer supplements. Still more education on the health and doping risks of dietary supplement products seems to be necessary for the protection of both athletes and the general public.
Stajic A., et al., 2017 [42]	Develop and validate the sensitive and reliable ultra-high pressure liquid chromatography tandem mass spectrometry (UHPLC/MS/MS) method for determination of higenamine in different dietary supplements.	Different dietary supplements of various compositions and pharmaceutical forms were collected. Among all collected supplements, 19 were of interest for higenamine analyses. Dietary supplements were purchased in sport shops, via the Internet or from the local pharmacy. Samples were taken from the original packages, adequately labeled and stored.	Higenamine	According to the results, most of the investigated supplements were free of higenamine, but on the other hand, the presence of higenamine was confirmed in some samples, while it was not declared on the label. Presence of higenamine, a banned substance, was confirmed in two investigated samples.	A sensitive and reliable UHPLC/MS/MS method for higenamine determination in various dietary supplements was developed and validated. This method was successfully applied for the analysis of 19 dietary supplements and, in this way, applicability of the method was confirmed.

Table 1. *Cont.*

Author/Year/Country	Aim	Sample	Selected Markers	Main Results	Conclusions
Kohler M., et al., 2010 [21]	Germany	Provides an overview the products that were analyzed in the Cologne Doping Control Laboratory in 2009 and gives an overview on the classes of substances and the astonishingly small number of products that contain exactly the labelled substance.	A number of different products were analyzed from various sources, such as customs, police, and national anti-doping authorities, or were bought over-the-counter as nutritional supplements. Most of the commodities contained protein- or peptide-based substances, many of which were not in agreement with their respective labels or contained poorly purified analogues or artefacts.	Long-R3-IGF-I, GHRP-2, Andarine (S-4)	The products analyzed during 2009 showed that black market products nowadays also include different peptide hormone-derived products rather than steroid hormone preparations only. From the confiscated products, only 4 out of 11 contained the substance and amount declared on their label, and long-growth factor 1 (R3-IGF-I) and human growth hormones were the proteins detected (or at least labelled) most frequently (three products each), which may indicate that they are also ordered and used very often. In contrast, the nutritional supplements containing Growth Hormone releasing Peptide-2 (GHRP-2) as well as the glass bottle with Andarine (S-4) were labelled with xenobiotic ingredients, although none of them are approved as regular therapeutic agents yet.	The awareness of new products on the black market and in nutritional supplements is of utmost importance for laboratories to develop detection methods accordingly and screen for new substances as early as possible.
Thomas A., et al., 2010 [43]	Germany	The qualitative identification and quantification of the approximate content of GHRP-2 in tablets offered as nutritional supplements by means of liquid chromatography coupled to high resolution/high accuracy mass spectrometry, is described.	Nutritional supplements in tablets	GHRP-2 and Hexarelin		The presented case report demonstrates the urgency of flexible analytics in doping controls. Although, to date no positive doping cases with GHRP-2 were reported, the fact that the bioactive compound is available as a nutritional supplement, indicates that analytical findings in routinely analyzed plasma or urine samples from elite sportsmen are possible.

Table 1. *Cont.*

Author/Year/Country	Aim	Sample	Selected Markers	Main Results	Conclusions
Kwiatkowska D., et al., 2015 [44]	Analyze urine samples to detecte stimulants and narcotics in anti-doping controls	The urine samples were taken from four athletes during in competition anti-doping control, and nutritional supplement NOXPUMP Pre-Training Formula (Fruit Punch)	Stimulants and narcotics	N,N-dimethyl-2-phenylpropan-1-amine (NN-DMPPA) is a possible new doping agent, detected and identified by the WADA-accredited laboratory in Warsaw (Poland) during routine anti-doping control. The presence of NN-DMPPA in several urine samples and in the supplement, NOXPUMP, was confirmed by GC-MS. In most of the athletes who failed urine drug tests because of the presence of NN-DMPPA, some other banned stimulants were also detected. NN-DMPPA was detected in the supplement NOXPUMP but we cannot exclude its presence in other supplements from the black market.	This suggests the use of supplements which are often mixtures of prohibited drugs which may not be listed on the label or even the use of several supplements containing various banned substances. The range of supplements available in stores is constantly growing and while many supplements contain materials (e.g., vitamins, proteins, minerals) with possible useful properties, many pose the risk of unintentional doping with designer agents. This is often caused by the lack of labelling of all contents and/or unusual naming of components on the supplement label. Improved legislation, dealing with the commercialization of the drugs banned for sport, should be enacted.

55

4. Discussion

Among the main findings of the present review is the presence of doping substances in studied dietary supplements or aids, which are not substances identified in the nutritional composition declared on the labeling, or whose amounts stated therein differ from their actual content. Among the substances found, but not listed, on the label are prohormones, anabolic steroids, mental enhancers, and 1,3-dimethylamylamine. All of these are substances that are prohibited by the WADA, which would give a positive doping test result for the athletes who have consumed these supplements or ergonutritional aids. Some of the studies analyzed the presence of contaminants in human subjects after the consumption of contaminated supplements or ergonutritional aids; in other studies, the products themselves were analyzed.

4.1. Consumption and Contamination of Ergonutritional Supplements

The consumption of ergonutritional supplements is one of the most common practices in the sports world; advertisements for such products claim that their use will prevent injuries or enhance performance [27]. They can be used by as many as 90% of participants, depending on the sport [28]. Linked to these high frequencies of consumption, we have found that one of the most serious and increasingly frequent problems regarding the intake of dietary supplements is unintentional doping. The consumption of these supplements forms part of the daily routine of most athletes, who must be completely sure of the efficacy and safety of any type of dietary supplement before its consumption, as well as of its detailed composition. The data reported by some studies are noteworthy; for instance, the rate of contamination in ergonutritional supplements varied from 12% to 58% in samples analyzed between 2002 and 2005, and in 216 cases, hormones were found in dietary supplements that should not have contained them [17,29,30]. To avoid this, the controls and legislative strategies related to these supplements need to be improved, to guarantee the safety of products that are freely available to the general population and athletes.

Specifically, in the present review, all the papers included showed the presence of substances that are prohibited by the WADA in some of the dietary supplements analyzed. The most frequently encountered components in these products were anabolic steroids (banned by the IOC since 1974 after the positives detected at the Commonwealth Games held in New Zealand), although other prohibited substances were also present—such as certain stimulants (ephedrine, nor-pseudoephedrine, sibutramine) [11,31,32]. In addition to the serious effects that the consumption of these contaminated substances can have on health—such as hepatotoxicity, cardiac and hormonal problems, carcinogenesis, and even death in some cases [4,31]—the following can be added: social damage, related to moral damage, loss of sponsors, and penalties (among others), deriving from possible detection in doping tests.

The presence of substances not listed on labeling and banned by the WADA is not the only problem derived from the consumption of supplements. The lack of precision in the labeling of these products, in terms of quantity, is another of the problems associated with the consumption of such substances, according to various studies [17,29,33–35].

This review of the literature indicated that the consumption of supplements occurs in a high percentage of athletes, mainly driven by coaches, relatives, and other athletes, with the aim of achieving better results. One of the most important studies regarding the consumption of supplements is the one made by Tscholl et al. in 2010 [9], in which the data of 3887 questionnaires were collected during the world championship of the International Association of Athletics Federations. This study showed the consumption of 6523 supplements (1.7 per athlete); the consumption was greatest in adults and in participants in outdoor competitions. A study of 567 Canadian athletes between the ages of 11 and 25 found daily intake of supplements by 28% of them, with the main goal being to improve the consumption of vitamins and minerals and to improve performance [36]. Another study, involving 292 Portuguese athletes, from 13 different federations, showed a consumption rate of 66%, with an average of four supplements per athlete, with acceleration of recovery (63%) and improvement of performance (62%) being the main reasons for consumption [45].

It was from the year 2000 when the problems caused by unintentional doping began to take on importance, and the first studies on the quality of nutritional supplements were carried out [17,46]. The contamination rate due to errors in labeling, either by omission of substances present in the product, or by errors in the quantification of the concentrations, is relatively high, according to the various studies carried out [4,10,12,46–48]. One of the most relevant studies, due to the number of supplements analyzed, which laid the groundwork for the determination of the contamination of nutritional supplements, is that performed by Geyer et al., in 2001, in Germany, where 634 non-hormonal supplements were analyzed in the search for testosterone and its prohormones, nandrolone and its prohormones, and boldenone [12]. The results showed that 15% of the samples contained hormones or prohormones that were not identified in the labeling. A similar study was conducted by Kamber et al., in 2001, in which the objective was the detection of anabolic steroids or stimulants, not indicated, or poorly described, on the label [17]. The study analyzed 75 products, of which 17 were prohormonal supplements, and all contained substances not described in the labeling. In 2004, a study was published, in which 103 supplements, purchased online, and divided into four categories (creatine, prohormones, mental enhancers, and branched-chain amino acids), were analyzed. In this case, the most common contaminant was testosterone and the products with the highest contamination rate were prohormones. The labeling error rate was 18%, whereas 20% of the products contained metabolites of different hormones not allowed by the WADA [49].

Many of the studies involving contamination in supplements are aimed at validating a precise method of analysis for the detection of compounds banned by entities, such as the World Anti-Doping Association. An example of this is the study by Martello et al., in which gas chromatography coupled to tandem mass spectrometry (GC–MS/MS) was used as a screening system to detect certain androgenic steroids and ephedrine in dietary supplements. Thus, 64 nutritional supplements, obtained from stores and by judicial procedures (and classified as four vitamins/mineral supplements, seven glutamine/creatine, nine amino acids, 12 protein, eight prohibited substances, 12 herbal extracts and four others) were analyzed. Through this method, anabolic steroids and ephedrine were detected in 12.5% of the analyzed samples [34].

Finally, the online expansion of the advertising and marketing of ergonutritional supplements for sportsmen and women on the Internet has begun to constitute a public health problem. This is due to the free sale of these products without the health authorities carrying out the necessary inspections of the distribution and marketing. A study published by Van Poucke in 2006 analyzed 19 dietary supplements obtained via the internet. Fifteen of these claimed, on the labeling, the presence of between one and five prohormones, but 11 supplements were suspected of containing at least one anabolic steroid. Liquid chromatography showed that all the suspect substances contained at least one anabolic steroid, with testosterone and b-boldenone being the banned substances with the highest rates of use [31].

As for the factors causing this contamination, there are two main causes: (1) cross-contamination and (2) intentional contamination. Cross-contamination occurs unintentionally, as described by Hon and Coumans, because the prohormone concentration is low, which would not produce a potentiating effect of the supplement [16]. This occurs mainly because the manufacturers of prohormones (sold legally as supplements in the United States until 2004) also make other nutritional supplements. Cross-contamination could be due to the lack of cleaning of the vitamin containers, since the same production line is used without sufficient cleaning of the machinery [4,10]. The consumption of supplements affected by cross-contamination, despite the low concentration of contaminants, can lead to cases of unintentional doping [17]. Intentional contamination occurs when high concentrations of prohormones are added to the supplement by the manufacturer, with the aim of enhancing its effects [46].

Geyer et al. analyzed the number of nutritional supplements subject to cross-contamination with prohormones in different countries, between 2001 and 2002. The United States and Germany were the countries with the highest production of supplements, although The Netherlands and Austria had the highest contamination rates in their products [48].

4.2. Anti-Doping Organizations

Because of this, mechanisms of action have been put in place to combat contamination in supplements. The purpose is to produce a reliable source of information in which the athlete can check the safety of the supplement to be consumed [50]. The WADA, one of the main bodies that deals with the detection and prevention of doping in athletes, has established a strict liability policy, which states that unintentional doping is the responsibility of the athlete. Therefore, even if the athlete had no intention of improving his/her performance through the use of prohibited substances, if a doping control proves positive due to the use of contaminated ergonutritional supplements, it is the athlete, not the manufacturer or the seller, on whom the established sanction would fall. To avoid this type of situation, the WADA publishes—via the internet—the novelties and adverse findings for the supplements analyzed by its accredited laboratories. Other entities, such as the Court of Arbitration for Sport (TAS) [51], make athletes aware of registered doping cases and provide information regarding the possible source of the prohibited substance. Contributions are also made by National Anti-Doping Organizations (NADOs), such as that of Australia (ASADA) [52]—which offers an online search tool (Global DRO) to athletes and support personnel, to find out whether the most commonly prescribed and over-the-counter medicines in Australia are permitted or prohibited in their sport. Two other organizations pursuing similar strategies are the UK Anti-Doping Authority (UKAD) [53] and the US Anti-Doping Agency (USADA) [54]. In addition, there are other ways to check the safety of ergonutritional supplements, unofficially and without being endorsed by the WADA or the respective NADO—such as the Anti-Doping Authority the Netherlands (NZVT) project in Holland [55], the Cologne List in Germany [56], Informed Sports in the UK [57], the NSF Certified for Sports program of the Canadian Center for Sports Ethics [58], the Drug-free Sport NZ application of the New Zealand Anti-Doping Agency [59], the Supplement 411 program of USADA [60], or the "Alerts" section of the website of the Spanish Agency for the Protection of Health in Sport (AEPSAD) [61].

4.3. Limitations

Some limitations of this review, inherent in the use of electronic searches and retrieval of documents, should be pointed out. One of the most important limitations is that not all papers included analyzed the same prohibited compounds neither the same kind of samples, so several prohibited substances not analyzed could be also present in those products.

5. Conclusions

The safety issue regarding dietary supplements is real and therefore an improvement of the current legislation regulating the market for dietary supplements is needed to ensure the safety, efficacy, potency, and legality of the available ergonutritional supplements. Hence, the awareness of both athletes and coaches of the possible consequences of the use of ergonutritional supplements is especially important, as are discussions of the advantages and disadvantages and the provision of information related to the safety, provenance, and effectiveness of any type of supplement, before its consumption. The use of supplements without a specific need, illness, or deficiency—in addition to not being recommended—is unnecessary, when the athlete is following a balanced and adapted diet. Despite the strategies implemented by different governmental agencies to avoid doping in athletes, some positive doping results might be non-intentional and caused by the consumption of dietary supplements contaminated with doping substances.

Likewise, the fact that, in these products, information is often omitted from the labeling is a reason for sanctioning the companies that manufacture these food substances—since they are providing inaccurate or incomplete data—in accordance with Spanish Law 28/2015, for the defense of food quality [62]. This shows non-compliance with food labeling legislation, intended to protect the quality, the regulator of which is the government.

Although our work shows the existence of several dietary supplements on sale containing prohibited substances, more comprehensive studies are needed to know the extent and the prevalence of this problem.

Therefore, the previously described factors that affect food quality could be considered as an avoidable public health problem that indicates the need for governments to establish control strategies for procedures throughout the food chain, to generate a high level of confidence in dietary supplements which are habitually consumed by athletes. Likewise, compliance with the general principle of veracity and demonstration of the information contained in the labeling of ergonutritional products, must be guaranteed.

Acknowledgments: We are grateful to David Walker (native English speaker) and for their reviews of the English grammar and style of the current report.

Author Contributions: José Miguel Martínez, Isabel Sospedra and Christian Mañas carried out the analytical processes and wrote and discussed the present paper. Eduard Baladia supervised the materials and methods section and helped with the review of the manuscript. Ángel Gil-Izquierdo and Rocio Ortiz Moncada designed, supervised, and discussed this research work.

Conflicts of Interest: This paper corresponds to a literature review and it isn't sent to another journal, besides this paper does not have present conflicts of interest and economic with institutions, organizations or authors. They are ceded to Nutrients, the exclusive rights to edit, publish, reproduce, distribute copies, prepare derivative works on paper, electronic or multimedia and include the article in national and international indices or databases.

Abbreviations

NSAIDs	Nonsteroidal anti-inflammatory drugs
WADA	World Anti-Doping Agency
IOC	International Olympic Committee
TAS	Court of Arbitration for Sport
NADO	National Anti-Doping Organization
ASADA	Australian Sports Anti-Doping Authority
UKAD	UK Anti-Doping Authority
USADA	United States Anti-Doping Agency
NZVT	Anti-Doping Authority the Netherlands
AEPSAD	Spanish Agency for Health Protection in Sport
DHEA	Dehydroepiandrosterone
DHT	Dihydrotestosterone
NMR	Magnetic resonance
N,α-DEPEA	N,alpha-Diethylphenylethylamine
SPE	Solid-phase extraction
PSA	Primary secondary amine
UHPLC /MS/MS	Ultra-high pressure liquid chromatography tandem mass spectrometry
R3-IGF I	Growth factor 1
GHRP-2	Growth hormone releasing peptide-2
S-4	Andarine

References

1. *Directive 2002/46/EC of the European Parliament and of the Council of 10 02 on the Approximation of the Laws of the Member States Relating to Food Supplements*; European Parliament and of the Council: Brussels, Belgium, 2002; pp. 51–57.

2. Gil-Antuñano, N.P.; Bonafonte, L.F.; Marqueta, P.M.; Manuz, B.; García, J.A.V. Consenso sobre bebidas para el deportista. Composición y pautas de reposición de liquidos. *Arch. Med. Deporte* **2008**, *25*, 245–258.

3. Wallace, T.C. Twenty Years of the Dietary Supplement Health and Education Act—How Should Dietary Supplements Be Regulated? *J. Nutr.* **2015**, *145*, 1683–1686. [CrossRef] [PubMed]

4. Maughan, R.J. Quality assurance issues in the use of dietary supplements, with special reference to protein supplements. *J. Nutr.* **2013**, *143*, 1843S–1847S. [CrossRef] [PubMed]

5. Van Thuyne, W.; Van Eenoo, P.; Delbeke, F.T. Nutritional supplements: Prevalence of use and contamination with doping agents. *Nutr. Res. Rev.* **2006**, *19*, 147–158. [CrossRef] [PubMed]

6. Burke, L. *Nutrition in Sport: A Practical. Approach*; Médica Panamericana: Madrid, Spain, 2009; 556p.

7. 2016 NBJ Sports Nutrition and Weight Loss Report. Available online: https://www.newhope.com/products/2016-nbj-sports-nutrition-and-weight-loss-report (accessed on 4 April 2017).

8. Casey, A.; Hughes, J.; Izard, R.M.; Greeves, J.P. Supplement use by UK-based British Army soldiers in training. *Br. J. Nutr.* **2014**, *112*, 1175–1184. [CrossRef] [PubMed]

9. Tscholl, P.; Alonso, J.M.; Dollé, G.; Junge, A.; Dvorak, J. The use of drugs and nutritional supplements in top-level track and field athletes. *Am. J. Sports Med.* **2010**, *38*, 133–140. [CrossRef] [PubMed]

10. Maughan, R.J. Contamination of dietary supplements and positive drug tests in sport. *J. Sports Sci.* **2005**, *23*, 883–889. [CrossRef] [PubMed]

11. World Anti-Doping Agency (WADA). World Anti-Doping Code. World Anti-Doping Agency, 2013. Available online: https://www.wada-ama.org/en/what-we-do/the-code (accessed on 15 May 2017).

12. Geyer, H.; Parr, M.K.; Mareck, U.; Reinhart, U.; Schrader, Y.; Schänzer, W. Analysis of non-hormonal nutritional supplements for anabolic-androgenic steroids—Results of an international study. *Int. J. Sports Med.* **2004**, *25*, 124–129. [PubMed]

13. Judkins, C.M.G.; Teale, P.; Hall, D.J. The role of banned substance residue analysis in the control of dietary supplement contamination. *Drug Test. Anal.* **2010**, *2*, 417–420. [CrossRef] [PubMed]

14. Ayotte, C.; Lévesque, J.F.; Clé roux, M.; Lajeunesse, A.; Goudreault, D.; Fakirian, A. Sport nutritional supplements: Quality and doping controls. *Can. J. Appl. Physiol. Rev. Can. Physiol. Appl.* **2001**, *26*, S120–S129. [CrossRef]

15. Pipe, A.; Ayotte, C. Nutritional supplements and doping. *Clin. J. Sport Med. Off. J. Can. Acad. Sport Med.* **2002**, *12*, 245–249. [CrossRef]

16. Green, G.A.; Catlin, D.H.; Starcevic, B. Analysis of over-the-counter dietary supplements. *Clin J. Sport Med. Off. J. Can. Acad. Sport Med.* **2001**, *11*, 254–259. [CrossRef]

17. Kamber, M.; Baume, N.; Saugy, M.; Rivier, L. Nutritional supplements as a source for positive doping cases? *Int. J. Sport Nutr. Exerc. Metab.* **2001**, *11*, 258–263. [CrossRef] [PubMed]

18. Starr, R.R. Too little, too late: Ineffective regulation of dietary supplements in the United States. *Am. J. Public Health* **2015**, *105*, 478–485. [CrossRef] [PubMed]

19. Dietary Supplement Health and Education (DSHEA) Act of 1994. Available online: https://ods.od.nih.gov/About/DSHEA_Wording.aspx (accessed on 14 May 2017).

20. Petroczi, A.; Taylor, G.; Naughton, D.P. Mission impossible? Regulatory and enforcement issues to ensure safety of dietary supplements. *Food Chem. Toxicol.* **2011**, *49*, 393–402. [CrossRef] [PubMed]

21. Kohler, M.; Thomas, A.; Geyer, H.; Petrou, M.; Schänzer, W.; Thevis, M. Confiscated black market products and nutritional supplements with non-approved ingredients analyzed in the Cologne Doping Control Laboratory 2009. *Drug Test. Anal.* **2010**, *2*, 533–537. [CrossRef] [PubMed]

22. What is Prohibited. World Anti-Doping Agency, 2016. Available online: https://www.wada-ama.org/en/prohibited-list (accessed on 24 April 2017).

23. Olympics I Olympic Games, Medals, Results, News I IOC. International Olympic Committee, 2017. Available online: https://www.olympic.org/ (accessed on 24 April 2017).

24. Ayotte, C. Significance of 19-norandrosterone in athletes' urine samples. *Br. J. Sports Med.* **2006**, *40* (Suppl. S1), i25–i29. [CrossRef] [PubMed]

25. Minuchin, P.S. *Manual of Nutrition Applied to the Sport*; Nobuko: Buenos Aires, Argentina, 2004; 274p.

26. ConsumerLab.com—Independent Tests and Reviews of Vitamin, Mineral, and Herbal Supplements. Available online: https://www.consumerlab.com/ (accessed on 24 April 2017).

27. Goel, D.P.; Geiger, J.D.; Shan, J.J.; Kriellaars, D.; Pierce, G.N. Doping-control urinalysis of a ginseng extract, Cold-FX, in athletes. *Int. J. Sport Nutr. Exerc. Metab.* **2004**, *14*, 473–480. [CrossRef] [PubMed]

28. Baume, N.; Mahler, N.; Kamber, M.; Mangin, P.; Saugy, M. Research of stimulants and anabolic steroids in dietary supplements. *Scand. J. Med. Sci. Sports* **2006**, *16*, 41–48. [CrossRef] [PubMed]

29. Martello, S.; Felli, M.; Chiarotti, M. Survey of nutritional supplements for selected illegal anabolic steroids and ephedrine using LC-MS/MS and GC-MS methods, respectively. *Food Addit. Contam.* **2007**, *24*, 258–265. [CrossRef] [PubMed]

30. Parr, M.K.; Koehler, K.; Geyer, H.; Guddat, S.; Schänzer, W. Clenbuterol marketed as dietary supplement. Biomed. Chromatogr. BMC **2008**, *22*, 298–300. [PubMed]

31. Van Poucke, C.; Detavernier, C.; Van Cauwenberghe, R.; Van Peteghem, C. Determination of anabolic steroids in dietary supplements by liquid chromatography-tandem mass spectrometry. *Anal. Chim. Acta* **2007**, *586*, 35–42. [CrossRef] [PubMed]

32. Parr, M.K.; Fusshöller, G.; Schlörer, N.; Opfermann, G.; Geyer, H.; Rodchenkov, G.; Schänzer, W. Detection of Δ6-methyltestosterone in a "dietary supplement" and GC-MS/MS investigations on its urinary metabolism. *Toxicol. Lett.* **2011**, *201*, 101–104. [CrossRef] [PubMed]

33. Watson, P.; Judkins, C.; Houghton, E.; Russell, C.; Maughan, R.J. Urinary nandrolone metabolite detection after ingestion of a nandrolone precursor. *Med. Sci. Sports Exerc.* **2009**, *41*, 766–772. [CrossRef] [PubMed]

34. Parr, M.K.; Geyer, H.; Hoffmann, B.; Köhler, K.; Mareck, U.; Schänzer, W. High amounts of 17-methylated anabolic-androgenic steroids in effervescent tablets on the dietary supplement market. *Biomed. Chromatogr. BMC* **2007**, *21*, 164–168. [CrossRef] [PubMed]

35. Thevis, M.; Thomas, A.; Beuck, S.; Butch, A.; Dvorak, J.; Schänzer, W. Does the analysis of the enantiomeric composition of clenbuterol in human urine enable the differentiation of illicit clenbuterol administration from food contamination in sports drug testing? *Rapid Commun. Mass Spectrom RCM* **2013**, *27*, 507–512. [CrossRef] [PubMed]

36. Monakhova, Y.B.; Ilse, M.; Hengen, J.; El-Atma, O.; Kuballa, T.; Kohl-Himmelseher, M.; Lachenmeier, D.W. Rapid assessment of the illegal presence of 1,3-dimethylamylamine (DMAA) in sports nutrition and dietary supplements using 1H NMR spectroscopy. *Drug Test Anal.* **2014**, *6*, 944–948. [CrossRef] [PubMed]

37. Abbate, V.; Kicman, A.T.; Evans-Brown, M.; McVeigh, J.; Cowan, D.A.; Wilson, C.; Coles, S.J.; Walker, C.J. Anabolic steroids detected in bodybuilding dietary supplements—A significant risk to public health. *Drug Test Anal.* **2015**, *7*, 609–618. [CrossRef] [PubMed]

38. Cooper, E.R.; McGrath, K.C.Y.; Li, X.; Heather, A.K. Androgen Bioassay for the Detection of Non-labeled Androgenic Compounds in Nutritional Supplements. *Int. J. Sport Nutr. Exerc. Metab.* **2017**, 1–26. [CrossRef] [PubMed]

39. Cohen, P.A.; Travis, J.C.; Venhuis, B.J. A methamphetamine analog (N,α-diethyl-phenylethylamine) identified in a mainstream dietary supplement. *Drug Test Anal.* **2014**, *6*, 805–807. [CrossRef] [PubMed]

40. Stepan, R.; Cuhra, P.; Barsova, S. Comprehensive two-dimensional gas chromatography with time-of-flight mass spectrometric detection for the determination of anabolic steroids and related compounds in nutritional supplements. *Food Addit. Contam. Part Chem. Anal. Control Expo. Risk Assess.* **2008**, *25*, 557–565. [CrossRef] [PubMed]

41. Parr, M.; Pokrywka, A.; Kwiatkowska, D.; Schänzer, W. Ingestion of designer supplements produced positive doping cases unexpected by the athletes. *Biol. Sport Inst. Sport* **2011**, *28*, 153–157. [CrossRef]

42. Stajić, A.; Anđelković, M.; Dikić, N.; Rašić, J.; Vukašinović-Vesić, M.; Ivanović, D.; Jančić-Stojanović, B. Determination of higenamine in dietary supplements by UHPLC/MS/MS method. *J. Pharm. Biomed. Anal.* **2017**, *146*, 48–52. [CrossRef] [PubMed]

43. Thomas, A.; Kohler, M.; Mester, J.; Geyer, H.; Schänzer, W.; Petrou, M.; Thevis, M. Identification of the growth-hormone-releasing peptide-2 (GHRP-2) in a nutritional supplement. *Drug Test Anal.* **2010**, *2*, 144–148. [CrossRef] [PubMed]

44. Kwiatkowska, D.; Wójtowicz, M.; Jarek, A.; Goebel, C.; Chajewska, K.; Turek-Lepa, E.; Pokrywka, A.; Kazlauskas, R. N,N-dimethyl-2-phenylpropan-1-amine—New designer agent found in athlete urine and nutritional supplement. *Drug Test Anal.* **2015**, *7*, 331–335. [CrossRef] [PubMed]

45. Striegel, H.; Vollkommer, G.; Horstmann, T.; Niess, A.M. Contaminated nutritional supplements—Legal protection for elite athletes who tested positive: A case report from Germany. *J. Sports Sci.* **2005**, *23*, 723–726. [CrossRef] [PubMed]

46. Stewart, B.; Outram, S. Smith ACT. Doing supplements to improve performance in club cycling: A life-course analysis. *Scand. J. Med. Sci. Sports* **2013**, *23*, e361–e372. [CrossRef] [PubMed]

47. Baume, N.; Avois, L.; Schweizer, C.; Cardis, C.; Dvorak, J.; Cauderay, M.; Mangin, P.; Saugy, M. [13C]Nandrolone excretion in trained athletes: Interindividual variability in metabolism. *Clin. Chem.* **2004**, *50*, 355–364. [CrossRef] [PubMed]

48. Bird, S.R.; Goebel, C.; Burke, L.M.; Greaves, R.F. Doping in sport and exercise: Anabolic, ergogenic, health and clinical issues. *Ann. Clin. Biochem.* **2016**, *53*, 196–221. [CrossRef] [PubMed]

49. Striegel, H.; Rössner, D.; Simon, P.; Niess, A.M. The World Anti-Doping Code 2003—Consequences for physicians associated with elite athletes. *Int. J. Sports Med.* **2005**, *26*, 238–243. [CrossRef] [PubMed]

50. Outram, S.; Stewart, B. Doping through supplement use: A review of the available empirical data. *Int. J. Sport Nutr. Exerc. Metab.* **2015**, *25*, 54–59. [CrossRef] [PubMed]

51. Tribunal Arbitral du Sport—Court of Arbitration for Sport. Available online: http://www.tas-cas.org/en/index.html (accessed on 17 May 2017).

52. Australian Sports Anti-Doping Authority—ASADA. 2016. Available online: https://www.asada.gov.au/ (accessed on 17 June 2017).

53. Anti-Doping Rule Violations. Available online: http://www.ukad.org.uk/anti-doping-rule-violations/about-adrvs (accessed on 14 January 2017).

54. U.S. Anti-Doping Agency—USADA. 2013. Available online: http://www.usada.org/ (accessed on 14 January 2017).

55. Dopingautoriteit. Available online: http://www.dopingautoriteit.nl/nzvt/disclaimer (accessed on 14 January 2017).

56. Kölner Liste. Available online: http://www.koelnerliste.com/no_cache/en/product-database.html (accessed on 14 January 2017).

57. Informed-Choice | Sports Supplement Banned Substance Testing. Available online: http://www.informed-choice.org/ (accessed on 14 January 2017).

58. NSF Certified for Sport: Certified Products. Available online: http://www.nsfsport.com/listings/certified_products.asp (accessed on 14 January 2017).

59. Drugfree Sport NZ. Available online: http://drugfreesport.org.nz/supplement-check (accessed on 14 January 2017).

60. High Risk List. Available online: http://www.supplement411.org/hrl/ (accessed on 14 January 2017).

61. Alertas-AEPSAD-Ministerio de Educación, Cultura y Deporte. Available online: http://www.aepsad.gob.es/aepsad/alertas.html (accessed on 14 January 2017).

62. Ministerio de la Presidencia y para las Administraciones Territoriales (España). Ley 28/2015, de 30 de julio, Para la Defensa de la Calidad Alimentaria. BOE» núm. 182, de 31/07/2015. Available online: http://www.boe.es/buscar/act.php?id=BOE-A-2015-8563 (accessed on 10 June 2017).

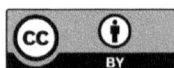

nutrients

MDPI

Review

Omega-3 Fatty Acids and Cardiovascular Disease: Summary of the 2016 Agency of Healthcare Research and Quality Evidence Review

Ethan M. Balk [1] and Alice H. Lichtenstein [2,*]

[1]   Center for Evidence Synthesis in Health, Brown University School of Public Health, Providence, RI 02912,
        USA; ethan_balk@brown.edu
[2]   Jean Mayer USDA Human Nutrition Research Center on Aging, Tufts University, Boston, MA 02111, USA
*   Correspondence: alice.lichtenstein@tufts.edu; Tel.: +1-(617)-556-3127

Received: 21 June 2017; Accepted: 4 August 2017; Published: 11 August 2017

Abstract: We summarize the 2016 update of the 2004 Agency of Healthcare Research and Quality's evidence review of omega-3 fatty acids and cardiovascular disease (CVD). The overall findings for the effects of marine oil supplements on intermediate CVD outcomes remain largely unchanged. There is high strength of evidence, based on numerous trials, of no significant effects of marine oils on systolic or diastolic blood pressures, but there are small, yet statistically significant increases in high density lipoprotein and low density lipoprotein cholesterol concentrations. The clinical significance of these small changes, particularly in combination, is unclear. The strongest effect of marine oils is on triglyceride concentrations. Across studies, this effect was dose-dependent and related to studies' mean baseline triglyceride concentration. In observational studies, there is low strength of evidence that increased marine oil intake lowers ischemic stroke risk. Among randomized controlled trials and observational studies, there is evidence of variable strength of no association with increased marine oil intake and lower CVD event risk. Evidence regarding alpha-linolenic acid intake is sparser. There is moderate strength of evidence of no effect on blood pressure or lipoprotein concentrations and low strength of evidence of no association with coronary heart disease, atrial fibrillation and congestive heart failure.

Keywords: omega-3 fatty acids; alpha-linolenic acid; eicosapentaenoic acid; docosahexaenoic acid; marine oil; cardiovascular disease; blood pressure; high density lipoprotein; low density lipoprotein cholesterol; triglyceride; systematic review; meta-analysis

1. Introduction

The relationship between high fish consumption and low cardiovascular mortality among Greenland Inuit was first reported in the late 1970s. Subsequently, numerous observational and intervention studies of fish and omega-3 fatty acids (*n*-3 FAs) intake have reported similar findings in many countries. The majority of the intervention trials have centered on cardiovascular disease (CVD) risk factors and intermediate markers. However, the beneficial effects on CVD risk factors and markers have not always been consistent with studies evaluating clinical CVD outcomes. Hence, the value of *n*-3 FA to decrease cardiovascular mortality and improve risk factors remains controversial.

The *n*-3 FAs are a group of long-chain and very-long-chain polyunsaturated fatty acids. The major *n*-3 FAs that are present in food are alpha-linolenic acid (ALA), occurring primarily in plants, and eicosapentaenoic acid (EPA) and docosahexaenoic acid (DHA), occurring primarily in marine life. Other *n*-3 FAs, including stearidonic acid (SDA) and docosapentaenoic acid (DPA), are present in very low amounts in the diet. The major dietary sources of ALA are soybean and canola oils, some nuts and flax seed. The major sources of EPA and DHA are oily fish and other marine life. Common dietary supplements of ALA are flax seed oil and some nut-derived oils. Common dietary supplements of EPA and DHA are fish oil, krill oil, and algae oil. There are no major commonly consumed sources of dietary SDA and DPA. However, SDA is relatively high in hemp oil and echium seed oil.

The term *n*-3 FAs is used to refer to a group of polyunsaturated fatty acids whose first double bond involves the third carbon counting from the methyl end of the fatty acid acyl chain. In contrast, the term omega-6 fatty acids (*n*-6 FA) is used to refer to a group of polyunsaturated fatty acids whose first double bond involves the sixth carbon counting from the methyl end of the fatty acid acyl chain. Both *n*-3 FAs and *n*-6 FAs are substrates for the synthesis of eicosanoids, a subcategory of oxylipins. As a group of bioactive molecules, they are signaling factors that affect a wide range of physiological systems. Depending on the substrate, eicosanoids can promote or inhibit immune responses, act as endocrine agents or have a broad range of other functions. The metabolic products of *n*-3 FAs and *n*-6 FAs tend to result in different and frequently opposite physiological effects. Metabolic products of *n*-3 FAs tend to be anti-inflammatory. In addition to being substrates for eicosanoid synthesis, *n*-3 FAs also serve as structural components of cell membranes, higher levels resulting in increased fluidity.

In 2002, the Institute of Medicine concluded that the evidence was inadequate to establish a Recommended Dietary Allowance for *n*-3 FAs. Instead, for healthy adults, they established an Adequate Intake for ALA of 1.1 g per day for females and 1.6 g per day for males [1,2]. On the basis of data for CVD and stroke, they further established an Acceptable Macronutrient Distribution Range for ALA of 0.6 to 1.2 percent of energy, with approximately 10 percent of this range contributed by EPA and/or DHA. To get an adequate *n*-3 FA intake, the 2015–2020 Dietary Guidelines for Americans recommends two fish meals, preferably oily fish, per week. This is consistent with prior editions of Dietary Guidelines for Americans and the American Heart Association's Diet and Lifestyle Recommendations [3,4]. While the intake of ALA in the U.S. is generally adequate, intakes of EPA and DHA tend to be low. Despite consistent recommendations to increase fish intake, from 1999–2000 to 2011–2012 estimated fish intake has only increased from 1.12 to 1.33 servings per week [5].

In 2004, evidence reviews of *n*-3 FA and CVD and CVD risk factors commissioned by the Agency of Healthcare Research and Quality (AHRQ) were published [6–10]. Since then, the evidence for a relationship between *n*-3 FA and CVD has continued to be inconsistent. In the past decade, there have been numerous secular trends that may have had an impact upon the potential effects of *n*-3 FA dietary intake and supplementation on CVD risk factors and outcomes. These include higher diagnosis rates of and pharmacologic treatment for CVD risk factors (e.g., statins, anti-hypertensive agents, and low dose aspirin), resulting in lower cardiovascular event rates. Smoking rates have also fallen [11], although obesity rates have remained stable [12]. These trends could lower the potential population level benefit of *n*-3 FAs because of a lower underlying risk, making comparisons with older studies somewhat tenuous.

For these reasons, the AHRQ commissioned an update of the earlier review on *n*-3 FA and CVD [13]. The updated review focused on clinically relevant CVD risk factors (lipoproteins and blood pressure (BP)) and CVD events. In addition, due to concerns about the accuracy of dietary *n*-3 FA intake estimates, the updated review added evaluations of associations between measures of nutrient biomarkers and clinical outcomes. The biomarkers of *n*-3 FA intake include fatty acid profiles of adipose tissue, erythrocytes, plasma, and plasma phospholipids, reflecting not only current intake but subsequent metabolism [14–16]. The results of the updated review are summarized below.

2. Materials and Methods

Standard systematic review methodology was employed to address three Key Questions on: (1) the efficacy or association of *n*-3 FA and CVD outcomes and risk factors; (2) differences in efficacy or association by patient characteristics, confounders, diet, and other factors on these outcomes and risk factors; and (3) adverse event data (Table 1). The Key Questions are summarized graphically in an Analytic Framework mapping linkages among populations of interest, exposures, modifying factors, and outcomes of interest (Figure 1). For each topic, the strength of evidence was rated as high,

Nutrients **2017**, *9*, 865

moderate, low, or insufficient, based on the number of studies, their limitations, consistency, precision, and other factors. Details about the study eligibility criteria and other methodology can be found in the full report [13].

Table 1. Key Questions.

Key Question	Question Text
1	What is the efficacy or association of *n*-3 FA (EPA, DHA, EPA+DHA, DPA, SDA, ALA, or total *n*-3 FA) exposures in reducing CVD outcomes (incident CVD events, including all-cause death, CVD death, nonfatal CVD events, new diagnosis of CVD, peripheral vascular disease, CHF, major arrhythmias, and hypertension diagnosis) and specific CVD risk factors (BP, key plasma lipids)?
1.1	What is the efficacy or association of *n*-3 FA in preventing CVD outcomes in people • Without known CVD (primary prevention) • At high risk for CVD (primary prevention), and • With known CVD (secondary prevention)?
1.2	What is the relative efficacy of different *n*-3 FA on CVD outcomes and risk factors?
1.3	Can the CVD outcomes be ordered by strength of intervention effect of *n*-3 FA?
2	*n*-3 FA variables and modifiers:
2.1	How does the efficacy or association of *n*-3 FA in preventing CVD outcomes and with CVD risk factors differ in subpopulations, including men, premenopausal women, postmenopausal women, and different age or race/ethnicity groups?
2.2	What are the effects of potential confounders or interacting factors—such as plasma lipids, body mass index, BP, diabetes, kidney disease, other nutrients or supplements, and drugs (e.g., statins, aspirin, diabetes drugs, hormone replacement therapy)?
2.3	What is the efficacy or association of different ratios of *n*-3 FA components in dietary supplements or biomarkers on CVD outcomes and risk factors?
2.4	How does the efficacy or association of *n*-3 FA on CVD outcomes and risk factors differ by ratios of different *n*-3 FA—DHA, EPA, and ALA, or other *n*-3 FA?
2.5	How does the efficacy or association of *n*-3 FA on CVD outcomes and risk factors differ by source (e.g., fish and seafood, common plant oils (e.g., soybean, canola), fish oil supplements, fungal-algal supplements, flaxseed oil supplements)?
2.6	How does the ratio of *n*-6 FA to *n*-3 FA intakes or biomarker concentrations affect the efficacy or association of *n*-3 FA on CVD outcomes and risk factors?
2.7	Is there a threshold or dose–response relationship between *n*-3 FA exposures and CVD outcomes and risk factors? Does the study type affect these relationships?
2.8	How does the duration of intervention or exposure influence the effect of *n*-3 FA on CVD outcomes and risk factors?
2.9	What is the effect of baseline *n*-3 FA status (intake or biomarkers) on the efficacy of *n*-3 FA intake or supplementation on CVD outcomes and risk factors?
3	Adverse events:
3.1	What adverse effects are related to *n*-3 FA intake (in studies of CVD outcomes and risk factors)?
3.2	What adverse events are reported specifically among people with CVD or diabetes (in studies of CVD outcomes and risk factors)?

Abbreviations: ALA = alpha-linolenic acid, BP = blood pressure, CHF = congestive heart failure, CVD = cardiovascular disease, DHA = docosahexaenoic acid, DPA = docosapentaenoic acid, EPA = eicosapentaenoic acid, *n*-3 FA = omega-3 fatty acid(s), *n*-6 FA = omega-6 fatty acid(s), SDA = stearidonic acid.

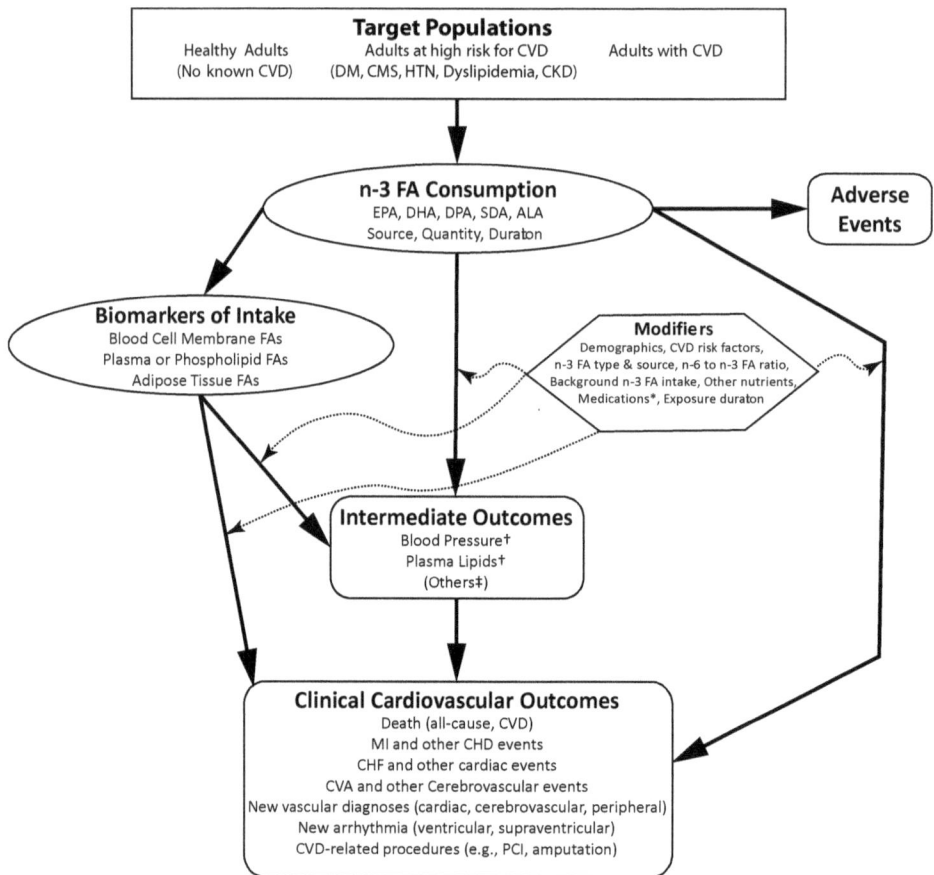

Figure 1. Analytic framework for omega-3 fatty acid exposure and cardiovascular disease. This framework concerns the effect of omega−3 fatty acid (*n*-3 FA) exposure (as a supplement or from food sources) on cardiovascular disease (CVD) events and risk factors. Populations of interest are noted in the top rectangle, exposure in the oval, outcomes in the rounded rectangles, and effect modifiers in the hexagon. * Specifically, cardiovascular medications, statins, anti-hypertensives, diabetes medications, hormone replacement regimens. [†] Systolic blood pressure, diastolic blood pressure, mean arterial pressure, high density lipoprotein cholesterol (HDL-c), low density lipoprotein cholesterol (LDL-c), total/HDL-C ratio, LDL-C /HDL-C ratio, triglycerides. [‡] Many other intermediate outcomes are likely in the causal pathway between n-3 FA intake and CVD outcomes, but only blood pressure and plasma lipids were included in the review. Other Abbreviations: ALA = alpha linolenic acid, CHD = coronary heart disease, CHF = congestive heart failure, CKD = non-dialysis-dependent chronic kidney disease, CMS = cardiometabolic syndrome, CVA = cerebrovascular accident (stroke), DHA = docosahexaenoic acid, DM = diabetes mellitus, DPA = docosapentaenoic acid, EPA = eicosapentaenoic acid, FA = fatty acid, HTN = hypertension, MI = myocardial infarction, *n*-6 = omega−6, PCI = percutaneous coronary intervention, SDA = stearidonic acid.

3. Results

In total, 147 articles met eligibility criteria, representing 61 randomized controlled trials (RCT, in 82 articles) and 37 longitudinal observational studies (in 65 articles). Across studies, there were few risk of bias concerns. The RCTs of clinical outcomes were almost all conducted in populations at increased risk of CVD, largely related to dyslipidemia, or with CVD. The RCTs that reported intermediate outcomes (BP and lipoproteins) were conducted in generally healthy, at-risk, and CVD populations. The observational studies, in contrast, were almost all conducted in general (unrestricted by CVD or risk factors) or healthy populations.

3.1. Key Question 1: Efficacy or Association of n-3 FA and CVD Outcomes or Risk Factors

Findings of effects or associations of increased *n*-3 FA intake on CVD outcomes or risk factors are summarized in Table 2. Findings of no effect or association are summarized in Table 3. Details about study results and summaries across studies can be found in the full report [13].

Table 2. Main findings of high, moderate, or low strength of evidence of significant effects or associations between omega-3 fatty acids and outcomes.

Effect or Association	Strength of Evidence	Finding	Study Types	Effect Sizes
Higher *n*-3 FA intake or biomarker levels with lower CVD risks or events	High	Marine Oil * Supplementation (Or Increased Intake) Raises HDL-C	RCTs (of mostly supplements)	Summary net change in HDL-C: 0.9 mg/dL (95% CI 0.2, 1.6)
	High	Marine oil supplementation (or increased intake) lowers Tg	RCTs (of mostly supplements)	Summary net change in Tg: −24 mg/dL (95% CI −31, −18)
	High	Marine oil supplementation (or increased intake) lowers TC/HDL-C ratio	RCTs (of mostly supplements)	Summary net change in TC/ HDL-C ratio: −0.17 (95% CI −0.26, −0.09)
	Low	Marine oil increased intake lowers risk of ischemic stroke	Observational studies (of total dietary intake)	By metaregression: 0.51 (95% CI 0.29, 0.89) per g/day
Higher *n*-3 FA intake or biomarker levels with higher CVD risk	High	Marine Oil Supplementation (Or Increased Intake) Raises LDL-C	RCTs (of mostly supplements)	Summary net change in LDL-C: 2.0 mg/dL (95% CI 0.4, 3.6)

* All statements about "marine oil" are based on all evidence of analyses of EPA+DHA+DPA, EPA+DHA, EPA, DHA, and DPA. Abbreviations: CHD = coronary heart disease (also known as coronary artery disease), CHF = congestive heart failure, CI = confidence interval, CVD = cardiovascular disease, DHA = docosahexaenoic acid, DPA = docosapentaenoic acid, EPA = eicosapentaenoic acid, HDL-C = high density lipoprotein cholesterol, HR = hazard ratio, LDL-C = low density lipoprotein cholesterol, *n*-3 FA = omega-3 fatty acids, RCT = randomized controlled trial, TC = total cholesterol, Tg = triglycerides.

3.1.1. Total *n*-3 FA

Overall, there is insufficient evidence regarding the effect of or association between total n-3 FA (combined ALA and marine oils) and most clinical and intermediate outcomes. There is low strength of evidence of no association between total *n*-3 FA intake and stroke death, and total (fatal and nonfatal) myocardial infarct, based on longitudinal observational studies of dietary intake.

Table 3. Main findings of high, moderate, or low strength of evidence of no significant effects or associations between omega-3 fatty acids and outcomes.

Strength of Evidence	Omega-3 Fatty Acid and Outcome	Study Types	Summary Effect Sizes
High	Marine oil* supplementation (or increased intake) and MACE	RCTs (of mostly supplements), supported by observational studies (of total dietary intake)	RCTs: 0.96 (95% CI 0.91, 1.02)
High	Marine oil intake and all-cause death	RCTs (of mostly supplements) and observational studies (of total dietary intake)	RCTs: 0.97 (95% CI 0.92, 1.03). Observational studies: 0.62 (95% CI 0.31, 1.25) per g/day
High	Marine oil intake and SCD	RCTs (of mostly supplements), supported by observational studies (of total dietary intake)	RCTs: 1.04 (95% CI 0.92, 1.17)
High	Marine oil intake and coronary revascularization	RCTs (of mostly supplements), supported by observational studies (of total dietary intake)	Not significant, not meta-analyzed
High	Marine oil intake and systolic or diastolic blood pressure	RCTs (of mostly supplements)	RCTs: summary net change in systolic blood pressure: 0.1 mg/dL (95% CI −0.2, 0.4); summary net change in diastolic blood pressure: −0.2 mg/dL (95% CI −0.4, 0.5)
Moderate	Marine oil intake and atrial fibrillation	RCTs (of mostly supplements) and observational studies (of total dietary intake)	Not significant, not meta-analyzed. Observational studies were inconsistent.
Moderate	Purified DHA supplementation and systolic or diastolic blood pressure	RCTs (of supplements)	Not significant, not meta-analyzed
Moderate	Purified DHA supplementation and LDL-C	RCTs (of supplements)	Not significant, not meta-analyzed
Moderate	ALA intake and systolic or diastolic blood pressure	RCTs (of mostly supplements)	Not significant, not meta-analyzed
Moderate	ALA intake and LDL-C, HDL-C, and Tg	RCTs (of mostly supplements)	Not significant, not meta-analyzed
Low	Total *n*-3 FA intake and stroke death	Observational studies (of total dietary intake and biomarkers)	Not significant, not meta-analyzed
Low	Total *n*-3 FA intake and myocardial infarction	Observational studies (of total dietary intake)	Not significant, not meta-analyzed
Low	Marine oil intake and CVD death	RCTs (of mostly supplements) and observational studies (of total dietary intake)	RCTs: 0.92 (95% CI 0.82, 1.02). Observational studies: 0.88 (95% CI 0.82, 0.95) per g/day
Low	Marine oil intake and CHD death	RCTs (of mostly supplements) and observational studies (of total dietary intake)	RCTs imprecise. Observational studies: 1.09 (95% CI 0.76, 1.57) per g/day
Low	Marine oil intake and CHD	Observational studies (of total dietary intake and biomarkers)	Observational studies: 0.94 (95% CI 0.81, 1.10) per g/day
Low	Marine oil intake and myocardial infarction	RCTs (of mostly supplements)	RCTs: 0.88 (95% CI 0.77, 1.02)
Low	Marine oil intake and angina pectoris	RCTs (of mostly supplements)	Not significant, not meta-analyzed

Table 3. *Cont.*

Strength of Evidence	Omega-3 Fatty Acid and Outcome	Study Types	Summary Effect Sizes
Low	Marine oil intake and CHF	RCTs (of mostly supplements) and observational studies (of total dietary intake)	RCTs not significant, not meta-analyzed. Observational studies: 0.76 (95% CI 0.58, 1.00) per g/day
Low	Marine oil intake and total stroke (fatal and nonfatal ischemic and hemorrhagic stroke)	RCTs (of mostly supplements) and observational studies (of total dietary intake)	RCTs: 0.97 (95% CI 0.83, 1.13). Observational studies: 0.68 (95% CI 0.53, 0.87) per g/day
Low	Marine oil intake and hemorrhagic stroke	Observational studies (of total dietary intake)	Observational studies: 0.61 (95% CI 0.34, 1.11) per g/day
Low	EPA intake and CHD	Observational studies (of total dietary intake)	Not significant, not meta-analyzed
Low	EPA biomarkers and atrial fibrillation	Observational studies (of biomarkers)	Not significant, not meta-analyzed
Low	DHA intake and CHD	Observational studies (of total dietary intake and biomarkers)	Not significant, not meta-analyzed
Low	DPA biomarkers and atrial fibrillation	Observational studies (of biomarkers)	Not significant, not meta-analyzed
Low	ALA intake and CHD death	Observational studies (of total dietary intake), supported by RCT (of supplementation) and observational study (of biomarkers)	Observational studies: 0.94 (95% CI 0.85, 1.03) per g/day
Low	ALA intake and CHD	Observational studies (of total dietary intake)	Observational studies: 0.97 (95% CI 0.92, 1.03) per g/day
Low	ALA intake and atrial fibrillation	Observational studies (of total dietary intake and biomarkers)	Not significant, not meta-analyzed
Low	ALA intake and CHF	Observational studies (of total dietary intake and biomarkers), supported by RCT (of supplementation)	Not significant, not meta-analyzed

* All statements about "marine oil" are based on all evidence of analyses of EPA+DHA+DPA, EPA+DHA, EPA, DHA, and DPA. Abbreviations: ALA = alphalinolenic acid, CHD = coronary heart disease, CHF = congestive heart failure, CI = confidence interval, DHA = docosahexaenoic acid, DPA = docosapentaenoic acid, EPA = eicosapentaenoic acid, HDL-C = high density lipoprotein cholesterol, LDL-C = low density lipoprotein cholesterol, MACE = major adverse cardiovascular event (including cardiac and stroke events and death; variously defined by studies), n-3 FA = omega-3 fatty acids, RCT = randomized controlled trial, SCD = sudden cardiac death, Tg = triglycerides.

3.1.2. Marine Oils

There is high strength of evidence of that marine oils (primarily EPA and DHA) statistically significantly lower triglyceride concentrations—possibly with greater effects with higher doses and in people with higher baseline triglyceride concentrations—and they statistically significantly raise high density lipoprotein cholesterol (HDL-C) and low density lipoprotein cholesterol (LDL-C) concentrations by similar amounts (2.0 and 0.9 mg/dL, respectively). There is also high strength of evidence that marine oils significantly lower the total cholesterol (TC)/HDL-C ratio (by −0.17). There is low strength of evidence that marine oils significantly lower risk of ischemic stroke (effect size per g/day = 0.51).

There is a high strength of evidence of no effect of marine oils on risk of major adverse cardiovascular events, all-cause death, sudden cardiac death, revascularization, and blood pressure (BP); moderate strength of evidence of no effect of marine oils on risk of atrial fibrillation; and low strength of evidence of no effect of marine oils on risk of CVD death, coronary heart disease (CHD) death, total CHD, myocardial infarction, angina pectoris, congestive heart failure, total stroke, and hemorrhagic stroke. There is insufficient evidence for other outcomes.

3.1.3. Specific Marine Oils

There is insufficient evidence regarding the effect of or association between oils high in EPA, DHA, or DPA (each marine oil individually) and most CVD clinical and intermediate outcomes. There is low strength of evidence of no association between EPA intake and CHD and between EPA biomarkers and atrial fibrillation. There is moderate strength of evidence of no effect of purified DHA supplementation on BP or LDL-C concentrations, and low strength of evidence of no association between DHA intake and incident CHD. There is low strength of evidence of no association between DPA biomarker levels and risk of atrial fibrillation.

There is insufficient evidence regarding effect of or association between SDA and CVD clinical and intermediate outcomes.

There is moderate strength of evidence of no significant effect of ALA intake on BP, or LDL-C, HDL-C, and triglyceride concentrations. There is low strength of evidence of no association between ALA intake or biomarker level and CHD or CHD death, atrial fibrillation, and congestive heart failure, each based on observational studies. There is insufficient evidence regarding other outcomes.

3.1.4. Sub-Questions

3.1.4.1. People with No Known CVD, At Increased Risk for CVD, and With Known CVD.

Almost all studies reporting CVD intermediate outcomes included study participants based on BP or lipoprotein concentrations; i.e., at increased risk for CVD, but no known CVD. Most observational studies evaluated general population registries or other large databases (for primary prevention). In contrast, RCTs with CVD event outcomes were conducted mostly in people with known history of CVD (for secondary prevention).

Based on the applicability of the different studies, in the population without known CVD, there is observational evidence of no association for major adverse cardiovascular events, CVD death, total stroke death, incident CHD, total stroke, ischemic stroke, hemorrhagic stroke, atrial fibrillation, and congestive heart failure. There is strong RCT evidence of no effect for BP (systolic and diastolic), mean arterial pressure, LDL-C and HDL-C concentrations, and strong RCT evidence for a significant effect on lowering triglyceride concentrations.

In people at increased risk for CVD, there is strong RCT evidence for no effect on major adverse cardiovascular events, all-cause death, BP (systolic and diastolic), LDL-C and HDL-C concentrations, TC/HDL-C ratio, and LDL-C/HDL-C ratio, and strong RCT evidence for a significant effect for lowering triglyceride concentrations.

In people with known CVD, there is RCT evidence of no effect for major adverse cardiovascular, CHD death, all-cause death, myocardial infarction, revascularization, total stroke, sudden cardiac death, atrial fibrillation, and congestive heart failure. There is strong RCT evidence of no effect on BP (systolic and diastolic) and LDL-C concentrations, and strong RCT evidence of a protective effect for HDL-C and triglyceride concentrations.

3.1.4.2. Relative Effect of Different *n*-3 FAs.

Based on studies that directly compared different n-3 FAs, there is low strength of evidence of no difference between EPA, DHA, and combined EPA+DHA. There is low strength of evidence of greater efficacy of marine oils over ALA.

3.1.4.3. Ordering of *n*-3 FAs by Strength of Effect.

Based on the summary effect sizes of meta-analyzed RCTs, marine oils had no statistically significant effect on CVD outcomes. The order of effect sizes (ignoring lack of statistical significance) of CVD outcomes with sufficient data to allow meta-analysis, was myocardial infarction, CVD death, major adverse cardiovascular events, all-cause death, total stroke, and sudden cardiac death.

3.2. Key Question 2: n-3 FA Variables and Modifiers

Sub-Questions

3.2.0.1. Subpopulations

There was insufficient evidence to assess the efficacy or association of *n*-3 FA in preventing CVD outcomes and with CVD risk factors in subgroups based on race/ethnicity and whether women were pre- or postmenopausal. Five studies (mostly observational) found no significant differences in association based on age, with cutoffs for subgroups ranging between 60 and 70 years of age. Two studies found no interaction with age as a continuous variable. One RCT found a significant difference in favor of women, two observational studies found a significant difference in favor of men, and nine studies (a mix of RCTs and observational) found no difference between men and women.

3.2.0.2. Confounders or Interacting Factors

There was evidence of no interactions with body mass index, hypertension status, diabetes status, and baseline TC/HDL-C ratio. There was inconsistent evidence for the following potential confounders or interacting factors: triglyceride concentrations, statin use, B-vitamin use, and baseline LDL-C concentrations. There was insufficient evidence to assess the following potential confounders or interacting factors: beta-blocker use, baseline HDL-C concentrations, insulin glargine use, nitrate use, digoxin use, diuretic use, estimated glomerular filtration rate, angiotensin-converting enzyme inhibitor use, anticoagulant use, total cholesterol concentrations, or use of fish oil supplements.

3–6. Different Ratios of n-3 FA Components, Different n-3 FA Sources, and n-6 FA to n-3 FA Ratio

There was insufficient information across studies to evaluate different ratios of *n*-3 FA components (e.g., EPA-to-DHA ratio) or to compare different ratios. Also, studies neither fully reported on *n*-3 FA source (e.g., soybean oil, canola oil) nor compared the different sources; therefore, there was insufficient evidence regarding differential effects based on source. No RCTs or observational studies directly evaluated *n*-6 FA to *n*-3 FA intake concentrations, and no differences across studies by this ratio was evident.

3.2.0.4. Threshold or Dose–Response Relationship

Among RCTs, for all clinical CVD outcomes, there is insufficient evidence regarding a dose–response relationship within or between RCTs. For BP, LDL-C and HDL-C concentrations, RCTs do not find significant differences in effect by marine oil dose either within or between RCTs. RCTs comparing marine oil doses mostly found no significant differences between higher and lower dose marine oils. However, a possible pattern could be discerned such that higher doses (3.4 or 4 g/day) reduced triglyceride concentrations by at least 30 mg/dL more than lower doses (1 to 2 g/day). By meta-regression, each increase of EPA+DHA dose by 1 g/day was associated with a greater net change triglyceride concentrations of -5.9 mg/dL (95% CI -9.9 to-2.0; $P = 0.003$); no inflection point was found above which the association plateaued. Meta-regressions of observational studies yielded the following conclusions. For all-cause death, there may be a ceiling effect at about 0.2 g/day, such that increasing marine oil intake up to this level may be associated with lower all-cause death, but increasing intake above this level may not be associated with further decreased risk. For total stroke, ischemic stroke, and congestive heart failure, at lower ranges of intake, there were statistically significant associations between higher marine oil intake level and lower risk of outcome, in contrast to associations found at higher ranges of intake. However, the associations at lower and higher doses were not statistically significantly different from each other. For ischemic stroke, associations between higher doses and risk of stroke were stronger and statistically significant across lower doses than at higher doses (with thresholds between lower and higher doses from 0.1 and 0.4 g/day) and the differences in associations between lower and higher doses were statistically significant. Any dose inflection point that may exist is likely to be beyond the range of testable thresholds (i.e., >0.4 g/day), based on available evidence. Similarly, for congestive heart failure, significant associations were found at lower doses, in contrast to at higher doses, with thresholds ranging from 0.1 to 0.5 g/day, and the differences were statistically significant at most thresholds. Any dose inflection point that may exist is likely to be beyond the range of testable thresholds (i.e., >0.5 g/day). For CVD death, CHD death, total CHD, and hemorrhagic stroke, there were no apparent differences in association between marine oil intake dose and outcome at lower or higher dose ranges. For CHD death and CHD, there were no apparent differences in association between ALA intake dose and outcome at lower or higher dose ranges.

3.2.0.5. Duration of Intervention or Exposure

None of the meta-regressions identified a significant interaction for follow-up time. No difference in effect was identified within studies at different durations of intervention. Observational studies did not evaluate differences in duration of exposure.

3.2.0.6. Effect of Baseline *n*-FA Status

The very few studies that investigated potential differential effects associated with baseline fish or *n*-3 FA intake found no significant differences.

3.3. Adverse Events

Sub-Questions

3.3.0.1. Adverse Events across All Studies

No serious or severe adverse events were related to *n*-3 FA intake (supplementation). Most reported adverse events were mild and gastrointestinal in nature. However, two of 25 RCTs reported statistically significant differences in adverse events between *n*-3 FA supplements and placebo.

3.3.0.2. Adverse Events among People with CVD or Diabetes

Among 10 RCTs of patients with CVD (9 with marine oil, 1 with total *n*-3 FA, 2 with ALA), either no adverse events or no significant difference between *n*-3 FA and placebo were reported. A single study reported adverse events from an RCT of people with diabetes, finding no significant differences in serious or non-serious adverse events between marine oil and placebo.

4. Discussion

The overall findings for the effects of marine oil supplements on intermediate CVD outcomes remain largely unchanged since a similar review in 2004 [7,13]. In summary, there is high strength of evidence, based on numerous trials, of no significant effects of marine oils (0.3–6 g/day) on systolic or diastolic BP, but small, yet statistically significant increases in HDL-C (0.9 mg/dL) and LDL-C (2.0 mg/dL) concentrations. However, the clinical significance of these small changes in both HDL-C and LDL-C concentrations on CVD outcomes, particularly in combination, is unclear. For both lipid outcomes, no differences in effect across studies were found by marine oil dose, follow-up duration, or population. The strongest effect of marine oils (0.3–6 g/day) was found on triglyceride concentrations. Across studies, this effect was dose-dependent and also dependent on the studies' mean baseline triglyceride concentrations. Recent genetic evidence from a wide range of investigations, including mutational analyses, genome-wide associations and Mendelian randomization, has linked triglycerides and triglyceride-rich lipoprotein particles in the causal pathway for CVD, possibly through promotion of low-grade inflammation [17,18].

In observational studies, there is a low strength of evidence that increased marine oil intake lowers the risk of ischemic stroke, but among both RCTs and observational studies there is evidence of variable strength of no association of increased marine oil intake with lower risks of a range of CVD events. Evidence regarding ALA intake is sparser. There is moderate strength of evidence of no effect of ALA on BP or lipoprotein concentrations, and low strength of evidence of no association with coronary heart disease, atrial fibrillation, and congestive heart failure.

The potential intake threshold-effects of *n*-3 FA on CVD events (the maximum dose above which no further benefit is attained) could not be determined from the RCTs; meta-analyses of observational studies found variable evidence of possible threshold effects. Most notably, intakes of EPA and DHA greater than 0.6 g/day do not provide additional benefit to lower risk of ischemic stroke than lower doses. Comparative differences in effects or associations of increased *n*-3 FA intake in different populations based on CVD risk, a question of particular interest, could not be adequately addressed because few RCTs were conducted in healthy populations (with normal CVD risk) and few observational studies were conducted in at-risk or CVD populations.

Of interest, the current National Institute for Health and Care Excellence (NICE) recommendations for CVD prevention concluded that the evidence does not support the use of omega-3 fatty acid supplements for people who are being treated for primary prevention or secondary prevention, and people with chronic kidney disease, type 1 diabetes, or type 2 diabetes [19].

5. Limitations

Overall, both RCTs and observational studies generally had few risk of bias concerns. However, as noted, the RCTs were mostly applicable to people with elevated BP or lipoprotein concentrations, without known CVD. In contrast, for clinical CVD outcomes, all but one of the RCTs was conducted in either high-risk individuals or people with existing CVD, but most observational studies were conducted in generally healthy populations. Furthermore, the doses of marine oil supplements in RCTs were often much higher than the highest intake reported for observational studies. Studies generally failed to account for differences in background diet or *n*-3 FA intake and did not fully characterize the *n*-3 FA under investigation.

While this report represents a complete systematic review, it does not encompass all trials or longitudinal observational studies that report on CVD and intermediate outcomes. Due to time and resource constraints, this review included only the largest RCTs of CVD risk factors and the largest observational studies. Smaller studies may have yielded more complete or conflicting findings.

6. Conclusions

In brief, there is high strength of evidence that marine oils have small effects on LDL-C and HDL-C concentrations, and a large, dose-dependent effect on triglyceride concentrations. In contrast, there is moderate strength of evidence that ALA has no significant effect on lipoprotein concentrations. Neither marine oils nor ALA have a significant effect on systolic or diastolic BP. There is moderate strength of evidence that marine oil supplementation lowers risk of major adverse cardiovascular events and CVD death, and low strength of evidence that higher marine oil intake is associated with lower risk of coronary heart disease and congestive heart failure. However, there is variable strength of evidence of no significant effect or association of marine oil intake and numerous different CVD outcomes.

The generalizability of specific findings to all populations is somewhat limited because studies tended to restrict their eligibility criteria. RCTs evaluating clinical outcomes included only people with known CVD while observational studies evaluated only databases of generally health populations (without known CVD). Furthermore, while there were few risk of bias concerns across the studies, very few studies fully characterized the *n*-3 FAs under investigation or attempted to account for differential effects in different populations or based on people's background diet or other characteristics. Also, few studies directly compared different *n*-3 FA components, ratios, doses, or duration of intake. Therefore, there was no or insufficient evidence to address most of the review's key questions.

Acknowledgments: This summary is based on Evidence Report/Technology Assessment Number 223, Omega-3 Fatty Acids and Cardiovascular Disease: An Updated Systematic Review, funded by a the Agency of Healthcare

Research and Quality (AHRQ), U.S. Department of Health and Human Services, Contract No. 290-2015-00002-I, and prepared by the Brown Evidence-based Practice Center, Providence, RI. The investigators were Ethan M. Balk, Gaelen P. Adam, M.L.I.S., Valerie Langberg, Christopher Halladay, B.A., Mei Chung, Lin Lin, M.A., Sarah Robertson, B.S., Agustin Yip, Dale Steele, Bryant T. Smith, Joseph Lau, Alice H. Lichtenstein, Thomas A. Trikalinos.

Author Contributions: E.M.B. and A.H.L. contributed equally to writing this review.

Conflicts of Interest: The authors declare no conflict of interest.

Disclaimer: The authors of this manuscript are responsible for its content. Statements in the manuscript should not be construed as endorsement by the AHRQ or the U.S. Department of Health and Human Services. AHRQ retains a license to display, reproduce, and distribute the data and the report from which this manuscript was derived under the terms of the agency's contract with the authors.

References

1. Scientific Report of the 2015 Dietary Guidelines Advisory Committee. 2015. Available online: http://health.gov/dietaryguidelines/2015-scientific-report/pdfs/scientific-report-of-the-2015-dietary-guidelines-advisory-committee.pdf (accessed on 7 August 2017).
2. Institute of Medicine. *Dietary Reference Intakes. Energy, Carbohydrate, Fiber, Fat Fatty Acids, Cholesterol, Protein and Amino Acids*; National Academy of Sciences: Washington, DC, USA, 2005.
3. Dietary Guidelines for Americans, 2010. Health. gov. Available online: https://health.gov/dietaryguidelines/dga2010/DietaryGuidelines2010.pdf (accessed on 7 August 2017).
4. Eckel, R.H.; Jakicic, J.M.; Ard, J.D.; Van Hubbard, S.; de Jesus, J.M.; Lee, I.-M.; Lichtenstein, A.H.; Loria, C.M.; Millen, B.E.; Miller, N.H.; et al. 2013 AHA/ACC Guideline on Lifestyle Management to Reduce Cardiovascular Risk: A Report of the American College of Cardiology/American Heart Association Task Force on Practice Guidelines. *J. Am. Coll. Cardiol.* **2014**, *63*, 3027–3028. [CrossRef] [PubMed]
5. Rehm, C.D.; Peñalvo, J.L.; Afshin, A.; Mozaffarian, D. Dietary Intake among US Adults, 1999–2012. *JAMA* **2016**, *315*, 2542–2553. [CrossRef] [PubMed]
6. Wang, C.; Chung, M.; Balk, E.; Kupelnick, B.; DeVine, D.; Lawrence, A.; Lichtenstein, A.; Lau, J. *Effects of Omega-3 Fatty Acids on Cardiovascular Disease*; Evidence Report/Technology Assessment No. 94 AHRQ Publication No. 04-E009-2; Agency for Healthcare Research and Quality: Rockville, MD, USA, 2004.
7. Balk, E.; Chung, M.; Lichtenstein, A.; Chew, P.; Kupelnick, B.; Lawrence, A.; DeVine, D.; Lau, J. *Effects of Omega-3 Fatty Acids on Cardiovascular Risk Factors and Intermediate Markers of Cardiovascular Disease*; Evidence Report/Technology Assessment No. 93 AHRQ Publication No. 04-E010-2; Agency for Healthcare Research and Quality: Rockville, MD, USA, 2004.
8. Wang, C.; Harris, W.S.; Chung, M.; Lichtenstein, A.H.; Balk, E.M.; Kupelnick, B.; Jordan, H.S.; Lau, J. n-3 Fatty acids from fish or fish-oil supplements, but not alpha-linolenic acid, benefit cardiovascular disease outcomes in primary- and secondary-prevention studies: A systematic review. *Am. J. Clin. Nutr.* **2006**, *84*, 5–17. [PubMed]
9. Balk, E.M.; Lichtenstein, A.H.; Chung, M.; Kupelnick, B.; Chew, P.; Lau, J. Effects of omega-3 fatty acids on serum markers of cardiovascular disease risk: A systematic review. *Atherosclerosis* **2006**, *189*, 19–30. [CrossRef] [PubMed]
10. Balk, E.M.; Lichtenstein, A.H.; Chung, M.; Kupelnick, B.; Chew, P.; Lau, J. Effects of omega-3 fatty acids on coronary restenosis, intima-media thickness, and exercise tolerance: A systematic review. *Atherosclerosis* **2006**, *184*, 237–246. [CrossRef] [PubMed]
11. Centers for Disease Control and Prevention. Cigarette Smoking Among Adults—United States, 2005–2015. *Morb. Mortal. Wkly. Rep.* **2016**, *65*, 1205–1211.
12. Flegal, K.M.; Carroll, M.D.; Kit, B.K.; Ogen, C.L. Prevalence of obesity and trends in the distribution of body mass index among US adults, 1999–2010. *JAMA* **2012**, *307*, 491–497. [CrossRef] [PubMed]
13. Balk, E.M.; Adam, G.P.; Langberg, V.; Halladay, C.; Chung, M.; Lin, L.; Robertson, S.; Yip, A.; Steele, D.; Smith, B.T.; Lau, J.; et al. *Omega-3 Fatty Acids and Cardiovascular Disease: An Updated Systematic Review*; Evidence Report/Technology Assessment No. 223 AHRQ Publication No. 16-E002-EF; Agency for Healthcare Research and Quality: Rockville, MD, USA, 2016.
14. Hodson, L.; Skeaff, C.M.; Fielding, B.A. Fatty acid composition of adipose tissue and blood in humans and its use as a biomarker of dietary intake. *Prog. Lipid Res.* **2008**, *47*, 348–380. [CrossRef] [PubMed]

15. Serra-Majem, L.; Nissensohn, M.; Øverby, N.C.; Fekete, K. Methods of assessment of *n*-3 long-chain polyunsaturated fatty acid status in humans: A systematic review. *Am. J. Clin. Nutr.* **2009**, *89*, 2070S–2084S.

16. Serra-Majem, L.; Nissensohn, M.; Øverby, N.C.; Fekete, K. Dietary methods and biomarkers of omega 3 fatty acids: A systematic review. *Br. J. Nutr.* **2012**, *107* (Suppl. 2), S64–S76. [CrossRef] [PubMed]

17. Budoff, M. Triglycerides and Triglyceride-Rich Lipoproteins in the Causal Pathway of Cardiovascular Disease. *Am. J. Cardiol.* **2016**, *118*, 138–145. [CrossRef] [PubMed]

18. Nordestgaard, B.G. Triglyceride-Rich Lipoproteins and Atherosclerotic Cardiovascular Disease: New Insights from Epidemiology, Genetics, and Biology. *Circ. Res.* **2016**, *118*, 547–563. [CrossRef] [PubMed]

19. National Institute for Heath and Care Excellence. Cardiovascular Disease: Risk Assessment and Reduction, Including Lipid Modification, 2014. National Institute for Health and Care Excellence. Available online: https://www.nice.org.uk/guidance/CG181 (accessed on 27 July 2017).

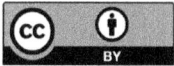

nutrients

Article

Developmental Outcomes at 24 Months of Age in Toddlers Supplemented with Arachidonic Acid and Docosahexaenoic Acid: Results of a Double Blind Randomized, Controlled Trial

Angela M. Devlin [1,*], Cecil M. Y. Chau [1], Roger Dyer [1], Julie Matheson [1], Deanna McCarthy [2], Karin Yurko-Mauro [2], Sheila M. Innis [1,†] and Ruth E. Grunau [1]

[1] Department of Pediatrics, University of British Columbia, BC Children's Hospital Research Institute, A4-194 950 West 28th Ave, Vancouver, BC V5Z 4H4, Canada; cchau@bcchr.ca (C.M.Y.C.); radyer@mail.ubc.ca (R.D.); jmatheson@bcchr.ca (J.M.); rgrunau@bcchr.ca (R.E.G.)
[2] DSM Nutritional Products, Columbia, MD 21045, USA; Deanna.McCarthy@dsm.com (D.M.); Karin.Yurko-Mauro@dsm.com (K.Y.-M.)
* Correspondence: adevlin@bcchr.ubc.ca; Tel.: +604-875-2000 (ext. 5378)
† Deceased.

Received: 25 July 2017; Accepted: 28 August 2017; Published: 6 September 2017

Abstract: Little is known about arachidonic acid (ARA) and docosahexaenoic acid (DHA) requirements in toddlers. A longitudinal, double blind, controlled trial in toddlers ($n = 133$) age 13.4 ± 0.9 months (mean $\pm$ standard deviation), randomized to receive a DHA (200 mg/day) and ARA (200 mg/day) supplement (supplement) or a corn oil supplement (control) until age 24 months determined effects on neurodevelopment. We found no effect of the supplement on the Bayley Scales of Infant and Toddler Development 3rd Edition (Bayley-III) cognitive and language composites and Beery–Buktenica Developmental Test of Visual–Motor Integration (Beery VMI) at age 24 months. Supplemented toddlers had higher RBC phosphatidylcholine (PC), phosphatidylethanolamine (PE), and plasma DHA and ARA compared to placebo toddlers at age 24 months. A positive relationship between RBC PE ARA and Bayley III Cognitive composite (4.55 (0.21–9.00), B (95% CI), $p = 0.045$) in supplemented boys, but not in control boys, was observed in models adjusted for baseline fatty acid, maternal non-verbal intelligence, and BMI z-score at age 24 months. A similar positive relationship between RBC PE ARA and Bayley III Language composite was observed for supplemented boys (11.52 (5.10–17.94), $p < 0.001$) and girls (11.19 (4.69–17.68), $p = 0.001$). These findings suggest that increasing the ARA status in toddlers is associated with better neurodevelopment at age 24 months.

Keywords: toddlers; long chain polyunsaturated fatty acids; arachidonic acid; docosahexaenoic acid; neurodevelopment

1. Introduction

The *n*-6 and *n*-3 long chain polyunsaturated fatty acids, arachidonic acid (20:4*n*-6, ARA), and docosahexaenoic acid (22:6*n*-3, DHA), are found at high concentrations in the brain, predominantly as components of phospholipids, and have important roles in brain development [1–3]. Brain DHA accumulation in phosphatidylethanolamine (PE) and phosphatidylcholine (PC) begins during gestation and is estimated to continue postnatally into childhood [4].

Considerable emphasis has been placed on dietary ARA and DHA requirements for infants under one year of age. Arachidonic acid and DHA can be synthesized from the dietary essential fatty acids, linoleic acid (18:2*n*-6, LA) and alpha linolenic acid (18:3*n*-3, ALA), respectively. However, studies in animals have reported that DHA from maternal diet is a more efficient source of DHA for the developing fetal and infant brain compared to ALA in maternal diet [5,6]. Randomized trials of DHA and ARA supplementation have reported that infants fed with formula supplemented with DHA and ARA from the first week after birth have better visual acuity at 12 months of age than infants consuming formula with no DHA or ARA [7], better attention at four and nine months of age [8], and higher cognitive scores at 18 months of age [9]. The long-term benefits of the DHA and ARA supplementation have also been reported. The infants that were fed the formulas supplemented with DHA and ARA performed better in executive function, vocabulary, and intelligence at 3–5 years of age compared to the infants that were fed the formula with no DHA and ARA [10]. Other studies have also reported beneficial effects of DHA and ARA supplementation during infancy on indicators of cognitive function at six years of age [11].

Less is known about requirements of DHA and ARA during the period from 12 to 24 months of age. This time point is one of rapid neurological and physical development, but also a time of great transition in diet and well-known vulnerability to nutrient deficiencies. Human milk is the recommended and best sole source of nutrition for infants from birth to six months of age, and provides the infant with ARA and DHA. Current Canadian infant feeding guidelines state that whole (homogenized, full-fat) cows' milk may be fed as a human milk alternate beginning at 9–12 months of age [12]. Cows' milk is a rich source of protein and calcium, but is low in *n*-6 and *n*-3 fatty acids and has negligible ARA and DHA. One randomized, controlled trial reported that the median daily intake of DHA in toddlers (18–36 months of age) was 13.3 mg and that those who received a formula supplemented with DHA for 60 days had fewer upper respiratory tract infections compared to toddlers that received no DHA supplementation [13]. This suggests some potential benefits of dietary DHA in this age group. The objective of the current study is to examine the effects of ARA and DHA supplementation in toddlers from 12 to 24 months of age compared to children following their usual diet on cognitive, language and visual-motor development, and biomarkers of ARA and DHA status.

2. Materials and Methods

2.1. Subjects and Study Design

This was a prospective, longitudinal double blind, randomized placebo-controlled trial of DHA and ARA supplementation. Healthy term (37–41 weeks gestation) toddlers (*n* = 133) born in 2009–2013 were recruited through advertisements at community centers and local family events, and Vancouver Coastal Health immunization clinics in Vancouver, Canada at 12–14 months of age. Inclusion criteria at the time of enrollment included the following: healthy 12–14 month ±7 days toddlers; appropriate weight for gestational age at birth (2500–4000 g); singleton birth; maternal age 20–40 years at delivery; English as the primary language in the home; non-smoking home environment; currently breast-fed ≤2 times per day or fed ≤236 mL/day infant formula containing ARA and DHA; primary source of milk for the toddler was cow's milk or other milk substitutes not containing ARA and DHA; and not received fish oil or other oil supplements and no intent to provide these during the duration of the study. Toddlers with known food allergies, metabolic, neurological, genetic, or immune disorders; and those that had been hospitalized for surgery, growth failure or any other event which was considered likely to impact the outcomes in this study were excluded. The recruitment and enrollment of toddlers in the study was completed under the direction of Dr. Sheila Innis and her staff at BC Children's Hospital Research Institute from January 2010 to September 2014.

Toddlers were randomized and assigned without bias to receive the DHA/ARA supplement (200 mg/day DHA from DHASCO®-S oil, 200 mg/day ARA from ARASCO® oil, DSM Nutritional Products) or control (400 mg/day corn oil), provided as sprinkles that were added to the toddlers' food daily, from baseline until 24 months of age. Home visits were scheduled to provide the nutrition supplements and to collect study diaries on infant feeding and health. Our goal was to provide a nutrition supplement of DHA + ARA to maintain DHA and ARA nutrition equivalent to what a toddler would receive if the mother were to continue breast-feeding the toddler from 12 to 24 months of age.

To avoid any possibility that participation in this study could lead to discontinuation of breast-feeding, only mothers and their toddlers in whom breast-feeding had stopped or were breast-feeding twice a day or less were enrolled. During the first week, the parents were contacted twice by phone to check for any problems and to answer questions. The parents were also contacted when the toddler was 15, 17, 19, 21 and 23 months of age to provide the nutrition supplements as needed and collect routine information on illnesses. Toddler assessments for development, growth and dietary intake occurred at baseline and when the infant was 18 and 24 months of age. The data collection sheets were kept in a locked cabinet in the Innis Lab at the BC Children's Hospital Research Institute.

Informed consent was provided by the child's parent/guardian for inclusion in the study before they participated. The study was conducted in accordance with the Declaration of Helsinki, and the protocol was approved by the Ethics Committee of the University of British Columbia Clinical Research Ethics Board and the Children's and Women's Health Centre of British Columbia Research Ethics Board (certificate number: H09-02028). Clinical Trial Registry: NCT01263912 at clinicaltrials.gov.

2.2. Supplements

The DHA is derived from DHASCO-S, an algal (*Schizochytrium* sp.) triglyceride oil, and the ARA is derived from ARASCO, a fungal (*Mortierella alpina*) triglyceride oil, and are regarded as safe for use in foods and supplements [14,15]. Details of the composition of the supplement and control are provided in Table 1.

Table 1. Composition of supplements.

	Supplement (mg/Package)	Control (mg/Package)
Fish Gelatin	325–460	325–460
Sucrose	325–460	325–460
Corn Starch	310–440	310–440
Sodium Ascorbate	75–105	75–105
DHA	100	0
ARA	100	0
Corn Oil	0	445–625

Abbreviations: ARA, arachidonic acid; DHA, docosahexaenoic acid; the source of DHA and ARA was DHASCO-S, algal (*Schizochytrium* sp.) triglyceride oil; ARASCO, fungal (*Mortierella alpina*) triglyceride oil.

The supplement and control were prepared in individual packages of sprinkles, about two grams each. Two packages were taken per day. The supplement provided 100 mg DHA and 100 mg ARA per package. In appearance, the sprinkles resembled skim milk powder and had a very faint odor similar to skim milk powder. The placebo sprinkles contained corn oil and no DHA or ARA. The amounts of saturated, monounsaturated and LA from the corn oil are insignificant relative to the usual intake of fat and these fatty acids in the usual diet.

The parents were instructed to give one full serving (one package) twice a day, at separate meals, preferably one in the morning and one in the afternoon. The parents were instructed to mix the entire contents of one package with milk, or food such as yogurt or cereal. Written instructions were provided and explained in-person at the beginning of the study. The parents were also instructed not to exceed two sachets a day; not to "catch-up" missed supplements on another day; and if the child spilled part of the milk, replacement supplements should not be given.

The parents were given a calendar for each month of the 12 months that they were in the study, with one line for each week, and each day having two check boxes for administering one for each of the two servings (packages) of sprinkles per day. The parents were asked to complete the calendar at the end of each day. The supplements and control were provided in a container to store in the fridge; containers for empty, unused or damaged packages were also provided. Empty supplement packages and unused supplements were kept and returned at the study visits and were used as a measure of compliance.

2.3. Randomization

Each subject was assigned a unique random code number system, with the codes held in opaque sealed envelopes. The random number subject code was used on all data collection forms and blood samples. If a toddler withdrew from the study, that toddler's unique random number code was not reassigned. Once the consent form was reviewed and signed, the random number code was opened. The supplement and control were prepared in identical packages, two identical supplement and two identical control packages, giving four groups each identified with a letter code, W, X, Y or Z. Each subject random number code was linked to one of the four potential study groups, W, X, Y, or Z. All research staff involved with the toddlers or with analyses of the samples were blinded to the group codes. The identity of the four codes was held in four separate sealed envelopes, in a locked cabinet, and opened at the completion of the study.

2.4. Measures of Nutritional Status

Venous blood (~10 mL) was collected from each toddler at baseline, enrolment at 12–14 months of age (±1 weeks); and at 24 months (±2 weeks) of age. For analyses of fatty acids status, plasma was separated from red blood cells by centrifugation, the buffy coat removed, and the plasma stored at $-70\,^{\circ}$C until later analysis. The red blood cells (RBC) were washed with saline two times to remove contaminating plasma, and stored at $-70\,^{\circ}$C until further analyses. Plasma and RBC lipids were extracted and lipid classes separated by HPLC, quantified with an evaporative light scattering detector, and recovered using a fraction collector. Fatty acids in the fractions of interest were converted to methyl esters, separated, and quantified by gas liquid chromatography as described previously [5,16].

2.5. Dietary Assessments

Dietary history information was collected using a food frequency questionnaire (FFQ). The FFQ included a diet history at baseline, and at ages 18 and 24 months to capture duration of breast-feeding, age of introduction and type of formula, dairy milks, milk substitutes and weaning foods. The FFQ was administered by interview with the parent or primary caregiver and covered the infant's intake for the previous 4 weeks. Information on the frequency with which a food was eaten, portion size, brand name, methods of preparation, and types of meat, fish, poultry, eggs, fish and seafood(s) were collected. Care was taken to guide parents to capture foods provided by daycares or given by other caregivers [17–19].

The 3-day food diary was completed at baseline, 18 months of age, and 24 months of age and included a written record of all beverages and foods consumed and vitamin and mineral supplements, and included questions on the infant's eating behavior, with the same format at each age. Food records were analyzed using Food Processor Nutrition Software (ESHA Research, Salem, OR) and the Canadian Nutrient File (Health Canada, CNF version 2007b) and USDA Nutrient File. Total fat, LA, ALA, ARA, and DHA intakes were determined.

2.6. Child Outcome Measures

The Bayley Scales of Infant and Toddler Development 3rd Edition (Bayley-III) is a standardized test of infant development based on age-referenced norms [20]. At age 24 months, Cognitive and Language scales of the Bayley-III were administered. The Beery–Buktenica Developmental Test of Visual–Motor Integration (5th Ed.) (Beery VMI) was administered at age 24 months and involved the child copying geometric designs arranged in order of increasing complexity [21].

Measures of attention during play with age appropriate toys are widely used [22]. At age 18 and 24 months, single object free play (5 min), multiple object free play (5 min), and a distractibility task (3 min) were given, following the methods of Columbo and colleagues [22,23]. The child was positioned on the parent's lap facing a table on which age appropriate toys were placed. Parents were asked to be quiet and avoid distracting or interacting with their child. The tester limited interaction to encouragement to play with the toy. Verbal communication with the child followed a standard script, and the sessions were timed with a stopwatch and recorded by a video camcorder, which also recorded elapsed time for detailed coding. In the distractibility task, show clips on a TV in the periphery of the play area were used as the distraction. All videos were viewed and analyzed by coders blinded to the infant's study group and all other information about the child and family. Videos were coded using Observer XT 12 (Noldus Information Technology). For the single-object task and the multiple-objects task, mean duration and total duration of looking at the toy, total number of looks to the toy and total number of inattention episodes were measured. For the distractibility task percentage of duration the child turned away from the toy, latency to turn from the toy to the distractor, and the duration of looking at the distractor were calculated.

2.7. Maternal Intelligence

The Test of Nonverbal Intelligence (TONI-3rd Ed.), a language-free measure, was used to assess mother's cognitive ability. The TONI-3 is a norm-referenced measure of intelligence, aptitude, abstract reasoning, and problem solving that requires no reading, writing, or speaking; subjects only have to point to indicate their response choice [24].

2.8. Statistical Analyses

Descriptive statistics were used to present baseline characteristics; group differences were determined by *t*-test for linear variables and by chi-squared test for categorical variables. Group differences in circulating *n*-6 and *n*-3 fatty acids and dietary intakes at baseline and age 24 months were determined by *t*-tests for linear variables and chi-squared test for categorical variables. The primary outcomes of the study were the Bayley-III Cognitive and Language composite scores and the Beery VMI. Differences in primary outcomes between supplement and control groups were determined by general linear models. Secondary outcomes of the study were the attention and distractibility scores. Generalized Linear Modeling (GZLM) and General Estimating Equations (GEE) were used to investigate the relationships between circulating ARA and DHA and primary outcomes.

3. Results

3.1. Baseline Characteristics of Subjects

A total of 133 toddlers were enrolled into the trial; $n = 68$ in the supplement group and $n = 65$ in the control group (Figure 1). Of these, 82.7% ($n = 110$) completed the trial. The dropout rate was 14.7% ($n = 10$) in the supplement group and 20.0% ($n = 13$) in the control group. There were no differences in baseline characteristics between subjects that completed the study and those that dropped out of the study.

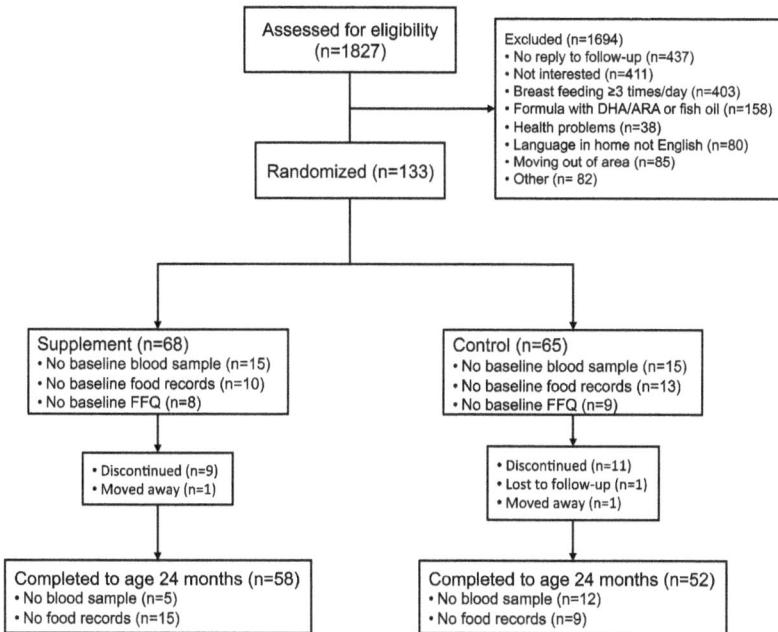

Figure 1. Flow chart illustrating the study subjects in the supplement and control group.

The baseline characteristics of the subjects are given in Table 2. All toddlers were healthy term-born babies with appropriate for gestational age birth weight. The majority of the toddlers were of European or Asian descent. There were no significant differences in the number of male subjects, gestational age, birth weight, age at baseline, zBMI at baseline and age 24 months, ethnicity, family income, maternal age at delivery, maternal education, and maternal nonverbal intelligence score (TONI-3) between the supplement group and the control group (Table 2).

3.2. Dietary Intakes at Baseline and Age 24 Months

At baseline, the supplement group had a greater percentage of toddlers (91.7%) that consumed fish compared to the control group (76.8%) (Table 3). There were no differences at baseline between the groups in the percentage of toddlers consuming eggs, poultry, or human milk. The supplement group also had a greater intake of ARA at baseline than the control group (Table 3). There were no differences in the intake of total dietary fat, LA, ALA, EPA or DHA. At age 24 months, there were no differences in dietary intake of any nutrients or food items.

Table 2. Participant characteristics at baseline.

	Supplement	Control	*p*
Male sex, *n* (%)	40 (59)	41 (63)	0.618
Gestational age, weeks	39.7 (1.4)	39.6 (1.2)	0.992
Birth weight, g	3396 (508)	3471 (440)	0.422
Child age at baseline, months	13.3 (0.9)	13.5 (0.8)	0.146
zBMI, baseline	0.6 (1.0)	0.5 (0.9)	0.958
zBMI, 24 months	0.9 (0.9)	0.9 (0.9)	0.898
Ethnicity			
Asian	19 (27.9)	14 (21.5)	
European	43 (63.2)	41 (63.1)	0.273
First Nations	0 (0)	2 (3.1)	
Missing	6 (8.8)	8 (12.3)	
Family Income, *n* (%)			
<$30,000/year	3 (5.1)	9 (17.6)	
$30,000/year–$50,000/year	8 (13.6)	5 (9.8)	0.079
>$50,000/year	46 (62.7)	32 (62.7)	
Not indicated	2 (3.4)	5 (9.8)	
Maternal age at delivery, years	32.2 (4.3)	32.6 (4.9)	0.606
Maternal Education, *n* (%)			
Did not finish high school	1 (1.5)	0 (0)	
High school	3 (4.4)	3 (4.6)	
College/vocational diploma	11 (16.2)	10 (15.4)	0.810
University undergraduate degree	20 (29.4)	22 (32.3)	
University graduate/professional degree	27 (39.7)	21 (86.2)	
Missing	6 (8.8)	9 (13.8)	
Maternal Nonverbal Intelligence (TONI-3)	110.2 (16.2)	112.9 (14.6)	0.404

Abbreviations: zBMI, BMI standardized for age and sex. Data presented as mean (standard deviation), unless otherwise stated.

3.3. Effect of the Supplement on Developmental Outcomes

The Bayley-III Cognitive and Language composite and Beery VMI scores at age 24 months showed no significant differences between the supplement and control groups in unadjusted models and models adjusted for baseline dietary ARA intakes (Table 4). Further separate analyses in girls and boys showed no effect of the supplement on developmental tests.

Inter-rater reliability for the attention tasks was assessed for look duration and episodes of attention on each task at each age (18 and 24 months) following Colombo et al. [22] using Cohen's Kappa on 25% of the coding, rather than percent agreement. Mean Kappa for the single-object task was: 0.93 at age 18 months and 0.88 at age 24 months, for the multi-object task 0.99 at age 18 months and 0.99 at age 24 months, and for distractibility was 0.94 at age 18 months and 0.94 at age 24 months. There were no significant differences on the single-object, multiple-object or distractibility tasks between the groups at 18 or 24 months (Table S1). We further used GEE to examine relationships between inattention at 18 months and 24 months of age in the multiple toys task by supplementation group and sex, adjusting for zBMI at birth, child age at first visit, and mother non-verbal intelligence (TONI-3) as covariates. In these models, we found that boys receiving the supplement had significantly fewer inattention episodes than boys receiving the control at 24 months of age (*p* = 0.042).

Table 3. Daily dietary intakes of children at baseline and age 24 months.

	Baseline				Age 24 Months		
	Supplement	Control	p		Supplement	Control	p
Total Fat, g	38.1 (12.7)	37.7 (11.9)	0.860	Total Fat, g	43.2 (12.7)	42.2 (14.4)	0.731
LA (18:2n-6), g	4.15 (2.0)	3.71 (1.5)	0.194	LA (18:2n-6), g	5.07 (2.3)	5.31 (2.9)	0.672
ALA (18:3n-3), g	0.59 (0.3)	0.54 (0.3)	0.386	ALA (18:3n-3), g	0.78 (0.5)	0.69 (0.4)	0.384
ARA (20:4n-6), mg	42.4 (35.4)	30.6 (22.0)	0.041	ARA (20:4n-6), mg	55.3 (40.0)	50.0 (32.5)	0.496
EPA (20:5n-3), mg	15.7 (37.5)	16.3 (47.3)	0.936	EPA (20:5n-3), mg	27.4 (67.1)	44.2 (77.8)	0.288
DHA (22:6n-3), mg	31.4 (51.8)	30.8 (66.1)	0.957	DHA (22:6n-3), mg	53.3 (98.9)	76.3 (115)	0.321
Fish in diet, n (%)	55 (91.7)	43 (76.8)	0.027	Fish in diet, n (%)	52 (89.7)	43 (82.7)	0.288
Egg in diet, n (%)	57 (95.0)	50 (89.3)	0.250	Eggs in diet, n (%)	54 (94.7)	47 (90.4)	0.384
Poultry in diet, n (%)	55 (91.7)	50 (90.9)	0.885	Poultry in diet, n (%)	54 (93.1)	47 (90.4)	0.603
Human milk, n (%)	13 (25.5%)	15 (25.9)	0.965	Human milk, n (%)	2 (4.7%)	1 (2.3)	0.557

Abbreviations: ALA, linolenic acid; ARA, arachidonic acid; DHA, docosahexaenoic acid; EPA, eicosapentaenoic acid; LA, linoleic acid. Data presented as mean (standard deviation), unless otherwise stated. Between group differences determined by t-tests for linear variables and chi-squared tests for categorical variables.

Table 4. Effect of ARA and DHA supplementation on developmental scores at age 24 months.

	Supplement	Control	Model 1	Model 2
Bayley-III Cognition Composite	103.9 (13.6)	103.7 (13.9)	$p = 0.932$	$p = 0.723$
Bayley-III Language Composite	105.6 (21.0)	106.9 (30.4)	$p = 0.742$	$p = 0.648$
Beery VMI	92.6 (21.2)	93.4 (11.0)	$p = 0.748$	$p = 0.471$

Abbreviations: ARA, arachidonic acid; Bayley-III, Bayley Scales of Infant and Toddler Development 3rd Edition; Beery VMI, Beery–Buktenica Developmental Test of Visual–Motor Integration (5th Ed.); DHA, docosahexaenoic acid. Data presented as mean (standard deviation). Between group comparisons by general linear models. Model 1, unadjusted. Model 2, adjusted for baseline dietary arachidonic acid intakes.

3.4. Circulating n-3 and n-6 Fatty Acid Status and Developmental Outcomes

We quantified the circulating status of LA, ALA, ARA, eicosapentaenoic acid (EPA, 20:5n-3), and DHA in plasma and RBC PC and PE in the toddlers at baseline and at age 24 months. Baseline RBC PE and PC ARA were higher in toddlers in the supplement group compared to those in the control group (Table 5). There were no differences at baseline in circulating levels of LA, ALA, EPA, and DHA in toddlers from the supplement group compared to those in the control group. As expected, at age 24 months, the supplement group had a greater percentage of ARA and DHA in plasma and RBC PE and PC, and in RBC PE EPA compared to the control group, after Bonferroni adjustment for multiple comparisons (Table 5). This was accompanied by a lower percentage of LA, oleic acid (18:1n-9) in RBC PE and plasma, and a higher percentage of stearic acid (18:0) in RBC PC in the supplement group compared to the control group at age 24 months (Table S2).

We further examined the relationships between circulating ARA, EPA, and DHA levels, and the Bayley-III Cognitive and Language composite. Separate GZLM models examined relationships between RBC PC and PE and plasma n-6 and n-3 fatty acids at age 24 months and the Bayley-III Cognitive and Language composite. Interactions between treatment group (supplement, control) and sex were examined, with adjustments for zBMI at age 24 months, fatty acid levels at baseline, and maternal nonverbal intelligence score (TONI-3). The overall omnibus test was significant ($\chi^2 = 18.23$, $p = 0.033$). There was a significant interaction between supplement group, sex, and ARA in RBC PE ($p = 0.019$, Wald $\chi^2 = 9.96$, Table 6). Interactions are illustrated in Figure 2A. Contrasts were performed to further understand the significant 3-way interaction. There was a significant contrast between boys in the supplement group compared to the control group ($p = 0.045$); boys in the supplement group had higher Bayley-III Cognitive scores than boys in the control group at age 24 months (Table 7; Figure 2A) in models adjusted for baseline fatty acid level, maternal non-verbal intelligence score (TONI), and zBMI at age 24 months. There was no significant difference between supplement and control groups for girls ($p = 0.092$) (Table 7).

The same GZLM models were used to assess Bayley-III language composite. The overall omnibus was significant (Omnibus $\chi^2 = 36.13$, $p \leq 0.001$). We observed a similar interaction between the supplement group, RBC PE ARA and sex ($p = 0.004$, Wald $\chi^2 = 13.11$, Table 6), as shown in Figure 2B. Both boys ($p = 0.0004$) and girls ($p = 0.003$) who received the supplement had higher Bayley-III Language composite compared to children in the control group.

Table 5. Circulating *n*-3 and *n*-6 fatty acids levels of children at baseline and age 24 months.

Fatty Acid	Baseline			Fatty Acid	Age 24 Months		
	Supplement	Control	*p*		Supplement	Control	*p*
Linoleic acid	Percent fatty acids	Percent fatty acids		Linoleic acid	Percent fatty acids	Percent fatty acids	
RBC PE	5.2 (0.8)	5.1 (0.9)	0.562	RBC PE	3.8 (0.8)	5.4 (1.0)	<0.001
RBC PC	20.0 (1.6)	20.3 (2.1)	0.370	RBC PC	17.5 (2.1)	20.9 (2.4)	<0.001
Plasma	22.2 (2.5)	23.2 (2.4)	0.058	Plasma	19.1 (3.3)	23.3 (2.6)	<0.001
Arachidonic acid				Arachidonic acid			
RBC PE	21.7 (1.0)	20.9 (1.6)	0.008	RBC PE	23.0 (1.1)	21.0 (1.5)	<0.001
RBC PC	6.0 (1.1)	5.6 (0.9)	0.024	RBC PC	8.3 (1.8)	5.5 (0.8)	<0.001
Plasma	8.2 (2.3)	7.9 (1.5)	0.448	Plasma	11.7 (2.7)	7.8 (1.3)	<0.001
α-Linolenic acid				Linolenic acid			
RBC PE	0.14 (0.04)	0.13 (0.04)	0.380	RBC PE	0.12 (0.04)	0.15 (0.04)	<0.001
RBC PC	0.21 (0.06)	0.19 (0.06)	0.184	RBC PC	0.20 (0.06)	0.21 (0.06)	0.222
Plasma	0.26 (0.09)	0.25 (0.09)	0.586	Plasma	0.22 (0.07)	0.23 (0.07)	0.589
Eicosapentaenoic Acid				Eicosapentaenoic Acid			
RBC PE	1.1 (0.5)	1.1(0.7)	0.531	RBC PE	0.9 (0.3)	1.1 (0.5)	0.001
RBC PC	0.4 (0.2)	0.4 (0.3)	0.502	RBC PC	0.4 (0.1)	0.4 (0.2)	0.294
Plasma	0.6 (0.4)	0.6 (0.4)	0.533	Plasma	0.6 (0.3)	0.5 (0.3)	0.692
Docosahexaenoic Acid				Docosahexaenoic Acid			
RBC PE	7.5 (1.7)	7.6 (2.0)	0.750	RBC PE	9.7 (1.6)	6.5 (1.8)	<0.001
RBC PC	2.0 (0.6)	1.9 (0.6)	0.823	RBC PC	3.0 (0.8)	1.7 (0.6)	<0.001
Plasma	2.8 (1.1)	2.7 (0.9)	0.660	Plasma	4.3 (1.3)	2.6 (0.9)	<0.001

Abbreviations: PC, phosphatidylcholine; PE, phosphatidylethanolamine. Data presented as mean (standard deviation). Between group differences determined by *t*-tests and Bonferroni correction for multiple comparison (*p* < 0.0028).

Table 6. Relationships between circulating ARA and DHA with developmental scores at age 24 months.

	Supplement Group × Sex × Fatty Acid Interaction		
	Bayley-III Cognitive	Bayley-III Language	Beery VMI
ARA (20:4n-6)			
RBC PE	9.96 (0.019)	13.11 (0.004)	NS
RBC PC	NS	4.75 (0.191)	NS
Plasma	NS	1.39 (0.707)	NS
DHA (22:6n-3)			
RBC PE	NS	2.43 (0.488)	NS
RBC PC	NS	1.35 (0.717)	NS
Plasma	NS	0.607 (0.895)	NS

Abbreviations: ARA, archidonic acid; DHA, docosahexaenoic acid; PC, phosphatidylcholine; PE, phosphatidylethanolamine. Relationships determined by separate general linear models adjusted for sex, zBMI at 24 months of age, baseline fatty acid, and maternal non-verbal intelligence (TONI-3). Supplement × sex × fatty acid interaction. Data presented as B (*p*-value).

Table 7. Relationships between RBC phosphatidylethanolamine arachidonic acid levels and Bayley-III developmental outcomes in boys and girls at age 24 months.

	Bayley-III Cognitive		Bayley-III Language	
	B (95% CI)	*p*	B (95% CI)	*p*
Boys				
RBC PE ARA × Supplement	4.55 (0.12–9.00)	0.045	11.52 (5.10–17.94)	0.0004
Girls				
RBC PE ARA × Supplement	3.86 (−0.64–8.350)	0.092	11.19 (4.69–17.68)	0.003

Abbreviations: ARA, archidonic acid; PE, phosphatidylethanolamine. Relationships determined by separate general linear models adjusted for zBMI at age 24 months, baseline fatty acid, and maternal non-verbal intelligence (TONI-3). Supplement × sex.

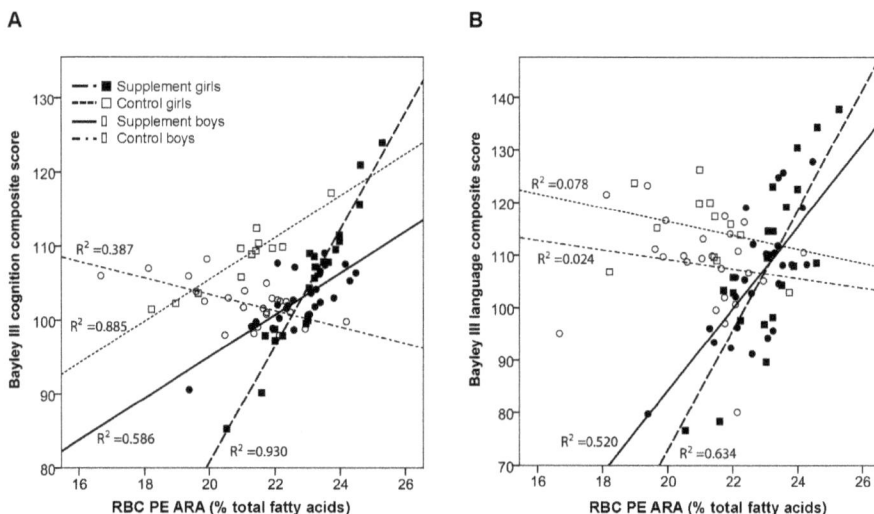

Figure 2. Relationship between RBC PE arachidonic acid (ARA) level and: (**A**) Bayley III cognitive composite scores; and (**B**) Bayley III language composite scores at age 24 months by supplement group and sex (supplement-treated girls (■); control-treated girls (□); supplement-treated boys (●); and control-treated boys (○).

4. Discussion

The objective of this prospective, longitudinal double blind, randomized controlled trial was to determine effects of supplementing toddlers with DHA and ARA from age 12 to 24 months on neurodevelopmental outcomes and biomarkers of ARA and DHA status. We found no differences between supplement and control-treated toddlers on BAYLEY-III cognition and language composite scores [20] and the Beery VMI [21], the primary outcomes of the study. As expected, the supplement increased circulating biomarkers of DHA and ARA status in RBC PE and PC and plasma from the toddlers. After adjusting for baseline fatty acid, zBMI at age 24 months, and mother's nonverbal IQ (TONI-3), we found a positive association between ARA status in RBC PE, the largest fraction of circulating ARA, and cognition but only for boys in the supplement group. No relationships were observed for girls. Similarly, RBC PE ARA was positively associated with language scores for both boys and girls in the supplement group but not for those in the control group. In contrast, no relationships were observed between supplement group, DHA status, and neurodevelopmental outcomes. Overall, these findings suggest that increasing the status of ARA in RBC PE in infants taking a supplement containing ARA (200 mg/day) and DHA (200 mg/day) from 12–24 months of age is associated with better cognition and language.

Interestingly, we found a positive relationship between RBC PE ARA and neurodevelopmental outcomes but only in supplemented toddlers. This suggests that increasing the status of ARA to levels observed in the supplemented toddlers has positive effects on neurodevelopment. The biological relevance of this relationship is not known and requires further investigation. A small trial in preterm infants (*n* = 45) reported better psychomotor development at age 24 months in infants that were fed a formula with 0.67% ARA/0.33% DHA compared to those fed a formula with 0.37% ARA/0.37% DHA suggesting a positive effect of higher ARA in the formula [25]. Similar findings of a positive effect of ARA and DHA on neurodevelopment of preterm infants were reported in the infants at age six months [26]. Arachidonic acid and PE are important during development; they are critical components of neural membranes [27] and are required for the synthesis of endocannabinoids, especially anandamide and 2-arachidonylglycerol [28]. The endocannabinoids play important roles in neurotransmission and behavior, functioning through the cannabinoid (CB) receptor, CB1, in the brain. A study in adult male rats reported higher levels of anandamide and 2-arachidonoylglycerol in the brain of rats supplemented with ARA compared to rats fed a palm oil diet despite no changes in brain phospholipid ARA [29]. It seems reasonable to predict that supplementing the infants with DHA and ARA may affect tissue levels of endocannibinoids, especially in the brain, and mediate the relationship between RBC PE ARA and neurodevelopmental scores that we observed in the supplemented infants.

Additional evidence supporting the importance of ARA during development has recently been described in a mouse model. Studies in male mice deficient in delta-6 desaturase (D6D, *Fads2* -/- mice), the enzyme required for the desaturation of LA and ALA to ARA and DHA, respectively, reported that D6D deficient mice were smaller, had reduced levels of motor activity and coordination, and reduced ARA and DHA levels in RBC and brain compared to wild-type mice [30]. Interestingly, supplementing the D6D deficient mice with ARA containing formula during the suckling period improved growth and motor activity but not motor coordination [30]. Beneficial effects on growth and motor coordination were also reported in the D6D deficient mice supplemented with DHA; but DHA supplementation did not improve motor activity [31]. Interestingly, D6D deficient mice supplemented with both ARA and DHA showed the greatest improvements in motor coordination compared to unsupplemented D6D deficient mice or those supplemented with just ARA or DHA [31]. However, in contrast to these studies, questions regarding the requirement for dietary ARA during infancy have been raised and the subject of some current reviews [3,32]. Further, a meta-analysis of randomized trials of long chain *n*-3 and *n*-6 polyunsaturated fatty acid supplementation of term infants reported no effects on growth, regardless of whether the formula contained ARA or not [33].

In contrast to what we predicted, this trial observed no effect of increasing DHA status in toddlers between ages 12 and 24 months on neurodevelopmental outcomes. The DHA levels in RBC phospholipids and plasma from the toddlers in the supplement group on average increased 30–50% from baseline to 24 months of age, whereas, in the control group, the levels of DHA slightly decreased between baseline and the end of the study, clearly demonstrating effects of the supplement on DHA status. This is in line with a small study (n = 86) that reported increases in DHA status of toddlers supplemented with either 43 mg/day DHA or 130 mg/day DHA for 60 days at 18–24 months of age [13]; fewer respiratory illnesses were also reported in the infants receiving 130 mg/day DHA compared to those receiving no DHA supplementation.

Little is known regarding the nutritional status of long chain polyunsaturated fatty acids and optimal intakes for toddlers between ages 12 and 24 months. The optimal levels of dietary intakes of DHA and ARA to support neurological development during this time period are not known. Most studies to date have focused on effects of prenatal (maternal) supplementation or supplementation during the first year after birth. Findings of these studies have been variable. A systematic review of 11 randomized controlled trials of 5272 participants found no effect of maternal DHA supplementation during pregnancy or during pregnancy and lactation on neurocognitive outcomes, except for a positive effect of DHA supplementation on IQ scores in children at 2–5 years of age [34].

Beneficial effects of DHA and ARA supplementation of infants during the first year of life on neurodevelopmental outcomes have been reported. The DIAMOND study was a multicenter, double-blind, randomized controlled trial (n = 244) conducted in Kansas City and Dallas that compared infants that were fed a formula with no ARA and DHA with infants fed formulas supplemented with ARA (34 mg/100 kcal) and DHA, at three different levels (17 mg/100 kcal, 34 mg/100 kcal, and 51 mg/100 kcal), from the first week of life to 12 months of age. The trial reported better visual acuity at 12 months of age in infants fed the DHA and ARA supplemented formulas compared to infants fed the formula with no ARA or DHA [7]. Further secondary analyses of infants in the trial reported that those fed the DHA supplemented formulas had better attention at four, six and nine months of age (n = 122) [8]. Follow-up studies reported no effect of the DHA/ARA supplementation during the first year of life on neurodevelopmental outcomes at 18 months of age in infants from Dallas (n = 117) [9] and in infants from Kansas City (n = 81) [8]. However, the children that received the DHA/ARA supplemented formula in infancy at the Kansas City site performed better on neurodevelopmental tests in a long term follow up study at 3–5 years of age (n = 81) [10] and showed differences in brain electrophysiology at 6 years of age (n = 69) [35]. Similarly, a multicenter European trial of DHA and ARA supplementation of infants (n = 147) during the first four months of life reported no effects of the supplementation on IQ at six years of age but did report that the supplemented children were faster at processing information than the unsupplemented children [11]. Together, these findings suggest long-term neurodevelopmental effects of supplementing infants in the first year of life with DHA and ARA. This raises question as to whether there may be, as yet unidentified, long-term benefits at later time points during childhood of supplementing toddlers with DHA and ARA between ages 12 and 24 months.

The supplement provided 200 mg/day of ARA and DHA, which is approximately six times higher than the levels found in the diet of the toddlers at baseline and at age 24 months. In addition to the ARA/DHA consumed from breast milk or formula during the first year of life, a large number of the toddlers in the study (>75%) consumed DHA and ARA containing foods, including fish, eggs, and poultry, at baseline and this number increased to >80% of the toddlers consuming these foods at age 24 months. The question remains as to what the optimal dietary intake levels are for children at this age and what are the best indicators of status and function. Providing 200 mg/day of DHA increased circulating biomarkers on average by 29–50% but this was not associated with any differences on indicators of neurodevelopment. In contrast, the 200 mg/day each of ARA and DHA, increased circulating RBC PE ARA by only 6% and this was associated with neurodevelopment outcomes. In contrast, the RBC PC ARA and DHA increased by 38% and 50%, respectively, and plasma ARA and DHA increased by 43% and 54%, respectively, but we found no relationships between these biomarkers of ARA and DHA status and neurodevelopment. It is possible that the neurodevelopmental tests used in this trial were not sensitive to changes in DHA status but that other functional endpoints might be affected. As mentioned above, no effect of supplementing infants with DHA/ARA during the first year of life on the Bayley (version 2) scores at age 18 months of age were reported by Columbo et al. [10]. Interestingly, maternal DHA levels have been associated with better infant attention at 12 and 18 months [22,23]. In the present study, we found that after adjusting for baseline fatty acid, zBMI at age 24 months, and mother's non-verbal IQ, boys in the supplementation group showed less inattention at age 24 months. Further research is needed to identify what markers of brain development and cognition are the best indicators of DHA and ARA function in toddlers during the age of 12–24 months.

Some limitations to the study must be considered when interpreting our results. Most importantly is whether the neurodevelopmental tests that were used in the trial, the Bayley-III, Beery VMI and attention tasks, are sensitive enough to detect effects of the DHA and ARA supplement on neurodevelopment. The sensitivity and limitations of these tests and appropriateness for nutritional interventions in healthy children have been raised [36]. Another limitation is the reliance on circulating concentrations of DHA and ARA as biomarkers of status. We have no other choice given we are studying young children. However, we do not know whether the circulating concentrations of fatty acids directly reflect levels that are found in tissues like the brain. It is reasonable to predict that uptake, incorporation, and use of fatty acids by tissues, is tissue and cell specific, and may not always reflect what is observed in circulation. We also cannot account for ARA and DHA stores that accrued in the toddlers prenatally and during the first year of life. There may also be genetic determinants of DHA and ARA metabolism that influence response of the infants to the DHA and ARA supplement. Prior studies have focused predominantly on variants in genes encoding enzymes required for the elongation and desaturation of essential fatty acids [37] but variants in other proteins governing the functional effects of DHA and ARA also warrant investigation. The sample size of the trial is also smaller than planned. The initial goal of the trial was to recruit 200 toddlers but enrollment of toddlers in the trial was slower than anticipated because of barriers relating to toddlers not meeting the inclusion criteria, such as breast-feeding <2 times per day; being fed <236 mL/day infant formula containing ARA and DHA; or taking fish oil or other oil supplements.

5. Conclusions

In summary, findings from this longitudinal, double-blind, randomized controlled trial of DHA and ARA supplementation of toddlers between 12 and 24 months of age found no effect on neurodevelopment. However, the study is limited because the cognitive tests that were used may not be sensitive enough to detect effects of DHA and ARA supplementation during this developmental period. A positive relationship between the status of ARA in RBC PE, in toddlers taking the supplement containing ARA (200 mg/day) and DHA (200 mg/day), and better neurodevelopment was observed. Further studies are required to determine the long-term effect of the supplement at later time points in childhood using more sensitive indicators of cognition.

Supplementary Materials: The following are available online at www.mdpi.com/2072-6643/9/9/975/s1. Table S1, Effect of ARA and DHA supplement on attention and distractibility measures at age 18 and 24 months; Table S2, Major fatty acids levels of children at baseline and age 24 months.

Acknowledgments: DSM Nutritional Products sponsored the study and provided the investigational products but had no role in the study design and data analyses. DM and KYM are employees of DSM Nutritional Products, a manufacturer of omega-3 and omega-6 fatty acids, vitamins and other nutrients. AMD and REG are supported by Investigator Grant Awards from the BC Children's Hospital Research Institute. We would like to acknowledge Sheila Innis (1953–2016) for her work and contributions to this project. We would like to acknowledge Glynis Siebert, Kelly Richardson, and Kelly Mulder for assistance with subject recruitment and data collection.

Author Contributions: S.M.I. designed the research; J.M., R.D., C.M.Y.C., A.M.D. and R.E.G. conducted the research and analyzed the data; C.M.Y.C. and A.M.D. wrote the manuscript; and all authors contributed to review and approval of the final manuscript.

Conflicts of Interest: The authors declare no conflict of interest.

References

1. Carlson, S.E.; Colombo, J. Docosahexaenoic acid and arachidonic acid nutrition in early development. *Adv. Pediatr.* **2016**, *63*, 453–471. [CrossRef] [PubMed]
2. Innis, S.M. Impact of maternal diet on human milk composition and neurological development of infants. *Am. J. Clin. Nutr.* **2014**, *99*, 734S–741S. [CrossRef] [PubMed]
3. Hadley, B.K.; Ryan, S.A.; Forsyth, S.; Gautier, S.; Salem, N. The essentiality of arachidonic acid in infant development. *Nutrients* **2016**, *8*, 216. [CrossRef] [PubMed]
4. Martínez, M.; Mougan, I. Fatty acid composition of human brain phospholipids during normal development. *J. Neurochem.* **1998**, *71*, 2528–2533. [CrossRef] [PubMed]
5. Arbuckle, L.D.; Innis, S.M. Docosahexaenoic acid is transferred through maternal diet to milk and to tissues of natural milk-fed piglets. *J. Nutr.* **1993**, *123*, 1668–1675. [PubMed]
6. Greiner, R.C.S.; Winter, J.; Nathanielsz, P.W.; Brenna, J.T. Brain docosahexaenoate accretion in fetal baboons: Bioequivalence of dietary [alpha]-linolenic and docosahexaenoic acids. *Pediatr. Res.* **1997**, *42*, 826–834. [CrossRef] [PubMed]
7. Birch, E.E.; Carlson, S.E.; Hoffman, D.R.; Fitzgerald-Gustafson, K.M.; Fu, V.L.N.; Drover, J.R.; Castañeda, Y.S.; Minns, L.; Wheaton, D.K.H.; Mundy, D.; et al. The DIAMOND (DHA intake and measurement of neural development) study: A double-masked, randomized controlled clinical trial of the maturation of infant visual acuity as a function of the dietary level of docosahexaenoic acid. *Am. J. Clin. Nutr.* **2010**, *91*, 848–859. [CrossRef] [PubMed]
8. Colombo, J.; Carlson, S.E.; Cheatham, C.L.; Fitzgerald-Gustafson, K.M.; Kepler, A.; Doty, T. Long-chain polyunsaturated fatty acid supplementation in infancy reduces heart rate and positively affects distribution of attention. *Pediatr. Res.* **2011**, *70*, 406–410. [CrossRef] [PubMed]
9. Drover, J.R.; Hoffman, D.R.; Castañeda, Y.S.; Morale, S.E.; Garfield, S.; Wheaton, D.H.; Birch, E.E. Cognitive function in 18-month-old term infants of the DIAMOND study: A randomized, controlled clinical trial with multiple dietary levels of docosahexaenoic acid. *Early Hum. Dev.* **2011**, *87*, 223–230. [CrossRef] [PubMed]
10. Colombo, J.; Carlson, S.E.; Cheatham, C.L.; Shaddy, D.J.; Kerling, E.H.; Thodosoff, J.M.; Gustafson, K.M.; Brez, C. Long-term effects of LCPUFA supplementation on childhood cognitive outcomes. *Am. J. Clin. Nutr.* **2013**, *98*, 403–412. [CrossRef] [PubMed]
11. Willatts, P.; Forsyth, S.; Agostoni, C.; Casaer, P.; Riva, E.; Boehm, G. Effects of long-chain PUFA supplementation in infant formula on cognitive function in later childhood. *Am. J. Clin. Nutr.* **2013**, *98*, 536S–542S. [CrossRef] [PubMed]
12. Infant Feeding Working Group. *Nutrition for Healthy Term Infants: Recommendations from Six to 24 Months*; Joint Statement of Health Canada, Canadian Pediatric Society, Dietitians of Canada, and Breastfeeding Committee for Canada; Health Canada, Ed.; Government of Canada: Ottawa, ON, Canada, 2014.
13. Minns, L.M.; Kerling, E.H.; Neely, M.R.; Sullivan, D.K.; Wampler, J.L.; Harris, C.L.; Berseth, C.L.; Carlson, S.E. Toddler formula supplemented with docosahexaenoic acid (DHA) improves DHA status and respiratory health in a randomized, double-blind, controlled trial of us children less than 3 years of age. *Prostaglandins Leukot. Essent. Fat. Acids* **2010**, *82*, 287–293. [CrossRef] [PubMed]
14. Food and Drug Administration Department of Health and Human Services. *Agency Response Letter GRAS Notice No. GRN 000137*; United States Government: College Park, MD, USA, 2004. Available online: https://www.fda.gov/Food/IngredientsPackagingLabeling/GRAS/NoticeInventory/ucm153961.htm (accessed on 5 September 2017).
15. Streekstra, H. On the safety of *Mortierella alpina* for the production of food ingredients, such as arachidonic acid. *J. Biotechnol.* **1997**, *56*, 153–165.
16. Mulder, K.A.; King, D.J.; Innis, S.M. Omega-3 fatty acid deficiency in infants before birth identified using a randomized trial of maternal DHA supplementation in pregnancy. *PLoS ONE* **2014**, *9*, e83764. [CrossRef] [PubMed]
17. Williams, P.L.; Innis, S.M. Food frequency questionnaire for assessing infant iron nutrition. *Can. J. Diet. Pract. Res.* **2005**, *66*, 176–182. [CrossRef] [PubMed]

18. Williams, P.L.; Innis, S.M.; Vogel, A.M.P.; Stephen, L. Factors influencing infant feeding practices of mothers in Vancouver. *Can. J. Public Health* **1999**, *90*, 114–119. [PubMed]

19. Williams, P.L.; Innis, S.M.; Vogel, A.M.P. Breastfeeding and weaning practices in Vancouver. *Can. J. Public Health* **1996**, *87*, 231–236. [PubMed]

20. Bayley, N. *Bayley Scales of Infant and Toddler Development*, 3rd ed.; Harcourt Assessment Inc.: San Antonio, TX, USA, 2006.

21. Beery, K.E.; Beery, N.A. *The Beery-Buktenica Developmental Test of Visual-Motor Integration (VMI)*, 5th ed.; NCS Pearson Inc.: Minneapolis, MI, USA, 2004.

22. Colombo, J.; Kannass, K.N.; Jill Shaddy, D.; Kundurthi, S.; Maikranz, J.M.; Anderson, C.J.; Blaga, O.M.; Carlson, S.E. Maternal DHA and the development of attention in infancy and toddlerhood. *Child Dev.* **2004**, *75*, 1254–1267. [CrossRef] [PubMed]

23. Kannass, K.N.; Colombo, J.; Carlson, S.E. Maternal DHA levels and toddler free-play attention. *Dev. Neuropsychol.* **2009**, *34*, 159–174. [CrossRef] [PubMed]

24. Brown, L.; Sherbenou, R.J.; Johnsen, S.K. *Manual of Test of Nonverbal Intelligence*, 3rd ed.; PRO-ED: Austin, TX, USA, 1997.

25. Alshweki, A.; Muñuzuri, A.P.; Baña, A.M.; de Castro, M.J.; Andrade, F.; Aldamiz-Echevarría, L.; de Pipaón, M.S.; Fraga, J.M.; Couce, M.L. Effects of different arachidonic acid supplementation on psychomotor development in very preterm infants; a randomized controlled trial. *Nutr. J.* **2015**, *14*, 101. [CrossRef] [PubMed]

26. Henriksen, C.; Haugholt, K.; Lindgren, M.; Aurvåg, A.K.; Rønnestad, A.; Grønn, M.; Solberg, R.; Moen, A.; Nakstad, B.; Berge, R.K.; et al. Improved Cognitive Development Among Preterm Infants Attributable to Early Supplementation of Human Milk With Docosahexaenoic Acid and Arachidonic Acid. *Pediatrics* **2008**, *121*, 1137–1145. [CrossRef] [PubMed]

27. Janssen, C.I.F.; Kiliaan, A.J. Long-chain polyunsaturated fatty acids (LCPUFA) from genesis to senescence: The influence of lcpufa on neural development, aging, and neurodegeneration. *Prog. Lipid Res.* **2014**, *53*, 1–17. [CrossRef] [PubMed]

28. Lu, H.-C.; Mackie, K. An introduction to the endogenous cannabinoid system. *Biol. Psychiatr.* **2016**, *79*, 516–525. [CrossRef] [PubMed]

29. Artmann, A.; Petersen, G.; Hellgren, L.I.; Boberg, J.; Skonberg, C.; Nellemann, C.; Hansen, S.H.; Hansen, H.S. Influence of dietary fatty acids on endocannabinoid and n-acylethanolamine levels in rat brain, liver and small intestine. *BBA Mol. Cell Biol. Lipid* **2008**, *1781*, 200–212. [CrossRef] [PubMed]

30. Hatanaka, E.; Harauma, A.; Yasuda, H.; Watanabe, J.; Nakamura, M.T.; Salem, N., Jr.; Moriguchi, T. Essentiality of arachidonic acid intake in murine early development. *Prostaglandin Leukot. Essent. Fat. Acids* **2016**, *108*, 51–57. [CrossRef] [PubMed]

31. Harauma, A.; Yasuda, H.; Hatanaka, E.; Nakamura, M.T.; Salem, N., Jr.; Moriguchi, T. The essentiality of arachidonic acid in addition to docosahexaenoic acid for brain growth and function. *Prostaglandin Leukot. Essent. Fat. Acids* **2017**, *116*, 9–18. [CrossRef] [PubMed]

32. Lauritzen, L.; Fewtrell, M.; Agostoni, C. Dietary arachidonic acid in perinatal nutrition: A commentary. *Pediatr. Res.* **2015**, *77*, 263–269. [CrossRef] [PubMed]

33. Makrides, M.; Gibson, R.A.; Udell, T.; Ried, K. International LCPUFA Investigators. Supplementation of infant formula with long-chain polyunsaturated fatty acids does not influence the growth of term infants. *Am. J. Clin. Nutr.* **2005**, *81*, 1094–1101. [PubMed]

34. Gould, J.F.; Smithers, L.G.; Makrides, M. The effect of maternal omega-3 (*n*-3) LCPUFA supplementation during pregnancy on early childhood cognitive and visual development: A systematic review and meta-analysis of randomized controlled trials. *Am. J. Clin. Nutr.* **2013**, *97*, 531–544. [CrossRef] [PubMed]

35. Liao, K.; McCandliss, B.D.; Carlson, S.E.; Colombo, J.; Shaddy, D.J.; Kerling, E.H.; Lepping, R.J.; Sittiprapaporn, W.; Cheatham, C.L.; Gustafson, K.M. Event-related potential differences in children supplemented with long-chain polyunsaturated fatty acids during infancy. *Dev. Sci.* **2016**. [CrossRef] [PubMed]

36. Colombo, J.; Carlson, S.E. Is the measure the message: The BSID and nutritional interventions. *Pediatrics* **2012**, *129*, 1166–1167. [CrossRef] [PubMed]

37. Glaser, C.; Lattka, E.; Rzehak, P.; Steer, C.; Koletzko, B. Genetic variation in polyunsaturated fatty acid metabolism and its potential relevance for human development and health. *Matern. Child Nutr.* **2011**, *7*, 27–40. [CrossRef] [PubMed]

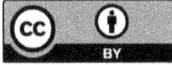

nutrients

MDPI

Article

Phytosterols and Omega 3 Supplementation Exert Novel Regulatory Effects on Metabolic and Inflammatory Pathways: A Proteomic Study

Carmen Lambert [1,†], Judit Cubedo [1,2,†], Teresa Padró [1,2], Joan Sánchez-Hernández [3,4], Rosa M. Antonijoan [5], Antonio Perez [4] and Lina Badimon [1,2,6,*]

[1] Cardiovascular Science Institute—ICCC IIB-Sant Pau, 08025 Barcelona, Spain; clambert@santpau.cat (C.L.); jcubedo@csic-iccc.org (J.C.); tpadro@csic-iccc.org (T.P.)
[2] Ciber CV, 28029 Madrid, Spain
[3] Ciber DEM, 28029 Madrid, Spain; jsanchezh@comb.cat
[4] Endocrinology Department, Hospital Sant Pau, IIB-Sant Pau, 08025 Barcelona, Spain; APerez@santpau.cat
[5] Medicament ResearchCenter (CIM), Hospital Sant Pau, IIB-Sant Pau, 08025 Barcelona, Spain; rantonijoana@santpau.cat
[6] Cardiovascular Research Chair UAB, 08025 Barcelona, Spain
[*] Correspondence:lbadimon@csic-iccc.org; Tel.: +34-93-556-5882
[†] These authors contributed equally to this study.

Received: 20 April 2017; Accepted: 8 June 2017; Published: 13 June 2017

Abstract: Cardiovascular disease (CVD) remains one of the major causes of death and disability worldwide. In addition to drug treatment, nutritional interventions or supplementations are becoming a health strategy for CVD prevention. Phytosterols (PhyS) are natural components that have been shown to reduce cholesterol levels; while poly-unsaturated fatty acids (PUFA), mainly omega-3 (ω3) fatty acids, have shown to reduce triglyceride levels. Here we aimed to investigate whether the proteins in the main lipoproteins (low density lipoproteins (LDL) and high density lipoproteins (HDL)) as well as proteins in the lipid free plasma fraction (LPDP) were regulated by the intake of PhyS-milk or ω3-milk, in overweight healthy volunteers by a proteomic based systems biology approach. The study was a longitudinal crossover trial, including thirty-two healthy volunteers with body mass index (BMI) 25–35 kg/m^2 (Clinical Trial: ISRCTN78753338). Basal samples before any intervention and after 4 weeks of intake of PhyS or ω3-milk were analyzed. Proteomic profiling by two dimensional electrophoresis (2-DE) followed by mass spectrometry-(MALDI/TOF), ELISA, Western blot, conventional biochemical analysis, and in-silico bioinformatics were performed. The intake of PhyS-milk did not induce changes in the lipid associated plasma protein fraction, whereas ω3-milk significantly increased apolipoprotein (Apo)- E LDL content ($p = 0.043$) and induced a coordinated increase in several HDL-associated proteins, Apo A–I, lecithin cholesterol acyltransferase (LCAT), paraoxonase-1 (PON-1), Apo D, and Apo L1 ($p < 0.05$ for all). Interestingly, PhyS-milk intake induced a reduction in inflammatory molecules not seen after ω3-milk intake. Serum amyloid P component (SAP) was reduced in the LPDP protein fraction ($p = 0.001$) of subjects taking PhyS-milk and C-C motif chemokine 2 (CCL2)expression detected by reverse transcription polymerase chain reaction (RT-PCR) analysis in white blood cells was significantly reduced ($p = 0.013$). No changes were observed in the lipid-free plasma proteome with ω3-milk. Our study provides novel results and highlights that the PhyS-milk induces attenuation of the pro-inflammatory pathways, whereas ω3-milk induces improvement in lipid metabolic pathways.

Keywords: phytosterols; omega 3; HDL; LDL; inflammation; lipid metabolism

1. Introduction

Cardiovascular disease (CVD) is a very common pathology that is the main cause of death and disability worldwide. The reduction of CVD risk is one of the major challenges of cardiovascular medicine.

Nowadays, the incidence of overweight and obesity is increasing, becoming an important risk factor for a number of diseases including atherosclerosis and CVD [1]. Moreover, several studies have demonstrated, and it is generally acknowledged, that lifestyle and nutritional habits are closely associated with the presentation of CVD [2–4].

A very common therapeutic strategy for the prevention of CVD is nutritional intervention or supplementation. The cardioprotective effects of poly-unsaturated fatty acids (PUFA) intake have been examined in several studies, which have established that diets enriched in omega 3 poly-unsaturated fatty acids (ω3-PUFA) from plants and fish have an important role in the prevention of CVD [5,6]. Some of the beneficial effects of PUFA rich foods include a reduced susceptibility to suffer from ventricular arrhythmia, antithrombogenic and antioxidant effects, retardation of atherosclerotic plaque growth, improved blood lipid and lipoprotein profile, and also anti-inflammatory and hypotensive effects. PUFA supplemented foods have been shown to reduce triglyceride (TG) levels [7]. Additionally, dietary supplementation with phytosterols (PhyS) has been shown to reduce the risk of CVD and it is a common nutritional strategy to reduce cholesterol levels [8].

Among the different lipid-associated plasma fractions, low-density lipoproteins (LDL) and high-density lipoproteins (HDL) are widely studied. In primary prevention, high levels of LDL-cholesterol (LDL-C) are related with a higher incidence of cardiovascular events in the continuum of CVD, whereas HDL-cholesterol (HDL-C) levels are commonly known as a risk-reducing factor [9]. It is now accepted that the importance of HDL in the progression of CVD, resides on their quality rather than their quantity, highlighting the importance of their composition, structure, and function [10–13]. Indeed, apolipoprotein A–I (Apo A–I), the major protein component of HDL, has cardiovascular protective properties [14,15]. Also, low levels of apolipoprotein E (Apo E) have been related to hyperlipidemia and atherosclerosis [16].

In addition to apolipoproteins, HDL-associated enzymes such as paraoxonase-1 (PON-1) and lecitin cholesterol acyltransferase (LCAT) exert antioxidant and cardioprotective effects [17]. In fact, the association of LCAT, PON-1, and Apo A–I have been shown to increase the time span of HDL protection against LDL oxidation [18].

Beside lipid metabolism, another key hallmark in the pathogenesis of atherosclerotic disease is inflammation. One of the main protein families involved in systemic inflammation are pentraxins [19]. Pentraxins are serum proteins with a relatively uncommon pentameric structure, which have a common amino acid domain in the C-terminal region (pentraxin signature), and besides their role in inflammation they also have a role in immunity and homeostasis [20,21]. Depending on the length of the amino acid chain, pentraxins are divided in two subfamilies, long pentraxins and short pentraxins. Members of the short pentraxins include C-reactive protein (CRP) and serum amyloid P component (SAP), which are acute-phase proteins secreted mainly by hepatocytes in response to pro-inflammatory stimuli. In fact, the role of CRP as a risk marker for atherosclerosis has been widely studied [21].

Our group has previously demonstrated that the intake of low fat milk supplemented with PhyS reduces plasma cholesterol levels; whereas ω3 supplementation reduces plasma TG and very-low density lipoprotein (VLDL) cholesterol levels [7]. Additionally, PhyS and ω3 supplementation induce a differential shift in the LDL lipidomic profile [7]. In the present study, we aimed to further characterize and extend PhyS and ω3 induced changes by analyzing the differential proteomic profile of the lipid-associated plasma protein fraction (LDL and HDL) and the soluble protein fraction of plasma (LPDP) in a subgroup of subjects of our previously reported study, in order to broaden our in-depth understanding of the effect of these food supplements and evidence further effects at a molecular level that could provide CVD protection.

2. Materials and Methods

2.1. Study Population

This is a sub-study of a previously reported double-blinded randomized two-arm longitudinal crossover trial [Clinical Trial: ISRCTN78753338] [7]. All subjects were submitted to two 28-day intervention periods in which volunteers were instructed to consume 250 mL of ω3-supplemented milk (131.25 mg EPA + 243.75 mg DHA/250 mL of milk) or PhyS-supplemented milk (1.6 g of plant sterols/250 mL of milk), separated by a 4 weeks wash-out period (Figure 1a). Both products were prepared by CAPSA Food (Spain) and with no identification of the product administrated. PhyS-milk was commercially available, whereas ω3-milk was prepared for the study. Before the initiation of the intervention, individuals were submitted to a 2 weeks run-in period. During the run-in and wash-out periods, participants received a commercially available plain low-fat milk (without PhyS or ω3), with the same composition to that used for preparing the PhyS- and ω3-enriched milks. These basal samples are used as self-control to avoid variability between volunteers. The trial demonstrated that milk-supplementation with 1.6 g of PhyS significantly reduces LDL-C and milk with 375 mg of ω3 significantly reduces TG levels [7].

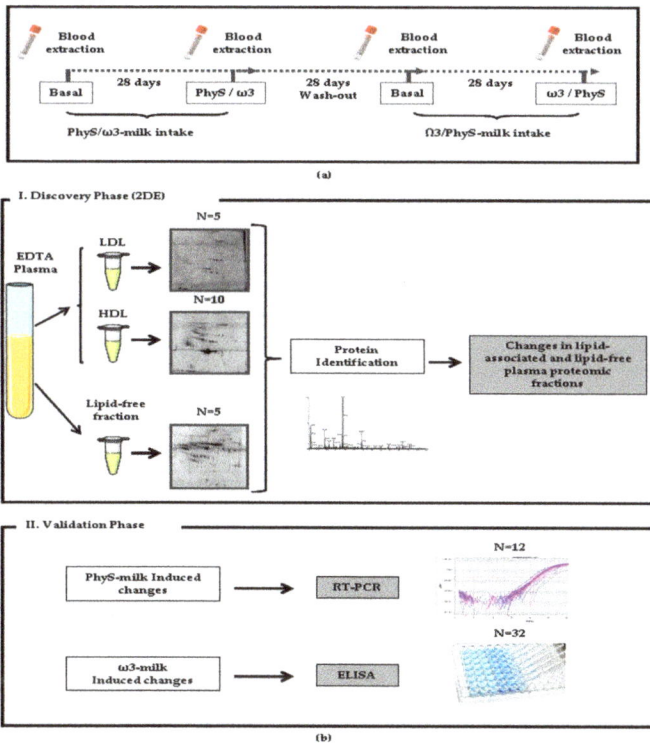

Figure 1. Study design. (**a**) Blood samples were obtained before and after the 28 day milk supplementation treatment period. A 28 day wash-out was made between treatments; (**b**) The study workflow of the present study comprised two phases: (**I**) the discovery phase in which a proteomic approach was used to identify changes in the proteomic profile of the different plasma fractions after the intake of supplemented milk (*N* = 5); and (**II**) the validation phase, where different selected proteins were validated by ELISA (*N* = 32) and inflammatory changes were analyzed by reverse transcription polymerase chain reaction (RT-PCR; *N* = 12).

Healthy volunteers between the ages of 25 and 70 years (N = 32), attending to regular medical controls, were eligible for participation if they had overweight or grade 1 obesity (BMI 25–35 kg/m^2; Table 1). Subjects were excluded if they reported existing chronic illnesses including cancer, overt hyperlipidemia, diabetes mellitus, hypertension, or heart, liver, or kidney disease. Volunteers were excluded if they were under anti-inflammatory medication or any blood thinning treatment during the study or during the 2-weeks run-in period. Other exclusion criteria were: use of lipid-lowering drugs, β-blockers, or diuretics, history of CVD, lactose intolerance, or being in a weight-loss program. To confirm health status, all subjects underwent a complete physical examination conducted by the physician of the study. Those consuming a PhyS-enriched spread and/or fish oil supplements or with strong aversion to milk derived products were also excluded. Compliance was controlled by telephone and personal interview and with a written formulary on each period. The Human Ethical Review Committee of the Hospital Sant Pau in Barcelona approved the study. Informed written consent was obtained from all participants. Reporting of the study conforms to the STROBE (strengthening the reporting of observational studies in epidemiology)-guidelines.

Table 1. Demographic and biochemical profile.

Product	PhyS-Milk		ω3-Milk	
Women/Men	19/13		19/13	
Age (Years)	50.5 ± 1.6		50.5 ± 1.6	
Parameter	Baseline	After PhyS-milk	Baseline	After ω3-milk
BMI	28.2 ± 0.7	28.1 ± 0.7	28.3 ± 0.7	28.2 ± 0.7
Ch (mg/dL)	216.0 ± 6.0	204.5 ± 5.6 *	216.4 ± 6.1	213.78 ± 5.9
TG (mg/dL)	110.2 ± 10.3	115.2 ±15.1	116.3 ± 14.3	99.5 ± 8.7 *
HDL-C (mg/dL)	54.5 ± 3.1	54.5 ± 3.0	57.0 ± 2.9	56.4 ± 2.8
LDL-C (mg/dL)	137.7 ± 4.9	127.2 ± 4.7 *	136.4 ± 5.0	137.7 ± 5.0
VLDL-C (mg/dL)	22.0 ± 2.0	23.0 ± 3.0	23.2 ± 2.9	19.8 ± 1.7 *
Non-HDL-C (mg/dL)	159.5 ± 5.8	150.0 ± 5.8 *	159.4 ± 6.0	157.3 ± 6.0

* Significant decrease after the intake of PhyS/ω3-milk (p < 0.05); Data are given as mean ± SEM. BMI = body mass index; Ch = cholesterol; HDL = high density lipoproteins; LDL = low density cholesterol; PhyS = phytosterols; TG = triglyceride; VLDL = very-low density lipoproteins.

2.2. Study Phases

The study was subdivided in two phases: (1) A discovery phase where the proteomic profile of the LDL fraction (N = 5), HDL fraction (N = 10) and lipid-free plasma fraction (N = 5) was investigated by bi-dimensional electrophoresis, followed by mass spectrometry (MS)identification (Figure 1b-I) in those subjects that showed the highest response in LDL-C and TG plasma levels after the intervention; and (2) a second phase in which the detected changes were validated by complementary methodologies (reverse transcription polymerase chain reaction (RT-PCR) and ELISA; Figure 1b-II).

Twelve hours fasting blood samples were collected on days 1 and 28 (baseline and endpoint of the first treatment period) and on days 56 and 84 (baseline and endpoint of the second treatment period), as previously described [7]. Blood samples were collected without anticoagulant or in EDTA-containing Vacutainer tubes for serum and plasma preparation, respectively. Serum and plasma fractions were separated by centrifugation at 3000× g for 20 min at 4 °C and stored at −80 °C until analysis.

2.3. Sample Preparation

Lipoprotein fractions were prepared in KBr density gradients (1.019–1.063 for LDL and 1.063–1.210 for HDL) [7,22–24]. Lipoprotein purity was routinely analyzed by electrophoresis (2 µL sample) in agarose gels using a commercial assay (SAS-MX Lipo 10 kit; Helena Biosciences, Gateshead, UK), as described by the providers. In addition, LDL purity was checked by analyzing the LDL profile in samples of randomly selected subjects (one subject per ultracentrifugation batch) by chromatography analysis by microgel filtration using a Superose 6 PC 3.2/30 column and an Agilent 1200 HPLC system, as previously described. Briefly, 10 µL of undiluted LDL sample fraction were loaded in the system and run with a constant flow of 100 µL/min. The retention time for the LDL fraction (130 min) was compared with that for HDL (134 min). The method of Karlsson et al. [25] was used for LDL protein mapping, with minor modifications as previously described [26]. Briefly, 1 mL of LDLs (1 g/L Apo B) was delipidated by mixing with 14 mL of ice-cold tributylphosphate:acetone:methanol (1:12:1) and incubating for 90 min at −20 °C, followed by centrifugation at 2800× g for 15 min. Protein pellets were washed sequentially with 1 mL of tributyl phosphate, acetone, and methanol, and then air dried. Precipitates were boiled in solution containing 0.325 M DTT, 4% chaps, and 0.045 M Tris for 3 min, cooled at room temperature, diluted (1:15) in urea/thiourea/chaps solution, and incubated at 35 °C for 15 min. For proteomic studies, HDL samples were prepared as previously described [22–24,26] by precipitation with pure ice-cold acetone and were solubilized in a urea/thiourea buffer (7 M urea, 2 M thiourea, 2% CHAPS).

In order to analyze only the soluble proteins present in plasma, microparticles were removed from LPDP samples by centrifugation at 25,000× g for 45 min at room temperature. For proteomic studies, LPDP was sonicated in ice and filtrated (0.22 µm) by centrifugation to avoid the presence of impurities. The 14 most abundant plasma proteins were depleted by using a specific affinity cartridge as reported by the providers (Multiple Affinity Removal Spin Cartridge, Agilent Technologies, Santa Clara, CA, USA). LPDP fractions were concentrated and de-salted by centrifugation with 5 kDa cutoff filter devices and sample buffer was exchange to a urea containing buffer (8 M urea, 2% CHAPS). Protein concentration was measured with 2D-Quant Kit (GE Healthcare, Little Chalfont, UK). All processed samples were stored at −80 °C until use.

2.4. Differential Proteomic Profiling Analysis

2.4.1. Two-Dimensional Gel Electrophoresis (2-DE)

A protein load of 100 µg (analytical gels) and 300 µg (preparative gels) of the urea/thiourea/chaps LDL or HDL extracts or of the urea/chaps LPDP extracts was applied to 17-cm dry strips (pH 4–7 linear range; BioRad, Hercules, CA, USA). The second dimension was resolved in 10–12% SDS-PAGE for LPDP and LDL or HDL samples, respectively. Gels were developed by fluorescent staining (Flamingo; BioRad, Hercules, CA, USA). For each independent experiment, 2-DE for protein extracts from baseline and post-PhyS/ω3-milk intake were processed in parallel to guarantee a maximum of comparability. Analysis for differences in protein extracts was performed with the PD-Quest 8.0 (BioRad, Hercules, CA, USA). Each spot was assigned a relative value (AU) that corresponds to the single spot volume compared to the volume of all spots in the gel, following background extraction and normalization between gels, as previously reported [22].

2.4.2. Mass Spectrometry Analysis

Proteins were identified after in-gel tryptic digestion and extraction of peptides from the gel pieces by matrix-assisted laser desorption/ionization time-of-flight (MALDI-TOF) using an AutoFlex III Smart beam MALDI-TOF/TOF (BrukerDaltonics, Billerica, MA, USA), as previously described [23,26]. Samples were applied to Prespotted Anchor Chip plates (BrukerDaltonics, Billerica, MA, USA) surrounding the calibrants provided on the plates. Spectra were acquired with flex control on reflector mode, (mass range: 850–4000 m/z, reflector 1:21.06 kV; reflector 2:9.77 kV; ion source 1 voltage: 19 kV; ion source 2:16.5 kV; detection gain: 2.37×) with an average of 3500 added shots at a frequency of 200 Hz. Each sample was processed with FlexAnalysis (version 3.0, BrukerDaltonics, Billerica, MA, USA) considering a signal-to-noise ratio over 3, applying statistical calibration and eliminating background peaks. For identification, peaks between 850 and 1000 m/z were not considered. After processing, spectra were sent to the interface BioTools (version 3.2, BrukerDaltonics, Billerica, MA, USA) and a MASCOT server search on the Swiss-Prot 57.15 database was done (Taxonomy: Homo Sapiens, Mass Tolerance 50 to 100, up to 2 trypsin miss cleavages, Global Modification: Carbamidomethyl (C),

Variable Modification: Oxidation (M)). Identified proteins were accepted when a mascot score higher than 50 was obtained by peptide mass fingerprint and confirmed by peptide fragmentation working in the reflection mode.

2.5. Western Blot Analysis

Protein extracts were resolved by 1-DE under reducing conditions and electrotransferred to nitrocellulose membranes in semi-dry conditions (Trans-Blot Turbo system; BioRad, Hercules, CA, USA). Serum amyloid P (SAP) detection was performed using a mouse monoclonal antibody against total SAP (ab27313, 1:200 dilution, abcam, Cambridge, UK). Band detection was performed using a chemiluminiscent substrate dye (Luminata Forte Western HRP Substrate, Merck Millipore, Billerica, MA, USA) and a molecular imager ChemiDoc XRS System, Universal Hood II (BioRad, Hercules, CA, USA). Band quantification was performed with Image Lab 4.0 software (BioRad Laboratories, Hercules, CA, USA). Protein load was normalized with total protein staining, as previously described [23].

2.6. Quantification of Total Protein Systemic Levels

Total Apo E, Apo A–I, and LCAT levels in the serum samples from the basal condition and after the intake of ω3-milk were measured by using a commercial sandwich-based ELISA kit in the whole cohort ($N = 32$; Table 1). The detection limit of the assays were: 1.5 ng/mL for Apo E (ELH-Apo E; Human Apo E ELISA Kit; RayBiotech, Norcross, GA, USA); 0.7 µg/mL for Apo A–I (EA5201-1; Human Apo A–I ELISA Kit; AssayPro, St. Charles, MO, USA); and 0.27 ng/mL for LCAT (RD191122200R; LCAT ELISA Kit; BioVendor, Brno-Řečkovice a MokráHora, Czech Republic).

2.7. Gene Expression Analyses

RNA was extracted from total blood samples in a randomly selected group of volunteers using a commercial kit (PreAnalytiX, PAX gene, Quiagen/BD Company, Hilden, Germany) and DNA synthesis was performed using a commercial RT First Strand kit. PAX gene tubes avoid RNA degradation during the transport and storage of blood samples. mRNA levels were analyzed by real-time PCR using TaqMan gene expression assays and the Prism 7900HT Sequence detection System (all from Thermo Fisher Scientific, Waltham, MA, USA) according to the manufacturer's instruction. All expression analyses were normalized with glyceraldehyde-3-phosphate dehydrogenase (GAPDH).

2.8. Bioinformatic Analysis

The statistically significant neural network and canonical pathway in which the identified proteins were involved were generated through the use of IPA (Ingenuity System, www.ingenuity.com).

2.8.1. Functional Analysis of a Network

The functional analysis of a network was used to identify the biological functions and/or diseases that were most significant to the molecules in the network. The network molecules associated with biological functions and/or diseases in the Ingenuity Knowledge Base were considered for the analysis. Right-tailed Fisher's exact test was used to calculate a *p*-value determining the probability that each biological function and/or disease assigned to that network is due to chance alone.

2.8.2. Canonical Pathway Analysis

Canonical pathway analysis was used to identify the pathways from the IPA library that were most significant to the data set. The significance of the association between the data set and the canonical pathway was measured in two ways: (1) a ratio of the number of molecules from the data set that maps to the pathway divided by the total number of molecules that maps to the canonical pathway is displayed; and (2) Fisher's exact test was used to calculate a *p*-value determining the probability that the association between the genes in the data set and the canonical pathway is explained by chance alone.

2.9. Statistical Analysis

Data are expressed as mean and standard error unless stated. N indicates the number of subjects tested. Statistical analysis was performed with Stat View 5.0.1 software (SAS Institute, Cary, NC, USA). Differences between the basal condition and after 4 weeks of intake of supplemented milk were tested using repeated measurements ANOVA analysis. A *p*-value ≤ 0.05 was considered significant.

3. Results

3.1. Four Weeks ω3-Milk Intake Induces Changes in the Proteomic Profile of the Lipoprotein Plasma Fraction

The intake of PhyS-milk did not induce any significant change in the LDL proteome (Supplementary Table S1). Only a trend to increased apolipoprotein A-IV (Apo A-IV) levels was observed (*p* = 0.080). On the contrary, the intake of ω3-milk (Supplementary Table S2) induced a 1.5-fold significant increase in the Apo E content in LDL (*p* = 0.043; Figure 2a). To analyze if the observed changes in Apo E in the LDL fraction were also found in total serum Apo E levels, a commercial ELISA was run in serum samples of the whole cohort of individuals (*N* = 32). No changes were observed in total Apo E serum levels (Figure 2b). However, a significant increase in Apo E serum levels was observed (*p* = 0.015; Figure 2c) only when individuals (*N* = 11) that showed a reduction in TG plasma levels (30.3% mean decrease) after the intake of ω3-milk were examined.

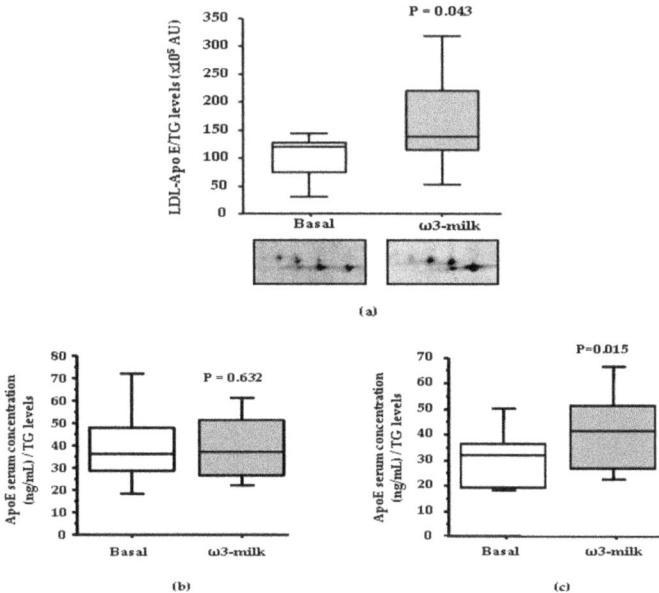

Figure 2. Changes in the apolipoprotein (Apo) E profile. (**a**) Box-Plot diagram and representative 2-DE images showing the low density lipoprotein (LDL)-associated Apo E proteomic profile before and after the intake of ω3-milk. A significant increase of Apo E levels (*p* = 0.043) is observed. Box-Plot diagrams showing serum Apo E levels (ng/mL) in basal conditions and after 4-weeks intervention with ω3-milk, measured by a commercial ELISA. No change was observed when all the volunteers were analyzed ((**b**); *N* = 32; *p* = 0.105). Apo E concentration of subjects with reduced triglyceride (TG) levels showed a significant increase after ω3-milk intake ((**c**); *N* = 11; *p* = 0.015).

The intake of ω3-milk induced a coordinated increase in the content of several key HDL protein components. Among the observed protein changes, ω3-milk induced a significant increase of the main HDL protein component, Apo A–I ($p = 0.009$; Figure 3a). Furthermore, there was a coordinated increase of two important enzymes involved in HDL metabolism, LCAT ($p = 0.044$; Figure 3b) and PON-1 ($p = 0.047$; Figure 3c). In addition, ω3-milk also increased the HDL content of Apo D ($p = 0.008$; Figure 3d) and Apo L1 ($p = 0.038$; Figure 3e). In silicobioinformatic analysis revealed that all the ω3-milk induced changes in the plasma proteome were related to HDL metabolism-related pathways (Supplementary Figure S1).

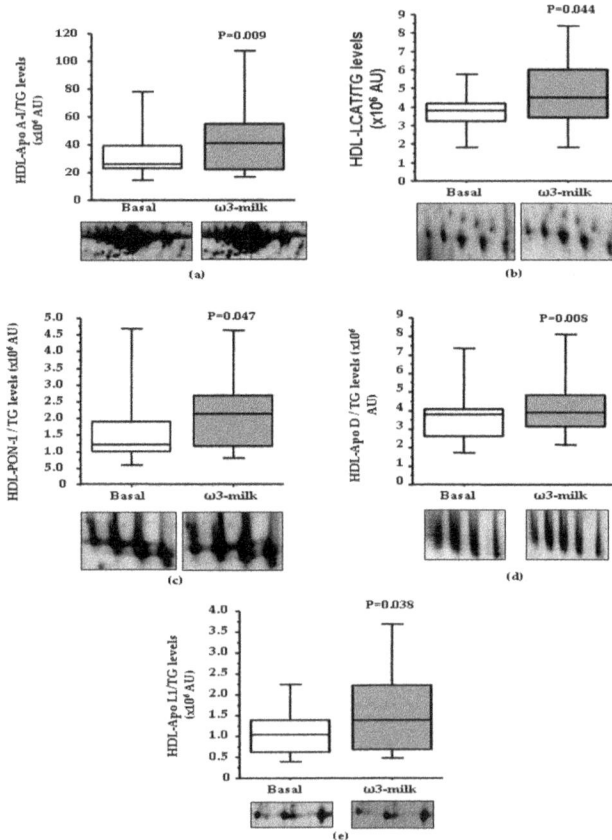

Figure 3. Impact of the intake of ω3-milk on the high density lipoprotein (HDL) profile. Box-Plots and 2-DE representative images showing the significant changes induced in HDL proteins by ω3-milk: (a) Apo A–I ($p = 0.009$); (b) lecitin cholesterol acyltransferase (LCAT) ($p = 0.044$); (c) paraoxonase-1 (PON-1) ($p = 0.047$); (d) Apo D ($p = 0.008$); and (e) Apo L1 ($p = 0.038$).

In order to analyze if the observed HDL-associated protein changes were translated into changes in total serum protein levels, Apo A–I and LCAT serum levels were measured with commercial ELISAs in the whole study population. This analysis revealed a lack of differences in both Apo A–I and LCAT (Figure 4a) total serum levels after ω3-milk intake when compared to basal levels. However, and as observed with Apo E, if only those subjects with a reduction on TG levels were analyzed, a non-significant trend to increased Apo A–I levels ($p = 0.099$) and a significant increase in LCAT levels ($p = 0.0397$; Figure 4b) after the intake of ω3-milk was observed. These results highlight that the changes observed on the lipid-associated plasma protein fraction after the intake of ω3-milk are associated to the changes on the HDL proteomic profile.

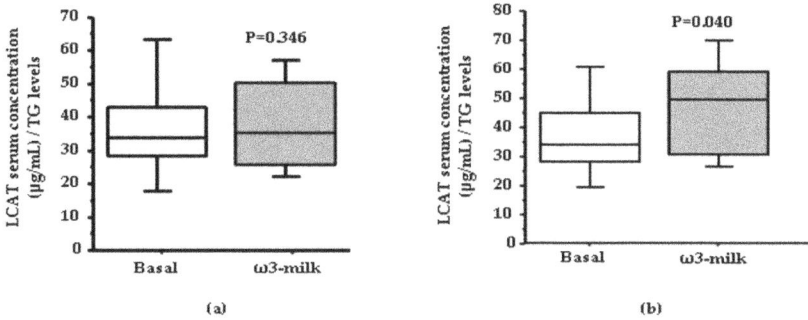

Figure 4. Changes on lecitin cholesterol acyltransferase (LCAT) serum levels after ω3-milk intake. Box-Plot diagrams showing LCAT concentration (µg/mL) in basal conditions and after the intake of ω3-milk, measured by a commercial ELISA. (**a**) No change was observed when all the volunteers were analyzed ($N = 32$; $p = 0.346$). (**b**) There was a significant increase in LCAT serum levels in subjects that showed a reduction in TG levels after ω3-milk intake ($N = 11$; $p = 0.0397$).

3.2. Inflammation Associated Changes after PhyS-Milk Intake

Proteomic analysis of the lipoprotein-depleted-plasma (LPDP) fraction revealed that the intake of PhyS-milk induced a non-significant decreasing trend in the levels of the pro-inflammatory protein SAP when compared to the basal samples ($p = 0.075$; Figure 5a; Supplementary Table S3). This result was confirmed after Western blot (WB) validation where a 1.21-mean fold decrease in SAP levels was detected in LPDP samples after the intake of PhyS-milk ($p = 0.001$; Figure 5b).

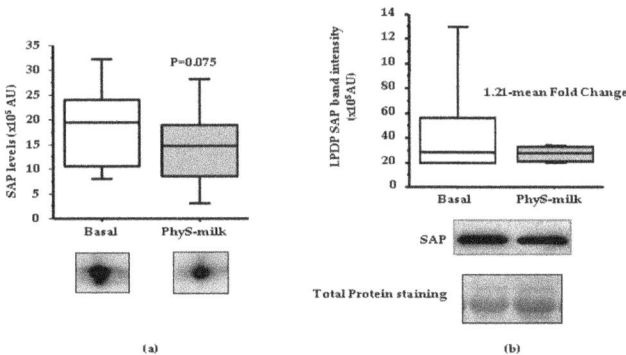

Figure 5. Serum amyloid P (SAP) proteomic profile. (**a**) Box-Plot diagram and 2-DE representative image showing a SAP decreasing trend in the soluble protein fraction of plasma (LPDP) proteomic profile after the intake of PhyS-milk ($p = 0.075$); (**b**) Box-Plot and representative western blot image showing changes in SAP in the LPDP samples after PhyS-milk intake ($N = 5$; 1.21-Fold change; $p = 0.001$).

On the contrary, no changes were observed in the LPDP fraction after the intake of ω3-milk (Supplementary Table S4).

Due to the observed changes in the inflammation-associated pentraxin SAP after the intake of PhyS-milk, we investigated if PhyS-milk could induce changes in the expression of the key pro-inflammatory chemokine in inflammatory cells, C-C motif chemokine 2 (CCL2). This analysis revealed a significant reduction of the CCL2 transcripts after the intake of PhyS-milk ($p = 0.03$; Figure 6). In addition, a trend towards increased expression levels of the Interleukin 10 receptor (IL-10R; $p = 0.06$) was also observed.

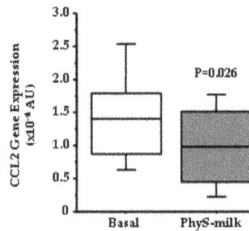

Figure 6. C-C motif chemokine 2 (CCL2) gene expression. Box-plot diagram showing the significant decrease in CCL2 gene expression after the intake of PhyS-milk in the peripheral blood leukocyte fraction of a randomly selected group of subjects ($N = 12$; $p = 0.026$).

4. Discussion

Nutritional intervention is a useful strategy for the prevention of many diseases, especially in those in which obesity is a risk factor [27]. Phytosterols (PhyS) are natural components derived from plants and vegetable oils with a similar structure to cholesterol that are not synthesized in humans [28]. Through their ability to interfere with cholesterol metabolism, PhyS have been shown to effectively reduce cholesterol levels, and possibly beneficially affect CVD risk prevention [29].

Our group and others have demonstrated that the intake of plant stanols and sterols, in different food-platforms, reduces serum levels of total cholesterol. However, controversy exists regarding plant sterols-mediated protection as some studies have suggested a potential deleterious effect in relation to cardiovascular risk [30–32]. The explanation of these contradictory results seems to be related to the amount of stanol supplementation. In fact, it has been shown that the increase in stanol supplementation beyond the maximum recommendable dose of 3 mg/day is not associated with a higher reduction of cholesterol levels [33]. Importantly, in our study, an intake of 1.6 g PhyS/day (value within the recommended dose range) with low fat milk for four weeks reduced total cholesterol, non-HDL-C, and LDL-C, and also reduced the susceptibility of LDL to oxidation [7]. It is important to highlight, that in the present study, each patient is his/her own control as all the analyzed variables have been compared to the baseline levels measured in each subject after a wash-out run-in period with plain low-fat milk. Indeed, the aim of the clinical trial was to compare the effects of both PhyS- and ω3-milk interventions. Although we cannot exclude a potential effect inherent to the participation in the study, the two-arm crossover design with the two bioactive products minimizes the potential influence of this effect in the results.

Here, we have observed a significant decrease in the pro-inflammatory pentraxin SAP in the soluble fraction of plasma (LPDP) of the healthy-overweight volunteers after the intake for four weeks of PhyS-milk. SAP plays an important role in innate immunity and in the atherosclerotic process [34]. Pentraxins have been detected within advanced human atherosclerotic plaques suggested to play an active role in atherogenesis [35]. Indeed, we have previously demonstrated an important increase in SAP levels in the early phase post acute myocardial infarction (AMI), and an even higher increase of this protein 3 days after the event [36]. SAP deficiency prevents atherosclerosis [37] and it is involved in other key biological processes for the cardiovascular system, such as inflammation, fibrosis, and coagulation [34,38]. Specifically, pentraxins have been shown to contribute to the chronic low-grade inflammatory state that characterizes obesity [39]. Therefore, the intake of PhyS-milk can reduce the cardiovascular risk associated to overweight and obesity by reducing the pro-inflammatory protein SAP.

Moreover, we have also found a significant decrease in the expression of the gene encoding for C-C motif chemokine 2 (CCL2), also known as monocyte chemotactic protein-1(MCP-1), and a trend to decreased the IL10-R, two important cytokines with pro- and anti-inflammatory properties respectively involved in CVD, after dietary intervention with PhyS-milk. In fact, it was shown that the intake of PhyS produces an anti-inflammatory reaction by acting on cytokines' activity [40]. CCL2/MCP-1 is a key driver of adipose tissue inflammation in obesity [41]. Indeed, it is directly implicated in the propagation of the chronic low-grade inflammatory state associated to obesity [42–44] through its role as a monocyte attractant, which is the major cell that differentiates into macrophages and foam cells in the atherosclerotic lesion [40]. On the other hand, IL-10 is an anti-inflammatory protein by suppressing the synthesis of pro-inflammatory cytokines and also by inhibiting the activation of macrophages [45]. Therefore, our results highlight that PhyS-milk consumption may induce a shift towards a decreased inflammatory state through its effect on two key cytokines, CCL2/MCP-1 and IL-10, having thus a potential effect in the context of obesity where inflammatory pathways are exacerbated.

The cardiovascular benefits of fish oils are well known and directly attributed to the effects of ω3 fatty acids (FA) [46]. Beneficial effects of ω3 and ω6 FA have been compared and the results suggest that higher levels of ω3 FA are protective against atherosclerosis. Therefore, modern western diets are directed towards a reduction of the ω6/ω3 FA ratio to protect against atherosclerosis [47,48]. Previous studies of our group have shown that the ingestion of this ω3-milk reduces the levels of triglycerides (TG) and palmitic acid [7]. Palmitic acid is a major component of the western diet and is associated with insulin resistance and glucose intolerance, becoming an important risk factor of diabetes and CVD [49]. Importantly, these metabolic alterations are often present in obese individuals. Our proteomic approach has shown that regular intake of ω3-milk results in a significant increase of Apo E protein level in LDL. It had been suggested that ω3 FA effects in reducing TG levels are dependent on Apo E [47]. Indeed, the beneficial effects of ω3 FA are partially blunted in Apo E deficient (Apo E$^{-/-}$) mice, suggesting that Apo E is necessary for the cardioprotective effects exerted by ω3 [50]. Accordingly, diverse studies have shown that *Apo E$^{-/-}$* mice suffer hypercholesterolemia and an association between Apo E levels and CVD has also been reported in humans [51,52]. Even more, it has been shown that in the absence of some isoforms of Apo E, the beneficial cardioprotective effect of ω3 PUFA may be partially lost [53,54]. Of note, our results highlight an association between Apo E increase in LDL and an improved TG profile in obese subjects after four weeks intervention with ω3-milk.

Importantly, herein we describe for the first time that the intake of ω3-milk induces a coordinated increase of several HDL associated proteins. Diverse studies show that the antioxidant effect of HDL is associated to a coordinated action of different proteins that allow HDL to protect LDL from oxidation for a longer period [18,55]. This correlates with the importance of HDL composition, emphasizing on HDL quality rather than HDL quantity. Apo A–I is the major protein component of HDL and therefore the cardioprotective benefits of HDL are often associated to this protein. High levels of Apo A–I are associated to a reduced vascular lesion and to an increase in the HDL plasma level [56]. It is widely known that Apo A–I is implicated on cholesterol transport from peripheral tissues to the liver for its clearance by the formation and stabilization of the HDL, but many additional proteins are also implicated in this process [9]. Lipid-free Apo A–I produces the nascent HDL particles and LCAT catalyzes HDL maturation by the esterification of free cholesterol (FC) into cholesteryl esters (CE), being both particles accumulated into the core of the HDL particle. Then, cholesterol ester transfer protein (CEPT) transfer CE particles for the mature form of HDL (HDL2) to VLDL and LDL to be finally excreted and eliminated [57,58]. LCAT is essential for cholesterol esterification, but also needs the presence of other proteins to be activated. Thus, Apo A–I and Apo E are the best LCAT activators in plasma and PON-1 protects LCAT from its inactivation [58]. PON-1 appears predominantly associated to HDL, especially to HDL3 and it is activated and stabilized by Apo A–I. PON-1 is an atheroprotective protein with an important role as an anti-oxidant [57]. Interestingly, in the present study we have found that ω3-milk intake significantly increases the HDL content of key proteins involved in HDL metabolism such as Apo A–I and LCAT. Those changes are specifically associated to a reduction in TG plasma levels after the intake of ω3-milk. Thus, it is conceivable that ω3 by increasing Apo A–I and LCAT levels enhances both cholesterol esterification and transport, significantly improving the lipoprotein profile (Figure 7). Furthermore, the ω3-milk-induced increase observed in PON1 could not only enhance LCAT activity but could also improve the anti-oxidant abilities of HDL particles. In addition, we observed an increase in Apo D HDL levels after the intake of ω3-milk. Apo D has been implicated in the reduction of TG plasma levels and also binds to LCAT improving its esterification activity [59]. Thus, the increase observed in Apo D after ω3-milk intake could contribute not only to the reduction in TG plasma levels but also to a decrease in VLDL-C levels (Figure 7). Furthermore, our study has shown that ω3-milk intake increases Apo L1 HDL content in overweight subjects. Apo L1 is mainly studied in chronic kidney disease, but studies in our group showed that a coordinated decrease in HDL content of both LCAT and Apo L1 seem to predispose to the presentation of acute ischemic events in hypercholesterolemia patients [24]. Therefore, the coordinated increase in both HDL-associated proteins after ω3-milk intake could reduce the CVD risk in high risk subjects such as those with overweight and metabolic syndrome.

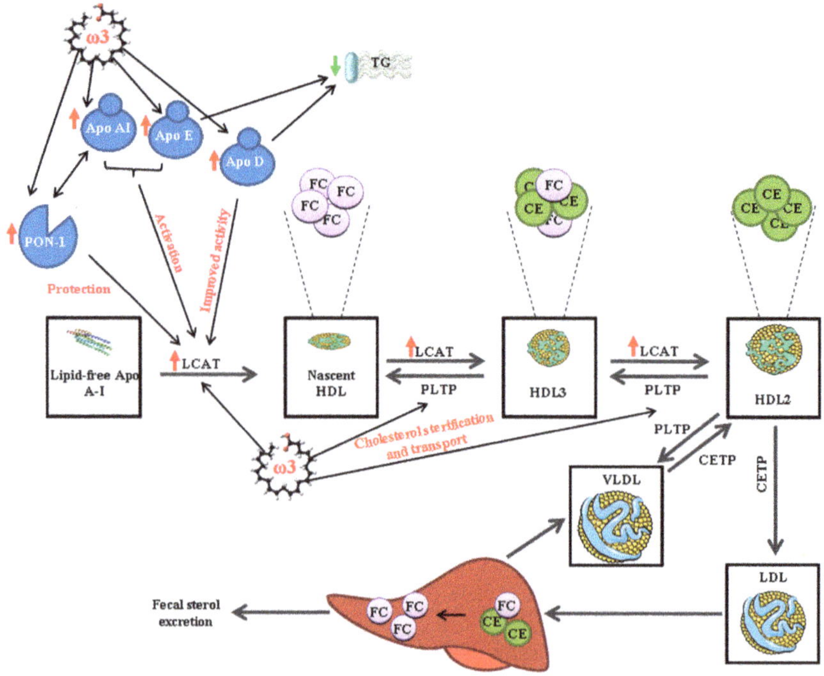

Figure 7. Simplified diagram of the lipid metabolism canonical pathway. Maturation of HDL and free cholesterol (FC) esterification are catalyzed by LCAT. Apo A–I and Apo E activate LCAT, and PON-I, which is also activated by Apo A–I, avoiding LCAT inactivation. Apo D binds to LCAT to improve its esterification activity. Finally, cholesterol is transported to the liver for its elimination by fecal excretion.

5. Conclusions

In summary, our study supports the concept of supplementing diets with ω3 FA and PhyS to prevent CVD by inducing a coordinated change of the lipid-associated plasma protein fraction profile and by reducing inflammation. These changes are then translated into a significant improvement of the lipid profile. This is of great importance in obese subjects, since they are more predisposed to suffer metabolic alterations and therefore increased risk of CVD. A healthy lifestyle and appropriate nutrition are key factors in the prevention of CVD, and the results of the present study support the notion that diet supplementation with PhyS and ω3 FA has beneficial effects against CVD in overweight and obese individuals by acting on two hallmarks of CVD progression, inflammation, and lipid metabolism.

Supplementary Materials: The following are available online at www.mdpi.com/2072-6643/9/6/599/s1, Figure S1: In silico analysis of HDL protein changes, Table S1: Lipid and inflammation proteins, Table S2: Lipid and inflammation proteins, Table S3: Protein composition in lipoprotein depleted plasma after PhyS-milk intake, Table S4: Protein composition in lipoprotein depleted plasma after ω3-milk intake.

Acknowledgments: The technical assistance of María Dolores Fernández and Ona Catot is gratefully acknowledged. Authors are indebted with Dra. Sandra Camino for the genomic support, and with María José Bartolomé and Montse Gómez-Pardo for their contribution during the clinical study. Finally, authors thank the study participants for their valuable contribution and CAPSA Food S.A., especially Marta Hernández, for providing the milk products used in the study. This work was supported by grants from CDTI Spanish Ministry of Competitiveness and Economy (MINECO) (CEN-20101016 (HENUFOOD) to L.B.); the Spanish Ministry of Economy and Competitiveness of Science (SAF2016-76819-R to L.B.); Institute of Health Carlos III, ISCIII (TERCEL RD16/00110018; and CB16/11/0041 to L.B.; and FIS PI16/01915 to T.P.); FEDER "UnaManera de Hacer Europa"; the Secretary of University and Research, Department of Economy and Knowledge of the Government of Catalonia (2014SGR1303 to L.B.); and "CERCA Programme/Generalitat de Catalunya" Spain. We thank FIC-FundacionJesús Serra, Barcelona, Spain, for their continuous support.

Author Contributions: C.L. designed and conducted the research; analyzed data and performed the statistical analysis; and wrote the manuscript. J.C. designed and conducted the research; analyzed data and performed the statistical analysis; and wrote the manuscript. T.P. designed and supervised the research; analyzed data and performed the statistical analysis; and wrote the manuscript. J.S.H. designed the research; provided essential reagents or provided essential materials; and analyzed data. R.M.A. designed the research; provided essential reagents or provided essential materials; and analyzed data. A.P. designed the research; provided essential reagents or provided essential materials; and analyzed data. L.B. designed and supervised the research; analyzed data and performed the statistical analysis; and wrote and revised the manuscript. All authors had primary responsibility for the final content and approved the final version of the manuscript.

Conflicts of Interest: The authors declare no conflict of interest.

References

1. Bastien, M.; Poirier, P.; Lemieux, I.; Despres, J.P. Overview of epidemiology and contribution of obesity to cardiovascular disease. *Prog. Cardiovasc. Dis.* **2014**, *56*, 369–381. [CrossRef] [PubMed]

2. Sayon-Orea, C.; Carlos, S.; Martínez-Gonzalez, M.A. Does cooking with vegetable oils increase the risk of chronic diseases: A systematic review. *Br. J. Nutr.* **2015**, *113*, S36–S48. [CrossRef] [PubMed]

3. Stefler, D.; Malyutina, S.; Kubinova, R.; Pajak, A.; Peasey, A.; Pikhart, H.; Brunner, E.J.; Bobak, M. Mediterranean diet score and total and cardiovascular mortality in Eastern Europe: The HAPIEE study. *Eur. J. Nutr.* **2015**, *56*, 1–9. [CrossRef] [PubMed]

4. Badimon, L.; Vilahur, G.; Padro, T. Nutraceuticals and atherosclerosis: Human trials. *Cardiovasc. Ther.* **2010**, *28*, 202–215. [CrossRef] [PubMed]

5. Ignarro, L.J.; Balestrieri, M.L.; Napoli, C. Nutrition, physical activity, and cardiovascular disease: An update. *Cardiovasc. Res.* **2007**, *73*, 326–340. [CrossRef] [PubMed]

6. Psota, T.L.; Gebauer, S.K.; Kris-Etherton, P. Dietary omega-3 fatty acid intake and cardiovascular risk. *Am. J. Cardiol.* **2006**, *98*, 3i–18i. [CrossRef] [PubMed]

7. Padro, T.; Vilahur, G.; Sanchez-Hernandez, J.; Hernandez, M.; Antonijoan, R.M.; Perez, A.; Badimon, L. Lipidomic changes of LDL in overweight and moderately hypercholesterolemic subjects taking phytosterol- and omega-3-supplemented milk. *J. Lipid Res.* **2015**, *56*, 1043–1056. [CrossRef] [PubMed]

8. Racette, S.B.; Lin, X.; Lefevre, M.; Spearie, C.A.; Most, M.M.; Ma, L.; Ostlund, R.E. Dose effects of dietary phytosterols on cholesterol metabolism: A controlled feeding study. *Am. J. Clin. Nutr.* **2010**, *91*, 32–38. [CrossRef] [PubMed]

9. Badimon, L.; Vilahur, G. LDL-cholesterol versus HDL-cholesterol in the atherosclerotic plaque: Inflammatory resolution versus thrombotic chaos. *Ann. N. Y. Acad. Sci.* **2012**, *1254*, 18–32. [CrossRef] [PubMed]

10. Vilahur, G.; Gutiérrez, M.; Casaní, L.; Cubedo, J.; Capdevila, A.; Pons-Llado, G.; Carreras, F.; Hidalgo, A.; Badimon, L. Hypercholesterolemia Abolishes High-Density Lipoprotein-Related Cardioprotective Effects in the Setting of Myocardial Infarction. *J. Am. Coll. Cardiol.* **2015**, *66*, 2469–2470. [CrossRef] [PubMed]

11. Schaefer, E.J.; Anthanont, P.; Asztalos, B.F. High-density lipoprotein metabolism, composition, function, and deficiency. *Curr. Opin. Lipidol.* **2014**, *25*, 194–199. [CrossRef] [PubMed]

12. Badimon, L.; Vilahur, G.; Cubedo, J. High density lipoproteins and kidney function: The friend turned foe? *J. Thorac. Dis.* **2016**, *8*, 2978–2981. [CrossRef] [PubMed]

13. Badimon, L.; Vilahur, G. HDL particles—More complex than we thought. *Thromb. Haemost.* **2014**, *112*, 857. [CrossRef] [PubMed]

14. Gao, F.; Ren, Y.; Shen, X.; Bian, Y.; Xiao, C.; Li, H. Correlation between the High Density Lipoprotein and its Subtypes in Coronary Heart Disease. *Cell. Physiol. Biochem.* **2016**, *38*, 1906–1914. [CrossRef] [PubMed]

15. Navab, M. Thematic review series: The Pathogenesis of Atherosclerosis: The oxidation hypothesis of atherogenesis: The role of oxidized phospholipids and HDL. *J. Lipid Res.* **2004**, *45*, 993–1007. [CrossRef] [PubMed]

16. Huang, N.F.; Kurpinski, K.; Fang, Q.; Lee, R.J.; Li, S. Proteomic identification of biomarkers of vascular injury. *Am. J. Transl. Res.* **2011**, *3*, 139–148. [PubMed]

17. Kassai, A.; Illyés, L.; Mirdamadi, H.Z.; Seres, I.; Kalmár, T.; Audikovszky, M.; Paragh, G. The effect of atorvastatin therapy on lecithin:cholesterol acyltransferase, cholesteryl ester transfer protein and the antioxidant paraoxonase. *Clin. Biochem.* **2007**, *40*, 1–5. [CrossRef] [PubMed]

18. Hine, D.; MacKness, B.; MacKness, M. Coincubation of PON1, APO A1, and LCAT increases the time HDL is able to prevent LDL oxidation. *IUBMB Life* **2012**, *64*, 157–161. [CrossRef] [PubMed]

19. Daigo, K.; Inforzato, A.; Barajon, I.; Garlanda, C.; Bottazzi, B.; Meri, S.; Mantovani, A. Pentraxins in the activation and regulation of innate immunity. *Immunol. Rev.* **2016**, *274*, 202–217. [CrossRef] [PubMed]

20. Du Clos, T.W. Pentraxins: Structure, function, and role in inflammation. *ISRN Inflamm.* **2013**, *2013*, 379040. [CrossRef] [PubMed]

21. Vilahur, G.; Badimon, L. Biological actions of pentraxins. *Vascul. Pharmacol.* **2015**, *73*, 38–44. [CrossRef] [PubMed]

22. Cubedo, J.; Padró, T.; García-Arguinzonis, M.; Vilahur, G.; Miñambres, I.; Pou, J.M.; Ybarra, J.; Badimon, L. A novel truncated form of apolipoprotein A–I transported by dense LDL is increased in diabetic patients. *J. Lipid Res.* **2015**, *56*, 1762–1773. [CrossRef] [PubMed]

23. Cubedo, J.; Padro, T.; Badimon, L. Glycoproteome of human apolipoprotein A–I: *N*- and *O*-glycosylated forms are increased in patients with acute myocardial infarction. *Transl. Res.* **2014**, *164*, 209–222. [CrossRef] [PubMed]

24. Cubedo, J.; Padró, T.; Alonso, R.; Mata, P.; Badimon, L. Apo L1 levels in HDL and cardiovascular event presentation in patients with familial hypercholesterolemia. *J. Lipid Res.* **2016**, *57*, 1059–1073. [CrossRef] [PubMed]

25. Karlsson, H.; Leanderson, P.; Tagesson, C.; Lindahl, M. Lipoproteomics I: Mapping of proteins in low-density lipoprotein using two-dimensional gel electrophoresis and mass spectrometry. *Proteomics* **2005**, *5*, 551–565. [CrossRef] [PubMed]

26. Cubedo, J.; Padró, T.; García-Moll, X.; Pintó, X.; Cinca, J.; Badimon, L. Proteomic signature of apolipoprotein J in the early phase of new-onset myocardial infarction. *J. Proteom. Res.* **2011**, *10*, 211–220. [CrossRef] [PubMed]

27. Juni, M.H. OBESITY: A Public Health Threats in Developing Countries. *Int. J. Public Health Clin. Sci.* **2015**, *2*, 2289–7577.

28. Richard, E.; Ostlund, J. Phytosterols in Human Nutrition. *Annu. Rev. Nutr.* **2002**, *22*, 533–549. [CrossRef] [PubMed]

29. Intake, P.; Meijer, L.; Zock, P.L.; Geleijnse, J.M.; Trautwein, E.A. Continuous Dose-Response Relationship of the LDL-Cholesterol—Lowering Effect of Phytosterol Intake. *J. Nutr.* **2009**, *139*, 271–284. [CrossRef] [PubMed]

30. Glueck, C.J.; Speirs, J.; Tracy, T.; Streicher, P.; Illig, E.; Vandegrift, J. Relationships of serum plant sterols (phytosterols) and cholesterol in 595 hypercholesterolemic subjects, and familial aggregation of phytosterols, cholesterol, and premature coronary heart disease in hyperphytosterolemic probands and their first-degree relatives. *Metabolism* **1991**, *40*, 842–848. [PubMed]

31. Assmann, G.; Cullen, P.; Erbey, J.; Ramey, D.R.; Kannenberg, F.; Schulte, H. Plasma sitosterol elevations are associated with an increased incidence of coronary events in men: Results of a nested case-control analysis of the Prospective Cardiovascular Munster (PROCAM) study. *Nutr. Metab. Cardiovasc. Dis.* **2006**, *16*, 13–21. [CrossRef] [PubMed]

32. Sudhop, T.; Gottwald, B.M.; von Bergmann, K. Serum plant sterols as a potential risk factor for coronary heart disease. *Metabolism* **2002**, *51*, 1519–1521. [CrossRef] [PubMed]

33. Weingärtner, O.; Böhm, M.; Laufs, U. Controversial role of plant sterol esters in the management of hypercholesterolaemia. *Eur. Heart J.* **2009**, *30*, 404–409. [CrossRef] [PubMed]

34. Bottazzi, B.; Inforzato, A.; Messa, M.; Barbagallo, M.; Magrini, E.; Garlanda, C.; Mantovani, A. The pentraxins PTX3 and SAP in innate immunity, regulation of inflammation and tissue remodelling. *J. Hepatol.* **2016**, *64*, 1–12. [CrossRef] [PubMed]

35. Li, X.A.; Hatanaka, K.; Ishibashi-Ueda, H.; Yutani, C.; Yamamoto, A. Characterization of Serum Amyloid P Component From Human Aortic Atherosclerotic Lesions. *Arter. Thromb. Vasc. Biol.* **1995**, *15*, 252–257. [CrossRef]

36. Cubedo, J.; Padró, T.; Badimon, L. Coordinated proteomic signature changes in immune response and complement proteins in acute myocardial infarction: The implication of serum amyloid P-component. *Int. J. Cardiol.* **2013**, *168*, 5196–5204. [CrossRef] [PubMed]

37. Zheng, L.; Wu, T.; Zeng, C.; Li, X.; Li, X.; Wen, D.; Ji, T.; Lan, T.; Xing, L.; Li, J.; et al. SAP deficiencymitigated atherosclerotic lesions in ApoE$^{-/-}$ mice. *Atherosclerosis* **2016**, *244*, 179–187. [CrossRef] [PubMed]

38. Xi, D.; Luo, T.; Xiong, H.; Liu, J.; Lu, H.; Li, M.; Hou, Y.; Guo, Z. SAP: Structure, function, and its roles in immune-related diseases. *Int. J. Cardiol.* **2015**, *187*, 20–26. [CrossRef] [PubMed]

39. Ogawa, T.; Kawano, Y.; Imamura, T.; Kawakita, K.; Sagara, M.; Matsuo, T.; Kakitsubata, Y.; Ishikawa, T.; Kitamura, K.; Hatakeyama, K.; et al. Reciprocal Contribution of Pentraxin 3 and C-Reactive Protein to Obesity and Metabolic Syndrome. *Obesity* **2010**, *18*, 1871–1874. [CrossRef] [PubMed]

40. Kanda, H.; Tateya, S.; Tamori, Y.; Kotani, K.; Hiasa, K.; Kitazawa, R.; Kitazawa, S.; Miyachi, H.; Maeda, S.; Egashira, K.; et al. MCP-1 contributes to macrophage infiltration into adipose tissue, insulin resistance, and hepatic steatosis in obesity. *J. Clin. Investig.* **2006**, *116*, 1494–1505. [CrossRef] [PubMed]

41. Panee, J. Monocyte Chemoattractant Protein 1 (MCP-1) in obesity and diabetes. *Cytokine* **2012**, *60*, 1–12. [CrossRef] [PubMed]

42. Badimon, L.; Cubedo, J. Adipose tissue depots and inflammation: Effects on plasticity and resident mesenchymal stem cell function. *Cardiovasc. Res.* **2017**. [CrossRef] [PubMed]

43. Wensveen, F.M.; Valentić, S.; Šestan, M.; Turk Wensveen, T.; Polić, B. The "Big Bang" in obese fat: Events initiating obesity-induced adipose tissue inflammation. *Eur. J. Immunol.* **2015**, *45*, 2446–2456. [CrossRef] [PubMed]

44. Han, M.S.; Jung, D.Y.; Morel, C.; Lakhani, S.A.; Kim, J.K.; Flavell, R.A.; Davis, R.J. JNK Expression by Macrophages Promotes Obesity-induced Insulin Resistance and Inflammation. *Science* **2013**, *339*, 1089–1098. [CrossRef] [PubMed]

45. Moore, K.W.; De Waal Malefyt, R.; Coffman, R.L.; O'garra, A. Interleukin-10 and the Interleukin-10 receptor. *Annu. Rev. Immunol.* **2001**, *19*, 683–765. [CrossRef] [PubMed]

46. Liang, S.; Steffen, L.M.; Steffen, B.T.; Guan, W.; Weir, N.L.; Rich, S.S.; Manichaikul, A.; Vargas, J.D.; Tsai, M.Y. APOE genotype modifies the association between plasma omega-3 fatty acids and plasma lipids in the Multi-Ethnic Study of Atherosclerosis (MESA). *Atherosclerosis* **2013**, *228*, 181–187. [CrossRef] [PubMed]

47. Wan, J.B.; Huang, L.L.; Rong, R.; Tan, R.; Wang, J.; Kang, J.X. Endogenously decreasing tissue *n*-6/*n*-3 fatty acid ratio reduces atherosclerotic lesions in apolipoprotein E-deficient mice by inhibiting systemic and vascular inflammation. *Arterioscler. Thromb. Vasc. Biol.* **2010**, *30*, 2487–2494. [CrossRef] [PubMed]

48. Simopoulos, A.P. An increase in the Omega-6/Omega-3 fatty acid ratio increases the risk for obesity. *Nutrients* **2016**, *8*, 128. [CrossRef] [PubMed]

49. Snook, J.T.; Park, S.; Williams, G.; Tsai, Y.-H.; Lee, N. Effect of synthetic triglycerides of myristic, palmitic, and stearic acid on serum lipoprotein metabolism. *Eur. J. Clin. Nutr.* **1999**, *53*, 597–605. [CrossRef] [PubMed]

50. Brown, A.L.; Zhu, X.; Rong, S.; Shewale, S.; Seo, J.; Boudyguina, E.; Gebre, A.K.; Alexander-Miller, M.A.; Parks, J.S. Omega-3 fatty acids ameliorate atherosclerosis by favorably altering monocyte subsets and limiting monocyte recruitment to aortic lesions. *Arterioscler. Thromb. Vasc. Biol.* **2012**, *32*, 2122–2130. [CrossRef] [PubMed]

51. Conway, V.; Allard, M.; Minihane, A.; Jackson, K.G.; Lovegrove, J.A.; Plourde, M. Postprandial enrichment of triacylglycerol-rich lipoproteins with omega-3 fatty acids: Lack of an interaction with apolipoprotein E genotype? *Lipids Health Dis.* **2014**, *13*, 148. [CrossRef] [PubMed]

52. Reilly, M.; Rader, D.J. Apolipoprotein E and coronary disease: A puzzling paradox. *PLoS Med.* **2006**, *3*, 736–738. [CrossRef] [PubMed]

53. Chouinard-watkins, R.; Plourde, M. Fatty Acid Metabolism in Carriers of Apolipoprotein E Epsilon 4 Allele: Is It Contributing to Higher Risk of Cognitive Decline and Coronary Heart Disease? *Nutrients* **2014**, *6*, 4452–4471. [CrossRef] [PubMed]

54. Kaneva, A.M.; Bojko, E.R.; Potolitsyna, N.N.; Odland, J.O. Plasma levels of apolipoprotein-E in residents of the European North of Russia. *Lipids Health Dis.* **2013**, *12*, 43. [CrossRef] [PubMed]

55. Daniels, J.-A.; Mulligan, C.; McCance, D.; Woodside, J.V.; Patterson, C.; Young, I.S.; McEneny, J. A randomised controlled trial of increasing fruit and vegetable intake and how this influences the carotenoid concentration and activities of PON-1 and LCAT in HDL from subjects with type 2 diabetes. *Cardiovasc. Diabetol.* **2014**, *13*, 16. [CrossRef] [PubMed]

56. White, C.R.; Garber, D.W.; Anantharamaiah, G.M. Anti-inflammatory and cholesterol-reducing properties of apolipoprotein mimetics: A review. *J. Lipid Res.* **2014**, *55*, 2007–2021. [CrossRef] [PubMed]

57. Gugliucci, A.; Menini, T. Paraoxonase 1 and HDL maturation. *Clin. Chim. Acta* **2015**, *439*, 5–13. [CrossRef] [PubMed]

58. Rousset, X.; Vaisman, B.; Amar, M.; Sethi, A.A.; Remaley, A.T. Lecithin: cholesterol acyltransferase: From biochemistry to role in cardiovascular disease. *Curr. Opin. Endocrinol. Diabetes Obes.* **2009**, *16*, 163–171. [CrossRef] [PubMed]

59. Ali, K.; Abo-Ali, E.M.; Kabir, M.D.; Riggins, B.; Nguy, S.; Li, L.; Srivastava, U.; Thinn, S.M.M. A Western-fed diet increases plasma HDL and LDL-cholesterol levels in ApoD$^{-/-}$ mice. *PLoS ONE* **2014**, *9*, 1–16. [CrossRef] [PubMed]

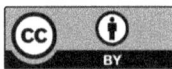

nutrients

MDPI

Review

Precision Nutrition and Omega-3 Polyunsaturated Fatty Acids: A Case for Personalized Supplementation Approaches for the Prevention and Management of Human Diseases

Floyd H. Chilton [1,*], Rahul Dutta [2], Lindsay M. Reynolds [3], Susan Sergeant [4], Rasika A. Mathias [5] and Michael C. Seeds [6]

[1] Department of Physiology and Pharmacology, Wake Forest School of Medicine, Winston-Salem, NC 27157, USA

[2] Department of Urology, Wake Forest School of Medicine, Winston-Salem, NC 27157, USA; rdutta@wakehealth.edu

[3] Department of Epidemiology and Prevention, Wake Forest School of Medicine, Winston-Salem, NC 27157, USA; lireynol@wakehealth.edu

[4] Department of Biochemistry, Wake Forest School of Medicine, Winston-Salem, NC 27157, USA; ssergean@wakehealth.edu

[5] GeneSTAR Research Program, General Internal Medicine, Johns Hopkins University School of Medicine, Baltimore, MD 21224, USA; rmathias@jhmi.edu

[6] Department of Internal Medicine, Section on Molecular Medicine, Wake Forest School of Medicine, Winston-Salem, NC 27157, USA; mseeds@wakehealth.edu

* Correspondence: schilton@wakehealth.edu; Tel.: +1-336-713-7106

Received: 6 September 2017; Accepted: 19 October 2017; Published: 25 October 2017

Abstract: Background: Dietary essential omega-6 (*n*-6) and omega-3 (*n*-3) 18 carbon (18C-) polyunsaturated fatty acids (PUFA), linoleic acid (LA) and α-linolenic acid (ALA), can be converted (utilizing desaturase and elongase enzymes encoded by *FADS* and *ELOVL* genes) to biologically-active long chain (LC; ≥20)-PUFAs by numerous cells and tissues. These *n*-6 and *n*-3 LC-PUFAs and their metabolites (ex, eicosanoids and endocannabinoids) play critical signaling and structural roles in almost all physiologic and pathophysiologic processes. Methods: This review summarizes: (1) the biosynthesis, metabolism and roles of LC-PUFAs; (2) the potential impact of rapidly altering the intake of dietary LA and ALA; (3) the genetics and evolution of LC-PUFA biosynthesis; (4) Gene–diet interactions that may lead to excess levels of *n*-6 LC-PUFAs and deficiencies of *n*-3 LC-PUFAs; and (5) opportunities for precision nutrition approaches to personalize *n*-3 LC-PUFA supplementation for individuals and populations. Conclusions: The rapid nature of transitions in 18C-PUFA exposure together with the genetic variation in the LC-PUFA biosynthetic pathway found in different populations make mal-adaptations a likely outcome of our current nutritional environment. Understanding this genetic variation in the context of 18C-PUFA dietary exposure should enable the development of individualized *n*-3 LC-PUFA supplementation regimens to prevent and manage human disease.

Keywords: omega-3 fatty acids; polyunsaturated fatty acids; gene-diet interaction; human disease; inflammation; fatty acid desaturase genes; arachidonic acid; eicosanoids; endocannabinoids

1. Introduction

Modern humans emerged from Africa ~200,000 years ago and spread across the earth over the past 100,000 years. During this time, available food sources created evolutionary pressure that drove genetic architecture which allowed our species to adapt, survive and proliferate; this was coupled with a rapid expansion in brain size (particularly gray matter in the cerebral cortex) and, with it, advancements in human intelligence, socialization, and innovation.

The modern Western diet (MWD) has dramatically changed the nutritional content of ingested foods in developed countries, and given the rapid nature of these nutritional transitions, mal-adaptations and related human diseases are a likely outcome of our current nutritional environment [1,2]. For example, up to 72% of dietary calories consumed presently in the MWD did not exist in hunter-gatherer diets [3]. Changes in food type (quality) and quantity in the MWD have been largely driven by technological changes in food production and processing to provide high-calorie and appealing food (high in sugars, refined grains and oils) to large urban populations [1,4]. These have led to detrimental shifts in nutrient metabolism leading to gene-diet interactions responsible for more obesity and localized and systemic inflammation [2]. In turn, this inflammation contributes to the pathogenesis of a variety of disease states, including cardiovascular disease, diabetes and insulin resistance, cancer, autoimmunity, hypersensitivity disorders such as asthma and allergies, chronic joint disease, skin and digestive disorders, dementia and Alzheimer's disease [5–14]. As challenging as these changes are for overall populations of developed countries such as the US, they are more negative for certain populations and ethnic groups [15–20], in whom a disproportionate burden of preventable disease, death, and disability now exists. However, the emergence of the field of precision nutrition that factors in individual- and population-based genetic variability in the context of human diets offers the promise to provide more specific and individualized dietary and supplement interventions that may prevent and mitigate many of the pro-inflammatory effects of the MWD [21].

With regard to fatty acid (FA) intake, there has been marked shift (due largely to recommendations from health agencies) to reduce levels of saturated fatty acids and replace them with polyunsaturated fatty acids (PUFAs) in an attempt to lower serum total cholesterol and LDL lipoproteins [22,23]. From a practical perspective, this meant a replacement of sources of saturated fat such as lard and butter with PUFA-containing vegetable oils (soybean, corn, and canola oils, as well as margarine and shortenings), which are rich in the 18 carbon (18C) omega-6 (*n*-6) PUFA linoleic acid (18:2*n*-6, LA) and poor in both the omega-3 (*n*-3) 18C-PUFA, α-linolenic acid (18:3*n*-3, ALA) and monounsaturated fatty acids. In fact, it has been estimated that soybean oil consumption alone (which contains 58 g LA/100 g oil) increased >1000-fold from 1909 to 1999 and now contributes to ~7% of daily energy of the MWD [1]. Over time, this progressive increase in the ingestion of vegetable oils has led to a 3-fold increase (to 6–8% energy) in dietary LA content of the MWD [1,3,24–26], as well as an estimated 40% reduction in total *n*-3 long chain ($\geq$20 carbon; LC-) PUFA levels, and a large shift in the ratio of dietary *n*-6/*n*-3 C18 PUFAs consumed from ~5:1 to >10:1 [1,27].

The objectives of this review are first to point out how lifestyle variables and specifically our current dietary PUFA exposure together with ancestral-based genetic variation in the LC-PUFA biosynthetic pathway gives rise to distinct molecular profiles (levels of LC-PUFAs, LC-PUFA metabolites, inflammatory and other disease biomarkers) that enhance disease risk for certain individuals and populations. These gene-diet interactions may be particularly important to health in western countries as dietary *n*-6 and *n*-3 18C PUFAs comprise almost 10% of daily calories in the MWD. The second objective of the review is to describe how an understanding of PUFA-based gene-diet interactions can provide a scientific basis for the development of specific dietary and supplement strategies with *n*-3 LC-PUFAs to prevent and manage human diseases.

2. Long Chain Polyunsaturated Fatty Acid Biosynthesis and Biological Activities

From the work of George and Mildred Burr almost 100 years ago [28,29], which was extended by the studies of Ralph Holman [30,31], it became clear that *n*-3 and *n*-6 18C-PUFAs were essential for human health. Furthermore, these 18C-PUFAs originated from the diet and were not synthesized from acetyl and malonyl CoA ester condensations catalyzed by fatty acid synthase. The two essential dietary PUFAs of shortest (18C) chain length, ALA and LA, are the key substrates that enter the biosynthetic pathways leading to biologically-active *n*-3 and *n*-6 LC-PUFAs, respectively. Figure 1 highlights the LC-PUFA biosynthetic pathway and genes known to encode for enzymes that play key roles in the two parallel and competing pathways that synthesize *n*-3 and *n*-6 LC-PUFAs. Two desaturation enzymes encoded by fatty acid desaturase 1 and 2 (*FADS1* and *FADS2*) and one elongation enzyme encoded by *ELOVL5* synthesize eicosapentaenoic acid (20:5*n*-3, EPA) and arachidonic acid (20:4*n*-6, ARA) from ALA and LA, respectively [32–36]. The *n*-3 LC-PUFA, docosapentaenoic acid (22:5*n*-3; DPA) and the *n*-6 LC-PUFA, adrenic acid (22:4*n*-6; ADA) can be generated from EPA and ARA, respectively, using an additional elongation enzyme (encoded by *ELVOL 5/2*), and finally docosahexaenoic acid (22:6*n*-3; DHA) can be produced from DPA with a Δ-4 desaturation enzyme also encoded by *FADS2* [37]. EPA may also be converted to DHA utilizing three additional biosynthetic steps (2 elongation, 1 desaturation and 1 β-oxidation). Smaller quantities of LC-PUFAs can be obtained directly from the diet. For example, preformed ARA is found in organ meats, eggs, poultry, and fish, and various types of seafood such as cold-water fish are rich in preformed *n*-3 LC-PUFAs, EPA, DPA and DHA [26].

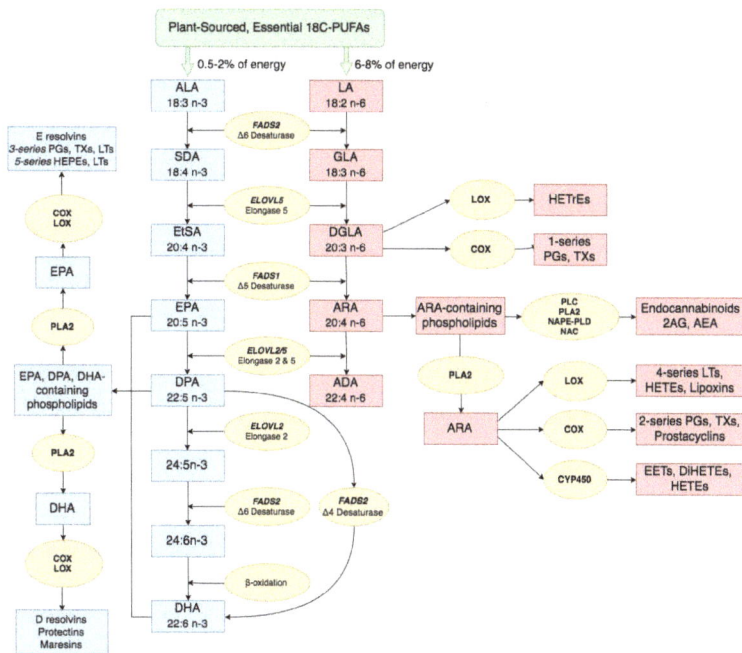

Figure 1. Polyunsaturated fatty acid biosynthesis. *n*-3 and *n*-6 LC-PUFA are synthesized from dietary intake of essential fatty acids ALA and LA, respectively, through a series of enzymatic desaturation (*FADS2* and *FADS1*) and elongation (*ELOVL2* and *ELOVL5*) steps. This pathway gives rise to primary *n*-3 LC-PUFAs and *n*-6 LC-PUFAs such as EPA, DPA, DHA and ARA. These LC-PUFAs (as free fatty acids or complex lipids) and their metabolites impact a wide ranges of physiologic and pathophysiologic processes. Abbreviations: *FADS1/2*, fatty acid desaturase 1/2; *ELOVL 2/5*, fatty acid elongase 2/5; ALA, α-linolenic acid; SDA, stearidonic acid; EtSA, eicosatetraenoic acid; EPA, eicosapentaenoic acid; DPA, docosapentaenoic acid; DHA, docosahexaenoic acid; LA, linoleic acid; GLA, γ-linolenic acid; DGLA, dihomo-γ-linolenic acid; ARA, arachidonic acid; ADA, adrenic acid; PG, prostaglandin; TX, thromboxane; LT, leukotriene; HEPE, hydroxyeicosapentaenoic acid; HETrE, hydroxyeicosatrienoic acid, HETE, hydroxyeicosatetraenoic acid; DiHETE, dihydroxyeicosatetraenoic acid; EET, epoxyeicosatetraenoic acid; 2AG, 2-arachidonoylglycerol; AEA, arachidonoyl ethanolamide/anandamide.

Once formed, LC-PUFAs have many roles as free fatty acids and esterified in complex lipids (Figure 1). These include biophysical properties essential for proper plasma membrane function, energy production by β-oxidation and specific biochemical roles as precursors of bioactive lipids [38,39]. For example, in the central nervous system, the *n*-3 LC-PUFA DHA is the most abundant FA in complex lipids constituting approximately 50% of the weight of neuronal plasma membranes. Its membrane status and signaling capacity directly impact brain development and function via several mechanisms, including maintaining membrane integrity, neurotransmission, neurogenesis, membrane receptor function and signal transduction [38,40–44].

Importantly, both *n*-6 and *n*-3 LC-PUFAs are also converted to a diverse family of metabolites including multiple forms of prostaglandins, thromboxanes, hydroxyeicosatetraenoic acids, epoxyeicosatrienoic acids, leukotrienes, lipoxins, resolvins, protectins, maresins and endocannabinoids (Figure 1) [45–52]. LC-PUFAs and their metabolites, along with their cellular receptors, are present in practically all cells and tissues of the body and act as potent signaling molecules that impact a wide range of physiologic and pathophysiologic processes [45–52].

Most evidence to date indicates that *n*-6 and *n*-3 LC-PUFAs and their metabolic products have not only different, but often opposing effects on immunity and inflammation [53–57]. In general, *n*-6 LC-PUFA metabolites and particularly ARA act as local hormones to promote acute and chronic inflammation [46,51,52]. In contrast to ARA, *n*-3 LC-PUFAs, such as EPA, DPA, and DHA, can be metabolized to anti-inflammatory mediators that have "pro-resolution" properties [47,58]. An exception to this principle are the ARA-derived lipoxins that exert anti-inflammatory, pro-resolution bioactions [59].

Over the past 20 years, one of the most fascinating areas of science has been the discovery of the pleiotropic effects of the endocannabinoid system [60–62]. Endocannabinoids have been shown to be complex lipids (such as 2-arachidonoyl glycerol and arachidonyl ethanolamine) derived from the *n*-6 LC-PUFA, ARA [60–62]. More recent studies have demonstrated that *n*-3 LC-PUFA derivatives of endocannabinoids also exist [63–65]. Endocannabinoid action via cannabinoid 1 and 2 receptors impacts a wide range of biological functions including energy balance and metabolism, mood, memory, sleep, reproduction, thermoregulation and immune function [63–75]. Endocannabinoids can also be metabolized by cyclooxygenases, lipoygenases, and p450 epoxygenases to form other biologically-active complex lipids [65,76,77].

It is clear from the aforementioned studies that *n*-6 and *n*-3 LC-PUFAs and their metabolites have structural and/or signaling roles throughout the human body (Figure 1). Additionally, maintaining a proper balance of *n*-6 and *n*-3 LC-PUFAs and their metabolites is critical to homeostasis in virtually every physiologic system. Consequently, environmental and genetic mechanisms that influence their levels and balance will impact human health and disease.

3. Impact of Dietary Linoleic Acid and α-Linolenic Acid Levels on *n*-3 LC-PUFA Biosynthesis

Several studies have warned against health and disease outcomes that could result from radical increases of dietary LA in the MWD in such a short period of time [26,78,79]. Given the shared enzymatic steps involved in the processing of LA and ALA, these *n*-6 and *n*-3 18C-PUFAs and their metabolic intermediates compete with each other in the liver and other tissues as substrates for synthetic enzymatic reactions that produce LC-PUFAs [80,81]. Additionally, there is an overall limited capacity of 18C-PUFAs that can be converted to LC-PUFAs [53]. As discussed in detail below, this biosynthetic limit in capacity is highly impacted at an individual level by genetic variation in the LC-PUFA biosynthetic pathway. Consequently, a dramatic increase in LA in the MWD observed over the past 75 years together with competition between *n*-6 and *n*-3 substrates within the pathway has been shown in animal models and humans to shift the pathway toward the biosynthesis of high levels *n*-6 LC-PUFAs and away from *n*-3 LC-PUFAs [53,82–87]. In 1992, Lands and colleagues described non-linear interactions between LA and ALA in forming LC-PUFAs utilizing a hyperbolic equation that fit for rats, mice and humans [53]. The equation points out the limitation of generating *n*-3

LC-PUFAs when *n*-3 ALA is ingested together with several-fold greater amounts of *n*-6 LA as is the case with the MWD. Wood and colleagues reviewed human studies that examined the effect of altering LA and ALA on *n*-6 and *n*-3 LC-PUFA biosynthesis and concluded that it is possible to increase *n*-3 LC-PUFAs by reducing LA or increasing ALA intake in humans [82]. However, LA levels need to be reduced to <2.5% energy before levels of DHA can be increased. Again, typical LA levels in the MWD reside between 6–8% energy; consequently, high levels of LA in the MWD would be predicted to markedly reduce, not increase DHA. In fact, it has been estimated that LA concentrations in the MWD have decreased the omega-3 index by 41%, from 6.51 to 3.84 [1].

A 1997 paper by Okuyama and colleagues made a compelling case that excess LA and the increase in the LA/ALA ratio as a result of moving away from traditional diets led to 'Omega-3 Deficiency Syndrome' in the elderly in Japan [84]. The paper summarized the "evidence which indicates that increased dietary LA and relative *n*-3 deficiency are major risk factors for western-type cancers, cardiovascular and cerebrovascular diseases and also for allergic hyper-reactivity." They also suggest that *n*-3 LC-PUFAs deficiency created by excess LA and LA/ALA ratios in the MWD affects human behavior patterns in industrialized countries. Certainly these assertions are supported by a large body of scientific literature in both animal models and human studies discussed throughout this review.

4. The Genetics and Evolution of LC-PUFA Biosynthesis

Through a better understanding of genetic variation associated with the utilization of specific nutrients, precision nutrition approaches offer the potential to predict the physiological and pathological consequences of the interaction of individual genetic differences and diet to prevent and/or manage adverse outcomes. Until recently, it was assumed that the metabolic capacity of the LC-PUFA biosynthetic pathway was limited and fairly uniform in all humans. This premise was supported by metabolic studies in European ancestry populations, which suggest that only a small proportion of ingested dietary 18C PUFAs (typically 2–3% energy) are converted into LC-PUFAs [81,88–90]. However, studies over the past decade have demonstrated common genetic and epigenetic variation in genes (including *FADS1*, *FADS2*, *ELOVL5* and *ELOVL2*) throughout the LC-PUFA biosynthetic pathway are highly associated with the levels of LC-PUFAs produced in human circulation, cells and tissues [91–116]. This body of evidence has challenged the concept that LC-PUFA biosynthesis from 18C-PUFAs is uniform among individuals and populations.

The desaturase enzymes within the pathway, encoded by the two genes (*FADS1*, *FADS2*) in the *FADS* cluster region (chr11: 61,540,615–61,664,170) have long been recognized as the rate-limiting steps in the conversion of 18C-PUFAs to LC-PUFA (Figures 1 and 2). Our laboratory initially demonstrated that there are marked differences between African and European ancestry populations in the circulating levels of *n*-6 and *n*-3 LC-PUFAs [100,106]. This work also showed that ~80% of African Americans carry two copies of *FADS* alleles associated with more efficient biosynthesis of LC-PUFAs, compared to only ~45% of European Americans and these genetic differences explained a large proportion of the variability in LC-PUFA levels between African and European Americans. Numerous other studies have also revealed strong genetic influences within the *FADS* cluster region on circulating, cellular and tissue levels of LC-PUFAs [2,36,117]. This region of association comprises a linkage disequilibrium (LD) block covering the promoter regions of both *FADS1* and *FADS2* (Figure 2). Importantly, the derived haplotype that includes numerous genetic variants with common allele frequencies (when compared to the ancestral haplotype) is associated with higher levels of LC-PUFAs and an increased efficiency (as determined by product to precursor ratios within the LC-PUFA biosynthetic pathway) by which LC-PUFAs are synthesized [117]. One of the most surprising aspects of these genetic studies is the observation that there are dramatic differences in the frequencies of the ancestral and derived haplotypes and thus the efficiency of LC-PUFA biosynthesis among diverse global populations. For example, the ancestral haplotype is most common (97%) in Native Americans and virtually absent in Africa, suggesting that Native Americans and individuals of Native American ancestry have a more limited capacity than Africans to synthesize LC-PUFAs [118]. The derived haplotype is observed at varying frequencies (25–50%) in Europe and East Asia [117,119]. As described in detail below, extensive evolution of the *FADS* cluster and thus changes in the efficiency of LC-PUFA biosynthesis took place as early humans adapted to local environments as they moved from Africa to the Americas. These are reflected in the dramatic differences in the *FADS* haplotype frequencies and LC-PUFA biosynthetic efficiencies observed in diverse modern populations.

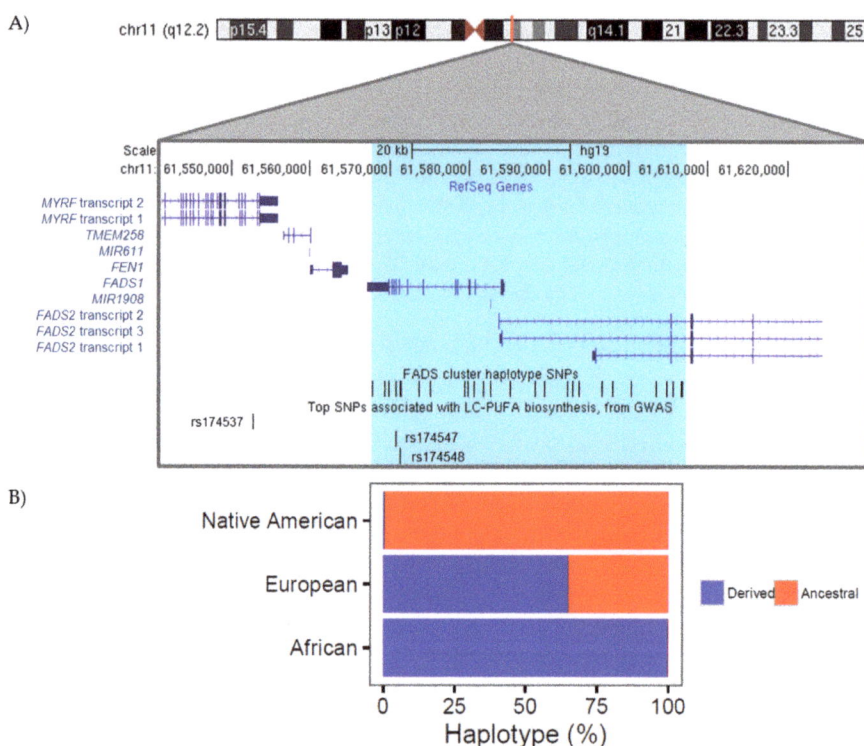

Figure 2. Genetic variation near the *FADS* gene cluster. (**A**) A expanded depiction of the *FADS* gene cluster on chromosome 11 illustrates the genomic location (build hg19) of: genes in this region (shown in dark blue, from RefSeq), the *FADS* cluster haplotype region and single nucleotide polymorphisms (SNPs) (region highlighted in light blue with SNPs shown as black vertical bars), and three individual SNPs identified as the most significantly associated genetic variants genome-wide with LC-PUFA levels (rs174537, rs174547, and rs174548); (**B**) The observed percentage of derived vs. ancestral *FADS* cluster haplotype varies by ethnicity.

Numerous individual genetic variants within the *FADS* cluster (as illustrated in Figure 2) have been identified by genome-wide association studies (GWAS) to be highly associated with LC-PUFA levels as well a wide variety of important molecular and clinical phenotypes. For instance, GWAS of plasma *n*-3 and *n*-6 LC-PUFA levels in Italian, European, and Chinese populations have identified single nucleotide polymorphisms (SNPs) such as rs174537 and rs174547 located near *FADS1*, which are the strongest signals genome-wide associating with levels of *n*-3 and *n*-6 LC-PUFAs such as ARA and EPA [94,101,120–122]. Genetic variants in the *FADS* cluster are also associated with numerous human phenotypes including inflammatory and cardiovascular disorders, blood lipid levels including low-density lipoprotein (LDL) and triglyceride levels, coronary artery disease, insulin resistance, perinatal depression, atopic diseases, attention/hyperactivity, intelligence and memory in children [36,92,96,99,102,105,109,111,116,123–128]. The strong associations between genetic variation in the *FADS* cluster, LC-PUFA levels, and important clinical phenotypes support the concept that genetically-induced alterations in LC-PUFA levels may play important roles in several human diseases. However, due to the high degree of LD observed between genetic variants in this region, it is difficult to determine which variants have a casual role in altering *FADS* activity thus the efficiency of LC-PUFA biosynthesis.

An important question from this work is: why are there such distinct ancestral-based genetic variation within the *FADS* cluster? It is important to understand that nutrients and genomes interact reciprocally. As described above, genetic variation confers differences in nutrient utilization. However, changes in nutrient exposure throughout human development also created adaptive pressures that led to selection of genetic variation that better fit nutritional environments. Our laboratory initially examined evolutionary forces shaping patterns of variation in the *FADS* cluster by examining geographically diverse populations representing 14 populations and focused on a 300 kb region centered on the *FADS* loci [119]. This work confirmed that there are marked global differences in allele frequencies of variants in the *FADS* gene cluster that are strongly associated with the efficiency of conversion of LA and ALA to ARA and DHA, respectively. This study also provided evidence that alleles associated with LC-PUFA biosynthesis were driven to near fixation in African populations by positive selection ~85,000 years ago. The selection of these *FADS* variants would have enhanced LC-PUFA synthesis from plant-sourced 18C-PUFAs. We postulate that this enhanced the capacity to synthesize LC-PUFAs and particularly *n*-3 LC-PUFAs such as DHA, and was therefore an important advantage that would have facilitated the movement of humans away from marine sources of LC-PUFAs in isolated geographic regions and concomitant rapid expansion and migration throughout the African continent 60,000–80,000 years ago. That same time, Ameur and colleagues described the *FADS* haplotype patterns (ancestral and derived), with the derived haplotype found in Africa, that were associated with more efficient conversion of 18C-PUFAs into LC-PUFAs [117].

However, it was unclear from these initial papers: (1) why human populations migrating out of Africa appeared to carry the ancestral haplotype; (2) why Eurasian populations are polymorphic; and (3) why the ancestral haplotype is at near fixation in Native American populations. Fumagalli and colleagues provided an important clue to this puzzle by carrying out a genome-wide scan for positive selection in the Greenlandic Inuit and showing that genetic variation in the *FADS* cluster to be the strongest signatures for cold adaptation [129]. Interestingly, the two most highly differentiated SNPs (rs7115739 and rs174570) were associated with lower levels of LC-PUFAs and higher levels of 18C-PUFAs precursors. It was also demonstrated that these *FADS* cluster alleles were associated with a decrease in weight, height, fasting serum insulin, and fasting serum LDL cholesterol [129]. These investigators posited that the challenging environmental conditions of the Arctic likely imposed strong selective pressures on the Inuit and their ancestors and these physical and molecular phenotypes were important to cold adaptation. However, the PUFA-related molecular mechanism responsible for physical phenotypes such as weight and height are not yet understood. Very recently, we have demonstrated that the ancestral haplotype frequency is also correlated to Siberian populations' geographic location, further suggesting the ancestral haplotype's role in cold weather adaptation [130]. Additionally, this likely explains the high haplotype frequency of the ancestral haplotype within Native American populations [118,130].

There are several other recently published papers which have focused on the role that evolution of the *FADS* cluster played in the capacity of humans to adapt to varying global nutritional environments containing fluctuating levels of LC-PUFAs. For example, Mathieson and colleague carried out a genome-wide scan for positive selection from ancient and present-day European genomes and demonstrated strong selection for derived alleles over the past 4000 years [131]. Kothapalli and colleagues studied genomes from populations in South Asia and showed positive selection for an indel in *FADS2* that is associated with more efficient LC-PUFA biosynthesis [132]. They suggest that this was an important adaptation as populations moved to more vegetarian diets with low levels of dietary LC-PUFAs [132]. Buckley and colleagues compared *FADS* sequencing data from present day to the Bronze Age and concluded that selection patterns in Europeans were driven by changes in dietary fat composition and specifically LC-PUFA levels following the transition to agriculture [133]. Taken together, all of these studies reflect the evolutionary importance for humans to regulate LC-PUFA biosynthesis. The complex interactions among local selective pressures in diverse local environments along global human migration patterns appears to have given rise to the global variation in frequencies of the derived and ancestral haplotypes that are observed today.

5. Anatomy of *n*-6 LC-PUFA Excesses and *n*-3 LC-PUFA Deficiencies

As outlined throughout this review, there are several components of the MWD and the diverse genetics of LC-PUFA biosynthesis among different human populations that could combine to create harmful gene-diet interactions, which in turn would impact levels of *n*-6 and *n*-3 LC-PUFAs, their metabolites and ultimately human disease (Figure 3). First, gene-diet interactions can arise when there is a major change in the exposure of a nutrient that is utilized by an important metabolic pathway. As discussed above, following recommendations to replace dietary saturated fatty acids with PUFAs, food production companies began replacing the saturated fatty acids, largely with *n*-6 18C-PUFAs, and this led to a dramatic increase (~3 fold) in the ingestion of LA. In contrast, the ingestion of the dietary *n*-3 18C-PUFA, ALA, has remained relatively constant [1]. This resulted in a significant change in not only LA exposure but also the ratio of dietary LA to ALA that enters the LC-PUFA biosynthetic pathway. As discussed above, LA and its *n*-6 metabolites directly compete with ALA and its *n*-3 metabolites in the synthesis of LC-PUFAs, and there is a limited capacity of the pathway to produce LC-PUFAs. Consequently, the ratio of LA to ALA has been altered by increasing dietary LA (to 6–8% of energy) and this dietary modification has shifted the pathway toward the biosynthesis of higher levels *n*-6 LC-PUFAs and away from *n*-3 LC-PUFAs.

A second component of potentially harmful gene-diet interactions is exemplified in some individuals or human populations that have a greater genetic capacity to more efficiently utilize/metabolize a specific nutrient than others. A well-recognized example of this situation are the variants near the *LCT* locus that codes for the lactase enzyme, which metabolizes lactose in milk [134–136]. Cattle domestication ~10,000 years ago induced strong selection to be able to utilize lactose, the primary carbohydrate in milk, as adults. In most humans, levels of the lactase enzyme decreases after weaning, but certain populations that traditionally depended on milk have variants near the *LTC* locus associated with high levels of lactase and thus retain the capacity to utilize lactose into adulthood.

Similarly, studies over the past decade show that diverse global populations have differences in their capacity to utilize 18C-PUFAs to synthesize LC-PUFAs, and there is now strong evidence that common *FADS* variants form ancestral and derived haplotypes that account for these pathway efficiency differences. It has been recently proposed that the derived haplotype played a crucial role in human evolution under circumstances when dietary LC-PUFAs, especially dietary *n*-3 LC-PUFA levels, were low [119,131–133]. This included movement away from *n*-3 LC-PUFA-rich marine sources during the 'great expansion' in Africa 60,000–80,000 years ago and the adaptation to largely vegetarian diets after the development of agriculture in Europe and Asia ~12,000 years ago. Consequently, African, African ancestry and some south Asian populations have high frequencies of a derived haplotype that is associated with efficient LC-PUFA biosynthesis [117,119]. Additionally, the MWD provides very high levels of LA to this genetically more efficient pathway resulting in significantly higher levels of the *n*-6 LC-PUFA, ARA, when compared to most European or European ancestry populations [100,106]. Figure 4 illustrates this point by demonstrating that there are significant differences between circulating LC-PUFAs, ARA and DHA, in African and European American populations. A major question that arises from the data in Figure 4 is; what are the biological consequences and specifically the risk of human disease for individuals who are either at the upper (excess ARA levels) or lower (depressed DHA levels) end extremes?

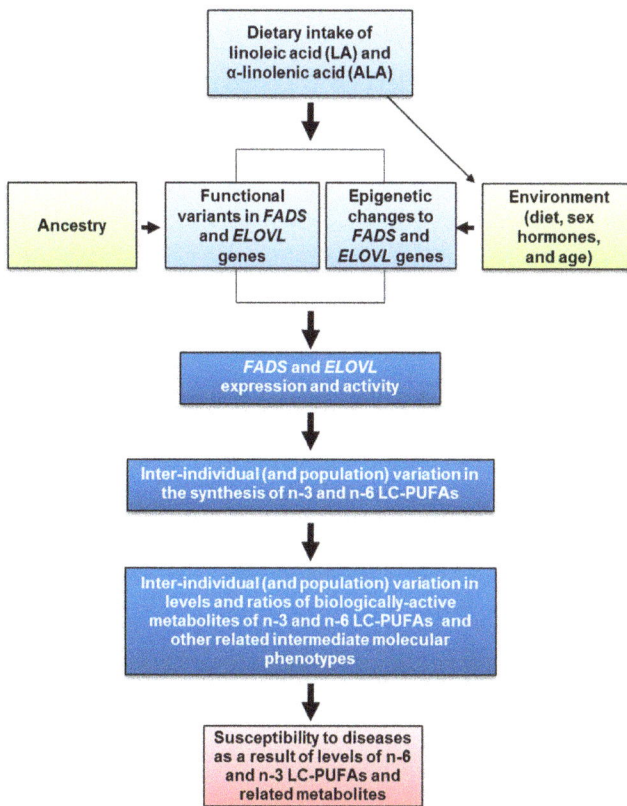

Figure 3. Anatomy of gene-diet interactions leading to *n*-6 LC-PUFA excesses and *n*-3 LC-PUFA deficiencies. Dietary intake of *n*-3 and *n*-6 18C-PUFAs, ALA and LA, respectively, interact with *FADS* or *ELOVL* genetic and epigenetic variation (that impacts *FADS* or *ELOVL* expression or resultant activity) to determine circulating and cellular levels of *n*-3 and *n*-6 LC-PUFAs. These interactions can result in an unhealthy balance of LC-PUFAs, with excess levels of *n*-6 LC-PUFAs or deficiencies of *n*-3 LC-PUFAs.

Numerous studies have addressed the issue of excess ARA or efficient LA to ARA conversion in the context of cardiovascular disease (CVD). For example, Martinelli and colleagues [116] examined associations among 13 *FADS* genotypes, desaturase activity (as determined by ARA/LA ratios), inflammation (C-reactive protein (CRP)), and coronary artery disease (CAD) in 876 individuals with (n = 610) and without (n = 266) CAD. Individuals carrying certain haplotypes (the derived haplotype) had higher ARA/LA ratios in red blood cell membranes, corresponding to enhanced desaturase activity. Importantly, the ARA/LA ratio was an independent risk factor for CAD (Odds Ratio 2.55, $p < 0.001$), Furthermore, the pro-inflammatory marker, CRP increased progressively across tertiles of ARA/LA. This study provided a powerful example of how variants in the *FADS* cluster alter molecular phenotypes, which in turn alter disease risk. Li and colleagues also examined the association of *FADS* genotypes and plasma fatty acids in control (n = 510) and CAD patients (n = 505) from a Chinese Han population [111]. They also showed that the ARA/LA ratio was higher in CAD patients and the low pathway efficiency T allele at rs174537 was associated with a lower risk of CAD (Odds Ratio 0.74, $p = 0.001$). Similarly, Kwak and colleagues [105] carried out a case-control study in a Korean cohort and discovered that minor T allele at rs174537 was associated with lower risk of CAD (Odds Ratio 0.75, $p = 0.006$), and T allele carriers had significantly lower pathway efficiency as measured by ARA/LA and ARA/DGLA ratios. The T allele was also associated with lower total-and LDL-cholesterol and lipid peroxides. Importantly, Lettre and colleagues performed a meta-analysis on five African American cohorts (*n* ~8,000) and confirmed the association of *FADS* SNPs with not only lipid phenotypes, but CAD itself [137].

Other studies have demonstrated that high levels of ARA in adipose tissue are associated with elevated risk of acute myocardial infarction (AMI) [138,139]. For example, Kark and colleagues showed that ARA in adipose tissue was positively associated with AMI (O.R. 2.12, *p* = 0.004). Our laboratory has demonstrated that the genotypes at the *FADS1* SNP, rs174537, which increases the efficiency of the LC-PUFA biosynthetic pathway, and thus circulating and cellular ARA levels, are also associated with higher levels of pro-inflammatory ARA-derived eicosanoids [140]. ARA-derived eicosanoids, such as urinary 8 epi-prostaglandin F(2α) that are independent risk factors for CAD, are also positively correlated with levels of ARA and ARA /LA ratios [105,141]. Together, these studies suggest that individuals and populations that have an enhanced genetic capacity to convert high levels of dietary LA to ARA are more likely to have high levels of ARA, ARA metabolites, inflammatory biomarkers, and diseases of inflammation such as CAD.

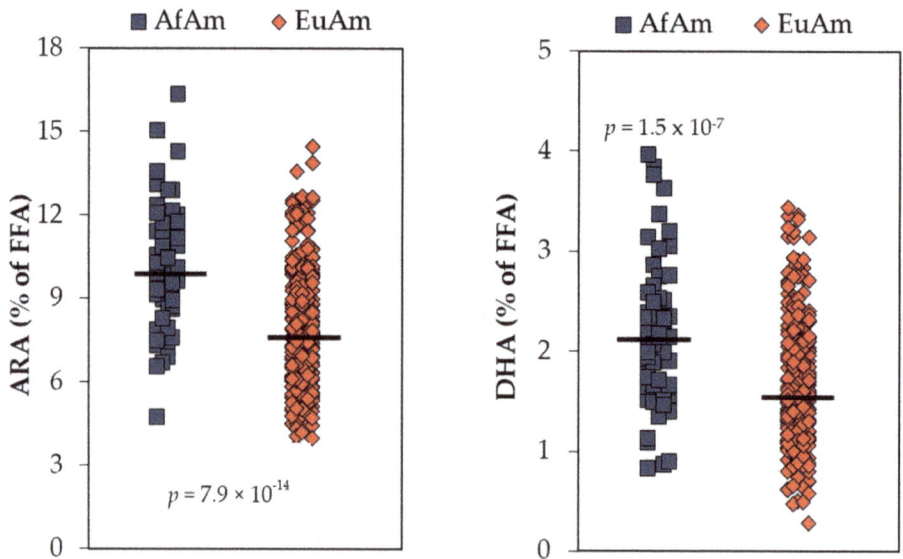

Figure 4. Serum Levels of ARA and DHA in African Americans (AfAm) and European Americans (EuAm). Both *n*-6 and *n*-3 LC-PUFAs (arachidonic acid, ARA; and docosahexaenoic acid, DHA) are elevated in serum from AfAm relative to EuAm from the same clinical diabetes study cohort [106].

Although the aforementioned findings show genetic variation in the *FADS* cluster to be cross-sectionally associated with LC-PUFA and LC-PUFA metabolite levels, biomarkers of inflammation and CAD risk, few studies have investigated whether genetic variation within the *FADS* cluster is a significant mediator of the relationship between PUFA intake and CVD risk. One longitudinal cohort study [142] with a mean follow-up of 14 years, which included 24,032 participants aged 44–74 years, reported a borderline significant interaction by genotype of the *FADS* SNP rs174546 on the incidence of CVD by PUFA intake levels. Particularly, the ALA-to-LA intake ratio was inversely associated with CVD risk only among participants homozygous for the T-allele of *FADS* SNP rs174546 (HR for quintile 5 vs. quintile 1 = 0.72; 95% CI: 0.50, 1.04; *p*-trend = 0.049). Additionally, ALA intake inversely associated with ischemic stroke only among rs174546 TT genotype carriers (HR for quintile 5 vs. quintile 1 = 0.50; 95% CI: 0.27, 0.94; *p*-trend = 0.02). This study provides some evidence, albeit weak, that genetic variation in the *FADS* cluster may mediate the associations between PUFA intake and CVD risk, and that high ALA intake and a high ALA-to-LA intake ratio may be preferable to help prevent CVD and ischemic stroke particularly among those that are homozygous for the minor T-allele of rs174546. In summary, accumulating evidence suggests that the *FADS* locus may be useful in stratification and targeting of LC-PUFA recommendations for prevention of CVD; however, further research is necessary to better understand how genetic variation within the *FADS* cluster modifies the relationship between PUFA intake and CVD risk [143].

What about individuals/populations with low levels of LC-PUFAs such as DHA? This would be expected in those individuals/populations with *FADS* variants that make up the ancestral haplotype associated with inefficient LC-PUFA biosynthesis. As discussed above, the ancestral haplotype appears to have played a crucial role in the adaptation of Arctic populations to cold environments under conditions where high levels of preformed *n*-3 LC-PUFAs were ingested from the abundant marine sources [129]. Importantly, very high frequencies of this ancestral haplotype are also observed in Native American populations [118,130]. This genetic architecture, together with the current levels of LA, ALA, preformed *n*-3 LC-PUFAs, and specifically low levels of DHA in the MWD raises vital questions of how modern populations with high Native American ancestry acquire DHA. Does the near fixation of the ancestral haplotype, with its limited capacity to synthesize LC-PUFAs in Native American ancestry individuals, together with the PUFA composition (high levels of LA and low levels of ALA and DHA) give rise to *n*-3 LC-PUFA deficiencies and resulting diseases/disorders in Native American populations? DHA is critical for brain function throughout the human life span, but its accumulation is especially important to healthy brain development during gestation and infancy [144–146]. Additionally, as described above, *n*-3 LC-PUFAs such as DHA, DPA and EPA and their metabolites have potent anti-inflammatory properties [47,58]. There are no studies to date that have compared circulating and cellular levels of LC-PUFAs in a Native American ancestry cohort to other human populations. Future studies will be necessary to determine the risk of *n*-3 LC-PUFA deficiency in this population and whether *n*-3 LC-PUFA supplementation could provide important health benefits to Native American ancestry populations.

Most European and Asian ancestry populations are polymorphic for derived and ancestral haplotypes and individual genetic variants within the *FADS* cluster that impact LC-PUFA biosynthesis. Consequently, these populations appear to be more diverse with respect to their capacity to synthesize LC-PUFAs. For example, we have demonstrated in three European ancestry cohorts that ~45% of individuals have the homozygous GG genotype at the *FADS1* SNP rs174537, which is associated with efficient LC-PUFA biosynthesis [36,97,100,106]. The TT genotype, which is associated with low efficiency LC-PUFA biosynthesis, is found in ~11% of the individuals in these cohorts and the balance (~44%) have the GT genotype. Similar to modern Native American ancestry populations, these studies raise important questions of how the 11% of individuals of European ancestry with the TT genotype and thus less efficient LC-PUFA biosynthesis acquire *n*-3 LC-PUFAs and particularly DHA when they are consuming a MWD.

Studies are just now beginning to emerge that indicate that epigenetics and specifically the methylation status of specific CpG sites within the *FADS* cluster (in a regulatory region between *FADS1* and *FADS2* that contains the *FADS1* and *FADS2* promoters and an regulatory enhancer) impacts the transcription of *FADS* cluster genes, LC-PUFA biosynthesis, and in one study, both immediate and delayed memory performance in toddlers [147,148]. A separate human study shows that previous PUFA exposure impacts the methylation status of GpG sites within this region [149]. We performed genome-wide allele-specific methylation (ASM) with the *FADS1* SNP, rs174537 in 144 human liver samples and identified highly significant ASM with CpG sites between *FADS1* and *FADS2* in a enhancer signature region [150], leading to the hypothesis that the associations of rs174537 with LC-PUFA levels may be impacted by the methylation status of that enhancer region. Additionally, a study in rats indicates that maternal fat intake alters ARA and DHA status and the epigenetic regulation of *FADS2* in offspring liver [151]. Although these studies are still early, collectively, they suggest that there are likely to be factors such as age, sex, pregnancy and prior PUFA exposure that impact epigenetic-mediated regulatory mechanisms of the *FADS* cluster leading to alterations in *FADS* gene transcription, LC-PUFA biosynthesis from 18C-PUFAs and ultimately LC-PUFA status [149]. Understanding the ramifications of these epigenetic modifications will likely be important in discerning how LC-PUFA levels are regulated both at individual and population levels.

6. Implications of Non-Uniform *n*-3 LC-PUFA Biosynthesis on the Efficacy of *n*-3 LC-PUFA Supplementation Trials

Pioneering studies 40 years ago showed that high dietary intake of *n*-3 LC-PUFA-enriched foods reduced mortality from myocardial infarction in Greenland Eskimos [152,153]. Since then, a growing body of evidence has shown that dietary *n*-3 LC-PUFAs may impact cardiovascular disease by numerous mechanisms including reducing circulating triglyceride concentrations, inflammatory processes, platelet aggregation and the incidence of arrhythmias and improving endothelial cell function [154]. Studies from predominantly secondary prevention trials and meta-analyses of observational studies in the 1980s through the early 2000s demonstrated a cardioprotective effect of fish consumption and *n*-3 PUFA supplementation [155–160]. Additionally, high circulating and dietary levels of *n*-3 LC-PUFAs were shown to associated with lower total mortality, especially deaths due to coronary artery disease [161,162]. However, more recent RCTs and meta-analyses indicate that supplementation with *n*-3 LC-PUFAs is not associated with lower risk of adverse outcomes such as all-cause mortality, cardiac death, sudden death, myocardial infarction, or stroke [163–167].

Similarly, several studies have shown associations between low levels of DHA and/or altered ratios of *n*-6 to *n*-3 LC-PUFAs and cognitive function (memory and Alzheimer's disease) as well as psychological disorders (attention-deficit/hyperactivity-ADHD, schizophrenia, autism spectrum and major depressive disorders) in children, adolescents or adults [168–180]. However, systematic reviews and meta-analyses reveal that RCTs show inconsistent results for the therapeutic benefit of *n*-3 LC-PUFAs [181–187]. This pattern of erratic clinical results with *n*-3 LC-PUFAs is also observed in several inflammatory diseases including asthma [188,189], rheumatoid arthritis [190,191] and cancer [192–195].

Together, these studies and the controversies stemming from them have led to great confusion among clinicians and consumers alike about the efficacy of *n*-3 LC-PUFAs for the prevention and treatment of human disease. These varying clinical results have been particularly difficult to comprehend in light of the vast numbers of studies that have examined the mechanism by which *n*-3 LC-PUFAs exert their effects and convincing in vivo data with LC-PUFAs in animal models. Recently, experts at the International Society for the Study of Fatty Acids and Lipids discussed experimental design issues that may contribute to inconsistent results with *n*-3 LC-PUFA interventions in cardiovascular studies and thus must be considered in future clinical designs [196]. These included: (1) the potential of current CVD drug treatments to hide *n*-3 LC-PUFA benefits; (2) the potential impact of high background intakes of LC-PUFAs; (3) small sample sizes; (4) short treatment durations; (5) insufficient dosages of *n*-3 LC-PUFAs; (6) increase in *n*-6 PUFA intake; and (7) failure to measure baseline *n*-3 status. This current review has emphasized the potential impact of the latter three.

First, as discussed in detail above, the dramatic increase in dietary levels of the *n*-6 18C-PUFA, LA, in the MWD has resulted in an imbalance of LA and ALA entering the LC-PUFA biosynthetic pathway (Figure 1). Because these 18C-PUFAs compete for the desaturase and elongase steps in the pathway, the imbalance in LA and ALA together with the limited capacity of the pathway results in a disproportionate synthesis of *n*-6 LC-PUFAs at the expense of *n*-3 LC-PUFAs. The other major consideration is the overall capacity of the pathway to synthesize LC-PUFAs, and a large body of evidence (summarized above) indicates that this pathway capacity is variable in individuals and diverse populations and strongly linked to ancestry. For example, African, African ancestry and most south Asian populations contain evolutionary-driven genetic variants, particularly in the *FADS* cluster, that are strongly associated with efficient LC-PUFA biosynthesis and thus high levels of LC-PUFAs and particularly ARA. We have demonstrated that genetic variants associated with elevated levels of ARA are also associated with the capacity to generate high concentrations of pro-inflammatory eicosanoids in whole blood [140]. Consequently, we hypothesize that the combination of a marked increase in dietary LA as a result of the MWD, together with an enhanced capacity to convert that LA to ARA gives rise to elevated levels of a diverse family of ARA-derived mediators, which promote obesity, inflammation and related diseases. In this case, it may be the excess in ARA and ARA-derived mediators, created by the aforementioned gene–diet interaction, that limits the capacity of *n*-3 LC-PUFAs to impact inflammatory diseases such as CVD and cancer.

On the other hand, individuals of Arctic and Native American ancestry as well as a significant percentage of European and Asian populations have evolutionary-driven *FADS* variants associated with a less efficient LC-PUFA biosynthetic pathway [130]. In this case, we postulate that high levels of LA (relative to ALA) in the MWD are converted to sufficient levels of *n*-6 LC-PUFAs such as ARA and ARA metabolites. However, because of the constraints of the less efficient LC-PUFA biosynthetic pathway, it would be predicted that low quantities of *n*-3 LC-PUFAs and specifically DHA and DHA metabolites would be generated from dietary ALA. Such gene–diet interactions in these individuals/populations could lead to *n*-3 LC-PUFA deficiency, and like other nutrient deficiencies, these may be the patients that most benefit from supplementation with *n*-3 LC-PUFAs. It is important to emphasize that this is a hypothetical scenario at this point in time, and future studies will be necessary to determine actual levels of *n*-3 LC-PUFAs in individuals/populations with the ancestral *FADS* haplotype.

Superko and colleagues reviewed clinical investigations that actually measured blood or plasma levels of *n*-3 LC-PUFAs [197]. Not surprising, their data suggest that diet and geography play a critical role in levels of *n*-3 LC-PUFAs. For example, the lowest 5th percentile of Japanese living in Japan had higher levels of *n*-3 LC-PUFAs than whites living in Pennsylvania and Japanese Americans living in Honolulu. In an analysis of nine studies, Hawkey and Nigg found lower overall blood levels of the *n*-3 LC-PUFAs, EPA and DHA, in individuals with ADHD versus controls [183]. They suggest that there may be "a disruption in the conversion process from ALA to EPA/DHA in the ADHD population". Several GWAS combined with metabolomics analyses have now examined associations between *FADS* variants and circulating levels of *n*-3 LC-PUFAs. Table 1 shows that *FADS1* variants (rs174547, rs174537, and rs174548) are strongly associated with *n*-3 LC-PUFAs, EPA, DPA or DHA either as free fatty acids or in complex lipids [198–200] and further suggest that much of the variation in background *n*-3 LC-PUFA levels is due to genetic variation within the *FADS* cluster.

In addition to blood levels, the review by Superko and colleagues also pointed out that there are marked differences in the impact of *n*-3 LC-PUFA supplementation on circulating levels of LC-PUFAs and altering ratios of *n*-3 to *n*-6 LC-PUFAs [197]. Consequently, large diverse RCTs typically have sizeable subsets of individuals with high, intermediate, and low blood levels of LC-PUFAs; and the degree to which these levels are altered appears highly variable. Thus, it is little wonder that RCTs with *n*-3 LC-PUFAs have yielded perplexing results. Providing individuals with *n*-3 LC-PUFA supplements who do not have LC-PUFA deficiencies, or diverse groups of individuals where diet–gene interactions have created markedly different *n*-6 to *n*-3 LC-PUFA levels and ratios is unlikely to provide clear results. Given the genetic diversity in the LC-PUFA biosynthetic pathway, it may be too much to expect that supplementation strategies that fail to stratify participants in some manner (ex, genetics, background *n*-3 LC-PUFA levels, or ratio of *n*-6 LC-PUFAs to *n*-3 LC-PUFAs) will show statistical efficacy for complex human diseases.

Table 1. Association of key FADS SNPS with serum LC-PUFAs.

n-3 PUFA/Metabolite	SNPs			Data Source
	rs174547 *p*-Value	rs174537 *p*-Value	rs174548 *p*-Value	
1-hexadecanoyl-2-docosapentaenoyl-GPC (16:0/22:5n3)	2.97×10^{-95}	3.83×10^{-93}	9.17×10^{-88}	Draisma et al. [198]
1-tetradecanoyl-2-docosapentaenoyl-GPC (14:0/22:5n3)	2.76×10^{-58}	1.94×10^{-57}	5.08×10^{-54}	Draisma et al. [198]
1-octadecanoyl-2-docosapentaenoyl-GPC (18:0/22:5n-3)	2.23×10^{-42}	4.61×10^{-41}	2.53×10^{-40}	Draisma et al. [198]
1-*O*-docosanyl-2-docosahexaenoyl-GPC (o-22:0/22:6n-3)	1.67×10^{-40}	6.03×10^{-40}	3.15×10^{-37}	Draisma et al. [198]
1-*O*-hexadecyl-2-docosahexaenoyl-GPC (o-16:0/22:6n-3)	1.35×10^{-25}	4.90×10^{-24}	1.36×10^{-23}	Draisma et al. [198]
1-eicosanoyl-2-docosahexaenoyl-GPC (20:0/22:6n-3)			2.19×10^{-23}	Draisma et al. [198]
eicosapentaenoate (EPA; 20:5n3)	1.12×10^{-21}	2.55×10^{-21}	3.71×10^{-22}	Shin et al. [199]
1-octadecanoyl-2-docosahexaenoyl-GPC (18:0/22:6n-3)	8.48×10^{-20}	3.88×10^{-19}	1.70×10^{-18}	Draisma et al. [198]
1-tetradecanoyl-2-docosahexaenoyl-GPC (14:0/22:6n-3)	9.86×10^{-18}	2.72×10^{-17}	1.38×10^{-15}	Draisma et al. [198]
1-octadecanoyl-2-docosahexaenoyl-GPC (18:0/22:5n3)	4.43×10^{-14}	9.83×10^{-14}	9.99×10^{-16}	Long et al. [200]
octadecatetraenoic acid (stearidonate) (18:4n3)	1.63×10^{-15}	1.07×10^{-15}	1.97×10^{-13}	Shin et al. [199]
1-*O*-octadecyl-2-docosahexaenoyl-GPC (o-18:0/22:6n-3)	2.02×10^{-15}	5.04×10^{-15}	1.47×10^{-14}	Draisma et al. [198]
1-hexadecanoyl-2-docosahexaenoyl-GPC 16:0/22:6	1.21×10^{-14}	4.16×10^{-14}	3.02×10^{-13}	Draisma et al. [198]
1-eicosatrienoyl-GPC (ETA; 20:3n-3)			1.30×10^{-14}	Shin et al. [199]
docosapentaenoate (DPA; 22:5n-3)	2.93×10^{-13}	5.07×10^{-13}		Shin et al. [199]
1-eicosapentaenoyl-GPC (20:5n-3)			1.59×10^{-12}	Long et al. [200]
1-octadecenoyl-2-eicosapentaenoyl-GPC (18:1/20:5n-3)			1.78×10^{-12}	Long et al. [200]
1-palmitoyl-2-eicosapentaenoyl-GPC (16:0/20:5n-3)			1.01×10^{-11}	Long et al. [200]

Association of three key *FADS* SNPS with levels of serum *n*-3 LC-PUFAs either as free fatty acids or esterified complex lipids. Serum levels of *n*-3 LC-PUFAs and glycerol-3-phosphocholine (GPC) containing *n*-3 LC-PUFAs were associated with three SNPS in *FADS1* gene region. Data are derived from SNiPA analysis [201] of studies by Draisma et al. [198]; Long et al. [200]; and Shin et al. [199]. Significant associations are shown for Bonferroni adjusted *p*-values for each of three representative studies.

7. Conclusions

A primary goal of the emerging field of precision nutrition is to have the capacity to predict physiological and pathological outcomes of human diets based on a better understanding of interacting parameters such as an individual's genetic capacity to utilize/metabolize certain dietary nutrients and that same individual's dietary nutrient exposure. Insights gained from such studies also offer the potential to tailor nutritional recommendations and interventions to individuals and populations throughout the life span. The *FADS* cluster and *ELOVL2/5* genes are highly polymorphic, with considerable ancestry-based variation in the frequencies of common variants. These variants are associated with different conversion efficiencies of ALA and LA to *n*-3 LC-PUFAs and *n*-6 LC-PUFAs, respectively, and also important molecular and clinical phenotypes linking them to the pathogenesis of numerous human diseases. Additionally, the imbalance of LA and ALA in the MWD alone has been demonstrated to induce higher levels of *n*-6 LC-PUFA relative *n*-3 LC-PUFAs in circulation, cells and tissues. Considering the high heritability of LC-PUFA biosynthetic capacity (i.e., the strong genetic regulation), marked epigenetic regulation (i.e., potential gene environment interplay in regulation) and differences in dietary PUFA intake (i.e., variability in the environment), it is highly likely that *n*-3 LC-PUFA supplementation efficacy is individualized with a complex interplay of genetics, epigenetics and environment.

What are the implications of all this genetic and dietary complexity from a practical application perspective? It is clear that there have been incredible increases in consumption of LA-containing oils, such as soybean oil, in the evolution of the MWD over the past 75 years, and that these dietary changes have led to dramatic increases in LA/ALA ratios and ARA-derived metabolites, and reductions in both circulating and tissue levels of *n*-3 LC-PUFAs. This has occurred during a time of marked increases in obesity and obesity-related inflammatory diseases. Indeed, the concept of 'Omega-3 Deficiency Syndrome' introduced by Okuyama and colleagues [84] as Japanese populations moved from their native to a Western diet, may apply to most individuals exposed to the MWD. Consequently, we believe it is safe to say that a reduction in the dietary intake of LA and ARA, together with an increase in *n*-3 LC-PUFAs would benefit most individuals. However, the fact that there are such individual- and population-based genetic differences in the metabolism of dietary 18C-PUFAs, resulting in high, intermediate, and low blood levels of *n*-6 and *n*-3 LC-PUFAs and LC-PUFA metabolites, suggests that some populations and individuals will respond to *n*-3 LC-PUFA supplementation better than others. Based on this premise, it is important for future investigations that focus on *n*-3 LC-PUFA supplementation for the prevention and management of human diseases to develop therapeutic strategies taking into consideration the genetic heterogeneity in their study populations.

Acknowledgments: Funding support includes National Institutes of Health grants, P50-AT002782 and R01-AT008621 (F.H.C.) and the WFHS Department of Urology.

Author Contributions: F.H.C. conceived and designed the review. M.C.S., R.D., L.M.R., S.S., R.A.M. and F.H.C. analyzed published data and wrote the paper.

Conflicts of Interest: The authors declare no conflict of interest.

References

1. Blasbalg, T.L.; Hibbeln, J.R.; Ramsden, C.E.; Majchrzak, S.F.; Rawlings, R.R. Changes in consumption of omega-3 and omega-6 fatty acids in the United States during the 20th century. *Am. J. Clin. Nutr.* **2011**, *93*, 950–962. [CrossRef] [PubMed]
2. Chilton, F.H.; Murphy, R.C.; Wilson, B.A.; Sergeant, S.; Ainsworth, H.; Seeds, M.C.; Mathias, R.A. Diet-gene interactions and pufa metabolism: A potential contributor to health disparities and human diseases. *Nutrients* **2014**, *6*, 1993–2022. [CrossRef] [PubMed]
3. Cordain, L.; Eaton, S.B.; Sebastian, A.; Mann, N.; Lindeberg, S.; Watkins, B.A.; O'Keefe, J.H.; Brand-Miller, J. Origins and evolution of the Western diet: Health implications for the 21st century. *Am. J. Clin. Nutr.* **2005**, *81*, 341–354. [PubMed]
4. Popkin, B.M. Global nutrition dynamics: The world is shifting rapidly toward a diet linked with noncommunicable diseases. *Am. J. Clin. Nutr.* **2006**, *84*, 289–298. [PubMed]
5. Ferrante, A.W., Jr. Obesity-induced inflammation: A metabolic dialogue in the language of inflammation. *J. Intern. Med.* **2007**, *262*, 408–414. [CrossRef] [PubMed]
6. Hamminga, E.A.; van der Lely, A.J.; Neumann, H.A.; Thio, H.B. Chronic inflammation in psoriasis and obesity: Implications for therapy. *Med. Hypotheses* **2006**, *67*, 768–773. [CrossRef] [PubMed]
7. Forsythe, L.K.; Wallace, J.M.; Livingstone, M.B. Obesity and inflammation: The effects of weight loss. *Nutr. Res. Rev.* **2008**, *21*, 117–133. [CrossRef] [PubMed]

8. Nguyen, X.-M.T.; Lane, J.; Smith, B.R.; Nguyen, N.T. Changes in inflammatory biomarkers across weight classes in a representative US population: A link between obesity and inflammation. *J. Gastrointest. Surg.* **2009**, *13*, 1205–1212. [CrossRef] [PubMed]

9. Calle, E.E.; Thun, M.J. Obesity and cancer. *Oncogene* **2004**, *23*, 6365–6378. [CrossRef] [PubMed]

10. Beuther, D.A.; Weiss, S.T.; Sutherland, E.R. Obesity and asthma. *Am. J. Respir. Crit. Care Med.* **2006**, *174*, 112–119. [CrossRef] [PubMed]

11. Naderali, E.K.; Ratcliffe, S.H.; Dale, M.C. Obesity and Alzheimer's disease: A link between body weight and cognitive function in old age. *Am. J. Alzheimers Dis. Other Demen.* **2009**, *24*, 445–449. [CrossRef] [PubMed]

12. Leveille, S.G.; Wee, C.C.; Iezzoni, L.I. Trends in obesity and arthritis among baby boomers and their predecessors, 1971–2002. *Am. J. Public Health* **2005**, *95*, 1607–1613. [CrossRef] [PubMed]

13. Serini, S.; Calviello, G. Reduction of oxidative/nitrosative stress in brain and its involvement in the neuroprotective effect of *n*-3 pufa in Alzheimer's disease. *Curr. Alzheimer Res.* **2016**, *13*, 123–134. [CrossRef] [PubMed]

14. Lee, Y.J.; Han, S.B.; Nam, S.Y.; Oh, K.W.; Hong, J.T. Inflammation and Alzheimer's disease. *Arch. Pharmcal Res.* **2010**, *33*, 1539–1556. [CrossRef] [PubMed]

15. Sankar, P.; Cho, M.K.; Condit, C.M.; Hunt, L.M.; Koenig, B.; Marshall, P.; Lee, S.S.; Spicer, P. Genetic research and health disparities. *JAMA* **2004**, *291*, 2985–2989. [CrossRef] [PubMed]

16. Sankar, P.; Cho, M.K.; Mountain, J. Race and ethnicity in genetic research. *Am. J. Med. Genet.* **2007**, *143A*, 961–970. [CrossRef] [PubMed]

17. Mensah, G.A.; Mokdad, A.H.; Ford, E.S.; Greenlund, K.J.; Croft, J.B. State of disparities in cardiovascular health in the United States. *Circulation* **2005**, *111*, 1233–1241. [CrossRef] [PubMed]

18. Krieger, N.; Chen, J.T.; Waterman, P.D.; Soobader, M.J.; Subramanian, S.V.; Carson, R. Geocoding and monitoring of US socioeconomic inequalities in mortality and cancer incidence: Does the choice of area-based measure and geographic level matter? The Public Health Disparities Geocoding Project. *Am. J. Epidemiol.* **2002**, *156*, 471–482. [CrossRef] [PubMed]

19. Braveman, P. Health disparities and health equity: Concepts and measurement. *Annu. Rev. Public Health* **2006**, *27*, 167–194. [CrossRef] [PubMed]

20. Kuzawa, C.W.; Sweet, E. Epigenetics and the embodiment of race: Developmental origins of US racial disparities in cardiovascular health. *Am. J. Hum. Biol.* **2009**, *21*, 2–15. [CrossRef] [PubMed]

21. De Toro-Martin, J.; Arsenault, B.J.; Despres, J.P.; Vohl, M.C. Precision Nutrition: A review of personalized nutritional approaches for the prevention and management of metabolic syndrome. *Nutrients* **2017**, *9*, 913. [CrossRef] [PubMed]

22. American Heart Association & American Stroke Association. 50 Years of American Heart Association Dietary Fats Recommendations. 2015. Available online: http://www.heart.org/idc/groups/heart-public/@wcm/@fc/documents/downloadable/ucm_475005.pdf (accessed on 9 February 2017).

23. Miller, M.; Stone, N.J.; Ballantyne, C.; Bittner, V.; Criqui, M.H.; Ginsberg, H.N.; Goldberg, A.C.; Howard, W.J.; Jacobson, M.S.; Kris-Etherton, P.M.; et al. Triglycerides and cardiovascular disease: A scientific statement from the American Heart Association. *Circulation* **2011**, *123*, 2292–2333. [CrossRef] [PubMed]

24. Nutrient Content of the U.S. Food Supply, 1909-99: A Summary Report. U.S. Department of Agriculture, Center for Nutrition Policy and Promotion 2002, Home Economics Research Report No. 55. Available online: https://www.cnpp.usda.gov/sites/default/files/nutrient_content_of_the_us_food_supply/FoodSupply1909-1999Report.pdf (accessed on 9 February 2017).

25. Eaton, S.B. Humans, lipids and evolution. *Lipids* **1992**, *27*, 814–820. [CrossRef] [PubMed]

26. Hibbeln, J.R.; Nieminen, L.R.; Blasbalg, T.L.; Riggs, J.A.; Lands, W.E. Healthy intakes of *n*-3 and *n*-6 fatty acids: Estimations considering worldwide diversity. *Am. J. Clin. Nutr.* **2006**, *83*, 1483S–1493S. [PubMed]

27. Simopoulos, A.P. Importance of the omega-6/omega-3 balance in health and disease: Evolutionary aspects of diet. *World Rev. Nutr. Diet.* **2011**, *102*, 10–21. [PubMed]

28. Burr, G.O.; Burr, M.M. A new deficiency disease produced by the rigid exclusion of fat from the diet. *J. Biol. Chem.* **1929**, *82*, 345–367. [CrossRef]

29. Burr, G.O.; Burr, M.M. On the nature and role of the fatty acids essential in nutrition. *J. Biol. Chem.* **1930**, *86*, 587–621. [CrossRef]

30. Holman, R.T. Essential fatty acids. *Nutr. Rev.* **1958**, *16*, 33–35. [CrossRef] [PubMed]

31. Holman, R.T. The slow discovery of the importance of omega 3 essential fatty acids in human health. *J. Nutr.* **1998**, *128*, 427S–433S. [PubMed]

32. Sprecher, H. Biochemistry of essential fatty acids. *Prog. Lipid Res.* **1981**, *20*, 13–22. [CrossRef]

33. Sprecher, H.; Luthria, D.L.; Mohammed, B.S.; Baykousheva, S.P. Reevaluation of the pathways for the biosynthesis of polyunsaturated fatty acids. *J. Lipid Res.* **1995**, *36*, 2471–2477. [PubMed]

34. Sprecher, H.; Chen, Q. Polyunsaturated fatty acid biosynthesis: A microsomal-peroxisomal process. *Prostaglandins Leukot. Essent. Fat. Acids* **1999**, *60*, 317–321. [CrossRef]

35. Park, W.J.; Kothapalli, K.S.; Lawrence, P.; Tyburczy, C.; Brenna, J.T. An alternate pathway to long-chain polyunsaturates: The *FADS2* gene product Delta8-desaturates 20:2n-6 and 20:3n-3. *J. Lipid Res.* **2009**, *50*, 1195–1202. [CrossRef] [PubMed]

36. Mathias, R.A.; Pani, V.; Chilton, F.H. Genetic variants in the *FADS* gene: Implications for dietary recommendations for fatty acid intake. *Curr. Nutr. Rep.* **2014**, *3*, 139–148. [CrossRef] [PubMed]

37. Park, H.G.; Park, W.J.; Kothapalli, K.S.; Brenna, J.T. The fatty acid desaturase 2 (*FADS2*) gene product catalyzes Delta4 desaturation to yield *n*-3 docosahexaenoic acid and *n*-6 docosapentaenoic acid in human cells. *FASEB J.* **2015**, *29*, 3911–3919. [CrossRef] [PubMed]

38. Spector, A.A. Plasma free fatty acid and lipoproteins as sources of polyunsaturated fatty acid for the brain. *J. Mol. Neurosci.* **2001**, *16*, 159–165. [CrossRef]

39. Lands, W.E.; Hart, P. Metabolism of glycerolipids.VI. Specificities of acyl coenzyme A: Phospolipid acyltransferases. *J. Biol. Chem.* **1965**, *240*, 1905–1911. [PubMed]

40. Gibson, R.A.; Muhlhausler, B.; Makrides, M. Conversion of linoleic acid and alpha-linolenic acid to long-chain polyunsaturated fatty acids (LCPUFAs), with a focus on pregnancy, lactation and the first 2 years of life. *Matern. Child Nutr.* **2011**, *7* (Suppl. 2), 17–26. [CrossRef] [PubMed]

41. McNamara, R.K.; Carlson, S.E. Role of omega-3 fatty acids in brain development and function: Potential implications for the pathogenesis and prevention of psychopathology. *Prostaglandins Leukot. Essent. Fat. Acids* **2006**, *75*, 329–349. [CrossRef] [PubMed]

42. McCann, J.C.; Ames, B.N. Is docosahexaenoic acid, an *n*-3 long-chain polyunsaturated fatty acid, required for development of normal brain function? An overview of evidence from cognitive and behavioral tests in humans and animals. *Am. J. Clin. Nutr.* **2005**, *82*, 281–295. [PubMed]

43. Weiser, M.J.; Butt, C.M.; Mohajeri, M.H. Docosahexaenoic acid and cognition throughout the lifespan. *Nutrients* **2016**, *8*, 99. [CrossRef] [PubMed]

44. Hibbeln, J.R.; Davis, J.M.; Steer, C.; Emmett, P.; Rogers, I.; Williams, C.; Golding, J. Maternal seafood consumption in pregnancy and neurodevelopmental outcomes in childhood (ALSPAC study): An observational cohort study. *Lancet* **2007**, *369*, 578–585. [CrossRef]

45. Node, K.; Huo, Y.; Ruan, X.; Yang, B.; Spiecker, M.; Ley, K.; Zeldin, D.C.; Liao, J.K. Anti-inflammatory properties of cytochrome P450 epoxygenase-derived eicosanoids. *Science* **1999**, *285*, 1276–1279. [CrossRef] [PubMed]

46. Smith, W.L. The eicosanoids and their biochemical mechanisms of action. *Biochem. J.* **1989**, *259*, 315–324. [CrossRef] [PubMed]

47. Serhan, C.N.; Chiang, N.; Van Dyke, T.E. Resolving inflammation: Dual anti-inflammatory and pro-resolution lipid mediators. *Nat. Rev. Immunol.* **2008**, *8*, 349–361. [CrossRef] [PubMed]

48. Di Marzoa, V.M.D.; Bisogno, T.; De Petrocellis, L. Endocannabinoids: Endogenous cannabinoid receptor ligands with neuromodulatory action. *Trends Neurosci.* **1998**, *22*, 521–528. [CrossRef]

49. Buczynski, M.W.; Dumlao, D.S.; Dennis, E.A. Thematic Review Series: Proteomics. An integrated omics analysis of eicosanoid biology. *J. Lipid Res.* **2009**, *50*, 1015–1038. [CrossRef] [PubMed]

50. Chilton, F.H.; Fonteh, A.N.; Surette, M.E.; Triggiani, M.; Winkler, J.D. Control of arachidonate levels within inflammatory cells. *Biochim. Biophys. Acta* **1996**, *1299*, 1–15. [CrossRef]

51. Smith, W.L.; DeWitt, D.L.; Garavito, R.M. Cyclooxygenases: Structural, cellular, and molecular biology. *Annu. Rev. Biochem.* **2000**, *69*, 145–182. [CrossRef] [PubMed]

52. Haeggstrom, J.Z.; Funk, C.D. Lipoxygenase and leukotriene pathways: Biochemistry, biology, and roles in disease. *Chem. Rev.* **2011**, *111*, 5866–5898. [CrossRef] [PubMed]

53. Lands, W.E.; Libelt, B.; Morris, A.; Kramer, N.C.; Prewitt, T.E.; Bowen, P.; Schmeisser, D.; Davidson, M.H.; Burns, J.H. Maintenance of lower proportions of (*n*-6) eicosanoid precursors in phospholipids of human plasma in response to added dietary (*n*-3) fatty acids. *Biochim. Biophys. Acta* **1992**, *1180*, 147–162. [CrossRef]

54. James, M.J.; Gibson, R.A.; Cleland, L.G. Dietary polyunsaturated fatty acids and inflammatory mediator production. *Am. J. Clin. Nutr.* **2000**, *71*, 343S–348S. [PubMed]

55. Lands, B. A critique of paradoxes in current advice on dietary lipids. *Prog. Lipid Res.* **2008**, *47*, 77–106. [CrossRef] [PubMed]

56. Lands, B. Omega-3 PUFAs lower the propensity for arachidonic acid cascade overreactions. *Biomed. Res. Int.* **2015**, *2015*, 285135. [CrossRef] [PubMed]

57. Schmitz, G.; Ecker, J. The opposing effects of *n*-3 and *n*-6 fatty acids. *Prog. Lipid Res.* **2008**, *47*, 147–155. [CrossRef] [PubMed]

58. Serhan, C.N. Novel pro-resolving lipid mediators in inflammation are leads for resolution physiology. *Nature* **2014**, *510*, 92–101. [CrossRef] [PubMed]

59. Romano, M.; Cianci, E.; Simiele, F.; Recchiuti, A. Lipoxins and aspirin-triggered lipoxins in resolution of inflammation. *Eur. J. Pharmacol.* **2015**, *760*, 49–63. [CrossRef] [PubMed]

60. Berghuis, P.; Rajnicek, A.M.; Morozov, Y.M.; Ross, R.A.; Mulder, J.; Urban, G.M.; Monory, K.; Marsicano, G.; Matteoli, M.; Canty, A.; et al. Hardwiring the brain: Endocannabinoids shape neuronal connectivity. *Science* **2007**, *316*, 1212–1216. [CrossRef] [PubMed]

61. Matias, I.; Di Marzo, V. Endocannabinoids and the control of energy balance. *Trends Endocrinol. Metab.* **2007**, *18*, 27–37. [CrossRef] [PubMed]

62. Batkai, S.; Pacher, P.; Osei-Hyiaman, D.; Radaeva, S.; Liu, J.; Harvey-White, J.; Offertaler, L.; Mackie, K.; Rudd, M.A.; Bukoski, R.D.; et al. Endocannabinoids acting at cannabinoid-1 receptors regulate cardiovascular function in hypertension. *Circulation* **2004**, *110*, 1996–2002. [CrossRef] [PubMed]

63. Brown, I.; Cascio, M.G.; Rotondo, D.; Pertwee, R.G.; Heys, S.D.; Wahle, K.W. Cannabinoids and omega-3/6 endocannabinoids as cell death and anticancer modulators. *Prog. Lipid Res.* **2013**, *52*, 80–109. [CrossRef] [PubMed]

64. Brown, I.; Cascio, M.G.; Wahle, K.W.; Smoum, R.; Mechoulam, R.; Ross, R.A.; Pertwee, R.G.; Heys, S.D. Cannabinoid receptor-dependent and -independent anti-proliferative effects of omega-3 ethanolamides in androgen receptor-positive and -negative prostate cancer cell lines. *Carcinogenesis* **2010**, *31*, 1584–1591. [CrossRef] [PubMed]

65. McDougle, D.R.; Watson, J.E.; Abdeen, A.A.; Adili, R.; Caputo, M.P.; Krapf, J.E.; Johnson, R.W.; Kilian, K.A.; Holinstat, M.; Das, A. Anti-inflammatory omega-3 endocannabinoid epoxides. *Proc. Natl. Acad. Sci. USA* **2017**, *114*, E6034–E6043. [CrossRef] [PubMed]

66. Araque, A.; Castillo, P.E.; Manzoni, O.J.; Tonini, R. Synaptic functions of endocannabinoid signaling in health and disease. *Neuropharmacology* **2017**, *124*, 13–24. [CrossRef] [PubMed]

67. Ashton, J.C.; Glass, M. The cannabinoid CB2 receptor as a target for inflammation-dependent neurodegeneration. *Curr. Neuropharmacol.* **2007**, *5*, 73–80. [CrossRef] [PubMed]

68. Skaper, S.D.; Di Marzo, V. Endocannabinoids in nervous system health and disease: The big picture in a nutshell. *Philos. Trans. R. Soc. Lond. B Biol. Sci.* **2012**, *367*, 3193–3200. [CrossRef] [PubMed]

69. Sloan, M.E.; Gowin, J.L.; Ramchandani, V.A.; Hurd, Y.L.; Le Foll, B. The endocannabinoid system as a target for addiction treatment: Trials and tribulations. *Neuropharmacology* **2017**, *124*, 73–83. [CrossRef] [PubMed]

70. Murillo-Rodriguez, E.; Poot-Ake, A.; Arias-Carrion, O.; Pacheco-Pantoja, E.; Fuente-Ortegon Ade, L.; Arankowsky-Sandoval, G. The emerging role of the endocannabinoid system in the sleep-wake cycle modulation. *Cent. Nerv. Syst. Agents Med. Chem.* **2011**, *11*, 189–196. [CrossRef] [PubMed]

71. Malek, N.; Starowicz, K. Dual-acting compounds targeting endocannabinoid and endovanilloid systems-a novel treatment option for chronic pain management. *Front. Pharmacol.* **2016**, *7*, 257. [CrossRef] [PubMed]

72. Lau, B.K.; Cota, D.; Cristino, L.; Borgland, S.L. Endocannabinoid modulation of homeostatic and non-homeostatic feeding circuits. *Neuropharmacology* **2017**, *124*, 38–51. [CrossRef] [PubMed]

73. Kruk-Slomka, M.; Dzik, A.; Budzynska, B.; Biala, G. Endocannabinoid system: The direct and indirect involvement in the memory and learning processes-a short review. *Mol. Neurobiol.* **2016**. [CrossRef] [PubMed]

74. Hedlund, P.; Gratzke, C. The endocannabinoid system—A target for the treatment of LUTS? *Nat. Rev. Urol.* **2016**, *13*, 463–470. [CrossRef] [PubMed]

75. Giaginis, C.; Lakiotaki, E.; Korkolopoulou, P.; Konstantopoulos, K.; Patsouris, E.; Theocharis, S. Endocannabinoid system: A promising therapeutic target for the treatment of haematological malignancies? *Curr. Med. Chem.* **2016**, *23*, 2350–2362. [CrossRef] [PubMed]

76. Fonseca, B.M.; Costa, M.A.; Almada, M.; Correia-da-Silva, G.; Teixeira, N.A. Endogenous cannabinoids revisited: A biochemistry perspective. *Prostaglandins Other Lipid Mediat.* **2013**, *102–103*, 13–30. [CrossRef] [PubMed]

77. Rouzer, C.A.; Marnett, L.J. Endocannabinoid oxygenation by cyclooxygenases, lipoxygenases, and cytochromes P450: Cross-talk between the eicosanoid and endocannabinoid signaling pathways. *Chem. Rev.* **2011**, *111*, 5899–5921. [CrossRef] [PubMed]

78. Ramsden, C.E.; Hibbeln, J.R.; Majchrzak, S.F.; Davis, J.M. *n*-6 fatty acid-specific and mixed polyunsaturate dietary interventions have different effects on CHD risk: A meta-analysis of randomised controlled trials. *Br. J. Nutr.* **2010**, *104*, 1586–1600. [CrossRef] [PubMed]

79. Ramsden, C.E.; Zamora, D.; Majchrzak-Hong, S.; Faurot, K.R.; Broste, S.K.; Frantz, R.P.; Davis, J.M.; Ringel, A.; Suchindran, C.M.; Hibbeln, J.R. Re-evaluation of the traditional diet-heart hypothesis: Analysis of recovered data from Minnesota Coronary Experiment (1968-73). *BMJ* **2016**, *353*, i1246. [CrossRef] [PubMed]

80. Lands, B. Dietary omega-3 and omega-6 fatty acids compete in producing tissue compositions and tissue responses. *Mil. Med.* **2014**, *179*, 76–81. [CrossRef] [PubMed]

81. Liou, Y.A.; King, D.J.; Zibrik, D.; Innis, S.M. Decreasing linoleic acid with constant alpha-linolenic acid in dietary fats increases (*n*-3) eicosapentaenoic acid in plasma phospholipids in healthy men. *J. Nutr.* **2007**, *137*, 945–952. [PubMed]

82. Wood, K.E.; Mantzioris, E.; Gibson, R.A.; Ramsden, C.E.; Muhlhausler, B.S. The effect of modifying dietary LA and ALA intakes on omega-3 long chain polyunsaturated fatty acid (*n*-3 LCPUFA) status in human adults: A systematic review and commentary. *Prostaglandins Leukot. Essent. Fat. Acids* **2015**, *95*, 47–55. [CrossRef] [PubMed]

83. Macintosh, B.A.; Ramsden, C.E.; Faurot, K.R.; Zamora, D.; Mangan, M.; Hibbeln, J.R.; Mann, J.D. Low-*n*-6 and low-*n*-6 plus high-*n*-3 diets for use in clinical research. *Br. J. Nutr.* **2013**, 1–10. [CrossRef] [PubMed]

84. Okuyama, H. Dietary fatty acids—The *N*-6/*N*-3 balance and chronic elderly diseases. Excess linoleic acid and relative *N*-3 deficiency syndrome seen in Japan. *Prog. Lipid Res.* **1996**, *35*, 409–457. [CrossRef]

85. Cleland, L.G.; James, M.J.; Neumann, M.A.; D'Angelo, M.; Gibson, R.A. Linoleate inhibits EPA incorporation from dietary fish-oil supplements in human subjects. *Am. J. Clin. Nutr.* **1992**, *55*, 395–399. [PubMed]

86. Blank, C.; Neumann, M.A.; Makrides, M.; Gibson, R.A. Optimizing DHA levels in piglets by lowering the linoleic acid to alpha-linolenic acid ratio. *J. Lipid Res.* **2002**, *43*, 1537–1543. [CrossRef] [PubMed]

87. Wood, K.E.; Lau, A.; Mantzioris, E.; Gibson, R.A.; Ramsden, C.E.; Muhlhausler, B.S. A low omega-6 polyunsaturated fatty acid (*n*-6 PUFA) diet increases omega-3 (*n*-3) long chain PUFA status in plasma phospholipids in humans. *Prostaglandins Leukot. Essent. Fat. Acids* **2014**, *90*, 133–138. [CrossRef] [PubMed]

88. Brenna, J.T.; Salem, N., Jr.; Sinclair, A.J.; Cunnane, S.C.; International Society for the Study of Fatty, Acids and Lipids, ISSFAL. alpha-Linolenic acid supplementation and conversion to *n*-3 long-chain polyunsaturated fatty acids in humans. *Prostaglandins Leukot. Essent. Fat. Acids* **2009**, *80*, 85–91. [CrossRef] [PubMed]

89. Arterburn, L.M.; Hall, E.B.; Oken, H. Distribution, interconversion, and dose response of *n*-3 fatty acids in humans. *Am. J. Clin. Nutr.* **2006**, *83*, 1467S–1476S. [PubMed]

90. Goyens, P.L.; Spilker, M.E.; Zock, P.L.; Katan, M.B.; Mensink, R.P. Conversion of alpha-linolenic acid in humans is influenced by the absolute amounts of alpha-linolenic acid and linoleic acid in the diet and not by their ratio. *Am. J. Clin. Nutr.* **2006**, *84*, 44–53. [PubMed]

91. Schaeffer, L.; Gohlke, H.; Muller, M.; Heid, I.M.; Palmer, L.J.; Kompauer, I.; Demmelmair, H.; Illig, T.; Koletzko, B.; Heinrich, J. Common genetic variants of the *FADS1 FADS2* gene cluster and their reconstructed haplotypes are associated with the fatty acid composition in phospholipids. *Hum. Mol. Genet.* **2006**, *15*, 1745–1756. [CrossRef] [PubMed]

92. Malerba, G.; Schaeffer, L.; Xumerle, L.; Klopp, N.; Trabetti, E.; Biscuola, M.; Cavallari, U.; Galavotti, R.; Martinelli, N.; Guarini, P.; et al. SNPs of the *FADS* gene cluster are associated with polyunsaturated fatty acids in a cohort of patients with cardiovascular disease. *Lipids* **2008**, *43*, 289–299. [CrossRef] [PubMed]

93. Xie, L.; Innis, S.M. Genetic variants of the *FADS1 FADS2* gene cluster are associated with altered (*n*-6) and (*n*-3) essential fatty acids in plasma and erythrocyte phospholipids in women during pregnancy and in breast milk during lactation. *J. Nutr.* **2008**, *138*, 2222–2228. [CrossRef] [PubMed]

94. Tanaka, T.; Shen, J.; Abecasis, G.R.; Kisialiou, A.; Ordovas, J.M.; Guralnik, J.M.; Singleton, A.; Bandinelli, S.; Cherubini, A.; Arnett, D.; et al. Genome-wide association study of plasma polyunsaturated fatty acids in the InCHIANTI Study. *PLoS Genet.* **2009**, *5*, e1000338. [CrossRef] [PubMed]

95. Rzehak, P.; Heinrich, J.; Klopp, N.; Schaeffer, L.; Hoff, S.; Wolfram, G.; Illig, T.; Linseisen, J. Evidence for an association between genetic variants of the fatty acid desaturase 1 fatty acid desaturase 2 (*FADS1 FADS2*) gene cluster and the fatty acid composition of erythrocyte membranes. *Br. J. Nutr.* **2009**, *101*, 20–26. [CrossRef] [PubMed]

96. Xie, L.; Innis, S.M. Association of fatty acid desaturase gene polymorphisms with blood lipid essential fatty acids and perinatal depression among Canadian women: A pilot study. *J. Nutrigenet. Nutrigenom.* **2009**, *2*, 243–250. [CrossRef] [PubMed]

97. Mathias, R.A.; Vergara, C.; Gao, L.; Rafaels, N.; Hand, T.; Campbell, M.; Bickel, C.; Ivester, P.; Sergeant, S.; Barnes, K.C.; et al. *FADS* genetic variants and omega-6 polyunsaturated fatty acid metabolism in a homogeneous island population. *J. Lipid Res.* **2010**, *51*, 2766–2774. [CrossRef] [PubMed]

98. Bokor, S.; Dumont, J.; Spinneker, A.; Gonzalez-Gross, M.; Nova, E.; Widhalm, K.; Moschonis, G.; Stehle, P.; Amouyel, P.; De, H.S.; et al. Single nucleotide polymorphisms in the *FADS* gene cluster are associated with delta-5 and delta-6 desaturase activities estimated by serum fatty acid ratios. *J. Lipid Res.* **2010**, *51*, 2325–2333. [CrossRef] [PubMed]

99. Rzehak, P.; Thijs, C.; Standl, M.; Mommers, M.; Glaser, C.; Jansen, E.; Klopp, N.; Koppelman, G.H.; Singmann, P.; Postma, D.S.; et al. Variants of the *FADS1 FADS2* gene cluster, blood levels of polyunsaturated fatty acids and eczema in children within the first 2 years of life. *PLoS ONE* **2010**, *5*, e13261. [CrossRef] [PubMed]

100. Mathias, R.A.; Sergeant, S.; Ruczinski, I.; Torgerson, D.G.; Hugenschmidt, C.E.; Kubala, M.; Vaidya, D.; Suktitipat, B.; Ziegler, J.T.; Ivester, P.; et al. The impact of FADS genetic variants on omega6 polyunsaturated fatty acid metabolism in African Americans. *BMC Genet.* **2011**, *12*, 50. [CrossRef] [PubMed]

101. Lemaitre, R.N.; Tanaka, T.; Tang, W.; Manichaikul, A.; Foy, M.; Kabagambe, E.K.; Nettleton, J.A.; King, I.B.; Weng, L.C.; Bhattacharya, S.; et al. Genetic loci associated with plasma phospholipid *n*-3 fatty acids: A meta-analysis of genome-wide association studies from the CHARGE Consortium. *PLoS Genet.* **2011**, *7*, e1002193. [CrossRef] [PubMed]

102. Morales, E.; Bustamante, M.; Gonzalez, J.R.; Guxens, M.; Torrent, M.; Mendez, M.; Garcia-Esteban, R.; Julvez, J.; Forns, J.; Vrijheid, M.; et al. Genetic variants of the *FADS* gene cluster and *ELOVL* gene family, colostrums LC-PUFA levels, breastfeeding, and child cognition. *PLoS ONE* **2011**, *6*, e17181. [CrossRef] [PubMed]

103. Lattka, E.; Rzehak, P.; Szabo, E.; Jakobik, V.; Weck, M.; Weyermann, M.; Grallert, H.; Rothenbacher, D.; Heinrich, J.; Brenner, H.; et al. Genetic variants in the *FADS* gene cluster are associated with arachidonic acid concentrations of human breast milk at 1.5 and 6 mo postpartum and influence the course of milk dodecanoic, tetracosenoic, and trans-9-octadecenoic acid concentrations over the duration of lactation. *Am. J. Clin. Nutr.* **2011**, *93*, 382–391. [PubMed]

104. Koletzko, B.; Lattka, E.; Zeilinger, S.; Illig, T.; Steer, C. Genetic variants of the fatty acid desaturase gene cluster predict amounts of red blood cell docosahexaenoic and other polyunsaturated fatty acids in pregnant women: Findings from the Avon Longitudinal Study of Parents and Children. *Am. J. Clin. Nutr.* **2011**, *93*, 211–219. [CrossRef] [PubMed]

105. Kwak, J.H.; Paik, J.K.; Kim, O.Y.; Jang, Y.; Lee, S.H.; Ordovas, J.M.; Lee, J.H. *FADS* gene polymorphisms in Koreans: Association with omega6 polyunsaturated fatty acids in serum phospholipids, lipid peroxides, and coronary artery disease. *Atherosclerosis* **2011**, *214*, 94–100. [CrossRef] [PubMed]

106. Sergeant, S.; Hugenschmidt, C.E.; Rudock, M.E.; Ziegler, J.T.; Ivester, P.; Ainsworth, H.C.; Vaidya, D.; Case, L.D.; Langefeld, C.D.; Freedman, B.I.; et al. Differences in arachidonic acid levels and fatty acid desaturase (*FADS*) gene variants in African Americans and European Americans with diabetes or the metabolic syndrome. *Br. J. Nutr.* **2012**, *107*, 547–555. [CrossRef] [PubMed]

107. Steer, C.D.; Hibbeln, J.R.; Golding, J.; Davey, S.G. Polyunsaturated fatty acid levels in blood during pregnancy, at birth and at 7 years: Their associations with two common *FADS2* polymorphisms. *Hum. Mol. Genet.* **2012**, *21*, 1504–1512. [CrossRef] [PubMed]

108. Porenta, S.R.; Ko, Y.A.; Gruber, S.B.; Mukherjee, B.; Baylin, A.; Ren, J.; Djuric, Z. Interaction of fatty acid genotype and diet on changes in colonic fatty acids in a Mediterranean diet intervention study. *Cancer Prev. Res.* **2013**, *6*, 1212–1221. [CrossRef] [PubMed]

109. Hong, S.H.; Kwak, J.H.; Paik, J.K.; Chae, J.S.; Lee, J.H. Association of polymorphisms in *FADS* gene with age-related changes in serum phospholipid polyunsaturated fatty acids and oxidative stress markers in middle-aged nonobese men. *Clin. Interv. Aging* **2013**, *8*, 585–596. [PubMed]

110. Harslof, L.B.; Larsen, L.H.; Ritz, C.; Hellgren, L.I.; Michaelsen, K.F.; Vogel, U.; Lauritzen, L. *FADS* genotype and diet are important determinants of DHA status: A cross-sectional study in Danish infants. *Am. J. Clin. Nutr.* **2013**, *97*, 1403–1410. [CrossRef] [PubMed]

111. Li, S.W.; Lin, K.; Ma, P.; Zhang, Z.L.; Zhou, Y.D.; Lu, S.Y.; Zhou, X.; Liu, S.M. *FADS* gene polymorphisms confer the risk of coronary artery disease in a Chinese Han population through the altered desaturase activities: Based on high-resolution melting analysis. *PLoS ONE* **2013**, *8*, e55869. [CrossRef] [PubMed]

112. Gillingham, L.G.; Harding, S.V.; Rideout, T.C.; Yurkova, N.; Cunnane, S.C.; Eck, P.K.; Jones, P.J. Dietary oils and *FADS1-FADS2* genetic variants modulate (13C)alpha-linolenic acid metabolism and plasma fatty acid composition. *Am. J. Clin. Nutr.* **2013**, *97*, 195–207. [CrossRef] [PubMed]

113. Freemantle, E.; Lalovic, A.; Mechawar, N.; Turecki, G. Age and haplotype variations within *FADS1* interact and associate with alterations in fatty acid composition in human male cortical brain tissue. *PLoS ONE* **2012**, *7*, e42696. [CrossRef] [PubMed]

114. Lattka, E.; Koletzko, B.; Zeilinger, S.; Hibbeln, J.R.; Klopp, N.; Ring, S.M.; Steer, C.D. Umbilical cord PUFA are determined by maternal and child fatty acid desaturase (*FADS*) genetic variants in the Avon Longitudinal Study of Parents and Children (ALSPAC). *Br. J. Nutr.* **2013**, *109*, 1196–1210. [CrossRef] [PubMed]

115. Tintle, N.L.; Pottala, J.V.; Lacey, S.; Ramachandran, V.; Westra, J.; Rogers, A.; Clark, J.; Olthoff, B.; Larson, M.; Harris, W.; et al. A genome-wide association study of saturated, mono- and polyunsaturated red blood cell fatty acids in the Framingham Heart Offspring Study. *Prostaglandins Leukot. Essent. Fat. Acids* **2015**, *94*, 65–72. [CrossRef] [PubMed]

116. Martinelli, N.; Girelli, D.; Malerba, G.; Guarini, P.; Illig, T.; Trabetti, E.; Sandri, M.; Friso, S.; Pizzolo, F.; Schaeffer, L.; et al. *FADS* genotypes and desaturase activity estimated by the ratio of arachidonic acid to linoleic acid are associated with inflammation and coronary artery disease. *Am. J. Clin. Nutr.* **2008**, *88*, 941–949. [PubMed]

117. Ameur, A.; Enroth, S.; Johansson, A.; Zaboli, G.; Igl, W.; Johansson, A.C.; Rivas, M.A.; Daly, M.J.; Schmitz, G.; Hicks, A.A.; et al. Genetic adaptation of fatty-acid metabolism: A human-specific haplotype increasing the biosynthesis of long-chain omega-3 and omega-6 fatty acids. *Am. J. Hum. Genet.* **2012**, *90*, 809–820. [CrossRef] [PubMed]

118. Amorim, C.E.; Nunes, K.; Meyer, D.; Comas, D.; Bortolini, M.C.; Salzano, F.M.; Hunemeier, T. Genetic signature of natural selection in first Americans. *Proc. Natl. Acad. Sci. USA* **2017**, *114*, 2195–2199. [CrossRef] [PubMed]

119. Mathias, R.A.; Fu, W.Q.; Akey, J.M.; Ainsworth, H.C.; Torgerson, D.G.; Ruczinski, I.; Sergeant, S.; Barnes, K.C.; Chilton, F.H. Adaptive evolution of the *FADS* gene cluster within africa. *PLoS ONE* **2012**, *7*, e44926. [CrossRef] [PubMed]

120. Dorajoo, R.; Sun, Y.; Han, Y.; Ke, T.; Burger, A.; Chang, X.; Low, H.Q.; Guan, W.; Lemaitre, R.N.; Khor, C.C.; et al. A genome-wide association study of *n*-3 and *n*-6 plasma fatty acids in a Singaporean Chinese population. *Genes Nutr.* **2015**, *10*, 53. [CrossRef] [PubMed]

121. Guan, W.; Steffen, B.T.; Lemaitre, R.N.; Wu, J.H.Y.; Tanaka, T.; Manichaikul, A.; Foy, M.; Rich, S.S.; Wang, L.; Nettleton, J.A.; et al. Genome-wide association study of plasma N6 polyunsaturated fatty acids within the cohorts for heart and aging research in genomic epidemiology consortium. *Circ. Cardiovasc. Genet.* **2014**, *7*, 321–331. [CrossRef] [PubMed]

122. Hu, Y.; Li, H.; Lu, L.; Manichaikul, A.; Zhu, J.; Chen, Y.D.; Sun, L.; Liang, S.; Siscovick, D.S.; Steffen, L.M.; et al. Genome-wide meta-analyses identify novel loci associated with *n*-3 and *n*-6 polyunsaturated fatty acid levels in Chinese and European-ancestry populations. *Hum. Mol. Genet.* **2016**, *25*, 1215–1224. [CrossRef] [PubMed]

123. Lattka, E.; Illig, T.; Heinrich, J.; Koletzko, B. Do *FADS* genotypes enhance our knowledge about fatty acid related phenotypes? *Clin. Nutr.* **2010**, *29*, 277–287. [CrossRef] [PubMed]

124. Chambers, J.C.; Zhang, W.; Sehmi, J.; Li, X.; Wass, M.N.; Van der Harst, P.; Holm, H.; Sanna, S.; Kavousi, M.; Baumeister, S.E.; et al. Genome-wide association study identifies loci influencing concentrations of liver enzymes in plasma. *Nat. Genet.* **2011**, *43*, 1131–1138. [CrossRef] [PubMed]

125. Mirkov, S.; Myers, J.L.; Ramirez, J.; Liu, W. SNPs affecting serum metabolomic traits may regulate gene transcription and lipid accumulation in the liver. *Metabolism* **2012**, *61*, 1523–1527. [CrossRef] [PubMed]

126. Dupuis, J.; Langenberg, C.; Prokopenko, I.; Saxena, R.; Soranzo, N.; Jackson, A.U.; Wheeler, E.; Glazer, N.L.; Bouatia-Naji, N.; Gloyn, A.L.; et al. New genetic loci implicated in fasting glucose homeostasis and their impact on type 2 diabetes risk. *Nat. Genet.* **2010**, *42*, 105–116. [CrossRef] [PubMed]

127. Burghardt, K.J.; Gardner, K.N.; Johnson, J.W.; Ellingrod, V.L. Fatty Acid desaturase gene polymorphisms and metabolic measures in schizophrenia and bipolar patients taking antipsychotics. *Cardiovasc. Psychiatry Neurol.* **2013**, *2013*, 596945. [CrossRef] [PubMed]

128. Standl, M.; Lattka, E.; Stach, B.; Koletzko, S.; Bauer, C.P.; von, B.A.; Berdel, D.; Kramer, U.; Schaaf, B.; Roder, S.; et al. FADS1 FADS2 gene cluster, PUFA intake and blood lipids in children: Results from the GINIplus and LISAplus studies. *PLoS ONE* **2012**, *7*, e37780. [CrossRef] [PubMed]

129. Fumagalli, M.; Moltke, I.; Grarup, N.; Racimo, F.; Bjerregaard, P.; Jorgensen, M.E.; Korneliussen, T.S.; Gerbault, P.; Skotte, L.; Linneberg, A.; et al. Greenlandic Inuit show genetic signatures of diet and climate adaptation. *Science* **2015**, *349*, 1343–1347. [CrossRef] [PubMed]

130. Harris, D.N.; Ruczinski, I.; Yanek, L.R.; Becker, L.C.; Guio, H.; Cui, T.; Chilton, F.H.; Mathias, R.A.; O'Conner, T. Evolution of hominim polyunsatruated fatty acid metabolism; from Africa to the New World. *BioRxiv* **2017**. [CrossRef]

131. Mathieson, I.; Lazaridis, I.; Rohland, N.; Mallick, S.; Patterson, N.; Roodenberg, S.A.; Harney, E.; Stewardson, K.; Fernandes, D.; Novak, M.; et al. Genome-wide patterns of selection in 230 ancient Eurasians. *Nature* **2015**, *528*, 499–503. [CrossRef] [PubMed]

132. Kothapalli, K.S.; Ye, K.; Gadgil, M.S.; Carlson, S.E.; O'Brien, K.O.; Zhang, J.Y.; Park, H.G.; Ojukwu, K.; Zou, J.; Hyon, S.S.; et al. Positive selection on a regulatory insertion-deletion polymorphism in FADS2 influences apparent endogenous synthesis of arachidonic acid. *Mol. Biol. Evol.* **2016**, *33*, 1726–1739. [CrossRef] [PubMed]

133. Buckley, M.T.; Racimo, F.; Allentoft, M.E.; Jensen, M.K.; Jonsson, A.; Huang, H.; Hormozdiari, F.; Sikora, M.; Marnetto, D.; Eskin, E.; et al. Selection in europeans on fatty acid desaturases associated with dietary changes. *Mol. Biol. Evol.* **2017**, *34*, 1307–1318. [CrossRef] [PubMed]

134. Sabeti, P.C.; Varilly, P.; Fry, B.; Lohmueller, J.; Hostetter, E.; Cotsapas, C.; Xie, X.; Byrne, E.H.; McCarroll, S.A.; Gaudet, R.; et al. Genome-wide detection and characterization of positive selection in human populations. *Nature* **2007**, *449*, 913–918. [CrossRef] [PubMed]

135. Enattah, N.S.; Sahi, T.; Savilahti, E.; Terwilliger, J.D.; Peltonen, L.; Jarvela, I. Identification of a variant associated with adult-type hypolactasia. *Nat. Genet.* **2002**, *30*, 233–237. [CrossRef] [PubMed]

136. Tishkoff, S.A.; Reed, F.A.; Ranciaro, A.; Voight, B.F.; Babbitt, C.C.; Silverman, J.S.; Powell, K.; Mortensen, H.M.; Hirbo, J.B.; Osman, M.; et al. Convergent adaptation of human lactase persistence in Africa and Europe. *Nat. Genet.* **2007**, *39*, 31–40. [CrossRef] [PubMed]

137. Lettre, G.; Palmer, C.D.; Young, T.; Ejebe, K.G.; Allayee, H.; Benjamin, E.J.; Bennett, F.; Bowden, D.W.; Chakravarti, A.; Dreisbach, A.; et al. Genome-wide association study of coronary heart disease and its risk factors in 8,090 African Americans: The NHLBI CARe Project. *PLoS Genet.* **2011**, *7*, e1001300. [CrossRef] [PubMed]

138. Kark, J.D.; Kaufmann, N.A.; Binka, F.; Goldberger, N.; Berry, E.M. Adipose tissue *n*-6 fatty acids and acute myocardial infarction in a population consuming a diet high in polyunsaturated fatty acids. *Am. J. Clin. Nutr.* **2003**, *77*, 796–802. [PubMed]

139. Baylin, A.; Campos, H. Arachidonic acid in adipose tissue is associated with nonfatal acute myocardial infarction in the central valley of Costa Rica. *J. Nutr.* **2004**, *134*, 3095–3099. [PubMed]

140. Hester, A.G.; Murphy, R.C.; Uhlson, C.J.; Ivester, P.; Lee, T.C.; Sergeant, S.; Miller, L.R.; Howard, T.D.; Mathias, R.A.; Chilton, F.H. Relationship between a common variant in the fatty acid desaturase (*FADS*) cluster and eicosanoid generation in humans. *J. Biol. Chem.* **2014**, *289*, 22482–22489. [CrossRef] [PubMed]

141. Park, J.Y.; Paik, J.K.; Kim, O.Y.; Chae, J.S.; Jang, Y.; Lee, J.H. Interactions between the APOA5-1131T>C and the FEN1 10154G>T polymorphisms on omega6 polyunsaturated fatty acids in serum phospholipids and coronary artery disease. *J. Lipid Res.* **2010**, *51*, 3281–3288. [CrossRef] [PubMed]

142. Hellstrand, S.; Ericson, U.; Gullberg, B.; Hedblad, B.; Orho-Melander, M.; Sonestedt, E. Genetic variation in *FADS1* has little effect on the association between dietary PUFA intake and cardiovascular disease. *J. Nutr.* **2014**, *144*, 1356–1363. [CrossRef] [PubMed]

143. O'Neill, C.M.; Minihane, A.M. The impact of fatty acid desaturase genotype on fatty acid status and cardiovascular health in adults. *Proc. Nutr. Soc.* **2017**, *76*, 64–75. [CrossRef] [PubMed]

144. Miller, L.R.; Jorgensen, M.J.; Kaplan, J.R.; Seeds, M.C.; Rahbar, E.; Morgan, T.M.; Welborn, A.; Chilton, S.M.; Gillis, J.; Hester, A.; et al. Alterations in levels and ratios of *n*-3 and *n*-6 polyunsaturated fatty acids in the temporal cortex and liver of vervet monkeys from birth to early adulthood. *Physiol. Behav.* **2016**, *156*, 71–78. [CrossRef] [PubMed]

145. Kitson, A.P.; Stark, K.D.; Duncan, R.E. Enzymes in brain phospholipid docosahexaenoic acid accretion: A PL-ethora of potential PL-ayers. *Prostaglandins Leukot. Essent. Fat. Acids* **2012**, *87*, 1–10. [CrossRef] [PubMed]

146. Kuipers, R.S.; Luxwolda, M.F.; Offringa, P.J.; Boersma, E.R.; Dijck-Brouwer, D.A.; Muskiet, F.A. Fetal intrauterine whole body linoleic, arachidonic and docosahexaenoic acid contents and accretion rates. *Prostaglandins Leukot. Essent. Fat. Acids* **2012**, *86*, 13–20. [CrossRef] [PubMed]

147. Cheatham, C.L.; Lupu, D.S.; Niculescu, M.D. Genetic and epigenetic transgenerational implications related to omega-3 fatty acids. Part II: Maternal *FADS2* rs174575 genotype and DNA methylation predict toddler cognitive performance. *Nutr. Res.* **2015**, *35*, 948–955. [CrossRef] [PubMed]

148. Lupu, D.S.; Cheatham, C.L.; Corbin, K.D.; Niculescu, M.D. Genetic and epigenetic transgenerational implications related to omega-3 fatty acids. Part I: Maternal *FADS2* genotype and DNA methylation correlate with polyunsaturated fatty acid status in toddlers: An exploratory analysis. *Nutr. Res.* **2015**, *35*, 939–947. [CrossRef] [PubMed]

149. Hoile, S.P.; Clarke-Harris, R.; Huang, R.C.; Calder, P.C.; Mori, T.A.; Beilin, L.J.; Lillycrop, K.A.; Burdge, G.C. Supplementation with *N*-3 long-chain polyunsaturated fatty acids or olive oil in men and women with renal disease induces differential changes in the DNA methylation of *FADS2* and *ELOVL5* in peripheral blood mononuclear cells. *PLoS ONE* **2014**, *9*, e109896. [CrossRef] [PubMed]

150. Howard, T.D.; Mathias, R.A.; Seeds, M.C.; Herrington, D.M.; Hixson, J.E.; Shimmin, L.C.; Hawkins, G.A.; Sellers, M.; Ainsworth, H.C.; Sergeant, S.; et al. DNA methylation in an enhancer region of the *FADS* cluster is associated with fads activity in human liver. *PLoS ONE* **2014**, *9*, e97510. [CrossRef] [PubMed]

151. Hoile, S.P.; Irvine, N.A.; Kelsall, C.J.; Sibbons, C.; Feunteun, A.; Collister, A.; Torrens, C.; Calder, P.C.; Hanson, M.A.; Lillycrop, K.A.; et al. Maternal fat intake in rats alters 20:4*n*-6 and 22:6*n*-3 status and the epigenetic regulation of *FADS2* in offspring liver. *J. Nutr. Biochem.* **2013**, *24*, 1213–1220. [CrossRef] [PubMed]

152. Bang, H.O.; Dyerberg, J.; Nielsen, A.B. Plasma lipid and lipoprotein pattern in Greenlandic West-coast Eskimos. *Lancet* **1971**, *1*, 1143–1145. [CrossRef]

153. Dyerberg, J.; Bang, H.O. Haemostatic function and platelet polyunsaturated fatty acids in Eskimos. *Lancet* **1979**, *2*, 433–435. [CrossRef]

154. Ander, B.P.; Dupasquier, C.M.; Prociuk, M.A.; Pierce, G.N. Polyunsaturated fatty acids and their effects on cardiovascular disease. *Exp. Clin. Cardiol.* **2003**, *8*, 164–172. [PubMed]

155. Burr, M.L.; Fehily, A.M.; Gilbert, J.F.; Rogers, S.; Holliday, R.M.; Sweetnam, P.M.; Elwood, P.C.; Deadman, N.M. Effects of changes in fat, fish, and fibre intakes on death and myocardial reinfarction: Diet and reinfarction trial (DART). *Lancet* **1989**, *2*, 757–761. [CrossRef]

156. Investigators, G.-P. Dietray supplementation with *n*-3 polyunsaturated fatty acids and vitamin E after myocardial infarction: Results of the GISSIPrevenzione trial. *Lancet* **1999**, *354*, 447–455.

157. Marchioli, R.; Barzi, F.; Bomba, E.; Chieffo, C.; Di Gregorio, D.; Di Mascio, R.; Franzosi, M.G.; Geraci, E.; Levantesi, G.; Maggioni, A.P.; et al. Early protection against sudden death by *n*-3 polyunsaturated fatty acids after myocardial infarction: Time-course analysis of the results of the Gruppo Italiano per lo Studio della Sopravvivenza nell'Infarto Miocardico (GISSI)-Prevenzione. *Circulation* **2002**, *105*, 1897–1903. [CrossRef] [PubMed]

158. Yokoyama, M.; Origasa, H.; Matsuzaki, M.; Matsuzawa, Y.; Saito, Y.; Ishikawa, Y.; Oikawa, S.; Sasaki, J.; Hishida, H.; Itakura, H.; et al. Effects of eicosapentaenoic acid on major coronary events in hypercholesterolaemic patients (JELIS): A randomised open-label, blinded endpoint analysis. *Lancet* **2007**, *369*, 1090–1098. [CrossRef]

159. Tavazzi, L.; Tognoni, G.; Franzosi, M.G.; Latini, R.; Maggioni, A.P.; Marchioli, R.; Nicolosi, G.L.; Porcu, M.; Investigators, G.-H. Rationale and design of the GISSI heart failure trial: A large trial to assess the effects of *n*-3 polyunsaturated fatty acids and rosuvastatin in symptomatic congestive heart failure. *Eur. J. Heart Fail.* **2004**, *6*, 635–641. [CrossRef] [PubMed]

160. He, K.; Song, Y.; Daviglus, M.L.; Liu, K.; Van Horn, L.; Dyer, A.R.; Greenland, P. Accumulated evidence on fish consumption and coronary heart disease mortality: A meta-analysis of cohort studies. *Circulation* **2004**, *109*, 2705–2711. [CrossRef] [PubMed]

161. Chowdhury, R.; Warnakula, S.; Kunutsor, S.; Crowe, F.; Ward, H.A.; Johnson, L.; Franco, O.H.; Butterworth, A.S.; Forouhi, N.G.; Thompson, S.G.; et al. Association of dietary, circulating, and supplement fatty acids with coronary risk: A systematic review and meta-analysis. *Ann. Intern. Med.* **2014**, *160*, 398–406. [CrossRef] [PubMed]

162. Del Gobbo, L.C.; Imamura, F.; Aslibekyan, S.; Marklund, M.; Virtanen, J.K.; Wennberg, M.; Yakoob, M.Y.; Chiuve, S.E.; Dela Cruz, L.; Frazier-Wood, A.C.; et al. Omega-3 polyunsaturated fatty acid biomarkers and coronary heart disease: Pooling project of 19 cohort studies. *JAMA Intern. Med.* **2016**, *176*, 1155–1166. [CrossRef] [PubMed]

163. Kromhout, D.; Giltay, E.J.; Geleijnse, J.M.; Alpha Omega Trial, G. *n*-3 fatty acids and cardiovascular events after myocardial infarction. *N. Engl. J. Med.* **2010**, *363*, 2015–2026. [CrossRef] [PubMed]

164. Rauch, B.; Schiele, R.; Schneider, S.; Diller, F.; Victor, N.; Gohlke, H.; Gottwik, M.; Steinbeck, G.; Del Castillo, U.; Sack, R.; et al. OMEGA, a randomized, placebo-controlled trial to test the effect of highly purified omega-3 fatty acids on top of modern guideline-adjusted therapy after myocardial infarction. *Circulation* **2010**, *122*, 2152–2159. [CrossRef] [PubMed]

165. Galan, P.; Kesse-Guyot, E.; Czernichow, S.; Briancon, S.; Blacher, J.; Hercberg, S.; Group, S.F.O.C. Effects of B vitamins and omega 3 fatty acids on cardiovascular diseases: A randomised placebo controlled trial. *BMJ* **2010**, *341*, c6273. [CrossRef] [PubMed]

166. Bosch, J.; Gerstein, H.C.; Dagenais, G.R.; Diaz, R.; Dyal, L.; Jung, H.; Maggiono, A.P.; Probstfield, J.; Ramachandran, A.; Riddle, M.C.; et al. *n*-3 fatty acids and cardiovascular outcomes in patients with dysglycemia. *N. Engl. J. Med.* **2012**, *367*, 309–318. [PubMed]

167. Roncaglioni, M.C.; Tombesi, M.; Avanzini, F.; Barlera, S.; Caimi, V.; Longoni, P.; Marzona, I.; Milani, V.; Silletta, M.G.; Tognoni, G.; et al. *n*-3 fatty acids in patients with multiple cardiovascular risk factors. *N. Engl. J. Med.* **2013**, *368*, 1800–1808. [PubMed]

168. Bourre, J.M. Roles of unsaturated fatty acids (especially omega-3 fatty acids) in the brain at various ages and during ageing. *J. Nutr. Health Aging* **2004**, *8*, 163–174. [PubMed]

169. Van Elst, K.; Bruining, H.; Birtoli, B.; Terreaux, C.; Buitelaar, J.K.; Kas, M.J. Food for thought: Dietary changes in essential fatty acid ratios and the increase in autism spectrum disorders. *Neurosci. Biobehav. Rev.* **2014**, *45*, 369–378. [CrossRef] [PubMed]

170. James, S.; Montgomery, P.; Williams, K. Omega-3 fatty acids supplementation for autism spectrum disorders (ASD). *Cochrane Database Syst. Rev.* **2011**. [CrossRef]

171. Gow, R.V.; Hibbeln, J.R. Omega-3 fatty acid and nutrient deficits in adverse neurodevelopment and childhood behaviors. *Child Adolesc. Psychiatr. Clin. N. Am.* **2014**, *23*, 555–590. [CrossRef] [PubMed]

172. Bondi, C.O.; Taha, A.Y.; Tock, J.L.; Totah, N.K.; Cheon, Y.; Torres, G.E.; Rapoport, S.I.; Moghaddam, B. Adolescent behavior and dopamine availability are uniquely sensitive to dietary omega-3 fatty acid deficiency. *Biol. Psychiatry* **2014**, *75*, 38–46. [CrossRef] [PubMed]

173. Kim, S.W.; Schafer, M.R.; Klier, C.M.; Berk, M.; Rice, S.; Allott, K.; Bartholomeusz, C.F.; Whittle, S.L.; Pilioussis, E.; Pantelis, C.; et al. Relationship between membrane fatty acids and cognitive symptoms and information processing in individuals at ultra-high risk for psychosis. *Schizophr. Res.* **2014**, *158*, 39–44. [CrossRef] [PubMed]

174. Meyer, B.J.; Grenyer, B.F.; Crowe, T.; Owen, A.J.; Grigonis-Deane, E.M.; Howe, P.R. Improvement of major depression is associated with increased erythrocyte DHA. *Lipids* **2013**, *48*, 863–868. [CrossRef] [PubMed]

175. Gillies, D.; Sinn, J.; Lad, S.S.; Leach, M.J.; Ross, M.J. Polyunsaturated fatty acids (PUFA) for attention deficit hyperactivity disorder (ADHD) in children and adolescents. *Cochrane Database Syst. Rev.* **2012**, *7*.

176. Lattka, E.; Klopp, N.; Demmelmair, H.; Klingler, M.; Heinrich, J.; Koletzko, B. Genetic variations in polyunsaturated fatty acid metabolism–implications for child health? *Ann. Nutr. Metab.* **2012**, *60* (Suppl. 3), 8–17. [CrossRef] [PubMed]

177. Horrobin, D.F.; Manku, M.S.; Hillman, H.; Iain, A.; Glen, M. Fatty acid levels in the brains of schizophrenics and normal controls. *Biol. Psychiatry* **1991**, *30*, 795–805. [CrossRef]

178. Assies, J.; Lieverse, R.; Vreken, P.; Wanders, R.J.; Dingemans, P.M.; Linszen, D.H. Significantly reduced docosahexaenoic and docosapentaenoic acid concentrations in erythrocyte membranes from schizophrenic patients compared with a carefully matched control group. *Biol. Psychiatry* **2001**, *49*, 510–522. [CrossRef]

179. McNamara, R.K.; Vannest, J.J.; Valentine, C.J. Role of perinatal long-chain omega-3 fatty acids in cortical circuit maturation: Mechanisms and implications for psychopathology. *World J. Psychiatry* **2015**, *5*, 15–34. [CrossRef] [PubMed]

180. Stevens, L.J.; Zentall, S.S.; Deck, J.L.; Abate, M.L.; Watkins, B.A.; Lipp, S.R.; Burgess, J.R. Essential fatty acid metabolism in boys with attention-deficit hyperactivity disorder. *Am. J. Clin. Nutr.* **1995**, *62*, 761–768. [PubMed]

181. Wu, S.; Ding, Y.; Wu, F.; Li, R.; Hou, J.; Mao, P. Omega-3 fatty acids intake and risks of dementia and Alzheimer's disease: A meta-analysis. *Neurosci. Biobehav. Rev.* **2015**, *48*, 1–9. [CrossRef] [PubMed]

182. Jiao, J.; Li, Q.; Chu, J.; Zeng, W.; Yang, M.; Zhu, S. Effect of *n*-3 PUFA supplementation on cognitive function throughout the life span from infancy to old age: A systematic review and meta-analysis of randomized controlled trials. *Am. J. Clin. Nutr.* **2014**, *100*, 1422–1436. [CrossRef] [PubMed]

183. Hawkey, E.; Nigg, J.T. Omega-3 fatty acid and ADHD: Blood level analysis and meta-analytic extension of supplementation trials. *Clin. Psychol. Rev.* **2014**, *34*, 496–505. [CrossRef] [PubMed]

184. Bloch, M.H.; Hannestad, J. Omega-3 fatty acids for the treatment of depression: Systematic review and meta-analysis. *Mol. Psychiatry* **2012**, *17*, 1272–1282. [CrossRef] [PubMed]

185. Cooper, R.E.; Tye, C.; Kuntsi, J.; Vassos, E.; Asherson, P. Omega-3 polyunsaturated fatty acid supplementation and cognition: A systematic review and meta-analysis. *J. Psychopharmacol.* **2015**, *29*, 753–763. [CrossRef] [PubMed]

186. Gould, J.F.; Smithers, L.G.; Makrides, M. The effect of maternal omega-3 (*n*-3) LCPUFA supplementation during pregnancy on early childhood cognitive and visual development: A systematic review and meta-analysis of randomized controlled trials. *Am. J. Clin. Nutr.* **2013**, *97*, 531–544. [CrossRef] [PubMed]

187. Shulkin, M.L.; Pimpin, L.; Bellinger, D.; Kranz, S.; Duggan, C.; Fawzi, W.; Mozaffarian, D. Effects of omega-3 supplementation during pregnancy and youth on neurodevelopment and cognition in childhood: A systematic review and meta-analysis. *FASEB J.* **2016**, *30* (Suppl. 295), 5.

188. Woods, R.K.; Thien, F.C.; Abramson, M.J. Dietary marine fatty acids (fish oil) for asthma in adults and children. *Cochrane Database Syst. Rev.* **2002**. [CrossRef]

189. Best, K.P.; Gold, M.; Kennedy, D.; Martin, J.; Makrides, M. Omega-3 long-chain PUFA intake during pregnancy and allergic disease outcomes in the offspring: A systematic review and meta-analysis of observational studies and randomized controlled trials. *Am. J. Clin. Nutr.* **2016**, *103*, 128–143. [CrossRef] [PubMed]

190. Fortin, P.R.; Lew, R.A.; Liang, M.H.; Wright, E.A.; Beckett, L.A.; Chalmers, T.C.; Sperling, R.I. Validation of a meta-analysis: The effects of fish oil in rheumatoid arthritis. *J. Clin. Epidemiol.* **1995**, *48*, 1379–1390. [CrossRef]

191. Goldberg, R.J.; Katz, J. A meta-analysis of the analgesic effects of omega-3 polyunsaturated fatty acid supplementation for inflammatory joint pain. *Pain* **2007**, *129*, 210–223. [CrossRef] [PubMed]

192. Leitzmann, M.F.; Stampfer, M.J.; Michaud, D.S.; Augustsson, K.; Colditz, G.C.; Willett, W.C.; Giovannucci, E.L. Dietary intake of *n*-3 and *n*-6 fatty acids and the risk of prostate cancer. *Am. J. Clin. Nutr.* **2004**, *80*, 204–216. [PubMed]

193. Chavarro, J.E.; Stampfer, M.J.; Li, H.; Campos, H.; Kurth, T.; Ma, J. A prospective study of polyunsaturated fatty acid levels in blood and prostate cancer risk. *Cancer Epidemiol. Biomark. Prev.* **2007**, *16*, 1364–1370. [CrossRef] [PubMed]

194. Sakai, M.; Kakutani, S.; Horikawa, C.; Tokuda, H.; Kawashima, H.; Shibata, H.; Okubo, H.; Sasaki, S. Arachidonic acid and cancer risk: A systematic review of observational studies. *BMC Cancer* **2012**, *12*, 606. [CrossRef] [PubMed]

195. Hooper, L.; Thompson, R.L.; Harrison, R.A.; Summerbell, C.D.; Ness, A.R.; Moore, H.J.; Worthington, H.V.; Durrington, P.N.; Higgins, J.P.; Capps, N.E.; et al. Risks and benefits of omega 3 fats for mortality, cardiovascular disease, and cancer: Systematic review. *BMJ* **2006**, *332*, 752–760. [CrossRef] [PubMed]

196. Rice, H.B.; Bernasconi, A.; Maki, K.C.; Harris, W.S.; von Schacky, C.; Calder, P.C. Conducting omega-3 clinical trials with cardiovascular outcomes: Proceedings of a workshop held at ISSFAL 2014. *Prostaglandins Leukot. Essent. Fat. Acids* **2016**, *107*, 30–42. [CrossRef] [PubMed]

197. Superko, H.R.; Superko, A.R.; Lundberg, G.P.; Margolis, B.; Garrett, B.C.; Nasir, K.; Agatston, A.S. Omega-3 fatty acid blood levels clinical significance update. *Curr. Cardiovasc. Risk Rep.* **2014**, *8*, 407. [CrossRef] [PubMed]

198. Draisma, H.H.M.; Pool, R.; Kobl, M.; Jansen, R.; Petersen, A.K.; Vaarhorst, A.A.M.; Yet, I.; Haller, T.; Demirkan, A.; Esko, T.; et al. Genome-wide association study identifies novel genetic variants contributing to variation in blood metabolite levels. *Nat. Commun.* **2015**, *6*, 7208. [CrossRef] [PubMed]

199. Shin, S.Y.; Fauman, E.B.; Petersen, A.K.; Krumsiek, J.; Santos, R.; Huang, J.; Arnold, M.; Erte, I.; Forgetta, V.; Yang, T.P.; et al. An atlas of genetic influences on human blood metabolites. *Nat. Genet.* **2014**, *46*, 543–550. [CrossRef] [PubMed]

200. Long, T.; Hicks, M.; Yu, H.C.; Biggs, W.H.; Kirkness, E.F.; Menni, C.; Zierer, J.; Small, K.S.; Mangino, M.; Messier, H.; et al. Whole-genome sequencing identifies common-to-rare variants associated with human blood metabolites. *Nat. Genet.* **2017**, *49*, 568–578. [CrossRef] [PubMed]

201. Arnold, M.; Raffler, J.; Pfeufer, A.; Suhre, K.; Kastenmuller, G. SNiPA: An interactive, genetic variant-centered annotation browser. *Bioinformatics* **2015**, *31*, 1334–1336. [CrossRef] [PubMed]

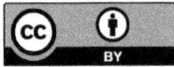

nutrients

MDPI

Article

Effect of Altering Dietary *n*-6:*n*-3 Polyunsaturated Fatty Acid Ratio with Plant and Marine-Based Supplement on Biomarkers of Bone Turnover in Healthy Adults

Sujatha Rajaram [1,*], Ellen Lan Yip [1], Rajneesh Reghunathan [2], Subburaman Mohan [2,3] and Joan Sabaté [1]

[1] Center for Nutrition, Healthy Lifestyle and Disease Prevention, School of Public Health, Loma Linda University, Loma Linda, CA 92350, USA; ellenlannguyen@gmail.com (E.L.Y.); jsabate@llu.edu (J.S.)
[2] Musculoskeletal Disease Center, Loma Linda VA Healthcare Systems, Loma Linda, CA 92357, USA; reghu.rajneesh@gmail.com (R.R.); subburaman.mohan@va.gov (S.M.)
[3] Department of Medicine, Loma Linda University, Loma Linda, CA 92350, USA
* Correspondence: srajaram@llu.edu; Tel.: +1-909-558-4598

Received: 1 September 2017; Accepted: 16 October 2017; Published: 24 October 2017

Abstract: Although there is accumulating evidence for a protective role of *n*-3 polyunsaturated fatty acids (*n*-3 PUFAs) on bone health, there are limited studies that examine the effect of altering dietary *n*-6:*n*-3 PUFA ratio with plant and marine sources of *n*-3 PUFA on bone health. Healthy adults ($n = 24$) were randomized into an eight-week crossover study with a four-week washout between treatments, with each subject consuming three of four diets. The four diets differed in the dietary *n*-6:*n*-3 PUFA ratios and either had an algal oil supplement added or not: (Control diet (10:1); α-linolenic acid (ALA) diet (2:1); Eicosapentaenoic acid/Docosahexaenoic acid (EPA/DHA) diet (10:1 plus supplement (S) containing EPA/DHA; Combination diet (2:1 + S)). The supplement was microalgae oil that provided 1 g EPA + DHA/day. Flaxseed oil and walnuts provided 8.6 g of ALA/day in the 2:1 diets. Serum levels of c-telopeptide (CTX), procollagen Type I N-terminal peptide, and osteocalcin showed significant correlation with age but none of the bone markers or peroxisomal proliferator-activated receptor-γ mRNA expression was significantly different between the diets. Serum CTX was negatively associated with red blood cell membrane linoleic acid and ALA and positively associated with membrane DHA. Neither altering dietary *n*-6:*n*-3 PUFA ratio from a 10:1 to a 2:1 ratio nor adding EPA/DHA supplement significantly changed bone turnover in the short term in healthy adults.

Keywords: dietary *n*-3 fatty acids; bone turnover; peroxisomal proliferator activated receptor γ; ALA; EPA/DHA

1. Introduction

N-3 polyunsaturated fatty acids (*n*-3 PUFAs) confer many health benefits including the prevention of cardiovascular, cardiometabolic, and other chronic diseases as well as the reduction of inflammation [1–3]. A limited number of human studies suggest that *n*-3 PUFAs play an important role in bone metabolism and may represent a potentially useful non-pharmacological therapeutic strategy to prevent bone loss and reduce the risk of osteoporosis [4,5]. The essential *n*-3 PUFA, α-linolenic acid (ALA) cannot be synthesized by humans, while eicosapentaenoic acid (EPA) and docosahexaenoic acid (DHA) can be generated from ALA, although the conversion rate is low. Western diets are low in *n*-3 PUFA and high in *n*-6 PUFA, which makes for a high dietary *n*-6:*n*-3 PUFA ratio. The health attributes of *n*-3 PUFA is due to the direct effects of ALA, or the conversion of ALA to EPA and DHA and/or the decrease in the *n*-6:*n*-3 PUFA ratio. Animal studies have demonstrated the protective role of fish oil in preventing bone loss in mice following ovariectomy [6,7], with a marked increase in mineral apposition rate. In many of these studies, *n*-3 fatty acids or a lower ratio of *n*-6:*n*-3 PUFA show a positive influence on bone. Accordingly, populations known to consume high amounts of *n*-3 PUFA-rich fish, such as the Japanese and Greenland Eskimos, have lower rates of osteoporosis [8]. *N*-3 PUFAs are thought to mediate their actions by regulating the fatty acid composition of skeletal cells [9,10]. Since the concentration of ALA in mammalian cell membranes is extremely low and makes up less than 0.5% of total fatty acids in plasma phospholipids, the specific functional and protective effects of ALA are attributed to its conversion to longer chain *n*-3 fatty acids, EPA and DHA [11–13].

Intervention trials with PUFAs in skeletal metabolism in humans are limited, and findings are controversial [14–17]. One potential explanation for this is that the skeletal effects of *n*-3 fatty acids may depend on the type, dose, and duration of treatment. Typical Western diets are associated with higher *n*-6:*n*-3 PUFA ratios, whereas, it is the low *n*-6:*n*-3 ratios that are correlated with optimal health and decreased risk of disease [4,5]. Griel et al. [4] showed that plant sources of *n*-3 PUFA lower bone resorption, especially when the background *n*-6:*n*-3 ratio is low (1.6:1). Studies investigating the role of marine *n*-3 PUFA (EPA/DHA) in the context of low and high *n*-6:*n*-3 PUFA ratios and comparing plant versus marine *n*-3 PUFAs in preventing bone loss in humans are sparse. Thus, the objective of this study was to examine the effect of altering the dietary *n*-6:*n*-3 PUFA ratio from 10:1 to 2:1 with and without adding a supplement of EPA/DHA.

2. Materials and Methods

2.1. Study Design

This study was part of a larger intervention trial assessing the changes in red blood cell (RBC) membrane fatty acid composition when the dietary *n*-6:*n*-3 fatty acid is altered from a ratio of 10:1 to 2:1 by adding plant- and marine-based supplements [18]. This aim of this study was to assess the effects of altering the dietary *n*-6:*n*-3 fatty acid ratio on biochemical markers of bone turnover and gene expression in healthy adults. This study was a single-blind, randomized, 4 × 3 incomplete crossover trial including four diets: (1) Control diet (*n*-6:*n*-3 ratio of 10:1, low in ALA, EPA/DHA); (2) EPA/DHA diet (10:1 plus supplement (S) of algal oil, low in ALA, high in EPA/DHA); (3) ALA diet (2:1, high ALA from walnuts and flaxseed oil, low EPA/DHA); and (4) Combination diet (2:1 + S, high in ALA and EPA/DHA). There was an initial one-week run-in phase to assess each participant's adherence to the dietary protocol. Study periods were eight weeks each and included a washout of four–six weeks between treatments. All meals were provided to the subjects and dietary compliance was assessed by the examination of individual participant diaries and through direct observation by research staff at each meal on campus. The complete study design and subject protocol have been previously published [18].

2.2. Subjects

The total number of participants completing all three diet periods was 24 (15 females and 9 males, age 42 ± 3 years). Participants were recruited from the Loma Linda area, including nearby hospitals and colleges. Participants that met all study criteria and received the highest commitment scores were selected. All selected subjects signed the informed consent approved by the Institutional Review Board at Loma Linda University (Loma Linda, CA, USA).

Subjects were included in the study if they had: (a) no prior affliction with hypertension, atherosclerosis, or other metabolic diseases; (b) serum cholesterol levels between 4.2–7.8 mmol/L; (c) serum triglyceride below 3.4 mmol/L; (d) body mass index below 30 kg/m^2; (e) stable weight within the past six months; (f) no intake of serum lipid-altering medications; (g) age range between 20 and 70 years; (h) no known food allergies to walnuts, flaxseed oil, or microalgae oil. All participants were non-smokers and maintained the same level of physical activity throughout the study as was established at their baseline.

2.3. Study Diets

There were four diets in all. Two diets had an *n*-6:*n*-3 fatty acid ratio of 10:1 (Control diet without supplement and EPA/DHA diet with supplementation, 1.40/5.04 g EPA/DHA from microalgae oil/week). There were two other diets with an *n*-6:*n*-3 fatty acid ratio of 2:1 (ALA diet, 42–49 g flaxseed oil/week + 10 g walnuts, 3 times/week and Combination diet with both ALA (42–49 g flaxseed oil/week + 10 g walnuts, 3 times/week) and supplementation, 1.40/5.04 g EPA/DHA/week). This was a rigorously controlled feeding study with all meals provided to participants by the research staff. Participants consumed dinners on the premises at Loma Linda University Campus, with all breakfast, lunch, and snacks provided as take out. All Saturday meals were packed and distributed to participants during Friday dinner. In order to increase dietary compliance, all dine-in meals were monitored by at least one senior investigator.

Menus were designed for seven levels of energy intake, ranging from 1500 to 3000 kcal/day to accommodate the eucaloric requirements of the subjects and has been described previously [18]. The main sources of *n*-3 fatty acid-rich foods were EPH/DHA-rich microalgae oil and ALA-rich flaxseed oil and walnuts. All menu plans adhered to a nine-day weekday and two-day weekend menu cycle with lacto-ovo vegetarian meals provided throughout the study.

2.4. Data Collection and Analyses

Each participant had fasting blood drawn at baseline and at the end of each diet period. Blood samples were collected at the standardized time of the day, i.e., 6:30 a.m. to 8:30 a.m. The variation between subjects was expected to be much higher than the minimal variation caused by sample collection in a 24-h time window [19]. Blood draw clinics were conducted at the Nutrition Assessment Laboratory and serum samples were stored at −80 °C. Lipomics Laboratory (Sacramento, CA, USA) measured RBC membrane fatty acid composition at the end of each treatment period.

Biochemical determination of all serum bone markers was carried out in duplicate runs after each experimental diet. Bone resorption marker c-telopeptide (CTX) was measured using the Serum Crosslaps ELISA Assay (Immunodiagnostic Systems Limited, Boldon, UK) that quantifies the degradation products of C-terminal telopeptides of Type 1 collagen in human serum. The intra- and inter-assay coefficients of variation were <6% and <10%, respectively. Bone formation marker procollagen type I N-terminal propeptide (P1NP) was measured using the UNiQ P1NP RIA (Orion Diagnostica, Espoo, Finland). This radioimmunoassay uses both labeled and unlabeled P1NP to competitively bind to limited sites located on polyclonal rabbit anti-P1NP antibody. The intra- and inter-assay coefficients of variation were 6.5–10.2% (12–173 µg/L) and 6.0–9.8% (12–167 µg/L), respectively. Bone formation marker osteocalcin (OC) was measured using N-MID Osteocalcin ELISA (Nordic Bioscience Diagnostics, Herlev, Denmark). This assay measures the N-Mid fragment region of OC in human serum. The intra- and inter-assay coefficients of variation were <4% and <7%, respectively. Insulin-like growth factor 1 (IGF-1) was measured using the assay IGF-1 ELISA (Immunodiagnostic Systems Limited, Boldon, UK), which quantifies the amount of this polypeptide in human serum. This assay uses a highly specific purified polyclonal sheep antibody and a high affinity labeled monoclonal anti-IGF-1 with horseradish peroxidase. The intra- and inter-assay coefficients of variation were <4% and <7%, respectively.

At the end of each diet period, samples of subcutaneous tissue were collected from the abdominal region and used for measurement of peroxisomal proliferator activated receptor-gamma (PPAR-γ) mRNA levels by real-time polymerase chain reaction (PCR) with actin as an internal standard.

2.5. Statistical Analyses

A trained statistician using SAS software, version 9.1 (SAS Institute Inc., Cary, NC, USA) performed the statistical analyses. Data are reported as least squares mean + standard error. A mixed-effect model was used that included a random-effect term for subjects nested in sequence, a fixed-effect term for period and treatment, and a covariate term representing the amount of specific *n*-3 fatty acids (ALA and/or EPA/DHA) in each respective diet. The Kenward-Roger method and Tukey-Kramer HSD tests were performed to estimate denominator degrees of freedom for tests of fixed effects and to evaluate significant pair-wise differences among the diets, respectively. A mixed model approach was also used to evaluate the association between bone markers (CTX, PINP, and OC) with individual RBC membrane fatty acids (Linoleic (LA), ALA, EPA, and DHA), adjusting for treatments and period effect. A pre-determined level of statistical significance was set at $p < 0.05$. The expression changes of PPARγ mRNA levels in different subjects were standardized to expression levels of the housekeeping gene, actin, and comparisons for different study diets made using student's *t*-test.

3. Results

3.1. Nutrient Analyses and Dietary Compliance

The nutrient composition of treatment diets from chemical analyses (Covance Laboratories, Madison, WI, USA) revealed that the percentage of total fat (≈30%), saturated fat (<10%), and trans fatty acids (<1%) were in the appropriate range [18]. The *n*-6:*n*-3 PUFA ratio for the ALA and combination diets was 2.5:1, and for the control and EPA/DHA diets was approximately 9.3:1. Both ratios were extremely close to the planned ratios of 2:1 and 10:1 for the ALA/combination diet and control/EPA+DHA diets, respectively [19]. Dietary compliance assessed through RBC fatty acid composition for each participant at the end of diet treatment indicated excellent adherence to dietary protocol as described previously [18].

3.2. N-3 Fatty Acids and Bone Markers

Mean serum CTX, PINP, and OC concentrations among the Control, EPA/DHA, ALA, and Combination diets are reported in Table 1. There was no significant diet effect or pair-wise differences among treatment diets, even after adjusting for age and gender ($p > 0.05$).

Table 1. Mean concentrations of serum bone markers at the end of each experimental diet [1].

	Bone Markers		
Diet	CTX (ng/mL)	PINP (µg/L)	OC (ng/mL)
Control (10:1) [2]	0.538 (0.041)	54.68 (2.96)	18.46 (1.13)
EPA/DHA (10:1 + S)	0.480 (0.041)	51.44 (2.96)	18.01 (1.13)
ALA (2:1)	0.588 (0.041)	50.10 (2.96)	16.34 (1.13)
Combination (2:1 + S)	0.583 (0.041)	50.89 (2.96)	16.91 (1.13)

[1] Least Square Mean (Standard Error). There was no significant diet effect among the experimental diets ($p > 0.05$). [2] *n*-6:*n*-3 ratio. CTX-C-telopeptide, PINP-procollagen type I N-terminal propeptide, OC-Osteocalcin, S-supplement containing microalgae oil that provided EPA/DHA of 1 g/day.

3.3. Correlation between Bone Markers, n-3 Fatty Acids, and Age

A mixed model approach was used to examine the association between bone markers (CTX, PINP, and OC) and individual *n*-3 fatty acids (Table 2). There was a significant negative association between serum CTX with RBC membrane LA ($p = 0.0143$) and ALA ($p = 0.0477$). There was a significant positive association with serum CTX and RBC membrane DHA ($p = 0.0385$). Even after adjusting for gender, results were significant.

A mixed model approach was also used to investigate an association between age and bone markers (CTX, PINP, and OC). There was a significant negative association between age and bone markers CTX ($p < 0.0001$), P1NP ($p = 0.0006$), and OC ($p = 0.0019$) (Table 2).

Table 2. Association between bone markers with individual *n*-3 fatty acids and age [1].

Bone Markers	*n*-3 Fatty Acid	Estimate	*p*-Value
	LA	−0.058 (0.023)	0.0143
	ALA	−0.419 (0.208)	0.0477
CTX	EPA	0.068 (0.133)	NS
	DHA	0.038 (0.018)	0.0385
	Age	−0.017 (0.00345)	<0.0001
	LA	0.083 (1.50)	NS
	ALA	11.18 (13.13)	NS
P1NP	EPA	−11.46 (8.19)	NS
	DHA	−1.50 (1.13)	NS
	Age	−0.909 (0.225)	0.0006
	LA	−0.903 (0.614)	NS
	ALA	−2.98 (5.32)	NS
OC	EPA	−1.81 (3.36)	NS
	DHA	−0.102 (0.463)	NS
	Age	−0.429 (0.122)	0.0019

[1] Even after adjusting for age and gender, results were still significant. NS-Not Significant.

3.4. Correlation between Bone Markers and IGF-1

After adjusting for age and gender, there were no significant associations between CTX, PINP, or OC and serum IGF-1 ($p > 0.05$). However, there was a significant negative association between serum IGF-1 and age ($p < 0.0001$) (Figure 1). The correlation coefficient between serum IGF-1 levels and age for the Control ($r^2 = 0.3459$), EPA/DHA ($r^2 = 0.5922$), ALA ($r^2 = 0.4174$), and Combination ($r^2 = 0.5382$) treatment diets in healthy adults are significant at $p < 0.001$ ($n = 24$).

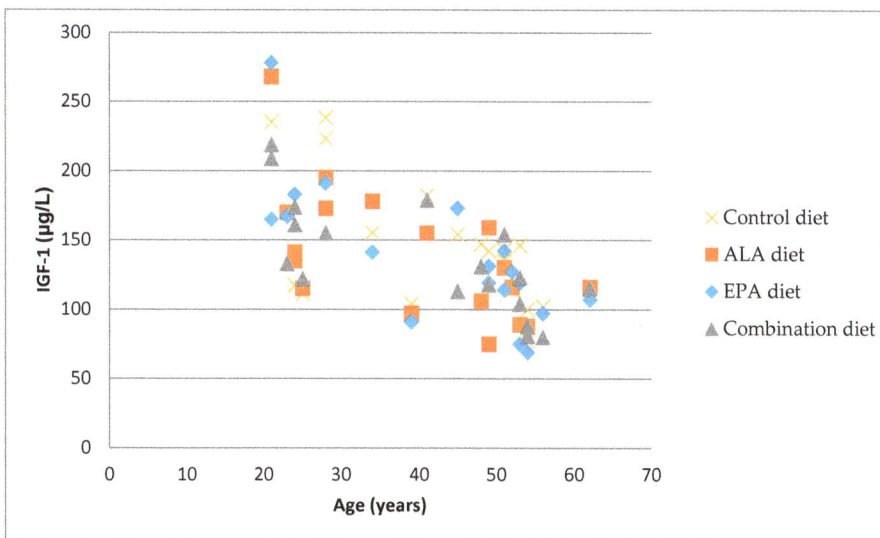

Figure 1. The association between serum IGF-1 levels and age in different diet groups.

3.5. Gene Expression

There were no significant changes in PPAR γ expression between the four different diets (Table 3).

Table 3. Expression of PPARγ mRNA in the subcutaneous tissue.

Diets	Fold Change ± SEM	p-Value
10:1 versus 2:1	1.72 ± 0.26	0.19
10:1 versus 10:1 + S	2.02 ± 0.32	0.11
10:1 versus 2:1 + S	2.20 ± 0.55	0.38
2:1 versus 10:1 + S	1.40 ± 0.22	0.55
2:1 versus 2:1 + S	1.52 ± 0.38	0.85
10:1 + S versus 2:1 + S	1.32 ± 0.33	0.55

Values are fold change versus actin mRNA levels. SEM-Standard error of the mean.

4. Discussion

We observed that altering the n-6:n-3 fatty acid ratio from 10:1 to 2:1 by increasing ALA (8.6 g of ALA) or by adding a supplement (1 g EPA + DHA/day) to either the 10:1 or 2:1 diet in the short term (eight weeks) did not alter serum bone markers or PPAR-γ gene expression in healthy adults. While these amounts promote cardioprotective effects [1,20], it appears that this dose may not be sufficient to influence bone turnover in healthy subjects. Previously, a six-week feeding trial by Griel et al. [4] providing a significantly higher dose (17 g ALA from walnuts and flaxseed oil) showed a significant reduction in bone resorption marker N-telopeptide. Lack of results from our cohort may be partly due to a lower ALA intake even in our 2:1 diet groups. Alternatively, the duration of intervention may have been too short to see changes in bone turnover markers in a relatively young, healthy adult cohort.

A low dietary ratio of n-6:n-3 PUFA has been correlated with increased bone mineral density in the hip in older adults and in the spine for healthy young men [5,21,22]. Weiler et al. [23] showed that diets with low n-6:n-3 ratios resulted in higher plasma DHA levels and decreased bone resorption in growing piglets. In our study, just altering the ratio from 10:1 to 2:1 did not increase RBC membrane DHA levels [18]. Although the 2:1 ALA diet had a high amount of ALA, conversion of ALA to DHA was poor. When the algal supplement containing EPA/DHA was added to the 2:1 diet (combination diet), then the DHA in RBC membrane increased significantly. It was still not sufficient to alter bone turnover markers. It appears that in healthy adults, the bone turnover rate is low and in order for diet-induced changes to occur, either a longer duration of intervention or a higher dose of intervention may be necessary.

The bone-protective effects observed with a low dietary n-6:n-3 ratio [4,5,21] may be attributed to a lower concentration of eicosanoids arising from the n-6 fatty acids pathway [24]. Evidence suggests that eicosanoids derived from arachidonic acid, a byproduct of n-6 fatty acid metabolism, have been linked to numerous inflammatory and autoimmune disorders [11]. We observed a significant negative association between serum CTX and RBC membrane LA and ALA. Other research also supports that lower dietary ratios of n-6:n-3 fatty acids protect bone [9]. The plausible mechanism by which tissue levels of ALA could influence bone resorption is via prostaglandin E2 (PGE2), a primary eicosanoid that affects bone metabolism and inhibits the activation of receptor-activated nuclear-kappa B ligand (RANKL), an important growth factor that promotes osteoclastogenesis [25]. In a nine-week animal study by Mollard et al. [26], ALA-rich flaxseed oil diet significantly reduced PGE2 levels. Dietary intake of ALA may exert an anabolic effect on bone through lowering concentrations of PGE2 [27]. Although the RBC ALA levels increased both by increasing ALA (2:1 diet) and by adding a supplement (10:1 + S and 2:1 + S diets) in our study, it is likely that it was insufficient to modify PGE2 or other inflammatory markers. Perhaps individuals with elevated inflammation at baseline may better respond to n-3 PUFA with respect to markers of bone formation and resorption. This needs to be explored in future studies.

Higher endogenous DHA helps reduce bone resorption. Serum phospholipid DHA levels were positively associated with total bone mineral density in healthy men between 16 and 22 years of age [21]. In animal studies, a high PUFA diet incorporating DHA-rich single cell oil supplementation increased femur bone mineral density and diets using lower ratios of n-6:n-3 fatty acids observed less bone resorption [27,28]. These findings suggest that high DHA supplementation may be beneficial and may help promote bone conservation. In contrast, we found a positive correlation between DHA levels and bone resorption, which could be due to the different age group of subjects used in this study. There was a significant negative association between age and bone markers CTX, P1NP, and OC. These findings are in agreement with other studies showing a biphasic effect of age on bone remodeling in specific age groups [29,30]. Bone resorption and formation markers decline with age, reaching their lowest levels between 30 and 50 years.

The majority of participants in this study were within this age range, with only 2 participants over 55 years of age (mean age = 42). After the age of 50, markers of both bone formation and resorption increase with resorption, exceeding the formation that is caused by lowering sex hormone levels [31]. There was also a significant negative association between age and IGF-1, which is in agreement with what others have observed [32]. Veldhuis et al. [33] showed that IGF-1 concentrations can actually decrease by more than 50% in healthy older adults. The effects of the different dietary PUFA ratios on serum IGF binding protein levels may be worth exploring.

Previously, it has been shown that *n*-3 fatty acids modulate the expression of PPARγ [34]. However, we did not find a significant difference in the subcutaneous tissue PPARγ among the four different diets. This lack of difference could be due to the use of subcutaneous rather than adipose tissue. While dietary fatty acids including *n*-3 PUFAs may have beneficial effects on bone, regulators of postprandial skeletal fatty acid flux need to be identified. One of the proposed regulators is lipoprotein lipase (LPL), involved in the metabolism of triglyceride-rich lipoproteins [35]. Since *n*-3 PUFAs are known to lower triglyceride levels through improved clearance of these lipids by activating LPL, future studies should consider exploring this relationship.

5. Conclusions

Epidemiological and intervention studies have shown that increasing *n*-3 PUFAs (ALA, EPA/DHA) and/or lowering the dietary *n*-6:*n*-3 PUFA ratio may have bone protective effects [4,17,21,22]. However, our study on healthy adults did not show any change in bone formation or resorption markers, even when the dietary *n*-6:*n*-3 PUFA ratio was altered from 10:1 to 2:1 using ALA-rich food sources or when a supplement containing EPA/DHA was added to the two diets. A low rate of bone turnover in these relatively young and healthy adults may be one of the reasons for the lack of favorable results. There is still merit to exploring the role of *n*-3 fatty acids on bone metabolism since these fatty acids clearly play a role in bone remodeling and bone microstructure. However, due consideration must be given to the type, dose, and duration of intervention and to the target population. Comparing the different sources of *n*-3 PUFAs is relevant since it will inform our dietary choices. From our current study, it is evident that incorporating plant sources of *n*-3 PUFA (ALA) can help reduce the dietary *n*-6:*n*-3 PUFA ratio and increase RBC EPA levels significantly. Whether or not these translate to protective effects on the bone metabolism of healthy adults' remains to be further explored.

Acknowledgments: This study was funded by the Center for Health and Nutrition Research, University of California, Davis. We would like to thank Joe Rung-Aroon for technical assistance and Keiji Oda for statistical support.

Author Contributions: S.R., E.L.Y. and J.S. conceived and designed the study, supervised data collection. E.L.Y. performed the biochemical analyses and wrote the first draft of the paper. S.M. supervised the biochemical analyses, contributed to the interpretation of the results and provided content for the results and discussion of the paper. R.R. contributed to the statistical analyses of the data, revising, and finalizing the paper. S.R., J.S. and E.L.Y. contributed to the interpretation and discussion of results. All authors read and approved the final contents of the paper.

Conflicts of Interest: The authors have no conflict of interest. The funding sponsors had no role in the design or conduct of the study, data collection, and analyses, interpretation, and on the writing of the paper and in the decision to publish the results.

References

1. Siscovick, D.S.; Barringer, T.A.; Fretts, A.M.; Wu, J.H.; Lichtenstein, A.H.; Costello, R.B.; Kris-Etherton, P.M.; Jacobson, T.A.; Engler, M.B.; Alger, H.M.; et al. Omega-3 polyunsaturated fatty acid (fish oil) supplementation and the prevention of clinical cardiovascular disease: A science advisory from the American heart association. *Circulation* **2017**, *135*, e867–e884. [CrossRef]

2. Chen, C.; Yu, X.; Shao, S. Effects of omega-3 fatty acid supplementation on glucose control and lipid levels in type 2 diabetes: A meta-analysis. *PLoS ONE* **2015**, *10*, e0139565. [CrossRef]

3. Sanders, T.A. Protective effects of dietary PUFA against chronic disease: Evidence from epidemiological studies and intervention trials. *Proc. Nutr. Soc.* **2014**, *73*, 73–79. [CrossRef]

4. Griel, A.E.; Kris-Etherton, P.M.; Hilpert, K.F.; Zhao, G.; West, S.G.; Corwin, R.L. An increase in dietary *n*-3 fatty acids decreases a marker of bone resorption in humans. *Nutr. J.* **2007**, *6*, 2. [CrossRef]

5. Weiss, L.A.; Barrett-Connor, E.; von Muhlen, D. Ratio of *n*-6 to *n*-3 fatty acids and bone mineral density in older adults: The Rancho Bernardo Study. *Am. J. Clin. Nutr.* **2005**, *81*, 934–938.

6. Sun, D.; Krishnan, A.; Zaman, K.; Lawrence, R.; Bhattacharya, A.; Fernandes, G. Dietary *n*-3 fatty acids decrease osteoclastogenesis and loss of bone mass in ovariectomized mice. *J. Bone Miner. Res.* **2003**, *18*, 1206–1216. [CrossRef] [PubMed]

7. Matsushita, H.; Barrios, J.A.; Shea, J.E.; Miller, S.C. Dietary fish oil results in a greater bone mass and bone formation indices in aged ovariectomized rats. *J. Bone Miner. Metab.* **2008**, *26*, 241–247. [CrossRef] [PubMed]

8. Pauneascu, A.C.; Ayotte, P.; Dewailly, E.; Dodin, S.; Pedersen, H.S.; Mulvad, G.; Côté, S. Polyunsaturated fatty acids and calcaneal ultrasound parameters among Inuit women from Nuuk (Greenland): A longitudinal study. *Int. J. Circumpolar Health* **2013**, *72*, 20988. [CrossRef] [PubMed]

9. Salari, P.; Rezaie, A.; Larijani, B.; Abdollahi, M. A systematic review of the impact of *n*-3 fatty acids in bone health and osteoporosis. *Med. Sci. Monit.* **2008**, *14*, RA37–RA44. [PubMed]

10. Watkins, B.A.; Li, Y.; Lippman, H.E.; Feng, S. Modulatory effect of omega-3 polyunsaturated fatty acids on osteoblast function and bone metabolism. *Prostaglandins Leukot. Essent. Fatty Acids* **2003**, *68*, 387–398. [CrossRef]

11. Albertazzi, P.; Coupland, K. Polyunsaturated fatty acids: Is there a role in postmenopausal osteoporosis prevention. *Maturitas* **2002**, *42*, 13–22. [CrossRef]

12. Burdge, G.C.; Calder, P.C. Conversion of α-linolenic acid to longer-chain polyunsaturated fatty acids in human adults. *Reprod. Nutr. Dev.* **2005**, *45*, 581–597. [CrossRef] [PubMed]

13. Baker, E.J.; Miles, E.A.; Burdge, G.C.; Yaqoob, P.; Calder, P.C. Metabolism and functional effects of plant-derived omega-3 fatty acids in humans. *Prog. Lipids Res.* **2016**, *64*, 30–56. [CrossRef] [PubMed]

14. Kruger, M.C.; Coetzer, H.; de Winter, R.; Gericke, G.; van Papendorp, D.H. Calcium, gamma-linolenic acid and eicosapentaenoic acid supplementation in senile osteoporosis. *Aging Clin. Exp. Res.* **1998**, *10*, 385–394. [CrossRef]

15. Van Papendrop, D.H.; Coetzer, H.; Kruger, M.G. Biochemical profile of osteoporotic patients on essential fatty acids supplementation. *Nutr. Res.* **1995**, *15*, 325–334. [CrossRef]

16. Martin-Bautista, E.; Muñoz-Torres, M.; Fonolla, J.; Quesada, M.; Poyatos, A.; Lopez-Huertas, E. Improvement of bone formation biomarkers after 1-year consumption with milk fortified with eicosapentaenoic acid, docosahexaenoic acid, oleic acid, and selected vitamins. *Nutr. Res.* **2010**, *30*, 320–326. [CrossRef] [PubMed]

17. Fonolla-Joya, J.; Reyes-Garcia, R.; Garcia-Martin, A.; Lopez-Huertas, E.; Munoz-Torres, M. Daily intake of milk enriched with *n*-3 fatty acids, oleic acid and calcium improves metabolic and bone biomarkers in postmenopausal women. *J. Am. Coll. Nutr.* **2016**, *35*, 529–536. [CrossRef] [PubMed]

18. Wien, M.; Rajaram, S.; Oda, K.; Sabaté, J. Decreasing the linoleic acid to alpha-linolenic acid diet ratio increases eicosapentaenoic acid in erythrocytes in adults. *Lipids* **2010**, *45*, 683–692. [CrossRef] [PubMed]

19. Redmond, J.; Fulford, A.J.; Jarjou, L.; Zhou, B.; Prentice, A.; Schoenmakers, I. Diurnal rhythms of bone turnover markers in three ethnic groups. *J. Clin. Endocrinol. Metab.* **2016**, *101*, 3222–3230. [CrossRef] [PubMed]

20. Rajaram, S.; Haddad, E.H.; Mejia, A.; Sabate, J. Walnuts and fatty fish influence different serum lipid fractions in normal to mildly hyperlipidemic individuals: A randomized controlled study. *Am. J. Clin. Nutr.* **2009**, *89*, 1657S–1663S. [CrossRef] [PubMed]

21. Hogstrom, M.; Nordstrom, P.; Nordstrom, A. *N*-3 Fatty acids are positively associated with peak bone mineral density and bone accrual in healthy men: The NO_2 Study. *Am. J. Clin. Nutr.* **2007**, *85*, 803–807. [PubMed]

22. Farina, E.K.; Kiel, D.P.; Roubenhoff, R.; Schaefer, E.J.; Cupples, L.A.; Tucker, K.L. Dietary intakes of arachidonic acid and α-linolenic acid are associated with reduced risk of hip fracture in older adults. *J. Nutr.* **2011**, *141*, 1146–1153. [CrossRef] [PubMed]

23. Weiler, H.A.; Fitzpatrick-Wong, S.C. Modulation of essential (*n*-6):(*n*-3) fatty acid ratios alters fatty acid status but not bone mass in piglets. *J. Nutr.* **2002**, *132*, 2667–2672. [PubMed]

24. Mangano, K.M.; Sahni, S.; Kerstetter, J.E.; Kenny, A.M.; Hannan, M.T. Polyunsaturated fatty acids and their relation to bone and muscle health in adults. *Curr. Osteoporos. Rep.* **2013**, *11*, 203–212. [CrossRef] [PubMed]

25. Coetzee, M.; Haag, M.; Kruger, M.C. Effects of arachidonic acid, docosahexaenoic acid, prostaglandin E(2) and parathyroid hormone on osteoprotegerin and RANKL secretion by MC3T3-E1 osteoblast-like cells. *J. Nutr. Biochem.* **2007**, *18*, 54–63. [CrossRef] [PubMed]

26. Mollard, R.C.; Gillam, M.E.; Wood, T.M.; Taylor, C.G.; Weiler, H.A. (*n*-3) fatty acids reduce the release of prostaglandin E2 from bone but do not affect bone mass in obese (fa/fa) and lean Zucker rats. *J. Nutr.* **2005**, *135*, 499–504. [PubMed]

27. Poulsen, R.C.; Moughan, P.J.; Kruger, M.C. Long-chain polyunsaturated fatty acids and the regulation of bone metabolism. *Exp. Biol. Med.* **2007**, *232*, 1275–1288. [CrossRef] [PubMed]

28. Watkins, B.A.; Li, Y.; Seifert, M.F. Dietary ratio of *n*-6/*n*-3 PUFAs and docosahexaenoic acid: Actions on bone mineral and serum biomarkers in ovariectomized rats. *J. Nutr. Biochem.* **2006**, *17*, 282–289. [CrossRef] [PubMed]

29. Pi, Y.Z.; Wu, X.P.; Liu, S.P.; Luo, X.H.; Cao, X.Z.; Xie, H.; Liao, E.Y. Age-related changes in bone biochemical markers and their relationship with bone mineral density in normal Chinese women. *J. Bone Miner. Metab.* **2006**, *24*, 380–385. [CrossRef] [PubMed]

30. Szulc, P.; Delmas, P.D. Biochemical markers of bone turnover in men. *Calcif. Tissue Int.* **2001**, *69*, 229–234. [CrossRef] [PubMed]

31. Claudon, A.; Vergnaud, P.; Valverde, C.; Mayr, A.; Klause, U.; Garnero, P. New automated multiplex assay for bone turnover markers in osteoporosis. *Clin. Chem.* **2008**, *54*, 1554–1563. [CrossRef] [PubMed]

32. Rajaram, S.; Baylin, D.J.; Mohan, S. Insulin-like growth factor binding proteins in serum and other biological fluids: Regulation and functions. *Endocr. Rev.* **1997**, *18*, 801–831. [CrossRef] [PubMed]

33. Veldhuis, J.D.; Iranmanesh, A.; Bowers, C.Y. Joint mechanisms of impaired growth-hormone pulse renewal in aging men. *J. Clin. Endocrinol. Metab.* **2005**, *90*, 4177–4183. [CrossRef] [PubMed]

34. Calder, P.C. Long-chain fatty acids and gene expression in inflammation and immunity. *Curr. Opin. Clin. Nutr. Metab. Care* **2013**, *16*, 425–433. [CrossRef] [PubMed]

35. Bartelt, A.; Koehne, T.; Todter, K.; Reimer, R.; Muller, B.; Behler-Janbeck, F.; Heeren, J.; Scheja, L.; Niemeier, A. Quantification of bone fatty acid metabolism and its regulation by adipocyte lipoprotein lipase. *Int. J. Mol. Sci.* **2017**, *18*, 1264. [CrossRef] [PubMed]

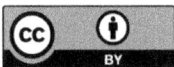

nutrients

Article

Effects of Marine Oils, Digested with Human Fluids, on Cellular Viability and Stress Protein Expression in Human Intestinal Caco-2 Cells

Cecilia Tullberg [1,*], Gerd Vegarud [2], Ingrid Undeland [1] and Nathalie Scheers [1,*]

[1]   Division of Food and Nutrition Science, Department of Biology and Biological Engineering, Chalmers University of Technology, Kemigården 4, 412 96 Gothenburg, Sweden; undeland@chalmers.se
[2]   Division of Food Proteins, Structure and Biological Function, Department of Chemistry, Biotechnology and Food Science, Norwegian University of Life Sciences, Chr. M. Falsens vei 1, 1432 Ås, Norway; gerd.vegarud@nmbu.no
*   Correspondences: cecilia.tullberg@chalmers.se (C.T.); nathalie.scheers@chalmers.se (N.S.); Tel.: +46-31-772-38-16 (C.T.); +46-31-772-38-21 (N.S.)

Received: 31 August 2017; Accepted: 1 November 2017; Published: 4 November 2017

Abstract: In vitro digestion of marine oils has been reported to promote lipid oxidation, including the formation of reactive aldehydes (e.g., malondialdehyde (MDA) and 4-hydroxy-2-hexenal (HHE)). We aimed to investigate if human in vitro digestion of supplemental levels of oils from algae, cod liver, and krill, in addition to pure MDA and HHE, affect intestinal Caco-2 cell survival and oxidative stress. Cell viability was not significantly affected by the digests of marine oils or by pure MDA and HHE (0–90 µM). Cellular levels of HSP-70, a chaperone involved in the prevention of stress-induced protein unfolding was significantly decreased (14%, 28%, and 14% of control for algae, cod and krill oil, respectively; $p \leq 0.05$). The oxidoreductase thioredoxin-1 (Trx-1) involved in reducing oxidative stress was also lower after incubation with the digested oils (26%, 53%, and 22% of control for algae, cod, and krill oil, respectively; $p \leq 0.001$). The aldehydes MDA and HHE did not affect HSP-70 or Trx-1 at low levels (8.3 and 1.4 µM, respectively), whilst a mixture of MDA and HHE lowered Trx-1 at high levels (45 µM), indicating less exposure to oxidative stress. We conclude that human digests of the investigated marine oils and their content of MDA and HHE did not cause a stress response in human intestinal Caco-2 cells.

Keywords: Caco-2; human digests; lipid oxidation; marine oil; HHE; MDA; Trx-1; HSP-70

1. Introduction

Intake of marine omega-3 fatty acids, i.e., the long-chain *n*-3 polyunsaturated fatty acids (LC *n*-3 PUFA) eicosapentaenoic acid (EPA), and docosahexaenoic acid (DHA), has been associated with beneficial health effects related to e.g., cardiovascular diseases [1,2]. Intake of marine oils high in EPA and DHA as dietary supplements, rather than ingesting them as a part of a complex seafood diet, has raised concerns regarding the stability of the pure oils, i.e., oils being separated from their native matrix. Marine oils are highly susceptible to peroxidation during storage and processing, and there are also indications of that the oils oxidize during gastrointestinal (GI) digestion [3–5], which is supported by several review [4,5], in vitro [3,6–9], and animal studies [10] of simulated GI digestion of marine oils.

Malondialdehyde (MDA) is one of the most well-known lipid oxidation products that is formed from PUFA. MDA is often used as a biomarker for lipid oxidation [11–14]. MDA has been attributed possible genotoxic features due to its ability to crosslink proteins and DNA, and it has also been associated with the development of cardiovascular disease, as reviewed by Del Rio et al. [15], and Uchida [16]. α,β-unsaturated aldehydes are thought to be more toxic than MDA, and are more reactive toward nucleophiles due to the hydroxyl-group, which is positioned close to the double bond [13,17]. One such aldehyde is 4-hydroxy-2-hexenal (HHE), which is derived from *n*-3 PUFAs [18,19], and is hence an important endpoint in the investigation of oxidative stability of marine oils.

Fish oil has been associated with anti-inflammatory properties, such as the down-regulation of inflammatory cytokines (e.g., TNF-α, IL-6), the increase of cellular membrane content of EPA and DHA, and the decrease of cellular membrane content of arachidonic acid (AA), all in healthy humans [20]. Also, EPA and DHA supplementation has led to decreased T-cell reactivity in cell and animal studies [20]. In murine models, high fat LC *n*-3 PUFA diets have been observed to decrease the levels of inflammation markers in plasma (IL-6 and MCP-1) [21] and in the spleen (NF-κB) [22], the same markers that increased in the study where mice were fed with an oxidized diet [10]. In another murine study, in which the mice were fed an oxidized LC *n*-3 PUFA diet, inflammatory markers such as NF-κB and glutathione peroxidase increased [10]. In addition, it was observed that HHE given orally to the mice was associated with an inflammatory response, as well as the formation of HHE-adducts. HHE in plasma increased significantly in mice given the oxidized LC *n*-3 PUFA diet [10]. In the search for sustainable LC *n*-3 PUFA rich substitutes to the traditional cod liver oil and fish oil [23,24], krill and microalgae oil (in this article referred to as algae oil) are two plausible candidates. Krill oil contains more EPA when compared to algae oil, while algae produce its own DHA, and therefore the oil is richer in this fatty acid (FA) [25]. They are both high in naturally occurring antioxidants, e.g., astaxanthin in krill oil [25,26], and phenolic compounds, flavonoids, sterols, and β-carotene in algae oil [27]. A specific feature of krill oil is that most of the LC *n*-3 PUFA are bound in phospholipids. In microalgae, fish muscle, and liver, the LC *n*-3 PUFA are incorporated in triacylglycerols (TG).

In this study, we investigated the effects of in vitro digests of three marine oils (cod liver oil, krill oil, and algae oil) generated with human digestive fluids on a cultured human intestinal epithelium (Caco-2 cell line). We measured the content of the secondary oxidation products MDA and HHE in the digests, and exposed the epithelium to pure MDA and HHE at these levels and above. We also measured the aldehyde levels in the basal medium. In addition, we examined stress-related protein levels in the Caco-2 cells with proteome profiler arrays to evaluate if the cells were exposed to stress during the various treatments.

2. Materials and Methods

2.1. Materials

The pre-cursor for MDA standard 1,1,3,3-tetraethoxypropane (TEP), 2,4-dinitrophenylhydrazine (DNPH), and reagents used for cell experiments were all purchased from Sigma-Aldrich (Schnelldorf, Germany). 4-hydroxy-2-hexenal (HHE), 4-hydroxy-2-nonenal (HNE), and 4-oxy-2-nonenal (ONE) standards were supplied from Cayman Chemicals (Ann Arbor, MI, USA). Media and supplements that were needed for cell culture maintenance were purchased from PAA (Pasching, Austria), and disposables in polystyrene used for cell cultivation and maintenance were bought from Corning (San Francisco, MA, USA). The human cell stress array kit was purchased from Bio-techne (Abingdon, UK).

2.2. Collection of Human Digestive Fluids

Saliva was collected from seven healthy fasting volunteers at Chalmers University of Technology (Gothenburg, Sweden) in November 2015. Saliva was collected in the morning by sterile straw pipets (Kemikalia; Skurup, Sweden) and volunteers were shown pictures of fish dishes to stimulate spontaneous drooling during collection. Saliva was pooled to eliminate individual effects, centrifuged, and stored at −80 °C.

Human gastric juice (HGJ) and human duodenal juice (HDJ) were aspirated from six healthy volunteers at Lovisenberg Diakonale Hospital (Oslo, Norway), as described by Ulleberg et al. [28], and Holm et al. [29]. The volunteers were semi-fasting using a stimulatory solution and aspiration was done using gastroscopy and a triple lumen tube (Maxter Catheters, Marseille, France), aspiration details are further described by Ulleberg et al. [28]. Aspirates were pooled, enzyme activities, and pH of the human GI fluids were recorded according to Minekus et al. [30], and the HGJ and HDJ were stored separately at $-80\,^\circ$C. All of the participants in the study were volunteers with informed consent, and the study was performed according to the Declaration of Helsinki. Ethical approval was received from the Norwegian Regional Ethics Committee (project no. 2012/2230, Biobank no. 2012/2210).

The human digestive fluids were characterized according to Minekus et al. [30], and enzymatic activities were measured in connection to the in vitro digestions. The pepsin activity of HGJ was 1200 U/mL, the gastric lipase activity in the HGJ was 16 U/mL, the pancreatic lipase activity in the HDJ was 48 U/mL, and the bile salt concentration in the HDJ was 0.230 mM. Ascorbic acid was analyzed by the method described by Lykkesfeldt et al. by ion chromatography followed by electrochemical detection [31], and approximately 0.3 ppm was detected in both HGJ and HDJ. Ca^{2+} was analyzed by an ion chromatograph couples with UV-vis according to Fredrikson et al. [32], and was found to be present in HGJ at 35 ppm and in HDJ at 16 ppm.

2.3. Marine Oils

Refined cod liver oil (*Gadus morhua*), without added antioxidants, was supplied by Lýsi hf (Reykjavík, Iceland). Unrefined algae oil from *Schizochytrium* sp. called Life's DHA S35-CO100 was supplied from DSM (Basel, Switzerland). Unrefined krill oil from Antarctic krill (*Euphausia superba*) called Superba™ Krill Oil (Aker Biomarine Antarctic AS, Oslo, Norway) was provided by Sanpharm AB (Gothenburg, Sweden). The LC *n*-3 PUFA profile of the oils, % as reported by Jónsdóttir et al. and according to the manufacturers specification [33], and quantitatively (mg FAME/g oil) measured in-house according to Cavonius et al. [34], can be found in the supplementary material (Table S1).

2.4. In Vitro Digestion with Human Digests

The three marine oils were digested in vitro in a static three-step digestion model, using the human digestive fluids. The model is based on the standardized InfoGest protocol with minor modifications [30]. The recommended daily intake (RDI) for supplemental oils are based on the consumption of EPA and DHA, and therefore the dose of each oil was normalized to its EPA and DHA content before the simulated GI digestion. For each oil, an amount providing 5 mg total LC *n*-3 PUFA, i.e., EPA+DHA, was used, which corresponds to 250 mg on a human level. Water was added to achieve samples of the same volume. In control digestions, oils were omitted and only water was used. In short, digestion was performed in darkness and the oil-water mixture was digested by one volume saliva, followed by HGJ addition (1:1, pH 6, 37 °C, 50 rpm, 120 min), including adjustment of pH to pH 3 after 60 min. Intestinal digestion was performed by the addition of HDJ (1:1, pH 7, 37 °C, 250 rpm, 90 min). Digested samples were flushed with N_2 gas (15 s) and stored in $-80\,^\circ$C until aldehyde analysis and cell experiments.

2.5. Cell Line

Caco-2 cells (HTB-37), passage 19, were obtained from the American Type Culture Collection (Rockville, MD, USA). The cells were cultured in an incubator at 37 °C/5% CO_2/95% humidified air. The medium used was EMEM (FBS; 10%) supplemented with Normocin™ (0.2%; Invivogen, San Diego, CA, USA). The medium was replaced every second or third day and passaging of cells was done at approximately 80% confluence. At passage 29–37, the cells were seeded in 12-well plates with Transwell® polycarbonate inserts (0.4 µm; Corning, San Francisco, MA, USA) at 60,000 cells/insert or without inserts (CellBiND®, polystyrene; Corning, Kennebunk, ME, USA) at 200,000 cells/well. All of the experiments were carried out 14 days post-seeding.

2.6. Cell Experiments

Cells (on inserts) were treated with in vitro digested marine oils and control digests (without oil), diluted 1:1 in the apical medium. The apical medium was added (0.5 mL) to the cells 24 h prior to the experiments to let the cells produce endogenous trypsin inhibitor. At the time of the experiment, 0.25 mL of the apical medium was replaced by 0.25 mL of the digests and were then left in the incubator for 2 h (37 °C). Controls with only medium were included, as well as standards with MDA in water and HHE in DMSO (DMSO at 0.01%), corresponding to the highest levels detected in digests; 16.6 and 2.8 μM, respectively. Standards were as digests diluted 1:1 in the apical medium, hence exposure of cells to MDA and HHE were 8.3 and 1.4 μM, respectively. From here on, these levels of MDA and HHE are referred to as "low" levels. To separately study the toxicity of the aldehydes at different levels, an experiment with cells in wells without inserts was performed. MDA levels tested were 8.3, 45, and 90 μM; HHE levels tested were 1.4, 45, and 90 μM. A mix (1:1) of the two aldehydes was also studied at (1) 45 μM each of MDA and HHE; (2) 22.5 μM each of MDA and HHE, and (3) 4.15 μM MDA and 0.7 μM HHE, to test combined, e.g., synergistic, effects. 90 μM of the individual aldehydes and 45 μM of each in a mix are from here on referred to as "high" levels. The highest aldehyde levels are in the same range, as previously used by Awada et al. [10], the levels in the middle are half of the highest levels, and in the same range as used by Alghazeer et al. [35]. Minimum Essential Medium Eagle, HEPES modification powder (14.2 g/L; Sigma-Aldrich, Schnelldorf, Germany) was used to be able to achieve high MDA concentrations without dilution, and mixed (1:1) with the ordinary medium that was used when studying the mixed effect of MDA and HHE. After the 2 h of incubation, the medium was aspirated and the cells were washed in PBS and lysed.

2.7. Harvesting of Caco-2 Cells and Protein Analysis

The medium was removed and the cells were washed in PBS prior to harvest. The basal medium was collected and the cells were lysed in RIPA (Sigma-Aldrich, Schnelldorf, Germany) with EDTA-free Pierce™ Protease and Phosphatase inhibitor (Thermo Fisher Scientific, Waltham, MA, USA). Total cellular protein content was measured by Pierce™ BCA Protein Assay Kit (Thermo Fisher Scientific, Waltham, MA, USA), following the instructions from the manufacturer. From the total protein content (which is proportional to cell number), cell viability/survival was estimated.

2.8. Analysis of Peroxide Value (PV) and Aldehydes (HHE & MDA)

Peroxide value (PV) was analysed prior to digestion in the crude oils by thiocyanate and ferric iron complexation, according to Undeland et al. [36].

HHE and MDA were analyzed, as described by Tullberg et al. [8]. Briefly, digests and basolateral media were acidified to precipitate proteins, followed by DNPH-derivatization and dichloromethane extraction. Samples were evaporated and re-suspended in MeOH, aldehydes were then determined in digests by detection on LC/APCI-MS (Agilent 1260 HPLC coupled with Agilent 6120 quadrupole; Agilent Technologies, Waldbron, Germany) in negative mode, using external standards for MDA and HHE. Analysis of the data was carried out using the software Agilent ChemStation (Agilent Technologies, Böblingen, Germany).

2.9. Human Cell Stress Array Analysis

The Human Cell Stress Array Kit (Bio-techne, Minneapolis, MN, USA) was used according to manufacturer's protocol. Briefly, membranes coated with 26 capture antibodies were blocked (1 h, RT). The blocking buffer was aspirated and the samples were adjusted by total cellular protein content were added (105 μg total protein; n = 3) together with a biotinylated antibody cocktail for detection (overnight, 130 rpm, 4 °C). Membranes were then washed in a wash buffer (10 min, repeated three times). Streptavidin-conjugated horseradish peroxidase (HRP) was added to the membranes (30 min, RT), and membranes were again washed (10 min, repeated 3 times). After the last washing step, a reaction mixture containing hydrogen peroxide and luminol (1:1) was added to the membranes, and was instantly analyzed with a detection system for chemiluminescence (Chemidoc XRS+, Bio-Rad), followed by software analysis of the images by ImageLab (Bio-Rad). See Table 1 for the specific analytes detected.

Table 1. Proteins detected by the Human Cell Stress Array Kit.

Nr	Analyte	Nr	Analyte
1	ADAMTS1	14	IDO
2	Bcl-2	15	Phospho-JNK PAN (T183/Y185)
3	Carbonic Anhydrase IX	16	NFκB1
4	Cited-2	17	p21/CIP1
5	COX-2	18	p27
6	Cytochrome C (Cyt C)	19	Phospho-p38a (T180/Y182)
7	Dickkopf-4 (Dkk-4)	20	Phospho-p53 (S46)
8	Fatty acid-binding protein 1 (FABP-1)	21	Paraoxonase-1 (PON-1)
9	HIF-1a	22	Paraoxonase-2 (PON-2)
10	HIF-2a	23	Paraoxonase-3 (PON-3)
11	Phospho-HSP27 (S78/S82)	24	Thioredoxin-1 (Trx-1)
12	Heat Shock Protein-60 (HSP-60)	25	Deacetylase Sirtuin 2 (SIRT2)
13	Heat Shock Protein-70 (HSP-70)	26	Superoxide dismutase 2 (SOD2)

2.10. Statistics

Calculated values are presented as mean values $\pm$ standard deviation (SD; $n = 3$) or when $n = 2$ as mean values $\pm$ (max $-$ min)/2. Digestion of oils with subsequent cell experiments were made in triplicates and repeated at three occasions, human stress arrays were done in duplicates and repeated 2–3 times. The significance of the difference between treatment and control was analyzed by Student's two-tailed, unpaired t test, and treatments were compared by a one- or two-way analysis of variance (ANOVA; Microsoft Office Excel, 2013), followed by treatment to treatment t test as above, whenever applicable. Differences were considered significant at $p \leq 0.05$. Significant levels are denoted in the graphs and tables when applicable; * = $p \leq 0.05$, ** = $p \leq 0.01$, *** = $p \leq 0.001$.

3. Results

3.1. MDA and HHE Formation during In Vitro Digestion with Human Digestive Fluids

The initial aldehyde levels prior to digesteion were 0.013 $\pm$ 0.01, 0.11 $\pm$ 0.05, and 0.38 $\pm$ 0.14 µM, for MDA, and 0.005 $\pm$ 0.009, 0.17 $\pm$ 0.02, and 0.04 $\pm$ 0.007 µM for HHE in the algae-, cod liver- and krill oil, respectively. The corresponding peroxide values (PV) in the crude oils were 0.18 $\pm$ 0.05 in algae-, 1.48 $\pm$ 0.06 in cod liver- and 1.00 $\pm$ 0.30 (mmol/kg oil) in the krill oil. According to the PV and HHE measurement, the cod liver oil was the most oxidized oil initially, however the krill oil contained a higher initial concentration of MDA. The aldehydes MDA and HHE both increased from start ($t = 0$ min) to end ($t = 210$ min) of the in vitro digestion. The levels of MDA and HHE detected in the digests were approximately 4 and 7–20 times higher in the cod liver oil as compared to the other oils, respectively (Table 2).

Table 2. Detected levels (μM) of 4-hydroxy-2-hexenal (HHE) and malondialdehyde (MDA) in in vitro digests ($t = 210$ min) using human digestive fluids. Data are shown as mean ± standard deviation (SD), $n = 3$.

Marine Oil	MDA μM ± SD	HHE μM ± SD
Algae oil	4.45 ± 1.81	0.13 ± 0.039
Cod liver oil	16.6 ± 7.74	2.77 ± 2.66
Krill oil	4.29 ± 0.70	0.38 ± 0.061

3.2. Cell Survival Was Not Significantly Affected by Either Oil Digests or HHE and MDA

There was no significant effect of digested oils on cell survival after 2 h of incubation and 22 additional hours with fresh medium (Figure 1). In a dose-response experiment with the oxidation products MDA and HHE, similar results were achieved with no adverse effect on cell viability (Figure 2). A minor increase was seen in protein levels when adding 45 μM of HHE, however this effect was within 2 SD:s and thus natural variation.

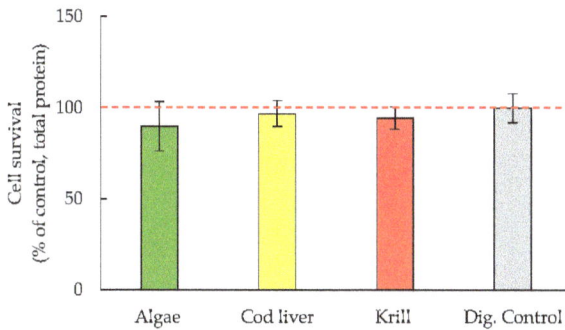

Figure 1. Cell survival estimated from the change in total protein level between untreated and treated cells, data are shown as mean % ± (max − min)/2, $n = 2$. Dig. Control = digests from digestion of only water.

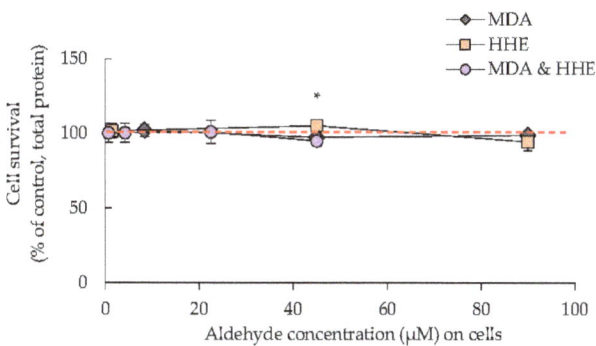

Figure 2. Cell survival in the presence of increasing concentrations of the aldehydes malondialdehyde (MDA) and 4-hydroxy-2-hexenal (HHE), data are shown as means ± (max − min)/2, $n = 2$, or $n = 4$ for the lowest concentrations of MDA (8.3 μM) and HHE (1.4 μM). Significant difference ($p \leq 0.05$). MDA and HHE is the combination of both aldehydes, at the lowest concentrations, 4.15 μM MDA and 0.7 μM HHE. * = $p \leq 0.05$.

3.3. Cellular Levels of HSP-70 and Trx-1 Were Decreased in the Presence of Digested Marine Oils

All of the digested oils significantly decreased the expression of HSP-70 and Trx-1 ($p \leq 0.001$), Figure 3. In addition, SOD2 levels were significantly lowered in the presence of algae and cod liver oil digests. Krill oil digests did not significantly affect SOD2 levels. HSP-70, Trx-1 and SOD2 are all a part of the anti-oxidative stress defense and are generally increased when the cells are exposed to oxidative stress [37,38]. HSP-70 is a chaperone protein that reduces oxidative damage by binding to proteins, which prevents unfolding and aggregation. Trx-1 is an oxidoreductase facilitating the reduction of oxidized proteins and SOD2 is a superoxide dismutase that eliminates superoxide radicals. The levels of HSP-60, coming from the same family as HSP-70, was significantly lowered in the presence of digested algae and krill oil, however not by digested cod liver oil.

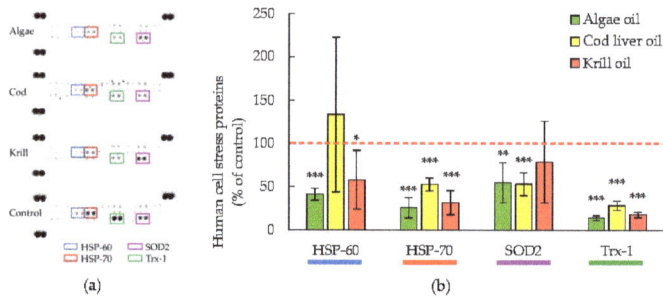

Figure 3. (**a**) Representative membranes showing the expression of human stress-related proteins (Proteome profiler™ arrays) in the presence of marine oils digested by human GI fluids.; (**b**) Bar graph representation of data for pooled triplicates of lysates ± SD, $n = 3$. * = $p \leq 0.05$, ** = $p \leq 0.01$, *** = $p \leq 0.005$. HSP-60= Heat Shock Protein-60; HSP-70= Heat Shock Protein-70; SOD2= Superoxide dismutase 2; Trx-1= Thioredoxin-1.

3.4. Cellular Hsp-70 and Trx-1 Levels Were Not Affected by Low MDA and HHE Levels (8.3 and 1.4 µM)

Low concentrations of MDA (8.3 µM) and HHE (1.4 µM), corresponding to the highest aldehyde levels in the marine oil digests, which the cells were exposed to, did not, or did only slightly, affect the cellular levels of HSP-70, TRX-1, SOD2, Figure 4. In addition, the HSP-70 family member, HSP-60, decreased significantly ($p = 0.043$) in the presence of low level HHE (1.4 µM).

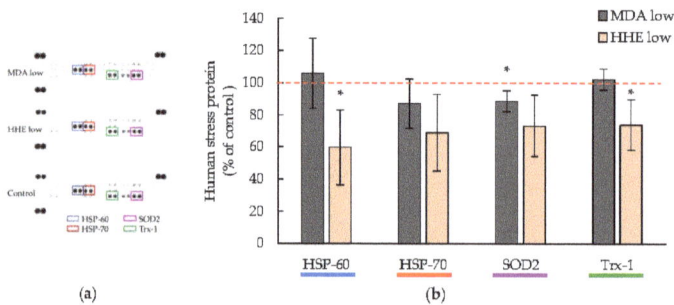

Figure 4. (**a**) Representative membrane showing the expression of human stress-related proteins (Proteome profiler™ arrays) in the presence of "low" aldehyde levels, 1.4 µM 4-hydroxy-2-hexenal (HHE) and 8.3 µM malondialdehyde (MDA), i.e., the levels found in cod liver oil digests; (**b**) Bar graph of the data for pooled triplicates of lysates ± (max − min)/2, $n = 2$. * = $p \leq 0.05$. HSP-60= Heat Shock Protein-60; HSP-70= Heat Shock Protein-70; SOD2= Superoxide dismutase 2; Trx-1= Thioredoxin-1.

3.5. High Levels (90 µM) of MDA and HHE Did Not Affect the Cellular Levels of HSP-70 and Trx-1

High concentrations of aldehydes (90 µM), did not significantly affect the cellular levels of HSP-70 and Trx-1, Figure 5. The stress proteins detected were even closer to 100% of the control as compared to the addition of low aldehyde levels to the cells, but HSP-60 significantly increased in the presence of high MDA concentrations ($p = 0.026$). Testing a combination of MDA and HHE, both at 45 µM, the result was a combined effect that was similar to the presence of isolated aldehydes at 90 µM. HSP-60 however, increased ($p = 0.0054$, MDA & HHE) when compared to control, and Trx-1 was significantly lower than the control when cells were exposed to the MDA and HHE mix ($p = 0.032$).

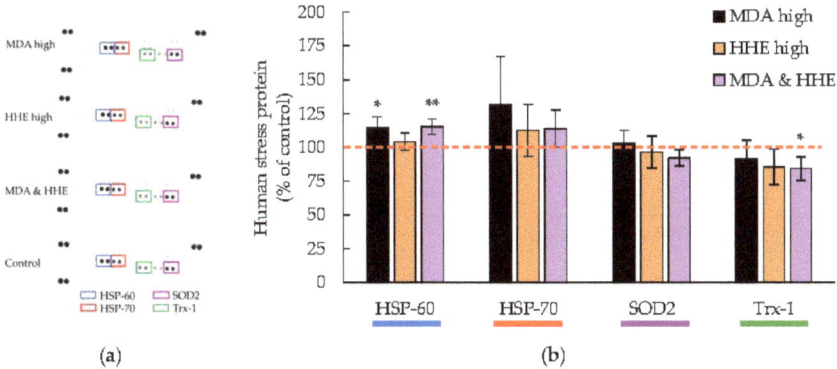

(a) (b)

Figure 5. (**a**) A representative membrane showing the expression of human stress-related proteins (Proteome profiler™ arrays) in the presence of high aldehyde levels (90 µM MDA; 90 µM HHE; 45 µM MDA & HHE); (**b**) Bar graph of the data for pooled triplicates of lysates of cells in the presence of MDA (90 µM), HHE (90 µM) and a mix of MDA and HHE (45 µM each), data are shown as means ± (max − min)/2, $n = 2$. * = $p \leq 0.05$, ** = $p \leq 0.01$. MDA= malondialdehyde; HHE= 4-hydroxy-2-hexenal; HSP-60= Heat Shock Protein-60; HSP-70= Heat Shock Protein-70; SOD2= Superoxide dismutase 2; Trx-1= Thioredoxin-1.

3.6. Levels of MDA and HHE on the Basal Side of the Epithelium

High concentrations of MDA and HHE were found in the basal medium after the incubation of Caco-2 cells with the oil digests (1.4, 2.1 and 0.8 µM MDA; 0.09, 0.2 and 0.06 µM HHE for algae, cod liver, and krill oil, respectively). The absolute amounts (nmol) in the apical versus the basal medium are presented in Figure 6. The medium with the algae oil digests contained significantly ($p \leq 0.05$) more MDA and HHE in the basal medium when compared to the apical medium. With the present experimental setup, we do not know if, or how much of, MDA and HHE that was actually transported across the intestinal epithelium. The decomposition of the digested oils is expected to be extensive, due to the elevated temperature (T = 37 °C), during the 2 h incubation time. This is expected to give increasing levels of aldehydes in the apical medium, and therefore a ratio of the basal concentration of MDA and HHE to the added sample concentration of MDA and HHE will not give an accurate measure of the transport. Thus, the bioavailability cannot be correctly estimated. Awada et al., who used deuterium labelling, estimated the basolateral transport of HHE in Caco-2/TC7 cells, which resulted in approximately 0.2% HHE transfer (100 µM, 24 h) [10]. This gives an indication of in which magnitude we should expect to find the transport. When we conducted a transport experiment with pure HHE, we found that HHE was transported across the epithelium at 1.14% when incubated with 1.4 µM HHE for 2 h. Corresponding data was 10.6% when using the lower concentration of HHE (0.65 µM, 2 h), Table 3.

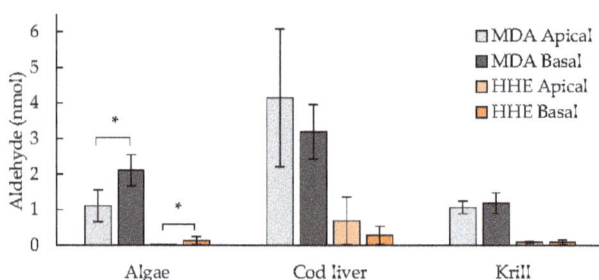

Figure 6. Aldehyde (nmol) added to the apical medium and detected in the basal medium of Caco-2 cells after incubation ($t = 2$ h). Data are shown as means $\pm$ standard deviation (SD), $n = 3$. * = $p \leq 0.05$. MDA= malondialdehyde; HHE= 4-hydroxy-2-hexenal.

Table 3. Absolute quantity of 4-hydroxy-2-hexenal (HHE; nmol) present in the apical and basal medium (BM), $n = 3$.

HHE (nmol) Added	HHE (nmol), BM
0.7	0.0080 ± 0.0042
0.0325	0.0035 ± 0.0011

4. Discussion

4.1. Oxidation of the Oils during In Vitro Digestion

Both MDA and HHE levels increased during in vitro digestion with human digestive fluids. These results are in agreement with results from studies where cod liver oil and salmon were subjected to in vitro digestion models, in which enzymes and bile have been of porcine or other animal origin [9,39,40]. Increase in aldehyde formation during digestion was also observed in our previous study, when digesting cod liver oil with human GI fluids [8].

4.2. Human Digests of Marine Oils and the Aldehydes MDA and HHE Had No Adverse Effect on the Epithelium

From these studies, we can conclude that the digested oils and their MDA/HHE content did not have a negative impact on the cells. The absence of effects of pure MDA and HHE (1.4–90 µM) on cell survival is supported by Awada et al. [10], in which no effect in TEER after incubating Caco-2 and T27 cells with similar levels of aldehydes (24 h, 0–100 µM) was observed. On the contrary, proteins associated with oxidative damage (Trx-1 and HSP-70) were down-regulated in the presence of all three digested marine oils, suggesting that the cells actually were experiencing less oxidative stress than in the absence of the digested oils. In addition, pure MDA and HHE, corresponding to the concentrations found in the oil digests, did not increase oxidative stress markers in the cells, HHE even significantly reduced the levels of Trx-1 in the cells, indicating that MDA and HHE had no harmful effect at the levels found after in vitro digestion of the three marine oils with human GI fluids. Hence, the lipid oxidation taking place during in vitro GI digestion in this study was not associated with harmful effects in human intestinal cells. Although it is not directly comparable with studies of digests in intestinal cell models, HHE has been shown to promote Nrf2 activation in HUVEC cells [41], and also, oxidized EPA has been shown to inhibit NF-κB activation in murine aortic endothelial cells [42]. In addition, a recent review by Roy et al. suggests that ROS play an important role for cellular redox homeostasis [43]. All of these data are in line with our findings. However, there are also some studies with digested marine oils showing opposite results to ours regarding lipid oxidation and effects on Caco-2 cells [7,10]. Different outcomes may in several cases be a direct cause of different experimental setups, such as exposing intestinal cells to undigested oils, exposing other cell types than intestinal cells to GI digests, using oils with a higher oxidation degree, using longer incubation time, or feeding a cell type of non-intestinal origin with oils. Even though we did not identify the adverse effects of MDA and HHE on the intestinal level, there may be potentially harmful systemic effects of lipid oxidation products, e.g., MDA protein adducts have been implicated in coronary artery disease development [44].

4.3. Comparison of the Different Marine Oils

In the crude oils, the concentration of EPA plus DHA was in the following order: algae > krill > cod liver oil. Digests with cod liver oil therefore contained the highest amount (mg/mL) of total oil per digest when compared to the other oils (10% more oil than krill oil, 50% more than algae oil). Algae oil contained mainly DHA, while the other two oils contained ratios between EPA and DHA that were 0.8 and 2.0 for cod liver oil and krill oil, respectively. The krill oil is unique in that it contains high levels of phospholipids and the antioxidant astaxhantin. The stability of the EPA/DHA-normalized samples differed between the oils during the GI digestion, and the cod liver oil was the one most oxidized after completed digestion (highest [MDA] and [HHE]). In the comparison of the different oil digests, blanks with pure digests without added oil, were always included as controls.

When comparing the effects of the digested oils on HSP-70 and Trx-1 levels, a significant difference between the cod liver oil and the other two oils was observed; but no significant difference was observed between algae and krill oil. Digested cod liver oil did not significantly affect HSP-60, while both the digested algae and krill oils had a reducing effect; indicating that a low oxidation degree, as in the algae and krill oils after digestion, could have a HSP-60 decreasing effect. However, this effect could also be due to the protective effects from the natural antioxidants in the algae and krill oils [24–26].

Krill oil digests did not significantly reduce the levels of the superoxide dismutase SOD2 as the other oils did. Krill oil digests also had a lower HHE to MDA ratio than cod liver and algae oil digests, but if there is a specific effect of HHE on the down-regulation of SOD2 levels is not known. Free fatty acids (FFA) extracted from krill oil was previously found to inhibit cell growth and induce apoptosis when added in undigested form to HCT-15, SW-480, and Caco-2 cells [45]. Our digests contain a mixture of FFA, as well as partially hydrolyzed TAG and phospholipids, but indeed the FFA could play a specific role. In another study, undigested whole krill oil was also found to have anti-inflammatory action, thus reducing the pro-inflammatory cytokines IL-8 and TNFα that was produced by Caco-2 and HT29 cells [46]. In a human trial, krill oil was found to have a positive effect on intestinal endothelial function, giving a mean EndoPAT Reactive Hyperemia Index of 2.16 after 17 weeks of supplementation, and the ingestion of krill oil also increased the serum levels of high-density lipoprotein [47], however it is not known whether these results had any connection to formation of lipid oxidation products in the krill oil during digestion.

In general, our results from comparing the three different oil digests indicate that krill oil, cod liver oil, and algae oil, have similar characteristics in regards to not being cytotoxic or stress-promoting to intestinal epithelial cells. The oil digest with the most reducing effect on HSP-60, HSP-70, and Trx-1 was that from algae oil. Algae oil differed from the other oils in that it had a different FA profile with a high content of DHA, a low content of the other FA, and also another antioxidant profile. Whether these factors played a role in reducing the oxidative stress response requires future work.

5. Conclusions

Exposing the Caco-2 cells with digests of marine oils and pure aldehydes did not affect cell survival. All of the digests significantly reduced the cellular expression of the human cellular stress proteins HSP-70 and Trx-1, indicating that the cells were experiencing less oxidative stress. Exposure (t = 2 h) to pure MDA at the same level that was present in the digests (8.3 μM) significantly lowered the expression of SOD2. Corresponding exposure of pure HHE at the level found in the digests (1.4 μM) decreased expression of HSP-60 and Trx-1. A mix of MDA and HHE (45 μM of each) significantly diminished the cellular expression of Trx-1, however, at high levels (90 μM) there was no change in Trx-1 expression. Altogether, the present aldehyde concentrations, relevant to aldehyde levels formed in vivo, did not increase the levels of the investigated stress-related proteins, indicating that physiological levels of these aldehydes may not induce intestinal cell stress.

Supplementary Materials: The following are available online at www.mdpi.com/2072-6643/9/11/1213/s1, Table S1: Amounts of EPA and DHA of algae oil, cod liver oil, and krill oil.

Acknowledgments: This study was funded by the Swedish Council for Environment, Agricultural Sciences and Spatial Planning, Formas (Grant no. 222-2012-1331).

Author Contributions: C.T., N.S. and I.U. conceived and designed the experiments; C.T. performed the experiments; C.T. and N.S. analyzed the data; N.S. contributed with expertise in cell studies and took an active part in the writing process; G.V. contributed with collection of human digests, design of in vitro digestion model and support during the writing process; I.U. contributed with expertise in the field of marine oils and lipid oxidation, and contributed with support during the writing process; C.T. was responsible for writing the paper.

Conflicts of Interest: The authors declare no conflict of interest.

References

1. Lavie, C.J.; Milani, R.V.; Mehra, M.R.; Ventura, H.O. Omega-3 polyunsaturated fatty acids and cardiovascular diseases. *J. Am. Coll. Cardiol.* **2009**, *54*, 585–594. [CrossRef] [PubMed]

2. Delgado-Lista, J.; Perez-Martinez, P.; Lopez-Miranda, J.; Perez-Jimenez, F. Long chain omega-3 fatty acids and cardiovascular disease: A systematic review. *Br. J. Nutr.* **2012**, *107* (Suppl. 2), S201–S213. [CrossRef] [PubMed]

3. Kanner, J.; Lapidot, T. The stomach as a bioreactor: Dietary lipid peroxidation in the gastric fluid and the effects of plant-derived antioxidants. *Free Radic. Biol. Med.* **2001**, *31*, 1388–1395. [CrossRef]

4. Turner, R.; McLean, C.H.; Silvers, K.M. Are the health benefits of fish oils limited by products of oxidation? *Nutr. Res. Rev.* **2006**, *19*, 53–62. [CrossRef] [PubMed]

5. Albert, B.B.; Cameron-Smith, D.; Hofman, P.L.; Cutfield, W.S. Oxidation of marine omega-3 supplements and human health. *Biomed. Res. Int.* **2013**, *2013*, 464921. [CrossRef] [PubMed]

6. Kristinova, V.; Storrø, I.; Rustad, T. Influence of human gastric juice on oxidation of marine lipids—In vitro study. *Food Chem.* **2013**, *141*, 3859–3871. [CrossRef] [PubMed]

7. Maestre, R.; Douglass, J.D.; Kodukula, S.; Medina, I.; Storch, J. Alterations in the intestinal assimilation of oxidized pufas are ameliorated by a polyphenol-rich grape seed extract in an in vitro model and caco-2 cells. *J. Nutr.* **2013**, *143*, 295–301. [CrossRef] [PubMed]

8. Tullberg, C.; Larsson, K.; Carlsson, N.G.; Comi, I.; Scheers, N.; Vegarud, G.; Undeland, I. Formation of reactive aldehydes (MDA, HHE, HNE) during the digestion of cod liver oil: Comparison of human and porcine in vitro digestion models. *Food Funct.* **2016**, *7*, 1401–1412. [CrossRef] [PubMed]

9. Larsson, K.; Harrysson, H.; Havenaar, R.; Alminger, M.; Undeland, I. Formation of malondialdehyde (MDA), 4-hydroxy-2-hexenal (HHE) and 4-hydroxy-2-nonenal (HHE) in fish and fish oil during dynamic gastrointestinal in vitro digestion. *Food Funct.* **2016**, *7*, 1176–1187. [CrossRef] [PubMed]

10. Awada, M.; Soulage, C.O.; Meynier, A.; Debard, C.; Plaisancie, P.; Benoit, B.; Picard, G.; Loizon, E.; Chauvin, M.A.; Estienne, M.; et al. Dietary oxidized *n*-3 PUFA induce oxidative stress and inflammation: Role of intestinal absorption of 4-HHE and reactivity in intestinal cells. *J. Lipid Res.* **2012**, *53*, 2069–2080. [CrossRef] [PubMed]

11. Gutteridge, J.M. Free-radical damage to lipids, amino acids, carbohydrates and nucleic acids determined by thiobarbituric acid reactivity. *Int. J. Biochem.* **1982**, *14*, 649–653. [CrossRef]

12. Frankel, E.N.; Neff, W.E. Formation of malonaldehyde from lipid oxidation-products. *Biochim. Biophys. Acta* **1983**, *754*, 264–270. [CrossRef]

13. Esterbauer, H.; Schaur, R.J.; Zollner, H. Chemistry and biochemistry of 4-hydroxynonenal, malonaldehyde and related aldehydes. *Free Radic. Biol. Med.* **1991**, *11*, 81–128. [CrossRef]

14. Ayala, A.; Muñoz, M.F.; Argüelles, S. Lipid peroxidation: Production, metabolism, and signaling mechanisms of malondialdehyde and 4-hydroxy-2-nonenal. *Oxid. Med. Cell. Longev.* **2014**, *2014*, 31. [CrossRef] [PubMed]

15. Del Rio, D.; Stewart, A.J.; Pellegrini, N. A review of recent studies on malondialdehyde as toxic molecule and biological marker of oxidative stress. *Nutr. Metab. Cardiovasc. Dis.* **2005**, *15*, 316–328. [CrossRef] [PubMed]

16. Uchida, K. Role of reactive aldehyde in cardiovascular diseases. *Free Radic. Biol. Med.* **2000**, *28*, 1685–1696. [CrossRef]

17. LoPachin, R.M.; Gavin, T. Molecular mechanisms of aldehyde toxicity: A chemical perspective. *Chem. Res. Toxicol.* **2014**, *27*, 1081–1091. [CrossRef] [PubMed]

18. Van Kuijk, F.J.; Holte, L.L.; Dratz, E.A. 4-hydroxyhexenal: A lipid peroxidation product derived from oxidized docosahexaenoic acid. *Biochim. Biophys. Acta* **1990**, *1043*, 116–118. [CrossRef]

19. Guichardant, M.; Bacot, S.; Moliere, P.; Lagarde, M. Hydroxy-alkenals from the peroxidation of *n*-3 and *n*-6 fatty acids and urinary metabolites. *Prostaglandins Leukot. Essent. Fat. Acids* **2006**, *75*, 179–182. [CrossRef] [PubMed]

20. Calder, P.C. Omega-3 polyunsaturated fatty acids and inflammatory processes: Nutrition or pharmacology? *Br. J. Clin. Pharmacol.* **2013**, *75*, 645–662. [CrossRef] [PubMed]

21. Awada, M.; Meynier, A.; Soulage, C.O.; Hadji, L.; Geloen, A.; Viau, M.; Ribourg, L.; Benoit, B.; Debard, C.; Guichardant, M.; et al. N-3 PUFA added to high-fat diets affect differently adiposity and inflammation when carried by phospholipids or triacylglycerols in mice. *Nutr. Metab. (Lond.)* **2013**, *10*, 23. [CrossRef] [PubMed]

22. Soni, N.K.; Ross, A.B.; Scheers, N.; Savolainen, O.I.; Nookaew, I.; Gabrielsson, B.G.; Sandberg, A.S. Splenic immune response is down-regulated in C57BL/6J mice fed eicosapentaenoic acid and docosahexaenoic acid enriched high fat diet. *Nutrients* **2017**, *9*, 50. [CrossRef] [PubMed]

23. Cicero, A.F.; Morbini, M.; Borghi, C. Do we need 'new' omega-3 polyunsaturated fatty acids formulations? *Expert Opin. Pharmacother.* **2015**, *16*, 285–288. [CrossRef] [PubMed]

24. Adarme-Vega, T.C.; Thomas-Hall, S.R.; Schenk, P.M. Towards sustainable sources for omega-3 fatty acids production. *Curr. Opin. Biotechnol.* **2014**, *26*, 14–18. [CrossRef] [PubMed]

25. Kassis, N.M.; Gigliotti, J.C.; Beamer, S.K.; Tou, J.C.; Jaczynski, J. Characterization of lipids and antioxidant capacity of novel nutraceutical egg products developed with omega-3-rich oils. *J. Sci. Food Agric.* **2012**, *92*, 66–73. [CrossRef] [PubMed]

26. Tou, J.C.; Jaczynski, J.; Chen, Y.C. Krill for human consumption: Nutritional value and potential health benefits. *Nutr. Rev.* **2007**, *65*, 63–77. [CrossRef] [PubMed]

27. Lv, J.; Yang, X.; Ma, H.; Hu, X.; Wei, Y.; Zhou, W.; Li, L. The oxidative stability of microalgae oil (*Schizochytrium aggregatum*) and its antioxidant activity after simulated gastrointestinal digestion: Relationship with constituents. *Eur. J. Lipid Sci. Technol.* **2015**, *117*, 1928–1939. [CrossRef]

28. Ulleberg, E.K.; Comi, I.; Holm, H.; Herud, E.B.; Jacobsen, M.; Vegarud, G.E. Human gastrointestinal juices intended for use in in vitro digestion models. *Food Dig.* **2011**, *2*, 52–61. [CrossRef] [PubMed]

29. Holm, H.; Krogdahl, A.; Hanssen, L.E. High and low inhibitor soybean meals affect human duodenal proteinase activity differently: In vitro comparison of proteinase inhibition. *J. Nutr.* **1988**, *118*, 521–525. [PubMed]

30. Minekus, M.; Alminger, M.; Alvito, P.; Ballance, S.; Bohn, T.; Bourlieu, C.; Carriere, F.; Boutrou, R.; Corredig, M.; Dupont, D.; et al. A standardised static in vitro digestion method suitable for food—An international consensus. *Food Funct.* **2014**, *5*, 1113–1124. [CrossRef] [PubMed]

31. Lykkesfeldt, J. Determination of ascorbic acid and dehydroascorbic acid in biological samples by high-performance liquid chromatography using subtraction methods: Reliable reduction with tris[2-carboxyethyl]phosphine hydrochloride. *Anal. Biochem.* **2000**, *282*, 89–93. [CrossRef] [PubMed]

32. Fredrikson, M.; Carlsson, N.G.; Almgren, A.; Sandberg, A.S. Simultaneous and sensitive analysis of Cu, Ni, Zn, Co, Mn, and Fe in food and biological samples by ion chromatography. *J. Agric. Food Chem.* **2002**, *50*, 59–65. [CrossRef] [PubMed]

33. Jónsdóttir, R.; Geirsdottir, M.; Hamaguchi, P.Y.; Jamnik, P.; Kristinsson, H.G.; Undeland, I. The ability of in vitro antioxidant assays to predict the efficiency of a cod protein hydrolysate and brown seaweed extract to prevent oxidation in marine food model systems. *J. Sci. Food Agric.* **2016**, *96*, 2125–2135. [CrossRef] [PubMed]

34. Cavonius, L.R.; Carlsson, N.-G.; Undeland, I. Quantification of total fatty acids in microalgae: Comparison of extraction and transesterification methods. *Anal. Bioanal. Chem.* **2014**, *406*, 7313–7322. [CrossRef] [PubMed]

35. Alghazeer, R.; Gao, H.; Howell, N.K. Cytotoxicity of oxidised lipids in cultured colonal human intestinal cancer cells (caco-2 cells). *Toxicol. Lett.* **2008**, *180*, 202–211. [CrossRef] [PubMed]

36. Undeland, I.; Hultin, H.O.; Richards, M.P. Added triacylglycerols do not hasten hemoglobin-mediated lipid oxidation in washed minced cod muscle. *J. Agric. Food Chem.* **2002**, *50*, 6847–6853. [CrossRef] [PubMed]

37. Hall, L.; Martinus, R.D. Hyperglycaemia and oxidative stress upregulate HSP60 & HSP70 expression in hela cells. *Springerplus* **2013**, *2*, 431. [CrossRef] [PubMed]

38. Leibowitz, G.; Ktorza, A.; Cerasi, E. The role of txnip in the pathophysiology of diabetes and its vascular complications: A concise review. *Medicographia* **2014**, *36*, 391–397.

39. Larsson, K.; Tullberg, C.; Alminger, M.; Havenaar, R.; Undeland, I. Malondialdehyde and 4-hydroxy-2-hexenal are formed during dynamic gastrointestinal in vitro digestion of cod liver oils. *Food Funct.* **2016**, *7*, 3458–3467. [CrossRef] [PubMed]

40. Steppeler, C.; Haugen, J.-E.; Rødbotten, R.; Kirkhus, B. Formation of malondialdehyde, 4-hydroxynonenal, and 4-hydroxyhexenal during in vitro digestion of cooked beef, pork, chicken, and salmon. *J. Agric. Food Chem.* **2016**, *64*, 487–496. [CrossRef] [PubMed]

41. Ishikado, A.; Morino, K.; Nishio, Y.; Nakagawa, F.; Mukose, A.; Sono, Y.; Yoshioka, N.; Kondo, K.; Sekine, O.; Yoshizaki, T.; et al. 4-hydroxy hexenal derived from docosahexaenoic acid protects endothelial cells via Nrf2 activation. *PLoS ONE* **2013**, *8*, e69415. [CrossRef] [PubMed]

42. Mishra, A.; Chaudhary, A.; Sethi, S. Oxidized omega-3 fatty acids inhibit NF-κb activation via a PPARα-dependent pathway. *Arterioscler. Thromb. Vasc. Biol.* **2004**, *24*, 1621–1627. [CrossRef] [PubMed]

43. Roy, J.; Galano, J.M.; Durand, T.; Le Guennec, J.Y.; Lee, J.C. Physiological role of reactive oxygen species as promoters of natural defenses. *FASEB J.* **2017**. [CrossRef] [PubMed]

44. Anderson, D.R.; Duryee, M.J.; Shurmur, S.W.; Um, J.Y.; Bussey, W.D.; Hunter, C.D.; Garvin, R.P.; Sayles, H.R.; Mikuls, T.R.; Klassen, L.W.; et al. Unique antibody responses to malondialdehyde-acetaldehyde (MAA)-protein adducts predict coronary artery disease. *PLoS ONE* **2014**, *9*, e107440. [CrossRef] [PubMed]

45. Jayathilake, A.G.; Senior, P.V.; Su, X.Q. Krill oil extract suppresses cell growth and induces apoptosis of human colorectal cancer cells. *BMC Complement. Altern. Med.* **2016**, *16*, 328. [CrossRef] [PubMed]

46. Costanzo, M.; Cesi, V.; Prete, E.; Negroni, A.; Palone, F.; Cucchiara, S.; Oliva, S.; Leter, B.; Stronati, L. Krill oil reduces intestinal inflammation by improving epithelial integrity and impairing adherent-invasive escherichia coli pathogenicity. *Dig. Liver Dis.* **2016**, *48*, 34–42. [CrossRef] [PubMed]

47. Lobraico, J.M.; DiLello, L.C.; Butler, A.D.; Cordisco, M.E.; Petrini, J.R.; Ahmadi, R. Effects of krill oil on endothelial function and other cardiovascular risk factors in participants with type 2 diabetes, a randomized controlled trial. *BMJ Open Diabetes Res. Care* **2015**, *3*, e000107. [CrossRef] [PubMed]

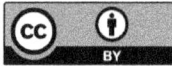

nutrients

MDPI

Article

Omega-3 Fatty Acids Supplementation Differentially Modulates the SDF-1/CXCR-4 Cell Homing Axis in Hypertensive and Normotensive Rats

Luiza Halmenschlager [1], Alexandre Machado Lehnen [1,2], Aline Marcadenti [1,3] and Melissa Medeiros Markoski [1,3,*]

[1] Postgraduate Program in Health Sciences: Cardiology, Institute of Cardiology of Rio Grande do Sul/ University Foundation of Cardiology (IC/FUC), Princesa Isabel Avenue, 370, Porto Alegre RS 90620-001, Brazil; luizahal@hotmail.com (L.H.); amlehnen@gmail.com (A.M.L.); alinemo@ufcspa.edu.br (A.M.)
[2] Laboratory of Biodynamics, Sogipa School of Physical Education, Benjamin Constant Avenue, 80, Porto Alegre RS 90550-003, Brazil
[3] Postgraduate Program in Nutrition Sciences, Federal University of Health Sciences of Porto Alegre (UFCSPA), Sarmento Leite Avenue, 245, Porto Alegre RS 90050-170, Brazil
* Correspondence: melissa.markoski@gmail.com; Tel.: +55-51-3223-2746

Received: 19 June 2017; Accepted: 27 July 2017; Published: 1 August 2017

Abstract: Background: We assessed the effect of acute and chronic dietary supplementation of ω-3 on lipid metabolism and cardiac regeneration, through its influence on the Stromal Derived Factor-1 (SDF-1) and its receptor (CXCR4) axis in normotensive and hypertensive rats. Methods: Male Wistar Kyoto (WKY) and spontaneously hypertensive rats (SHR) were allocated in eight groups (of eight animals each), which received daily orogastric administration of ω-3 (1 g) for 24 h, 72 h or 2 weeks. Blood samples were collected for the analysis of the lipid profile and SDF-1 systemic levels (ELISA). At the end of the treatment period, cardiac tissue was collected for CXCR4 expression analysis (Western blot). Results: The use of ω-3 caused a reduction in total cholesterol levels ($p = 0.044$), and acutely activated the SDF-1/CXCR4 axis in normotensive animals ($p = 0.037$). In the presence of the ω-3, after 72 h, SDF-1 levels decreased in WKY and increased in SHR ($p = 0.017$), and tissue expression of the receptor CXCR4 was higher in WKY than in SHR ($p = 0.001$). Conclusion: The ω-3 fatty acid supplementation differentially modulates cell homing mediators in normotensive and hypertensive animals. While WKY rats respond acutely to omega-3 supplementation, showing increased release of SDF-1 and CXCR4, SHR exhibit a weaker, delayed response.

Keywords: ω-3 fatty acid; spontaneously hypertensive rats; Wistar Kyoto rats; cell homing; hypertension; Stromal Derived Factor-1; CXCR4 receptor

---

1. Introduction

Hypertension (HTN) is the leading cause of cardiovascular disease [1] and strongly contributes to worldwide mortality [2]. Although dietary interventions have been related to the control of blood pressure levels [3,4] and reduced incidence of cardiovascular disease [5], all possible underlying molecular and cellular mechanisms involved in these interactions are still unknown.

The World Health Organization (WHO)'s guidelines on the prevention of cardiovascular diseases [6] point out that the consumption of fish and fish oils is associated with decreased cardiovascular risks, something which is also defended by the so-called Mediterranean Diet (MeDiet) [7]. In this way, the intake of marine omega-3 (ω-3) polyunsaturated fatty acids (PUFA), EPA (eicosapentaenoic) and DHA (docosahexaenoic) acids, has been related to the prevention of heart disease by a variety of mechanisms, including management of atrial fibrillation [8], blood pressure control [9,10], modulation of the lipid profile [11], and coronary heart disease prevention [12,13]. Such effects of ω-3 PUFA can be related to their anti-inflammatory activities, which inhibit the release of pro-inflammatory cytokines and the formation of platelets [14,15]. In addition, ω-3 PUFA influence eicosanoid metabolism, nuclear factor kappa B (NF-κB) gene expression, intercellular communication, cell membrane phospholipid fatty acid composition, which also depends on the amount of dietary PUFA intake [16]. Despite all benefits, the role of ω-3 PUFA in regenerative medicine, especially in the process of stem cell homing, including migration, proliferation, differentiation, and engrafting of cells, is unknown.

Stem cells are able to multiply while maintaining their undifferentiated state (self-renewal capability) and actively replacing damaged cells in tissues, and may also differentiate into various cell types. Therefore, it is believed that adult stem cells, present in different tissues, have a regenerative role when they are exposed to injury [17,18]. The stromal cell-derived factor-1 (SDF-1), a chemokine secreted in situations of tissue stress, and its receptor CXCR4 (CXC-Chemokine Receptor Type 4), anchored to the outer membrane of stem cells and some immune system cells, are the main elements involved in cell homing [19].

The expression and release of SDF-1 by damaged tissue acts as a positive allosteric modulator, promoting the migration of progenitor cells from the bone marrow and different organs towards the SDF-1 gradient, and hence to the site of the lesion [20]. Thus, physiologically, the SDF-1/CXCR-4 axis is also responsible for organogenesis and replacement of apoptotic or senescent cells in healthy tissues [21]. Both processes can be influenced by eating habits.

The aim of this study was to investigate the effects of ω-3 PUFA supplementation on cell homing, precisely on the expression of SDF-1 and its receptor CXCR4 in spontaneously hypertensive rats (SHR) and normotensive Wistar-Kyoto (WKY) rats in different time intervals, to test the acute, subacute and the chronic effects of the supplemented diet.

2. Materials and Methods

All procedures were carried out according to the National Institute of Health Guide for the Care and Use of Laboratory Animals [22] and to the Brazilian College of Animal Experimentation (COBEA). This study was approved by the Committee of Ethics of Instituto de Cardiologia do Rio Grande do Sul (protocol UP4503/10).

2.1. Sample Groups, Treatments and Blood Collection

Male WKY and SHR aged 90 days were used in this study. The animals were obtained from laboratory animal house of Fundacao Estadual de Producao em Pesquisa em Saude (FEPPS), Porto Alegre, Brazil. The average values of pressure for these animals, at 3 months old, were 123.16 ± 12.86 mmHg (WKY) and 183.50 ± 14.27 (SHR) in the baseline and 120.20 ± 11.51 mmHg (WKY) and 179.80 ± 13.91 mmHg (SHR) at the end of 2 weeks (for groups that receive ω-3). The rats were kept in plastic cages with wire floors, at 22–24 °C, 12 h light/dark cycle, and fed ad libitum with water and a commercial rat chow (Nuvilab, Colombo, Brazil) containing 19.0% of protein, 56.0% of carbohydrate, 3.5% of lipids, 4.5% cellulose, 5.0% of vitamins and minerals and 17.03 kJ/g of energy. Rats were treated with 1 g/day of marine ω-3 (fish oil), containing 180 mg of EPA and 120 mg of DHA by gastric gavage. The administrations were carried out early in the morning and blood collection and/or euthanasia occurred 24 h (acute effect), 72 h (subacute effect) or 14 days (chronic effect) after. The marine ω-3 was acquired commercially (Confiare, Porto Alegre, Brazil) in form of gelatin capsules (free from any microbe contamination) that were aseptically opened for oil removing on each day of administration. The dosage is safe for rats [23] and compatible with the recommended amount of fish oil for humans [24]. For both animal models (WKY and SHR), we used 8 animals per group, distributed in: control group (Gc), animals that received only water (1 mL) by gastric gavage; 24 h group (G24h); 72 h group (G72h); and 2 weeks group (G2w). All animals were euthanized immediately after the treatment period (24 h, 72 h or 2 weeks).

The animals were weighed every day and subjected to blood collection (100 µL, by puncture of tail vein) at baseline, under anesthesia with 0.2 mL/100 g of ketamine (50 mL/kg and xylazine (20 mL/kg), and at the moment of euthanasia (2 mL by cardiac puncture), also under anesthesia (same as described above). The G2w rats also had a blood collection in the middle of treatment, after 1 week of fatty acid administration. This sample and the baseline sample of the control group were respectively named "G1w" and "Baseline". The biological tests were carried out according to the Guide for the Care and Use of Laboratory Animals [22] and the Brazilian legislation (law number 11794) for the care and use of laboratory animals.

2.2. Recovery of Biological Materials

All blood samples were centrifuged at 2000 rpm for 10 min, and the plasma were aliquoted and stored at −20 °C until use. After euthanasia, the hearts were removed, immediately weighed, placed into cryogenic tubes and immersed in liquid nitrogen. After freezing, the samples were transferred and stored at −80 °C. The tissues were homogenized in 5 mL of buffer (pH 7.4, 0.6057 mmol/L Tris-base, Invitrogen; 0.18612 mmol/L Ethylenediamine tetraacetic acid (EDTA), Invitrogen; and 42.79 mmol/L sucrose, Synth), using a mechanical homogenizer (Polytron, Marconi, Piracicaba, Brazil), as described by Mori et al. (2008) [25]. The homogenized samples were transferred to 50 mL tubes and centrifuged at 1700 rpm, for 10 min at 4 °C. The supernatant (~3 mL), containing total protein extracts, was collected and stored at −20 °C until use.

2.3. Biochemical Analysis of Metabolic Markers

Concentrations of total cholesterol (COL), high-density lipoproteins (HDL-cholesterol) and triglycerides (TGL) were determined by colorimetric assay using commercial kits (Labtest Diagnostica SA, Lagoa Santa, Brazil). Optical densities were measured by spectrophotometry (Spectramax M2e, Molecular Devices, Sunnyvale, CA, USA) at 500–505 nm. Baseline measurements were obtained by comparing the optical densities of the samples with the respective standards, available in the kits. Data were expressed in milligrams per deciliter (mg/dL).

2.4. ELISA and Western Blot Analysis

Systemic levels of SDF-1α were determined by enzyme-linked immunosorbent assay (ELISA) using a commercial kit (Cusabio, Wuhan, China), in accordance with the manufacturer's instructions. The optical densities were measured in a spectrophotometer (Spectramax M2e) at 450 nm and 25 °C, with background subtraction at 570 nm. Baseline measurements were obtained by linear regression of the 4 parameters. Data were expressed in picograms of protein per milliliter (pg/mL).

Protein concentration of the samples was determined by the Bradford method [26]. Samples containing 100 µg of total protein extract were mixed with NuPage transfer buffer (Invitrogen, Carlsbad, CA, USA), denatured by incubation at 100 °C for 5 min, and separated on a 12% denaturing polyacrylamide gel electrophoresis. Later, proteins were transferred to nitrocellulose membrane Hybond ECL (GE Healthcare, Cleveland, OH, USA) using a semi-dry system (Amersham Biosciences, Little Chalfont, UK), in the same buffer with 20% methanol (Merck, Kenilworth, NJ, USA), at 100 mA for 3 h at room temperature. After the transfer, the membranes were stained with Ponceau, photographed and washed in phosphate-buffered saline (1X PBS) to remove the dye. The membranes were blocked with non-fat dried milk, and subjected to immunodetection using anti-CXCR4 antibody (Santa Cruz Biotech, Dallas, TX, USA). The membranes were incubated with 100 mg of secondary antibody (anti-rabbit IgG, Millipore, Billerica, MA, USA; titration of 1:5000) diluted in 20 mL of 5% casein solution for 16 h at 4 °C, followed by an additional incubation for 3 h at 37 °C under agitation. For chemiluminescence detection, the membranes were incubated for 3 min with a solution containing hydrogen peroxide and luminol (ECL kit, GE Healthcare, Cleveland, OH, USA). The membranes were then exposed to X-ray film (Ge Healthcare, Cleveland, OH, USA) for 1 min, 5 min, 15 min, 30 min or 2 h in the dark. The films were then scanned and quantified by optical densitometry with the software

Scion Image (Scion Corporation, Frederick, MD, USA). The results were expressed as *arbitrary units* (AU) and related to the total sample volume, weight of the tissue and weight of the animal.

2.5. Statistical Analysis

The normality of the variables' distribution was analyzed by the Shapiro-Wilk test. Data with normal distribution were represented as means and standard deviation, and those with non-normal distribution as median and interquartile range. The differences among groups were tested using Kruskall Wallis with Student–Newman-Keuls post-test (non-normal distribution variables) or a generalized estimating equation (GEE) followed by Bonferroni's post-hoc test (normal distribution variable). Correlations were analyzed by Spearman's rank correlation. The significance level used for all tests was 5%. Analyses were performed using the software BioEstat version 5.3 [27] and the Statistical Package for the Social Sciences (SPSS) version 23 (IBM).

3. Results

3.1. Omega-3 Supplementation Does not Cause Changes in Body Weight but Modifies the Lipid Profile

After two weeks of treatment, the effect of ω-3 PUFA supplementation on body weight was compared between the WKY and SHR (Table 1), and no significant changes were observed in both groups. The initial and final body weights (WKY and SHR) were 268.97 ± 26.22 g and 283.03 ± 22.68 g, respectively ($p = 0.073$). Nevertheless, daily ω-3 PUFA supplementation caused reduction in COL levels in SHR animals after 72 h of treatment, as compared with the G24h ($p = 0.044$), and WKY rats ($p = 0.001$) (Figure 1A). Although changes in triglycerides and HDL-cholesterol levels were also observed (Figure 1B,C), they were not statistically significant.

Table 1. Body weight of animals that received supplementation with water (control) or ω-3 in the initial phase and ending of the treatment (2 weeks).

Model	Treatment	Initial Weight (g)	Final Weight (g)	*p*-Value
WKY	water	274.38 ± 12.35	297.00 ± 16.00	0.116
WKY	ω-3	232.63 ± 33.51	250.25 ± 30.40	0.221
SHR	water	273.63 ± 46.24	285.50 ± 49.49	0.410
SHR	ω-3	295.25 ± 16.20	299.38 ± 16.78	0.775

WKY, Wistar-Kyoto rats; SHR, spontaneously hypertensive rats.

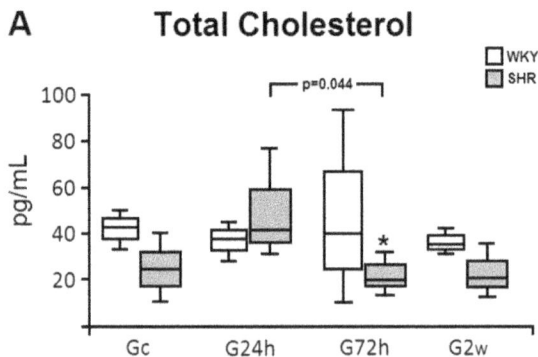

Figure 1. *Cont.*

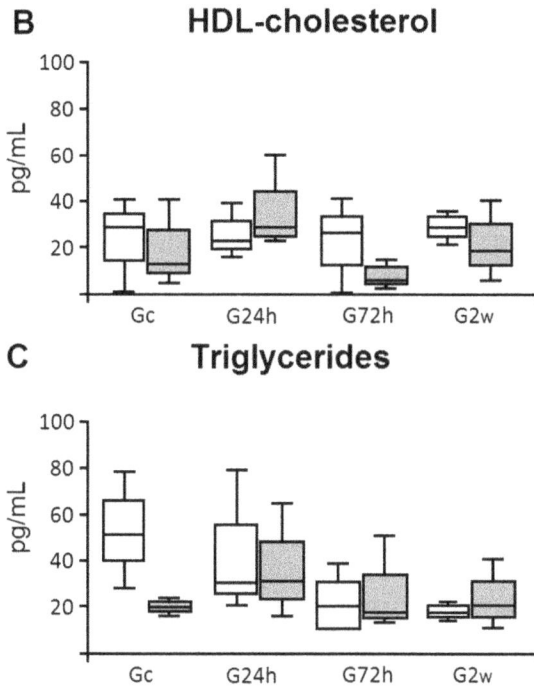

Figure 1. Lipid profile of normotensive and hypertensive rats after daily supplementation with omega-3 (ω-3). The levels of total cholesterol (**A**), cholesterol-HDL (**B**) and triglycerides (**C**) were quantified after 24 h, 72 h and 2 weeks of ω-3 supplementation and after 2 weeks of water intake in normotensive (WKY) and hypertensive (SHR) animals. The *p* values for comparisons between models at a specific time are shown in the panel. * *p* = 0.001, G72h SHR vs. G72h WKY. HDL, High-Density Lipoprotein; Gc, Control group; G24h, 24 h group; G72h, 72 h group; G2w, 2 weeks group.

3.2. ω-3 PUFA Reduced the Release of SDF-1 in Normotensive Rats and Increased in Hypertensive Rats

Significant differences in SDF-1α concentrations were found between treatment groups ($p = 0.017$) (Figure 2). The animal models showed different behaviors in relation to cytokine release in response to ω-3 PUFA supplementation: WKY rats showed a greater reduction in SDF-1α release when compared to SHR rats at 72 h (16.8%, $p = 0.001$) and after one week (14.3%, $p = 0.006$) of treatment. When the period of ω-3 PUFA supplementation was analyzed by group, a decrease in SDF-1 release was detected in WKY rats after 24 h (55–51 pg/mL), and remained decreased after one week, and returned to basal levels after two weeks (50–55 pg/mL) with similar concentrations of those in the Gc (56 pg/mL). On the other hand, SHR rats showed a small increase in SDF-1 levels after 72 h of supplementation (56–59 pg/mL), similar to the control group, but this effect was not maintained after the two-week period (54 pg/mL) (Figure 2).

3.3. CXCR4 Expression in Cardiac Tissue Was Differentially Modulated by ω-3 PUFA Supplementation in Normotensive and Hypertensive Rats

The expression of the CXCR4 receptor was compared between WKY and SHR throughout the two-week treatment period (Figure 3). Normotensive rats showed high expression of the receptor in the early period (G24h vs. Gc, $p = 0.001$), which returned to basal levels at the end of the protocol (G24h vs. G2w, $p = 0.005$). In contrast, SHR showed a significant, gradual increase in CXCR4 expression in cardiac tissue as compared with the Gc, which remained increased after two weeks (G24h, $p = 0.003$;

G72h, p = 0.016; G2w, p = 0.014). CXCR4 expression was higher in SHR than in WKY animals in both acute (p = 0.001) and chronic period (p = 0.04). Thus, SDF-1 receptor expression is differently modulated by ω-3 PUFA supplementation in the heart tissue of SHR and WKY rats.

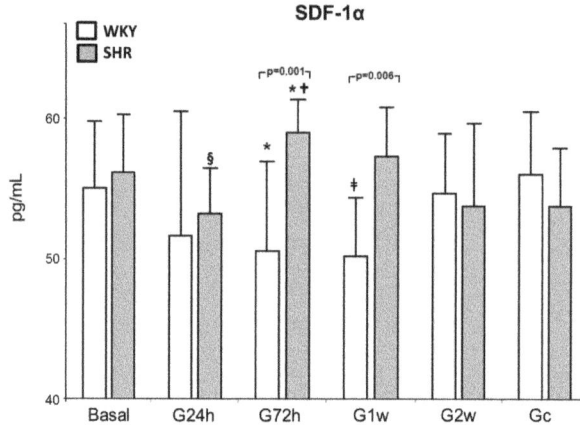

Figure 2. Systemic release of SDF-1 in normotensive and hypertensive rats after daily supplementation with ω-3. Normotensive (WKY) and hypertensive (SHR) animals had plasma collected in basal period and after 24 h, 72 h, 1 and 2 weeks of ω-3 supplementation and after 2 weeks of water intake. Data are expressed in picograms/milliliter (pg/mL). The p values for comparisons between models at a specific time are shown in the panel. * p < 0.05 vs. Gc; § p < 0.05 vs. G2w; † p < 0.05 vs. G24h; ‡ p < 0.05 vs. Basal. SDF-1, Stromal-Derived Factor-1; Gc, Control group; G24h, 24 h group; G72h, 72 h group; G1w, 1 week group; G2w, 2 weeks group.

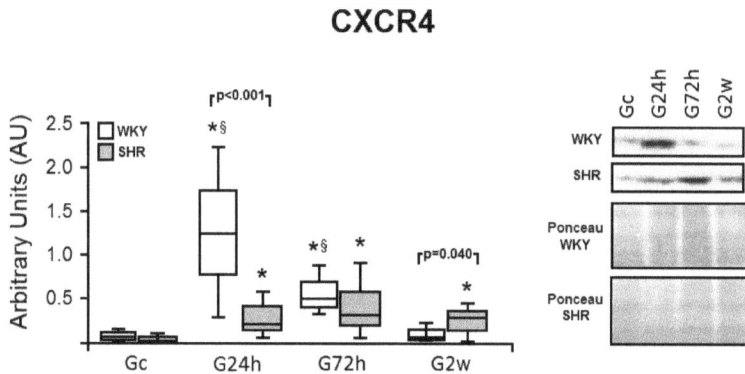

Figure 3. Cardiac tissue expression of CXCR4 in normotensive and hypertensive rats after daily supplementation with ω-3. Normotensive (WKY) and hypertensive (SHR) animals were submitted to CXCR-4 protein analysis in the heart tissue after 24 h, 72 h and 2 weeks of ω-3 supplementation and after 2 weeks of water intake. Data obtained by densitometry were compared to heart and animal weight, ponceau staining and are expressed in Arbitrary Units (AU). The right panel shows representative *blots* and reference bands (stained with Ponceau red) for all groups. The p values for comparisons between models at a specific time are shown in the figure. * p < 0.05 vs. Gc; § p < 0.05 vs. G2w. CXCR4, C-X-C chemokine receptor type 4; Gc, Control group; G24h, 24 h group; G72h, 72 h group; G2w, 2 weeks group.

3.4. Activation of the SDF-1/CXCR-4 Axis Was Influenced by Acute Administration of ω-3 PUFA and Was Not Dependent on Changes of Cardiovascular Dynamics

To analyze the influence of PUFA and blood pressure on the activation of the SDF-1/CXCR4 axis, we compared the results of the systemic release of SDF-1 and the cardiac tissue expression of its receptor between the animal models. The WKY rats showed a high correlation ($r = 0.9$; $p = 0.037$) between these parameters after the first 24 h of ω-3 PUFA supplementation (Figure 4). These results show that ω-3 PUFA supplementation had an acute, transient effect on the activation of homing molecules in normotensive animals.

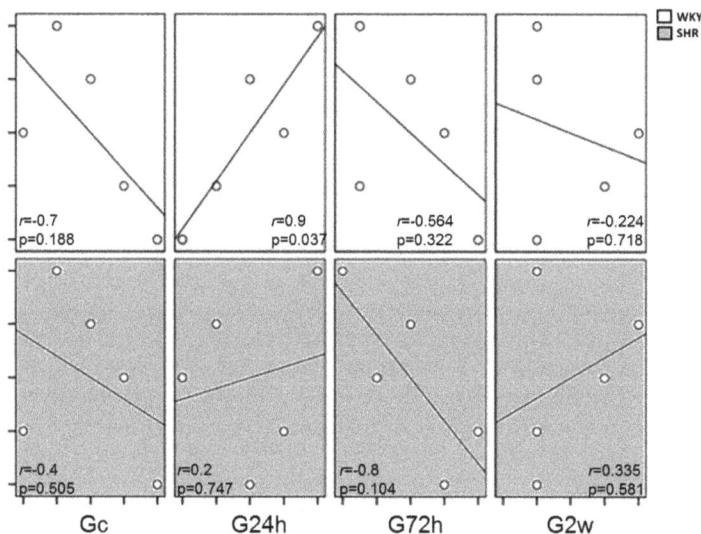

Figure 4. Correlations between the SDF-1 release and the tissue expression of CXCR-4 in normotensive and hypertensive rats after daily supplementation with ω-3. The normotensive (WKY) and hypertensive (SHR) animals were compared as the SDF-1/CXCR-4 axis activation during the time interval of dietary supplementation with ω-3. r = Spearman's coefficient. The p values are indicated in the panel. Gc, Control group; G24h, 24 h group; G72h, 72 h group; G2w, 2 weeks group.

4. Discussion

The present study showed the effects of dietary supplementation with ω-3 PUFA on cell homing in the setting of HTN, compared with normal blood pressure. Here, we noticed that ω-3 PUFA acutely induced CXCR4 expression in the cardiac tissue of normotensive animals (24 h after supplementation). In SHR rats, despite increased release of the ligand SDF-1 in response to ω-3 PUFA supplementation, only a small increase on the receptor expression was detected after 72 h of treatment.

The supplementation with ω-3 PUFA did not promote weight gain, which reflected a pattern of weight gain expected for healthy young rats. Indeed, it has been postulated that diets with high contents of marine ω-3 PUFA may decrease fat synthesis, contribute to body fat reduction, and be used for the treatment of obesity [28]. Also, ω-3 PUFA may positively influence the immune system and reduce low-grade inflammation [29,30]. Moreover, the control groups were treated with water instead of other vehicles to ensure that the control supplementation was inert on the activation of any biochemical mechanism or weight gain.

It was also reported that ω-3 PUFA modulates the expression of genes involved in lipid metabolism and adipogenesis, acting as ligand to important transcription factors, such as the peroxisome proliferator-activated receptors (PPAR) [16]. In this context, we also evaluated the influence of ω-3 PUFA on lipid profile. The supplementation with ω-3 PUFA had a positive effect in reducing COL levels in hypertensive animals after 72 h of supplementation. Since we did not detect important reductions in HDL-cholesterol levels in both groups, the reduction in COL levels may have been due to a decrease in low density lipoprotein (LDL-cholesterol) levels, which were not measured in this study. Many hypotheses about the mechanism by which PUFA decrease blood cholesterol levels have been considered, by increasing the formation of bile acid promoting a redistribution of cholesterol in the tissues, and by increasing LDL receptors in the liver, leading to a decrease in cholesterol plasma concentrations [31]. Lombardo et al. (2013) [32] have indicated that ω-3 PUFA have an effect in cholesterol reduction, which corroborates the fact that the decrease in COL levels in both normotensive and hypertensive rats in our study was due to the ω-3 PUFA supplementation. However, it is important to mention that the SHR model presents polymorphisms in the gene that encodes the epoxide hydrolase (EPHX2), an enzyme related to renal metabolism of arachidonic acid, transient states of anorexia and imbalances in cholesterolemic levels after ingestion of fatty acids. We believe this slight initial increase (after ingestion of omega-3) could be resultant of an action of this and its consequent regulation [33]. Studies that evaluated the effect of EPA and DHA on the lipid profile have shown, in general, a reduction of LDL-cholesterol [34], triglyceridemia [35], apolipoproteins, and an increase in lipoprotein lipase activity [36], an enzyme that hydrolyzes triglycerides. Lipid and lipoprotein metabolism changes significantly with the regular consumption of fish or nutritional supplementation with marine ω-3 PUFA, and doses lower than 2 g/day are sufficient to produce such effects [37]. In addition, Colussi et al. (2004) showed that ω-3 PUFA administered to hypertensive subjects (1 g/day by 6 months or 4 g/day by 1 month) were able to decrease plasma levels of Lipoprotein (a), a similar LDL particle identified as a risk factor for atherosclerotic disease [38]. Therefore, we believe that the amounts of ω-3 PUFA used in this study were able, at least in part, to positively influence the metabolism of lipids, which, for humans, may be beneficial in the prevention and treatment of HTN and other cardiovascular risk factors.

Regarding the effect of ω-3 PUFA supplementation on cell homing in normotensive and hypertensive animals, the intervention induced a pronounced increase in CXCR4 expression in the cardiac tissue and a decrease in systemic SDF-1 levels in WKY animals in the acute phase, possibly due to recruitment of the ligand by CXCR4$^+$ cells. However, such effect was not sustained in the chronic phase, maybe due to the absence of cooperative signaling from inflammation, oxidative stress and hypoxia response. The opposite occurred in the SHR, who showed a signaling response that promotes the expression of cytokines in response to the injury [39] and enhances cell homing, mainly during the chronic phase of ω-3 PUFA supplementation. In fact, marine ω-3 PUFA activates PPAR [40], that triggers the immune response, as well as chronic inflammatory cytokines, reactive oxygen species and transcription factors like the hypoxia inducible factor 1 (HIF-1) and NF-kB, which lead to the activation of SDF-1. Both DHA and EPA also exert anti-inflammatory properties [41], allowing a balance between anti-inflammatory molecules and pro-inflammatory cytokines involved in cell homing.

The chemokine SDF-1 is primarily expressed in high levels by bone marrow stromal cells [42] and several studies have been carried out to evaluate the action of this ligand and its receptor CXCR4 on tissue regeneration [43–45], acting in both physiological cell replacement and also under lesion or injury [45–47]. In cardiac tissue, the increase in SDF-1 levels stimulates the recruitment of cells to the site of injury (niche), which promote tissue repair and display positive paracrine effects on cardiomyocyte survival and cardiac function [48–50]. Our study is the first to show the relationship between HTN and the activity of SDF-1/CXCR4 axis that may be modulated by functional nutrients. It is worth mentioning that neither the cytokine levels nor its receptor expression were changed in the control group, which received only water.

Recently, it has been reported that the SDF-1 is an important regulator of the sympathetic nervous system and hemodynamic function in normal or pathological conditions, and it may contribute to neural and humoral activation in heart failure [51], the main pathological consequence of HTN.

The ω-3 PUFA was able to sustain the expression of this molecule during the entire period of protocol in hypertensive animals, probably through the maintenance of common signaling pathways that lead to the release of SDF-1 as inflammatory cytokines. Although the dietary intake of ω-3 PUFA in the form of food-sources like fish oil has no direct effect on the treatment to cardiovascular diseases [52], it may be related to the secondary prevention of heart failure [53,54]. However, the mechanisms involved in the effects of cardioprotective substances or functional foods on the homing of stem cells still require further investigations. We found a differential influence of the ω-3 fatty acid from fish oil on cell homing, mediated by an acute modulation of the SDF-1/CXCR4 axis activity in normotensive animals, and a late response in those with altered cardiovascular dynamics as in HTN. Additional studies with different experimental models are needed for a better understanding of specific mechanisms and mediators involved in cell homing in cardiovascular disease. This information can be used to develop targeted interventions involving nutritional factors aimed at the prevention and treatment of this condition.

5. Conclusions

This study shows that omega-3 polyunsaturated fatty acids can modulate molecules involved in cell homing in a time-dependent manner and according to blood pressure conditions. While normotensive animals respond acutely (72 h) to omega-3 supplementation, showing increased release of the chemokine SDF-1 and its receptor CXCR4, hypertensive rats exhibit a weaker, delayed response. Understanding how functional foods can affect cell response and their contributions to prevention/regulation of HTN can support effective therapeutic interventions. Additionally, clarifying the mechanisms that regulate stem-cell homing may help the management of cell therapy protocols, not only for cardiovascular diseases, but also for other conditions involving tissue regeneration and repair.

Acknowledgments: This study was supported by Fundo de Apoio do Instituto de Cardiologia/Fundacao Universitaria de Cardiologia a Ciencia e Cultura (FAPICC). L. H. was recipiente of Coordenacao de Aperfeicoamento de Pessoal de Nivel Superior (CAPES). We thank to Patricia Sesterheim for support regarding animal strains, Graziela Pinto and Thiago Peres for their excellent technical assistance, and Sergio Kato for support in statistical analysis.

Author Contributions: Luiza Halmenschlager developed the study, and drafted the manuscript. Alexandre Machado Lehnen performed data and statistical analyses. Aline Marcadenti helped in data analysis and revised the manuscript. Melissa Medeiros Markoski designed and supervised the study and revised the manuscript. All authors read and approved the final manuscript.

Conflicts of Interest: The authors declare no conflict of interest.

References

1. Yusuf, S.; Hawken, S.; Ounpuu, S.; Dans, T.; Avezum, A.; Lanas, F.; McQueen, M.; Budaj, A.; Pais, P.; Varigos, J.; et al. Effect of potentially modifiable risk factors associated with myocardial infarction in 52 countries (the INTERHEART study): Case-control study. *Lancet* **2004**, *364*, 937–952. [CrossRef]
2. Lewington, S.; Clarke, R.; Qizilbash, N.; Peto, R.; Collins, R.; Studies, C.P. Age-specific relevance of usual blood pressure to vascular mortality: A meta-analysis of individual data for one million adults in 61 prospective studies. *Lancet* **2002**, *360*, 1903–1913. [CrossRef]
3. Roel, J.P.; Hildebrant, C.L.; Grimm, R.H., Jr. Quality of life with nonpharmacologic treatment of hypertension. *Curr. Hypertens. Rep.* **2001**, *3*, 466–472. [CrossRef] [PubMed]
4. Law, M.R.; Morris, J.K.; Wald, N.J. Use of blood pressure lowering drugs in the prevention of cardiovascular disease: Meta-analysis of 147 randomised trials in the context of expectations from prospective epidemiological studies. *BMJ* **2009**, *338*, b1665. [CrossRef] [PubMed]
5. Estruch, R.; Ros, E.; Salas-Salvadó, J.; Covas, M.I.; Corella, D.; Arós, F.; Gómez-Gracia, E.; Ruiz-Gutiérrez, V.; Fiol, M.; Lapetra, J.; et al. Primary prevention of cardiovascular disease with a Mediterranean diet. *N. Engl. J. Med.* **2013**, *368*, 1279–1290. [CrossRef] [PubMed]

6. Organization, W.H. *Diet, Nutrition, and Prevention of Chronic Diseases*; WHO Prevention of Noncommunicable Diseases: Geneva, Switzerland, 2003.

7. Anand, S.S.; Hawkes, C.; de Souza, R.J.; Mente, A.; Dehghan, M.; Nugent, R.; Zulyniak, M.A.; Weis, T.; Bernstein, A.M.; Krauss, R.M.; et al. Food consumption and its impact on cardiovascular disease: Importance of solutions focused on the globalized food system: A report from the workshop convened by the world heart federation. *J. Am. Coll. Cardiol.* **2015**, *66*, 1590–1614. [CrossRef] [PubMed]

8. Christou, G.A.; Christou, K.A.; Korantzopoulos, P.; Rizos, E.C.; Nikas, D.N.; Goudevenos, J.A. The current role of omega-3 fatty acids in the management of atrial fibrillation. *Int. J. Mol. Sci.* **2015**, *16*, 22870–22887. [CrossRef] [PubMed]

9. Mori, T.A.; Burke, V.; Puddey, I.B.; Shaw, J.E.; Beilin, L.J. Effect of fish diets and weight loss on serum leptin concentration in overweight, treated-hypertensive subjects. *J. Hypertens.* **2004**, *22*, 1983–1990. [CrossRef] [PubMed]

10. Miller, P.E.; Van Elswyk, M.; Alexander, D.D. Long-chain omega-3 fatty acids eicosapentaenoic acid and docosahexaenoic acid and blood pressure: A meta-analysis of randomized controlled trials. *Am. J. Hypertens.* **2014**, *27*, 885–896. [CrossRef] [PubMed]

11. Jacobson, T.A. Role of n-3 fatty acids in the treatment of hypertriglyceridemia and cardiovascular disease. *Am. J. Clin. Nutr.* **2008**, *87*, 1981S–1990S. [PubMed]

12. Colussi, G.; Catena, C.; Baroselli, S.; Nadalini, E.; Lapenna, R.; Chiuch, A.; Sechi, L.A. Omega-3 Fatty Acids: From Biochemistry to their Clinical Use in the Prevention of Cardiovascular Disease. *Recent. Pat. Cardiovasc. Drug Discov.* **2007**, *2*, 13–21. [CrossRef] [PubMed]

13. Sala-Vila, A.; Guasch-Ferré, M.; Hu, F.B.; Sánchez-Tainta, A.; Bulló, M.; Serra-Mir, M.; López-Sabater, C.; Sorlí, J.V.; Arós, F.; Fiol, M.; et al. Dietary α-Linolenic Acid, Marine ω-3 Fatty Acids, and Mortality in a Population with High Fish Consumption: Findings From the PREvención con DIeta MEDiterránea (PREDIMED) Study. *J. Am. Heart Assoc.* **2016**, *5*, e002543. [CrossRef] [PubMed]

14. Uauy, R.; Valenzuela, A. Marine oils: The health benefits of n-3 fatty acids. *Nutrition* **2000**, *16*, 680–684. [CrossRef]

15. Hu, F.B.; Manson, J.E.; Willett, W.C. Types of dietary fat and risk of coronary heart disease: A critical review. *J. Am. Coll. Nutr.* **2001**, *20*, 5–19. [CrossRef] [PubMed]

16. Jump, D.B. The biochemistry of n-3 polyunsaturated fatty acids. *J. Biol. Chem.* **2002**, *277*, 8755–8758. [CrossRef] [PubMed]

17. Fodor, W.L. Tissue engineering and cell based therapies, from the bench to the clinic: The potential to replace, repair and regenerate. *Reprod. Biol. Endocrinol.* **2003**, *1*, 102. [CrossRef] [PubMed]

18. Lapidot, T.; Petit, I. Current understanding of stem cell mobilization: The roles of chemokines, proteolytic enzymes, adhesion molecules, cytokines, and stromal cells. *Exp. Hematol.* **2002**, *30*, 973–981. [CrossRef]

19. Sharma, M.; Afrin, F.; Satija, N.; Tripathi, R.P.; Gangenahalli, G.U. Stromal-derived factor-1/CXCR4 signaling: Indispensable role in homing and engraftment of hematopoietic stem cells in bone marrow. *Stem. Cells Dev.* **2011**, *20*, 933–946. [CrossRef] [PubMed]

20. Da Silva Meirelles, L.; Chagastelles, P.C.; Nardi, N.B. Mesenchymal stem cells reside in virtually all post-natal organs and tissues. *J. Cell. Sci.* **2006**, *119*, 2204–2213. [CrossRef] [PubMed]

21. Hoggatt, J.; Scadden, D.T. The stem cell niche: Tissue physiology at a single cell level. *J. Clin. Invest.* **2012**, *122*, 3029–3034. [CrossRef] [PubMed]

22. Guide for the Care and Use of Laboratory Animals. *The National Academies Collection: Reports Funded by National Institutes of Health*, 8th ed.; National Academies Press: Washington, DC, USA, 2011.

23. Gaíva, M.H.; Couto, R.C.; Oyama, L.M.; Couto, G.E.; Silveira, V.L.; Ribeiro, E.B.; Nascimento, C.M. Diets rich in polyunsaturated fatty acids: Effect on hepatic metabolism in rats. *Nutrition* **2003**, *19*, 144–149. [CrossRef]

24. Diniz, Y.S.; Cicogna, A.C.; Padovani, C.R.; Santana, L.S.; Faine, L.A.; Novelli, E.L. Diets rich in saturated and polyunsaturated fatty acids: Metabolic shifting and cardiac health. *Nutrition* **2004**, *20*, 230–234. [CrossRef] [PubMed]

25. Mori, R.C.; Hirabara, S.M.; Hirata, A.E.; Okamoto, M.M.; Machado, U.F. Glimepiride as insulin sensitizer: Increased liver and muscle responses to insulin. *Diabetes Obes. Metab.* **2008**, *10*, 596–600. [CrossRef] [PubMed]

26. Bradford, M.M. A rapid and sensitive method for the quantitation of microgram quantities of protein utilizing the principle of protein-dye binding. *Anal. Biochem.* **1976**, *72*, 248–254. [CrossRef]

27. Ayres, M.; Ayres, M., Jr.; Ayres, D.L.; Santos, A.A. *BIOESTAT—Aplicacoes Estatisticas nas Areas das Ciencias Biomedicas*; Ong Mamiraua: Belem, Brazil, 2007.

28. Kim, H.J.; Takahashi, M.; Ezaki, O. Fish oil feeding decreases mature sterol regulatory element-binding protein 1 (SREBP-1) by down-regulation of SREBP-1c mRNA in mouse liver. A possible mechanism for down-regulation of lipogenic enzyme mRNAs. *J. Biol. Chem.* **1999**, *274*, 25892–25898. [CrossRef] [PubMed]

29. Shephard, R.J.; Shek, P.N. Heavy exercise, nutrition and immune function: Is there a connection? *Int. J. Sports Med.* **1995**, *16*, 491–497. [CrossRef] [PubMed]

30. Monk, J.M.; Liddle, D.M.; De Boer, A.A.; Brown, M.J.; Power, K.A.; Ma, D.W.; Robinson, L.E. Fish-oil-derived *n*-3 PUFAs reduce inflammatory and chemotactic adipokine-mediated cross-talk between co-cultured murine splenic CD8+ T cells and adipocytes. *J. Nutr.* **2015**, *145*, 829–838. [CrossRef] [PubMed]

31. Eritsland, J. Safety considerations of polyunsaturated fatty acids. *Am. J. Clin. Nutr.* **2000**, *71*, 197S–201S. [PubMed]

32. Lombardo, F.; Lunghi, R.; Pallotti, F.; Palumbo, A.; Senofonte, G.; Cefaloni, A.C.; Gandini, L.; Lenzi, A. Effects of a dietary supplement on cholesterol in subjects with moderate hypercholesterolemia. *Clin. Ther.* **2013**, *164*, e147–e150. [CrossRef]

33. Fornage, M.; Hinojos, C.A.; Nurowska, B.W.; Boerwinkle, E.; Hammock, B.D.; Morisseau, C.H.; Doris, P.A. Polymorphism in soluble epoxide hydrolase and blood pressure in spontaneously hypertensive rats. *Hypertension* **2002**, *40*, 485–490. [CrossRef] [PubMed]

34. Castro, I.A.; Barroso, L.P.; Sinnecker, P. Functional foods for coronary heart disease risk reduction: A meta-analysis using a multivariate approach. *Am. J. Clin. Nutr.* **2005**, *82*, 32–40. [PubMed]

35. Schuchardt, J.P.; Neubronner, J.; Block, R.C.; von Schacky, C.; Hahn, A. Associations between Omega-3 Index increase and triacylglyceride decrease in subjects with hypertriglyceridemia in response to six month of EPA and DHA supplementation. *Prostaglandins Leukot. Essent. Fatty Acids* **2014**, *91*, 129–134. [CrossRef] [PubMed]

36. Park, Y.; Harris, W.S. Omega-3 fatty acid supplementation accelerates chylomicron triglyceride clearance. *J. Lipid. Res.* **2003**, *44*, 455–463. [CrossRef] [PubMed]

37. Kris-Etherton, P.M.; Harris, W.S.; Appel, L.J.; Association AHANCAH. Omega-3 fatty acids and cardiovascular disease: New recommendations from the American Heart Association. *Arterioscler. Thromb. Vasc. Biol.* **2003**, *23*, 151–152. [CrossRef] [PubMed]

38. Colussi, G.L.; Baroselli, S.; Sechi, L. ω-3 polyunsaturated fatty acids decrease plasma lipoprotein(a) levels in hypertensive subjects. *Clin. Nutr.* **2004**, *23*, 1246–1247. [CrossRef] [PubMed]

39. Schiffrin, E.L. The immune system: Role in hypertension. *Can. J. Cardiol.* **2013**, *29*, 543–548. [CrossRef] [PubMed]

40. Unoda, K.; Doi, Y.; Nakajima, H.; Yamane, K.; Hosokawa, T.; Ishida, S.; Kimura, F.; Hanafusa, T. Eicosapentaenoic acid (EPA) induces peroxisome proliferator-activated receptors and ameliorates experimental autoimmune encephalomyelitis. *J. Neuroimmunol.* **2013**, *256*, 7–12. [CrossRef] [PubMed]

41. Hofmanova, J.; Strakova, N.; Vaculova, A.H.; Tylichova, Z.; Safarikova, B.; Skender, B.; Kozubík, A. Interaction of dietary fatty acids with tumour necrosis factor family cytokines during colon inflammation and cancer. *Mediat. Inflamm.* **2014**, *2014*, 848632. [CrossRef] [PubMed]

42. Xu, X.; Zhu, F.; Zhang, M.; Zeng, D.; Luo, D.; Liu, G.; Cui, W.; Wang, S.; Guo, W.; Xing, W.; et al. Stromal cell-derived factor-1 enhances wound healing through recruiting bone marrow-derived mesenchymal stem cells to the wound area and promoting neovascularization. *Cells Tissues Organs* **2013**, *197*, 103–113. [CrossRef] [PubMed]

43. Ghadge, S.K.; Muhlstedt, S.; Ozcelik, C.; Bader, M. SDF-1alpha as a therapeutic stem cell homing factor in myocardial infarction. *Pharmacol. Ther.* **2011**, *129*, 97–108. [CrossRef] [PubMed]

44. Saito, Y.; Shimada, M.; Utsunomiya, T.; Ikemoto, T.; Yamada, S.; Morine, Y.; Imura, S.; Mori, H.; Arakawa, Y.; Kanamoto, M.; et al. Homing effect of adipose-derived stem cells to the injured liver: The shift of stromal cell-derived factor 1 expressions. *J. Hepatobiliary Pancreat. Sci.* **2014**, *21*, 873–880. [CrossRef] [PubMed]

45. Brzoska, E.; Kowalewska, M.; Markowska-Zagrajek, A.; Kowalski, K.; Archacka, K.; Zimowska, M.; Grabowska, I.; Czerwińska, A.M.; Czarnecka-Góra, M.; Stremińska, W.; et al. Sdf-1 (CXCL12) improves skeletal muscle regeneration via the mobilisation of Cxcr4 and CD34 expressing cells. *Biol. Cell* **2012**, *104*, 722–737. [CrossRef] [PubMed]

46. Kaplan, R.N.; Psaila, B.; Lyden, D. Niche-to-niche migration of bone-marrow-derived cells. *Trends Mol. Med.* **2007**, *13*, 72–81. [CrossRef] [PubMed]

47. Hwang, H.D.; Lee, J.T.; Koh, J.T.; Jung, H.M.; Lee, H.J.; Kwon, T.G. Sequential Treatment with SDF-1 and BMP-2 Potentiates Bone Formation in Calvarial Defects. *Tissue Eng. Part A* **2015**, *21*, 2125–2135. [CrossRef] [PubMed]

48. Zhang, M.; Mal, N.; Kiedrowski, M.; Chacko, M.; Askari, A.T.; Popovic, Z.B.; Koc, O.N.; Penn, M.S. SDF-1 expression by mesenchymal stem cells results in trophic support of cardiac myocytes after myocardial infarction. *FASEB J.* **2007**, *21*, 3197–3207. [CrossRef] [PubMed]

49. Tang, J.M.; Wang, J.N.; Zhang, L.; Zheng, F.; Yang, J.Y.; Kong, X.; Guo, L.Y.; Chen, L.; Huang, Y.Z.; Wan, Y.; et al. VEGF/SDF-1 promotes cardiac stem cell mobilization and myocardial repair in the infarcted heart. *Cardiovasc. Res.* **2011**, *91*, 402–411. [CrossRef] [PubMed]

50. Sullivan, K.E.; Quinn, K.P.; Tang, K.M.; Georgakoudi, I.; Black, L.D., 3rd. Extracellular matrix remodeling following myocardial infarction influences the therapeutic potential of mesenchymal stem cells. *Stem Cell Res. Ther.* **2014**, *5*, 14. [CrossRef] [PubMed]

51. Wei, S.G.; Zhang, Z.H.; Yu, Y.; Weiss, R.M.; Felder, R.B. Central actions of the chemokine stromal cell-derived factor 1 contribute to neurohumoral excitation in heart failure rats. *Hypertension* **2012**, *59*, 991–998. [CrossRef] [PubMed]

52. Enns, J.E.; Yeganeh, A.; Zarychanski, R.; Abou-Setta, A.M.; Friesen, C.; Zahradka, P.; Taylor, C.G. The impact of omega-3 polyunsaturated fatty acid supplementation on the incidence of cardiovascular events and complications in peripheral arterial disease: A systematic review and meta-analysis. *BMC Cardiovasc. Disord.* **2014**, *14*, 70. [CrossRef] [PubMed]

53. Nestel, P.; Clifton, P.; Colquhoun, D.; Noakes, M.; Mori, T.A.; Sullivan, D.; Thomas, B. Indications for Omega-3 Long Chain Polyunsaturated Fatty Acid in the Prevention and Treatment of Cardiovascular Disease. *Heart Lung Circ.* **2015**, *24*, 769–779. [CrossRef] [PubMed]

54. Wu, C.; Kato, T.S.; Ji, R.; Zizola, C.; Brunjes, D.L.; Deng, Y.; Akashi, H.; Armstrong, H.F.; Kennel, P.J.; Thomas, T.; et al. Supplementation of L-Alanyl-L-Glutamine and Fish Oil Improves Body Composition and Quality of Life in Patients With Chronic Heart Failure. *Circ. Heart Fail.* **2015**, *8*, 1077–1087. [CrossRef] [PubMed]

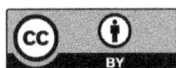

nutrients

Review

Vitamin D: Moving Forward to Address Emerging Science

Christine L. Taylor [1,*] , Christopher T. Sempos [1], Cindy D. Davis [1] and Patsy M. Brannon [2]

[1]   Office of Dietary Supplements, National Institutes of Health, Room 3B01, 6100 Executive Boulevard, Bethesda, MD 20892, USA; SemposCH@nih.gov (C.T.S.); DavisCI@nih.gov (C.D.D.)
[2]   Division of Nutritional Sciences, 225 Savage Hall, Cornell University, Ithaca, NY 14853, USA; pmb22@cornell.edu
*   Correspondence: TaylorCL3@od.nih.gov; Tel.: +1-301-435-2920

Received: 20 September 2017; Accepted: 27 November 2017; Published: 1 December 2017

Abstract: The science surrounding vitamin D presents both challenges and opportunities. Although many uncertainties are associated with the understandings concerning vitamin D, including its physiological function, the effects of excessive intake, and its role in health, it is at the same time a major interest in the research and health communities. The approach to evaluating and interpreting the available evidence about vitamin D should be founded on the quality of the data and on the conclusions that take into account the totality of the evidence. In addition, these activities can be used to identify critical data gaps and to help structure future research. The Office of Dietary Supplements (ODS) at the National Institutes of Health has as part of its mission the goal of supporting research and dialogues for topics with uncertain data, including vitamin D. This review considers vitamin D in the context of systematically addressing the uncertainty and in identifying research needs through the filter of the work of ODS. The focus includes the role of systematic reviews, activities that encompass considerations of the totality of the evidence, and collaborative activities to clarify unknowns or to fix methodological problems, as well as a case study using the relationship between cancer and vitamin D.

Keywords: vitamin D; data evaluation; cancer; assay standardization; dietary reference values; vitamin D standardization program

1. Introduction

Vitamin D remains a major research focus. No doubt there is great interest in the question of vitamin D, ranging from the reason for the presence of its receptors in many body cell types, to the relationship between intake and overall health outcomes. Vitamin D is a component of the diet, but it is a unique nutrient in that it functions as a prohormone, which may be endogenously produced under conditions of sun exposure. Regardless if whether obtained from food, supplements, or sun exposure, it functions similarly in the body and must undergo further processing by the body in order to become the physiologically active hormone (1,25-dihyroxyvitamin D). The active hormone has potent cell signaling abilities and is tightly regulated at the tissue level.

Table 1 lists examples of health conditions for which vitamin D involvement has been suggested. The PubMed search engine identifies more than 71,000 publications on vitamin D in general, and at least 14,000 publications that are related to vitamin D and health specifically [1]. Approximately 3000 publicly and privately supported vitamin D clinical studies are listed within the United States (U.S.) government's Web-based registry of clinical trials [2].

Table 1. Health/disease conditions suggested as linked to vitamin D [1].

- Cancer/neoplasms including breast, colorectal, prostate
- Cardiovascular diseases and hypertension
- Type 2 diabetes
- Metabolic syndrome (obesity)
- Falls and physical performance
- Immune responses including asthma, autoimmune (eczema, type 1 diabetes, inflammatory bowel and Crohn's disease, multiple sclerosis, rheumatoid arthritis, systemic lupus erythematosus), and mortality due to infectious diseases including tuberculosis and influenza/upper respiratory infections
- Neuropsychological functioning including autism, cognitive function, and depression
- Preeclampsia of pregnancy, preterm birth, low birth weight, and infant mortality
- Skeletal health

---

[1] Modified from IOM, 2011 [3], Table 4-1; reproduced with permission.

Yet, there remains considerable uncertainty surrounding vitamin D—a nutrient that is characterized by emerging science. Despite much conjecture about its role beyond bone health, the science does not reflect an agreed-upon trajectory for many conclusions about vitamin D. Some have identified vitamin D as a notable nutrient that is responsible for many benefits that are associated with reducing chronic disease risk, and some advocate for greater health through a increased consumption of vitamin D. Yet, others conclude that the interest surrounding vitamin D may be similar to an earlier experience, which is referred to as the "beta carotene phenomenon", in which supplementation with beta carotene (a precursor of the nutrient vitamin A, and quite distinct from vitamin D) was initially purported to be beneficial and widely recommended. Subsequently—after clinical trials—beta carotene was found to have unanticipated detrimental effects or a spurious benefit. In any case, it is evident that the science surrounding vitamin D is far from settled. At the same time, research continues to accumulate. A key question is how such data are evaluated, enhanced, synthesized, and incorporated into scientific conclusions and related recommendations about vitamin D so that these are reasonably stable over time and ensure public confidence in health guidance.

The Office of Dietary Supplements (ODS) at the National Institutes of Health (NIH) has a mission to foster dialogue and research related to scientific uncertainties. During recent years it has worked to address vitamin D, both as a supplement and within the context of total exposure. The underlying interest of the office is to encourage the development of systematic reviews along with consideration of the totality of the evidence when reviewing the science surrounding vitamin D. An additional ODS focus has been collaborative activities to support research and foster improved methodologies and scientific understandings. These activities reflect the types of efforts that help to deal with uncertain data, identify knowledge gaps to be addressed, and work to move the science to the next step.

2. Promoting Consideration of the Totality of the Evidence

2.1. Systematic Reviews Underpin the Totality of Evidence

The systematic review process within the field of nutrition has been described by others [4,5]. Briefly, a systematic review is a structured process to comprehensively identify, examine, compare, and synthesize available literature. As such, a systematic review is likely the single best approach to surveying literature in anticipation of drawing conclusions that are based on current evidence. It begins with an analytic framework to guide the formulation and refinement of the questions to be asked of the systematic review. These questions are central to ensuring that the completed systematic review meets the needs of its intended users. An example question might be: "What is the efficacy or association of vitamin D intake levels in preventing incidence CVD (cardiovascular disease) outcomes in people without known CVD (i.e., primary prevention) and with known CVD (i.e., secondary prevention)?" Question formulation is followed by the development of a search strategy, specification of the appropriate inclusion and exclusion criteria for the studies to be examined, and then the determination of a grading system to rate studies based on methodological quality and bias. The systematic review comes to a close at the point when data are extracted and summarized in tables. The final step is the compilation of an evidence report.

Systematic reviews evolved from the field of clinical medicine, for which questions tend to be more straightforward than issues related to nutritional topics. Nutritional questions are by their nature more complex because there is often a high degree of uncertainty as well as considerable variability among nutrition studies. In short, there may be considerable data on a specific nutrient, but cumulatively the data do not lend themselves to merging for increased statistical power [5]. For these reasons, approaches to developing systematic reviews for nutrition questions, including vitamin D, have required some specification to facilitate a better understanding of the challenges involved and the relevance of the review. Between 2009 and 2013, ODS supported efforts by the Agency for Healthcare Research and Quality (AHRQ) to develop six technical reviews that outlined the application of systematic review methodologies to the field of nutrition [6]. Specifically, for vitamin D, ODS co-funded a 2007 systematic review [7] that focused on bone health that examined specified subpopulations and total exposure levels accounting for vitamin D exposures from diet and synthesis in the skin. This systematic review incorporated intermediate biomarkers and surrogate health outcomes and took into account measures of serum 25(OH)D. A 2009 systematic review on vitamin D that was also co-funded by ODS [8] focused on a range of health outcomes in addition to bone health, again including both RCT and observational studies. It was based on two analytic frameworks—one that addressed deficiency and adequacy relative to the nutrient and the health outcomes, and one that focused on adverse outcomes relative to vitamin D excess or toxicity. In preparation for a 2014 special dialogue about vitamin D [9], ODS funded an update of the 2009 systematic in order to determine whether newer data had changed the conclusions of the 2009 systematic review; the conclusions remained stable when the newer data were taken into account [10]. These systematic reviews have provided a useful platform not only for recommendations about the nature of strength of the relationship between vitamin D and certain health conditions, but also as a way to identify and focus research needs. Table 2 contains examples of the types of data limitations that present challenges in carrying out systematic reviews for vitamin D.

Table 2. Notable evidence gaps for vitamin D.

• Many study protocols administer combination of vitamin D and calcium, reducing ability to determine effects of vitamin D independently
• Data are lacking to examine effects of graded doses to elucidate dose-response relationships
• Elucidation of mechanisms related to adequate calcium intake diminishing need for vitamin D for bone health
• Study protocols to address vitamin D as a prohormone with feedback loops related to health effects
• Additional studies to address effects and nature of sun exposure and ability to integrate sun exposure with intake
• Determination of the validity of serum 25(OH)D measures as biomarkers of effect
• Characterization of the variability surrounding measures of serum 25(OH)D concentrations due to different analytical methodologies used
• Clarification of non-linear relationship between serum 25(OH)D concentrations and increasing vitamin D exposure

Abbreviations: 25(OH)D, 25-hydroxyvitamin D.

2.2. Incorporating the Totality of the Evidence

The development of nutrient reference values illustrates the nature of the steps that are necessary to ensure that the totality of the evidence is taken into account when making scientific conclusions or underpinning public health recommendations, an approach that is central to the ODS perspective on addressing emerging science. In the United States and Canada, reference values, known as Dietary Reference Intakes (DRIs), are established by expert committees that are convened by the Institute of Medicine (IOM), now the National Academy of Medicine. The approach used by the IOM to establish vitamin D reference values demonstrates a process that takes into account the totality and strength of the evidence [3,11]. The values have key roles in public health policy as well as research activities.

In 2008, ODS and other federal sponsors co-funded IOM's efforts to convene an IOM committee to establish DRIs for vitamin D, as well as calcium, with a final report being issued in 2011 [3]. The committee carried out a number of steps to ensure the needed consideration of the totality of the evidence. At the beginning of the IOM committee's work, it outlined the intended evaluation process, as shown in Table 3. To determine the health outcome that would serve as the basis for the DRI for vitamin D, it next considered the overall literature regardless of the nature of the evidence, including those relationships that are listed in Table 1. The available systematic reviews on vitamin D, as outlined above, were a critical initial aspect of surveying the totality and strength of the available evidence. The committee also recognized that useful studies had been published after the completion of these reviews and that several relevant studies for the committee's interests did not meet the inclusion criteria for the AHRQ analyses and had not been reviewed. The committee added such data to its deliberations. As a general matter, the committee determined that RCTs provided the greatest level of confidence, but it also considered the outcomes from observational studies. The comprehensive examination of the entire dataset required an evaluation of data quality and strength, identification of consistency of effect, and searches for confounding factors.

Table 3. Evidence evaluation components [1]: Dietary Reference Intake review for calcium and vitamin.

• Full review of all purported health outcomes
• Focus on risk reduction in generally healthy populations
• Consideration of totality of the evidence
  ○ Evidence maps as qualitative consideration
  ○ Summary tables of data arrays
  ○ Forest plots as appropriate

• Strength of evidence to be based on analytic approach, target population, study design and overall quality
  ○ Consistency of effect
  ○ Confounding factors
  ○ Randomized controlled trials reflective of primary outcomes reflect strongest evidence and establish causality and therefore offer higher confidence
  ○ Lower confidence in observational studies but these are taken into account as confirmatory and to ensure consistency of data.

[1] Based on discussions in IOM, 2011 [3].

For ease of its consideration of the totality and strength of the evidence, data can be arrayed in a variety of ways. Figure 1A is an example of a forest plot, in this case showing the relationship between vitamin D and colorectal cancer risk, and reflects the nature of the inconsistent results. Figure 1B illustrates an evidence map for vitamin D and immune outcomes, and indicates the limited number of trials. Through this type of detail-oriented approach, the committee determined that the evidence was insufficient to establish a causal link between vitamin D and health outcomes other than bone health. This insufficiency reflected—on balance given the totality of the evidence—three limitations of the evidence: the data failed to demonstrate causality, research outcomes were contradictory, and that the effects were inconsistent across studies [3]. For the identified bone health outcome, the committee integrated the following measures: calcium absorption, bone accretion (including bone mineral content/density and rickets), bone maintenance (including bone mineral density and osteomalacia), and bone loss (including fracture risk).

Using fractures as an example of integration, the types of summaries from systematic evidence-based reviews that were important to the committee's conclusions are highlighted in Table 4. The evidence for fractures was rated as good, but it could not be characterized as strong. Other evidence that was gleaned by the committee from the AHRQ reviews indicated that calcium absorption was enhanced only when serum 25(OH)D levels were quite low (<12.5 nmol/L); a linear relationship between serum 25(OH)D and calcium absorption could not be demonstrated; relationship between parathryroid hormone and serum 25(OH)D concentrations was too inconsistent to be useful; and, bone mineral content clearly increases with vitamin D exposure in children, but the relationship is not strongly demonstrated in adults.

Table 4. Evidence for relationship between vitamin D exposure and fractures: Example of good-but-not-strong evidence [1].

Outcome	Evidence
Dose-response for fractures	No data
Incidence total fractures: Vitamin D ± calcium vs. placebo	14 RCTs: OR = 0.90 (0.80–1.20)
Incidence total fractures: Vitamin D + calcium vs. placebo	8 non-RCTs: OR = 0.87 (0.76–1.00)
Incidence hip fractures: Vitamin D + calcium vs. placebo	8 non-RCTs: OR = 0.87 (0.76–1.00)

[1] Compiled from data presented in Chung et al., 2009 [8]. Abbreviations: RCT, randomized controlled trial; OR, odds ratio.

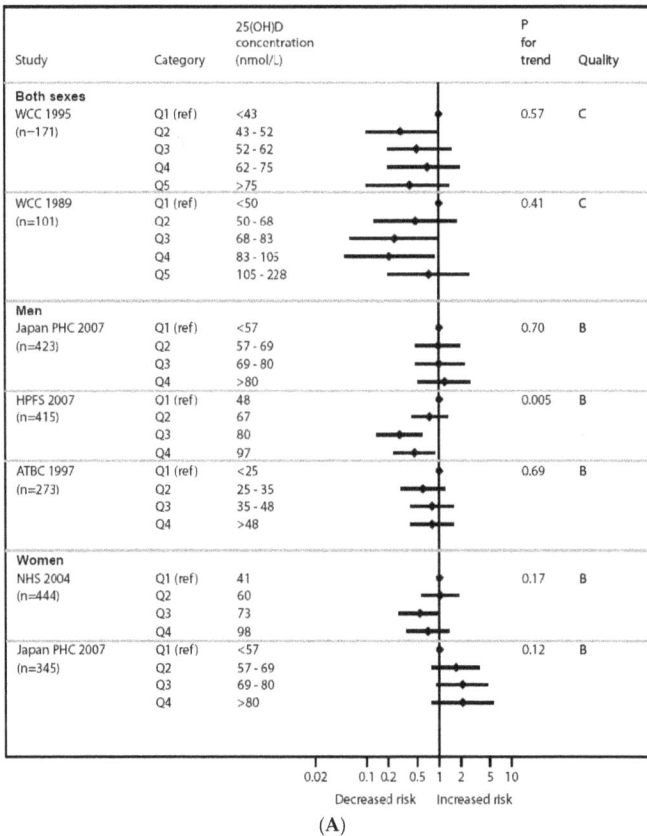

Figure 1. *Cont.*

				Randomized Trials	
Indicator	Mechanistic Data	Animal Data	Observational Studies	Primary Outcome	Secondary or non-Prespecified Outcomes
Vitamin D					
Asthma	√[1]	√	√	√	---[2]
Diabetes (Type 1)	√	√	√	√	---
Irritable Bowel and Crohn's Disease	√	√	√	√	---
Multiple Sclerosis	√	√	√	√	---
Rheumatoid Arthritis	√	---	√	√	√
Systemic Lupus Erythematosus	√	√	√	√	---
Tuberculosis	√	√	√	√	√
Influenza/Upper Respiratory Infections	√	√	√	√	---
Allergic Rhinitis	---	---	√	√	---

[1] √ = published evidence.
[2] --- = no evidence published.

(B)

Figure 1. Illustration of data arrays to evaluate totality of the evidence. (**A**) Forest plot for colon cancer risk stratified by vitamin D concentration (from Chung et al., 2009 [8], Figure 9); (**B**) Evidence map for vitamin D and immune outcomes (modified and updated based on IOM, 2011 [3], Table E-5; reproduced with permission). Abbreviations: WCC = Washington County Cohort, Women's Health Initiative; PHS = Public Health Centers; HFPS = Health Facilities Program Section; ATBC = α-Tocopherol, β-Carotene Cancer Prevention Study; NHS = National Health Survey.

The committee next focused on specifying a dose-response relationship between serum 25(OH)D concentrations and bone health based on the identified measures. Compiling and integrating data led the IOM committee to conclude that the strongest evidence linked a concentration of 16 ng/mL (40 nmol/L) serum 25(OH)D to an average requirement for bone health (Figure 2), the value that was established as the Estimated Average Requirement or EAR. The committee had no reason to assume that the requirement for vitamin D was not normally distributed. Therefore, based on a two-standard-deviation calculation, the level that surpassed the need for 97.5% of the population was 20 ng/mL (50 nmol/L), the value established as the Recommended Dietary Allowance or RDA. Although some studies may have suggested a higher average requirement and some studies a lower one, the weight of the totality of the evidence rested on a 16 ng/mL (40 nmol/L) concentration. As an aside, it is worth noting the efforts that are made to make clear that the RDA value of 20 ng/mL (50 nmol/L) does not reflect a clinical cut-point for deficiency, as it is at times misunderstood to be [12].

Finally, the committee specified the total dietary intake that is needed to achieve the EAR- and RDA-linked values for serum 25(OH)D concentrations [3]. Newer studies have enabled linkages to be made between vitamin D intakes and changes in serum 25(OH)D concentrations under conditions of minimal sun exposure, thereby mitigating issues that may be confounded by endogenous production of the substance. These were informative in estimating a dose-response of total vitamin D intake with achieved 25(OH)D concentrations.

A goal of DRI development is to ensure that the conclusions can stand the test of time. That is, reference values should be based on endpoints with data that are not likely to be quickly reversed with a few additional studies. As an example of this concern, at the time of the committee's work efforts to link the relationship between reduced risk of falls in older individuals and high doses of vitamin D (presumably due to improvements in muscle strength and lower extremity function), was gaining momentum that was based on both observational data and clinical trials. The committee considered that the available evidence was derived from small, underpowered randomized trials, and appeared to be contradictory among the observational data [3,13]. In 2016, well after the committee's deliberations, a report was published on a trial that was designed to increase concentrations of serum 25(OH)D to 30 ng/mL among home-dwelling seniors (70+ years) to reduce the risk for a repeat fall [14]. It showed the opposite outcome, falls appeared to increase with supplementation. The study concluded that high monthly doses of vitamin D might not be warranted in seniors with a prior fall because of a potentially deleterious effect on falls.

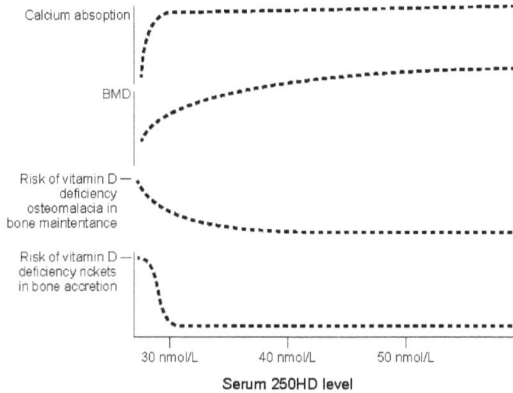

Figure 2. Conceptualization of integrated bone health outcomes and vitamin D exposure (from Institute of Medicine (IOM), 2011 [3], Figure 5-1; reproduced with permission).

Reference values are also established by authoritative bodies in other countries, including the Scientific Advisory Committee on Nutrition (SACN) in the United Kingdom and the European Union's European Food Safety Authority (EFSA). Comparison of the IOM outcomes for vitamin D with those from SACN [15] and EFSA [16] underscores the value of a comprehensive review relative to providing sustainable and consistent conclusions. The three authoritative bodies, using the same available research findings, established reference values that are comparable (or slightly lower) than those that are specified by IOM (Table 5). These expert panels were each charged with considering the totality of the evidence, yet worked independently to use systematic reviews, integrate data, select viable health outcomes related to bone health, conduct special analyses of intake data concomitant with minimal sun exposure, and link a specified dietary requirement to a serum 25(OH)D concentration. The estimates of dose-response and the distribution of serum concentrations of 25(OH)D reflective of bone health were notably consistent and underscored the value of systematic reviews and of incorporating the totality of the evidence.

Table 5. Comparison of vitamin D reference values and reported approach: Institute of Medicine [1], Scientific Advisory Committee on Nutrition (United Kingdom) [2] and European Food Safety Authority [3].

	IOM	SACN	EFSA
Serum-linked reference value [4]	EAR: 16 ng/mL RDA: 20 ng/mL	EAR (cannot establish) RNI $\geq$ 10 ng/mL	AR (cannot establish) PRI (cannot establish) AI: 20 ng/mL
Intake reference value [4]	EAR: 400 IU (10 µg) RDA: 600 IU (15 µg)	RNI: 400 IU (10 µg)	AI: 600 IU (15 µg)
Selected Outcome	Skeletal health	Musculoskeletal health	Musculoskeletal health
Components of Selected Outcome	Integrated BMC/BMD, rickets, osteomalacia, calcium absorption, fractures	Rickets, osteomalacia, bone health indicators, fractures, falls, muscle health	Consideration of increased risk of adverse musculoskeletal outcomes

Table 5. *Cont.*

	IOM	SACN	EFSA
Other Health Outcomes Reviewed But Not Selected	Cancer, diabetes, CVD, falls, immune function, infectious disease, neuropsychological outcomes, pregnancy outcomes	Pregnancy/lactation outcomes, cancer, CVD, hypertension, all-cause mortality, immune modulation, neuropsychological outcomes, oral health, macular degeneration	Pregnancy outcomes, cancer, CVD, immune function, neuropsychological function
Rationale for Non-Selection	Contradictory, inconclusive, lack of causality	Weak, inconclusive	Inconclusive, weak or lacking causality

[1] IOM, 2011 [3]; [2] SACN, 2016 [15]; [3] EFSA, 2016 [16]; [4] Persons 1–70 years. Abbreviations: IOM, Institute of Medicine; SACN, Scientific Advisory Committee on Nutrition; EFSA, European Food Safety; EAR, Estimated Average Requirement; AR, Average Requirement; RDA, Recommended Dietary Allowance; RNI, Reference Nutrient Intake; PRI, Population Reference Intake; AI, Adequate Intake.

Finally, the effort to establish DRIs highlighted data gaps in the field of vitamin D research that are particularly germane to the process of establishing nutrient requirements. Examples of these are shown in Table 6. Notable among them is the need for better dose-response data for vitamin D, an effort to design studies that allow for the effect of vitamin D to be determined separately from the effect of calcium intake, focused research related to the effect of excessive vitamin D and its adverse effects, and further elucidation as to the appropriateness of serum 25(OH)D as a biomarker of effect. Concomitant with these interests is the need to develop methodologies that enhance approaches to conducting systematic reviews that make the best use and appropriate integration of a wide array of data including epidemiological reports, clinical trials and mechanistic studies.

Table 6. Examples of research gaps identified during development of Dietary Reference Intakes for vitamin D [1].

Research Topic Area	Research Needs
Health outcomes and related conditions	• Clarify threshold effects of vitamin D on skeletal health outcomes by life stage and for different racial/ethnic groups. • Elucidate inter-relationship between calcium and vitamin D, and specify independent effect(s) of each. • Elucidate effect of genetic variation, including that among racial/ethnic groups, and epigenetic regulation of vitamin D on development outcomes.
Adverse effects, toxicity, and safety	• Develop innovative methodologies to identify and assess adverse effects of excess vitamin D. • Elucidate adverse effects of long-term, high-dose vitamin D. • Further explore nature of vitamin D toxicity.
Basic physiology and molecular pathways	• Examine the influence of calcium and phosphate on the regulation of vitamin D activation and catabolism through parathyroid hormone and fibroblast-like growth factor 23. • Clarify 25(OH)D distribution in body pools including storage and mobilization from adipose tissue. • Clarify extent to which differences exist between vitamin D_2 and D_3.
Synthesizing evidence and research methodology	• Explore enhanced methodologies for data synthesis. • Identify approaches to better weight potential health outcomes.
Dose-response relationship	• Conduct studies to identify specific health outcomes in relation to graded and fully measured intakes of vitamin D and calcium. • Clarify influence of age, body weight, and body composition on 25(OH)D levels in response to intake/exposure.
Sun exposure	• Investigate whether a minimal-risk ultraviolet B radiation exposure relative to skin cancer exists that also enables vitamin D production. • Clarify how physiological factors such as skin pigmentation, genetics, age, body weight, and body composition influence vitamin D synthesis. • Clarify how environmental factors such as sunscreen use affect vitamin D synthesis.
Intake assessment	• Enhance dietary assessment methods for vitamin D and calcium intake, and methods for measurement of in foods and supplements. • Investigate food and supplement sources for bioequivalence, bioavailability, and safety. • Improve standardization of assay for serum 25(OH)D.

[1] Based on discussions in IOM, 2011 [3].

2.3. Cancer and Vitamin D: Illustration of Why Further Research Is Worthwhile

Science, of course, continues to advance. An important factor in arguing for further research relative to vitamin D is the notable expansion of interest in the topic given the many receptors in the human body coupled with the mixed nature of available data to date, the number of health benefits that have been hypothesized, the numerous confounding factors that complicate interpretation of the data, and its unique role as a nutrient that is also a hormone. The topic of cancer and vitamin D illustrates the continued progression of understandings that have evolved following the development of DRIs and the need for further research, and, in turn, it serves to reflect similar needs for other vitamin D health relationships.

The hypothesis that vitamin D might exert cancer protective effects was first suggested 30 years ago by ecologic or geographic correlation studies, which demonstrated lower cancer mortality in regions with greater exposure to solar UV-B radiation [17,18]. Because ultraviolet radiation can result in vitamin D formation in the skin, this led to the hypothesis that vitamin D or one of its metabolites (25(OH)D or 1,25(OH)$_2$D) may be protective against cancer. To date, preclinical studies usually have demonstrated the protective effects of vitamin D against cancer through the modulation of many different molecular targets and biological processes that are dysregulated during carcinogenesis, including cell proliferation, apoptosis, inflammation, cell differentiation, angiogenesis, invasion, and metastasis [19]. Similarly, epidemiological studies have generally demonstrated an inverse association of plasma 25(OH)D concentrations with colorectal cancer incidence and mortality [20,21]. In contrast, the association between vitamin D intake and incidence of colorectal cancer is conflicting [21], and the relationship between plasma 25(OH)D concentrations and other cancers is less clear [19].

This disparity between the preclinical literature on vitamin D supplementation and cancer and the epidemiologic literature on vitamin D status and cancer can best be resolved by randomized controlled trials investigating the relationship between vitamin D supplementation and cancer. A Cochrane review was conducted to assess the beneficial and harmful effects of vitamin D supplementation for the prevention of cancer in adults [22]. Eighteen randomized trials with 50,623 participants were included in the analyses. Cancer occurrence was observed in 1927/25,275 (7.6%) recipients of vitamin D versus 1943/25,348 (7.7%) recipients of control interventions (RR 1.00 (95% confidence interval (CI) 0.94 to 1.06); p = 0.88). The authors of this analysis concluded "There is currently no firm evidence that vitamin D supplementation decreases or increases cancer occurrence in predominantly elderly community-dwelling women [22]." However, the authors also concluded, "We need more trials on vitamin D supplementation, assessing the benefits and harms among younger participants, men, and people with low vitamin D status, and assessing longer duration of treatments as well as higher dosages of vitamin D".

Internationally, four large (>10,000 participants) randomized controlled trials that are investigating the effect of vitamin D supplementation on the primary prevention of cancer can be found in clinical trial registries (Table 7) [23–26]. While both *VIT*amin D and Omeg*A*-3 Tria*L* (VITAL) and D-Health have been successful in recruitment [23,24], the Finnish Vitamin D Trial (FIND) was only able to recruit 2500 subjects [25], and it is not clear that the Vitamin D and Longevity (VIDAL) trial is being continued beyond the feasibility study [26].

The VITAL study [23], which was funded by a number of federal agencies, including ODS, highlights how a clinical trial can be used to answer multiple questions and gaps in the literature. VITAL is a randomized double-blind, placebo-controlled 2 × 2 factorial trial of vitamin D and omega-3 fatty acid supplementation for the primary prevention of cancer and cardiovascular disease in a nationwide cohort of 25,874 U.S. adults. This trial includes 5107 African Americans, making it the most racially diverse of the ongoing large randomized controlled trials of vitamin D.

At baseline, 16,956 participants or 65.5% of the total study population provided blood samples [23]. Blood samples will also be collected at trial years 1–4 from a randomly selected subset of these participants (~6000 subjects). Based on "lessons learned" from the ODS vitamin D standardization program discussed below, the VITAL study investigators are working with two different laboratories that are participating in the CDC vitamin D standardization program to calibrate their assays and analyze the samples for serum 25(OH)D. Moreover, these archived blood samples will serve as a valuable resource to allow for the assessment of effect modification by baseline 25(OH)D concentrations, changes in biomarkers over time, and future genetic analysis.

Table 7. Current Randomized-Controlled Trials with >10,000 Participants Investigating Vitamin D Supplementation and Cancer Listed in Clinical Trial Registries.

Trial	Location	Sample Size	Treatment Duration (Year)	Vitamin D Intervention	Primary Endpoints	Trial Registry No.
*VIT*amin D and Omeg*A*-3 Tria*L* (VITAL) [23]	The United States	25,874	5	2000 IU/day	Cancer, Cardiovascular	NCT 01169259
D-Health [24]	Australia	21,315	5	60,000 IU/month	Total mortality, Cancer	ACTRN 1263000743763
Finnish Vitamin D Trial (FIND) [25]	Finland	18,000 [1]	5	1600 or 3200 IU/day	Cancer, Cardiovascular	NCT 01463813
Vitamin D and Longevity [26] (VIDAL)	United Kingdom	20,000 [2]	5	100,000 IU/month	Total mortality, Cancer	ISRCTN 46328341

[1] Projected sample; final randomized sample = 2495; [2] Projected sample; status of trial is pending.

In addition to assessing total 25(OH)D concentrations of subjects, the VITAL study is also assessing other potential 25(OH)D-related measures of vitamin D status. The VITAL study investigators plan to use a nested case-control study to measure vitamin D binding protein and free 25(OH)D and to calculate the bioavailable 25(OH)D. It will comprise 2000 incident cases of cancer and cardiovascular disease and 1000 controls, and will assess whether baseline levels of these emerging measures are related to the risk of these outcomes or modify the effect of the vitamin D intervention. Thus, as an important example of efforts to advance understandings about vitamin D, the VITAL study should clarify a number of gaps in the literature, such as whether vitamin D supplementation is protective for the primary prevention of cancer, whether there are ethnic differences in the relationship between vitamin D supplementation and cancer risk, what is the relationship between baseline vitamin D status and the response to vitamin D supplementation and subsequent cancer risk, and what is the utility of evolving biomarkers of vitamin D status.

3. Promoting Research and Collaborative Activities

3.1. ODS Research Portfolio

Efforts both to clarify the basic biological activities of vitamin D and to enhance the applicability of the existing research are often at the forefront of discussions about vitamin D. As funding allows and in collaboration with the institutes and centers at NIH, ODS supports research on topics related to dietary supplements, including vitamin D. Proposals from interested parties are solicited via program announcements, requests for applications, and other mechanisms. A complete listing of ODS co-funded grants can be found on the ODS website [27]. As illustrated by the listing, the topics that are focused on vitamin D are diverse and range from the effect of the nutrient on hyaluronic acid signaling in women with triple negative breast cancer to the effect of vitamin D supplementation on the prevention of falls in the elderly. Grant applications are subjected to a competitive process and are funded on the basis of merit and design quality [28].

Although such grants help to build an important foundation for conclusions about vitamin D, ODS also works to enhance the multiplier effect, which expands and enhances collaborative and follow-on research and activities. This includes dialogues to identify and increase awareness of research needs and knowledge gaps, such as a 2014 conference on evidence-based decision making for vitamin D in primary care [9], as well as long term collaborative projects, such as the program that is focused on standardizing vitamin D measurements as described directly below.

3.2. Vitamin D Assay Standardization

Leveraging expertise is an important component of addressing uncertainties, especially given the reality of limited resources. One such ODS-driven collaborative activity is the Vitamin D Standardization Program (VDSP). Currently, there is an international debate regarding the interpretation of serum 25(OH)D concentrations, especially related to questions of dose-response and to determining status [3,15,29]. An important factor contributing to the debate has been assay variability in the measurement of 25(OH)D [30,31]. The lack of standardized assay has made it difficult to pool results from different research studies, which has confounded the development of guidelines for interpreting the concentration of 25(OH)D. These challenges have been a major focus of ODS because serum 25(OH)D is considered to be the best measure of vitamin D exposure and status used to define clinical states, e.g., deficiency, sufficiency, and overload, in nutrition guidelines.

To address the problem of assay variation, ODS established VDSP in 2010 with the objective to promote the standardized measurement of 25(OH)D worldwide [32]. The VDSP is a public/private partnership that was initiated in collaboration with the Centers for Disease Control and Prevention (CDC), the National Institute for Standards and Technology (NIST), Ghent University, the College of American Pathologists (CAP), the Vitamin D External Quality Assessment Scheme (DEQAS), the ACCC and the International Federation of Clinical Chemistry and Laboratory Medicine (IFCC), national health surveys in Australia, Canada, Germany, Ireland, Mexico, Korea, the United Kingdom, and the US and collaborators from around the world.

A standardized laboratory measurement is one that is accurate and comparable over time, location, and laboratory procedure. In this context, the standardized measurement of 25(OH)D is one in which all of the laboratories using different assays at different times and in different locations obtain the same results—within specified statistical criteria—for the same sample [33]. Moreover, it would be the true concentration as measured by the NIST, Ghent University, and CDC reference measurement procedures (RMP) [34–36]. The effect of standardization is that research results from different studies can be pooled—all based on the true concentration of 25(OH)D. This helps to promote the development of evidenced-based guidelines and informed decision making by physicians, policy makers, and patients.

To accomplish the goals of standardization, the VDSP, sponsored by NIH/ODS, has worked with its collaborators to assemble a set of tools that can be used to standardize 25(OH)D measurements now and in the future [33]. Those tools include the NIST, Ghent University and CDC RMPs, NIST Standard Reference Materials (SRMs), the CDC Vitamin D Standardization Certification Program (VDSCP), the CAP Accuracy-Based Vitamin D (ABVD) Survey, DEQAS, and statistical criteria to define where standardization exists. SRMs include serum-based materials with target values that are assigned using the NIST RMP and calibration solutions in ethanol (Table 8) [37]. Sets of single donor serum samples with RMP target values can be used in a CDC VDSCP program to standardize commercial assays and large commercial laboratories. In addition, accuracy-based performance testing schemes of the CAP ABVD and DEQAS use materials with RMP target values assigned. The basic steps to the standardization are then to use the tools that are listed to establish a chain of calibration from the RMPs/SRMs to commercial assay manufacturers and then to individual laboratories (Figure 3). Finally, laboratories participating in the CAP ABVD and DEQAS individual laboratories can test if an assay in their use is properly calibrated to the RMPs or traceable. With this VDSP system, individual laboratories can be standardized, again, through a series of calibration steps so that the assay measures the true concentration of 25(OH)D.

STEPS   **TOOLS**

| Develop reference measurement system | Reference methods
NIST SRMs
CDC certification program
Accuracy-based PT/EQA |

| Calibrate commercial assay systems to reference methods | NIST SRMs
Single donor serum panels
CDC certification program |

| Calibrate individual clinical and research laboratory assays to reference methods | NIST SRMs
CAP ABVD samples
DEQAS samples |

| Verify "end-user" test performance | Consistency across assays
CAP ABVD
DEQAS |

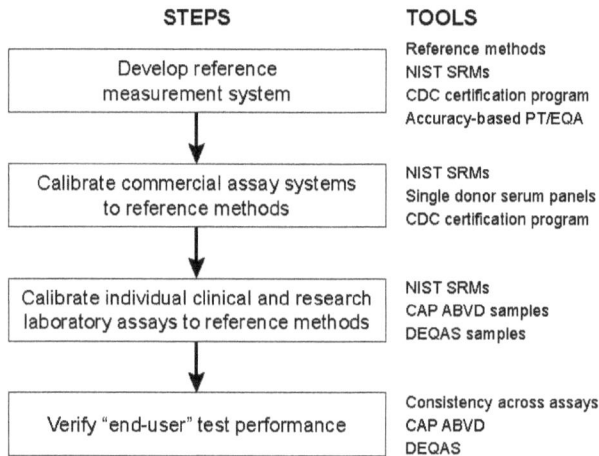

Figure 3. Standardization process for assays of serum 25-hydroxyvitamin D.

Table 8. Standard Reference Materials from the National Institute for Standards and Technology.

- Vitamin D metabolites in human serum/plasma
  - SRM 972a Vitamin D Metabolites in Frozen Human Serum
  - SRM 1950 Metabolites in Human Plasma
  - SRM 968e Fat Soluble Vitamins, Carotenoids, and Cholesterol in Human Serum
  - SRM 2973 Vitamin D Metabolites in Frozen Human Serum

- 25-hydroxyvitamin D calibrating solutions in ethanol
  - SRM 2972a

At these point standardization programs nearly always stop. However, given the wealth of published data, ODS and its collaborators considered it important to standardize 25(OH)D data from national health surveys, clinical trials, and other key completed studies where properly banked serum samples exist [38,39]. Thus, the VDSP has developed methods that can be used to standardize 25(OH)D measurements from completed studies. Those methods have been successfully used to standardize national nutrition survey data from Ireland [40], Canada [41], and Nordic countries [42], as well as the US NHANES [43]. Newer more cost-effective methods for standardizing completed studies were recently suggested by Jakab et al. [44]. Those new methods are based using small subsets of DEQAS and CAP ABVD materials to determine an equation to calibrate the original 25(OH)D values to NIST-Ghent-CDC RMP standardized or true values [45]. Over time, it is hoped that data from key clinical trials and other research studies will be standardized and added to the pool of true results.

4. Implications

In any field of study, emerging science with its surrounding uncertainties will offer an array of challenges relative to interpretation and application in the public health arena. Perhaps one of the most important lessons to be learned in addressing emerging science is the need to be clear about its nature—its strengths and weaknesses—and to be clear about what is needed to clarify the questions that it raises. The natural tendency to rush to strong conclusions should be avoided when based on limited or contradictory data that are available or on data that are appealing. Rather, the goal should be to make the best conclusions given the totality of the evidence that is appropriately caveated and presented in a transparent manner. Likewise, the desirable research strategy is to actively identify the specific data gaps and systematically work to close them. Vitamin D—and the work of the ODS—offers examples of how such strategies can be employed.

Nutrients **2017**, *9*, 1308

In addition to those data gaps identified in Table 6, there are larger questions, such as how multiple environmental and/or genetic risk factors may interact to produce specific diseases, and, in turn, the relevance to questions of vitamin D in such a scenario. As another example, given the complexity of chronic disease considerations, there is interest in a focus on the cumulative effects of poor health or other disease conditions. Others have noted that the relationship between serum 25(OH)D and rickets due to vitamin D deficiency is used to define cut-points for vitamin D deficiency, or more generally, hypovitaminosis D. This approach is limited by the fact that there are currently inconsistent case definitions of vitamin D in the context of nutritional rickets, measurement is not standardized, and there is inconsistent evaluation of other possible risk factors for nutritional rickets. It may be worth pursuing the establishment of a rickets registry to correct these problems and model the risk of nutritional rickets as a multifactorial disease that is similar in concept to coronary heart disease. Further, research is needed that is related to life-long exposure to vitamin D versus considerations of so-called "snap shot" status measures. Of special interest in order to ensure accurate and relevant measurement of vitamin D—which in turn assists with the ability to combine data from a variety of research sources and to determine status—is the continued focus of the VDSP. For instance, the metabolized and free forms of vitamin D are currently the subject of intense research to determine their role in assessing vitamin D status. Their measurement in vitamin D research should be standardized and harmonized to prevent a recurrence of the problems due to assay variation that has been historically experienced with serum 25(OH)D.

Acknowledgments: Funded as a staff project by the National Institutes of Health, Bethesda, MD, USA.

Author Contributions: C.L.T. drafted the manuscript with contributions from C.T.S., C.D.D. and P.M.B.

Conflicts of Interest: The authors declare no conflict of interest.

References

1. U.S. National Library of Medicine National Institutes of Health. PubMed Vitamin D Search Results. Available online: https://www.ncbi.nlm.nih.gov/pubmed/?term=vitamin+D (accessed on 8 September 2017).
2. U.S. National Institutes of Health. ClinicalTrials.gov. Available online: https://clinicaltrials.gov/ (accessed on 8 September 2017).
3. Institute of Medicine (US). Committee to Review Dietary Reference Intakes for Vitamin D and Calcium. In *Dietary Reference Intakes for Calcium and Vitamin D*; National Academies Press: Washington, DC, USA, 2011.
4. Brannon, P.M.; Taylor, C.L.; Coates, P.M. Use and applications of systematic reviews in public health nutrition. *Annu. Rev. Nutr.* **2014**, *34*, 401–419. [CrossRef] [PubMed]
5. Lichtenstein, A.H. Evaluating the evidence for DRI development: What are the issues in applying systematic evidence-based review approaches to DRI development? In *The Development of DRIs, 1994–2004: Lessons Learned and New Challenges*; National Academies Press: Washington, DC, USA, 2008.
6. Agency for Healthcare Research and Quality (AHRQ). Nutritional Research Series. Available online: https://www.ahrq.gov/research/findings/evidence-based-reports/tr17-series.html (accessed on 15 July 2017).
7. Cranney, A.; Horsley, T.; O'Donnell, S.; Weiler, H.; Puil, L.; Ooi, D.; Atkinson, S.; Ward, L.; Moher, D.; Hanley, D.; et al. Effectiveness and safety of vitamin D in relation to bone health. *Evid. Rep. Technol. Assess.* **2007**, *158*, 1–235.
8. Chung, M.; Balk, E.M.; Brendel, M.; Ip, S.; Lau, J.; Lee, J.; Lichtenstein, A.; Patel, K.; Raman, G.; Tatsioni, A.; et al. *Vitamin D and Calcium: Systematic Review of Health Outcomes*; Evidence Report/Technology Assessment No. 183 (Prepared by Tufts Evidence-based Practice Center under Contract No. 290-2007-10055-I); Agency for Healthcare Research and Quality: Rockville, MD, USA, 2009.
9. NIH Office of Dietary Supplements. Vitamin D: Moving Toward Evidence-Based Decision Making in Primary Care Conference, 2–3 December 2014. Available online: https://ods.od.nih.gov/Research/VitaminDConference2014.aspx (accessed on 8 September 2017).

10. Newberry, S.J.; Chung, M.; Shekelle, P.G.; Booth, M.S.; Liu, J.L.; Maher, A.R.; Motala, A.; Cui, M.; Perry, T.; Shanman, R.; et al. *Vitamin D and Calcium: A Systematic Review of Health Outcomes (Update)*; Evidence Report/Technology Assessment No. 217 (Prepared by the Southern California Evidence-based Practice Center under Contract No. 290-2012-00006-I); Agency for Healthcare Research and Quality: Rockville, MD, USA, 2014.

11. Institute of Medicine. *Dietary Reference Intakes: The Essential Guide to Nutrient Requirements*; National Academies Press: Washington, DC, USA, 2006.

12. Manson, J.E.; Brannon, P.M.; Rosen, C.J.; Taylor, C.L. Vitamin D deficiency—Is there really a pandemic? *N. Engl. J. Med.* **2016**, *375*, 1817–1820. [CrossRef] [PubMed]

13. Rosen, C.J.; Taylor, C.L. Vitamin D supplementation and fall risk. *Lancet Diabetes Endocrinol.* **2014**, *2*, 532–534. [CrossRef]

14. Bischoff-Ferrari, H.A.; Dawson-Hughes, B.; Orav, E.J.; Staehelin, H.B.; Meyer, O.W.; Theiler, R.; Dick, W.; Willett, W.C.; Egli, A. Monthly high-dose vitamin D treatment for the prevention of functional decline: A randomized clinical trial. *JAMA Intern. Med.* **2016**, *176*, 175–183. [CrossRef] [PubMed]

15. Scientific Advisory Committee on Nutrition (SACN). *SACN Vitamin D and Health Report*; Public Health England: London, UK, 2016.

16. EFSA Panel on Dietetic Products Nutrition and Allergies (NDA). Dietary reference values for vitamin D. *Eur. Food Saf. Auth. J.* **2016**, *14*, 4547.

17. Garland, C.F.; Garland, F.C. Do sunlight and vitamin D reduce the likelihood of colon cancer? *Int. J. Epidemiol.* **1980**, *9*, 227–231. [CrossRef] [PubMed]

18. Hanchette, C.L.; Schwartz, G.G. Geographic patterns of prostate cancer mortality. Evidence for a protective effect of ultraviolet radiation. *Cancer* **1992**, *70*, 2861–2869. [CrossRef]

19. Bandera Merchan, B.; Morcillo, S.; Martin-Nunez, G.; Tinahones, F.J.; Macias-Gonzalez, M. The role of vitamin D and VDR in carcinogenesis: Through epidemiology and basic sciences. *J. Steroid Biochem. Mol. Biol.* **2017**, *167*, 203–218. [CrossRef] [PubMed]

20. Ekmekcioglu, C.; Haluza, D.; Kundi, M. 25-Hydroxyvitamin D status and risk for colorectal cancer and type 2 diabetes mellitus: A systematic review and meta-analysis of epidemiological studies. *Int. J. Environ. Res. Public Health* **2017**, *14*, 127. [CrossRef] [PubMed]

21. Dou, R.; Ng, K.; Giovannucci, E.L.; Manson, J.E.; Qian, Z.R.; Ogino, S. Vitamin D and colorectal cancer: Molecular, epidemiological and clinical evidence. *Br. J. Nutr.* **2016**, *115*, 1643–1660. [CrossRef] [PubMed]

22. Bjelakovic, G.; Gluud, L.L.; Nikolova, D.; Whitfield, K.; Krstic, G.; Wetterslev, J.; Gluud, C. Vitamin D supplementation for prevention of cancer in adults. *Cochrane Database Syst. Rev.* **2014**, *6*, CD007469.

23. Bassuk, S.S.; Manson, J.E.; Lee, I.M.; Cook, N.R.; Christen, W.G.; Bubes, V.Y.; Gordon, D.S.; Copeland, T.; Friedenberg, G.; D'Agostino, D.M.; et al. Baseline characteristics of participants in the VITamin D and OmegA-3 TriaL (VITAL). *Contemp. Clin. Trials* **2016**, *47*, 235–243. [CrossRef] [PubMed]

24. Neale, R.E.; Armstrong, B.K.; Baxter, C.; Duarte Romero, B.; Ebeling, P.; English, D.R.; Kimlin, M.G.; McLeod, D.S.; RL, O.C.; van der Pols, J.C.; et al. The D-Health Trial: A randomized trial of vitamin D for prevention of mortality and cancer. *Contemp. Clin. Trials* **2016**, *48*, 83–90. [CrossRef] [PubMed]

25. ClinicalTrials.gov. Finnish Vitamin D Trial (FIND). Available online: https://clinicaltrials.gov/ct2/show/NCT01463813 (accessed on 8 September 2017).

26. ISRCTN Registry. Vitamin D and Longevity (VIDAL) Trial: Randomised Feasibility Study. Available online: http://www.isrctn.com/ISRCTN46328341 (accessed on 8 September 2017).

27. NIH Office of Dietary Supplements. ODS Research Portfolio. Available online: https://ods.od.nih.gov/Funding/Grants_Contracts.aspx (accessed on 8 September 2017).

28. NIH Office of Dietary Supplements. General NIH Funding Guidance. Available online: https://ods.od.nih.gov/Research/General_NIH_Funding_Guidance.aspx (accessed on 8 September 2017).

29. Holick, M.F.; Binkley, N.C.; Bischoff-Ferrari, H.A.; Gordon, C.M.; Hanley, D.A.; Heaney, R.P.; Murad, M.H.; Weaver, C.M. Evaluation, treatment, and prevention of vitamin D deficiency: An Endocrine Society clinical practice guideline. *J. Clin. Endocrinol. Metab.* **2011**, *96*, 1911–1930. [CrossRef] [PubMed]

30. Binkley, N.; Krueger, D.; Cowgill, C.S.; Plum, L.; Lake, E.; Hansen, K.E.; DeLuca, H.F.; Drezner, M.K. Assay variation confounds the diagnosis of hypovitaminosis D: A call for standardization. *J. Clin. Endocrinol. Metab.* **2004**, *89*, 3152–3157. [CrossRef] [PubMed]

31. Le Goff, C.; Cavalier, E.; Souberbielle, J.C.; González-Antuña, A.; Delvin, E. Measurement of circulating 25-hydroxyvitamin D: A historical review. *Pract. Lab. Med.* **2015**, *2*, 1–14. [CrossRef] [PubMed]

32. Sempos, C.T.; Vesper, H.W.; Phinney, K.W.; Thienpont, L.M.; Coates, P.M. Vitamin D status as an international issue: National surveys and the problem of standardization. *Scand. J. Clin. Lab. Investig.* **2012**, *72* (Suppl. S243), 32–40.

33. Binkley, N.; Sempos, C.T. Standardizing vitamin D assays: The way forward. *J. Bone Miner. Res.* **2014**, *29*, 1709–1714. [CrossRef] [PubMed]

34. Tai, S.S.; Bedner, M.; Phinney, K.W. Development of a candidate reference measurement procedure for the determination of 25-hydroxyvitamin D3 and 25-hydroxyvitamin D2 in human serum using isotope-dilution liquid chromatography-tandem mass spectrometry. *Anal. Chem.* **2010**, *82*, 1942–1948. [CrossRef] [PubMed]

35. Stepman, H.C.; Vanderroost, A.; Van Uytfanghe, K.; Thienpont, L.M. Candidate reference measurement procedures for serum 25-hydroxyvitamin D3 and 25-hydroxyvitamin D2 by using isotope-dilution liquid chromatography-tandem mass spectrometry. *Clin. Chem.* **2011**, *57*, 441–448. [CrossRef] [PubMed]

36. Mineva, E.M.; Schleicher, R.L.; Chaudhary-Webb, M.; Maw, K.L.; Botelho, J.C.; Vesper, H.W.; Pfeiffer, C.M. A candidate reference measurement procedure for quantifying serum concentrations of 25-hydroxyvitamin D(3) and 25-hydroxyvitamin D(2) using isotope-dilution liquid chromatography-tandem mass spectrometry. *Anal. Bioanal. Chem.* **2015**, *407*, 5615–5624. [CrossRef] [PubMed]

37. National Institute of Standards and Technology (NIST). Standard Reference Materials. Available online: https://www.nist.gov/srm (accessed on 8 September 2017).

38. Sempos, C.T.; Durazo-Arvizu, R.A.; Binkley, N.; Jones, J.; Merkel, J.M.; Carter, G.D. Developing vitamin D dietary guidelines and the lack of 25-hydroxyvitamin D assay standardization: The ever-present past. *J. Steroid Biochem. Mol. Biol.* **2016**, *164*, 115–119. [CrossRef] [PubMed]

39. Binkley, N.; Dawson-Hughes, B.; Durazo-Arvizu, R.; Thamm, M.; Tian, L.; Merkel, J.M.; Jones, J.C.; Carter, G.D.; Sempos, C.T. Vitamin D measurement standardization: The way out of the chaos. *J. Steroid Biochem. Mol. Biol.* **2016**, *173*, 117–121. [CrossRef] [PubMed]

40. Cashman, K.D.; Kiely, M.; Kinsella, M.; Durazo-Arvizu, R.A.; Tian, L.; Zhang, Y.; Lucey, A.; Flynn, A.; Gibney, M.J.; Vesper, H.W.; et al. Evaluation of Vitamin D Standardization Program protocols for standardizing serum 25-hydroxyvitamin D data: A case study of the program's potential for national nutrition and health surveys. *Am. J. Clin. Nutr.* **2013**, *97*, 1235–1242. [CrossRef] [PubMed]

41. Sarafin, K.; Durazo-Arvizu, R.; Tian, L.; Phinney, K.W.; Tai, S.; Camara, J.E.; Merkel, J.; Green, E.; Sempos, C.T.; Brooks, S.P. Standardizing 25-hydroxyvitamin D values from the Canadian Health Measures Survey. *Am. J. Clin. Nutr.* **2015**, *102*, 1044–1050. [CrossRef] [PubMed]

42. Cashman, K.D.; Dowling, K.G.; Skrabakova, Z.; Kiely, M.; Lamberg-Allardt, C.; Durazo-Arvizu, R.A.; Sempos, C.T.; Koskinen, S.; Lundqvist, A.; Sundvall, J.; et al. Standardizing serum 25-hydroxyvitamin D data from four Nordic population samples using the Vitamin D Standardization Program protocols: Shedding new light on vitamin D status in Nordic individuals. *Scand. J. Clin. Lab. Investig.* **2015**, *75*, 549–561. [CrossRef] [PubMed]

43. Schleicher, R.L.; Sternberg, M.R.; Lacher, D.A.; Sempos, C.T.; Looker, A.C.; Durazo-Arvizu, R.A.; Yetley, E.A.; Chaudhary-Webb, M.; Maw, K.L.; Pfeiffer, C.M.; et al. A method-bridging study for serum 25-hydroxyvitamin D to standardize historical radioimmunoassay data to liquid chromatography-tandem mass spectrometry. *Natl. Health Stat. Rep.* **2016**, *93*, 1–16.

44. Jakab, E.; Kalina, E.; Petho, Z.; Pap, Z.; Balogh, A.; Grant, W.B.; Bhattoa, H.P. Standardizing 25-hydroxyvitamin D data from the HunMen cohort. *Osteoporos. Int.* **2017**, *28*, 1653–1657. [CrossRef] [PubMed]

45. Sempos, C.T.; Durazo-Arvizu, R.A.; Carter, G.D. Cost effective measures to standardize serum 25(OH)D values from completed studies. *Osteoporos. Int.* **2017**, *28*, 1503–1505. [CrossRef] [PubMed]

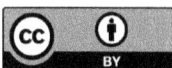

nutrients

MDPI

Article

Association of Sun Exposure, Skin Colour and Body Mass Index with Vitamin D Status in Individuals Who Are Morbidly Obese

Clare F. Dix [1],*, Judith D. Bauer [1], Ian Martin [2], Sharon Rochester [2], Briony Duarte Romero [3], Johannes B. Prins [4] and Olivia R. L. Wright [1]

[1] School of Human Movement and Nutrition Sciences, The University of Queensland, Brisbane, QLD 4076, Australia; j.bauer1@uq.edu.au (J.D.B.); o.wright@uq.edu.au (O.R.L.W.)
[2] Wesley Hospital, Auchenflower, Brisbane, QLD 4066, Australia; Ian.Martin@uchealth.com.au (I.M.); smrochester01@gmail.com (S.R.)
[3] QIMR Berghofer Medical Research Institute, Brisbane, QLD 4029, Australia; bduarteromero@hotmail.com
[4] Mater Research Institute, South Brisbane, QLD 4101, Australia; john.prins@mater.uq.edu.au
*   Correspondence: clare.dix@uqconnect.edu.au; Tel.: +61-7-3365-6313

Received: 30 August 2017; Accepted: 28 September 2017; Published: 4 October 2017

Abstract: Vitamin D deficiency is a common issue, particularly in obese populations, and is tested by assessing serum 25(OH)D concentrations. This study aimed to identify factors that contribute to the vitamin D status in fifty morbidly obese individuals recruited prior to bariatric surgery. Data collected included serum 25(OH)D concentrations, dietary and supplement intake of vitamin D, sun exposure measures, skin colour via spectrophotometry, and genotype analysis of several single nucleotide polymorphisms in the vitamin D metabolism pathway. Results showed a significant correlation between serum 25(OH)D concentrations and age, and serum 25(OH)D and ITAC score (natural skin colour). Natural skin colour accounted for 13.5% of variation in serum 25(OH)D, with every $10°$ increase in ITAC score (i.e., lighter skin) leading to a 9 nmol/L decrease in serum 25(OH)D. Multiple linear regression using age, ITAC score, and average UV index in the three months prior to testing, significantly predicted serum 25(OH)D concentrations (R^2 = 29.7%). Single nucleotide polymorphisms for all vitamin D genes tested, showed lower serum 25(OH)D for those with the rare genotype compared to the common genotype; this was most pronounced for *fok1* and rs4588, where those with the rare genotype were insufficient (<50 nmol/L), and those with the common genotype were sufficient ($\geq$50 nmol/L). Assessing vitamin D status in individuals with morbid obesity requires testing of 25(OH)D, but potential risk factors for this population include natural skin colour and age.

Keywords: vitamin D; morbid obesity; sun exposure; skin colour; biomarkers; micronutrients

1. Introduction

Vitamin D refers to a group of fat-soluble secosteroids that act as a hormone in the body. There are five forms of vitamin D, of which vitamin D_2 and vitamin D_3 are physiologically important. Classical physiological roles for vitamin D include calcium homeostasis and bone metabolism [1], but in recent years, a more varied role for vitamin D has been identified [2,3]. The majority of vitamin D_3 is produced endogenously in the skin from dehydro-cholesterol after exposure to ultraviolet B (UVB) rays. vitamin D_2 and vitamin D_3 are also found in supplements and some food sources. Vitamin D is transported in the blood, attached to a binding protein, and is metabolised in the liver to 25-hydroxyvitamin D (25(OH)D), and in the kidneys to 1α,25-dihydroxyvitamin D (1,25(OH)$_2$D). The majority of the active form of vitamin D, 1,25(OH)$_2$D, is produced in the kidneys, although almost all tissues in the body have the ability to produce it [4]. $1,25(OH)_2D$ has both genomic and non-genomic effects, through either a nuclear or membrane receptor [5–8].

Assessing an individual's vitamin D status is a difficult task; currently, serum 25(OH)D concentration is used as a biomarker for vitamin D status. There are many definitions for sufficiency. The Endocrine Society define deficiency as <50 nmol/L (<20 ng/mL), and insufficiency as 52.5–72.5 nmol/L (21–29 ng/mL) [9]. In Australia, serum 25(OH)D concentrations ≥50 nmol/L are considered sufficient for the general population, with graded concentrations of insufficiency; mild (49–30 nmol/L), moderate (29–12.5 nmol/L), and severe (<12.5 nmol/L) [10]. Higher concentrations are recommended for specific sub-groups, e.g., >60 nmol/L for falls prevention in the elderly [11], and >82.5 nmol/L for reducing colorectal cancer risk [2]. In Australia, deficiency affects around 6% of the population in summer and around 49% of the population in winter [12]. In the USA, around 32% of the population are classified as deficient [13]. There are many issues to consider when assessing a persons' vitamin D status, including age, gender, physical activity levels, sun exposure, skin colour, diet, and supplement intake. The influence of individual genetics of the person assayed may also affect their status. Single nucleotide polymorphisms (SNPs) in the genes that encode for the vitamin D receptor (VDR) [14–16] and vitamin D binding protein (DBP) [17,18] have the potential to influence the activity of $1,25(OH)_2D$.

The majority of vitamin D comes from endogenous production that requires exposure of the skin to UVB rays from sunlight. In assessing a person's vitamin D status, information regarding sun exposure can help identify those at risk of deficiency. Several questionnaires have been developed to assess sun exposure using a combination of questions about clothing, time spent outdoors, sunscreen use and skin colour [19,20]. Those with darker skin colour appear to require long periods of UV exposure to reach sufficient serum 25(OH)D concentrations [21]. Conversely, those with very light skin are also at risk due to increased sun protective behaviours [22]. Previously, measures of natural and tanned skin colour using spectrophotometry have identified associations with vitamin D status [23]. It has been postulated that tanned skin colour is an important determinant of 25(OH)D status [23]. This suggests that the natural skin colour of a person is not as important as the amount of sun exposure they receive when assessing vitamin D status.

Vitamin D deficiency is very common in obese populations, including bariatric patients [24,25]. There is an inverse correlation between obesity and low vitamin D status, but it is not clear whether vitamin D is a cause or a consequence of obesity. Strengthening the link between the two are the associations between vitamin D deficiency and many of the co-morbidities associated with obesity [26–29]. There are several theories on the link between vitamin D deficiency and obesity. One of these is volumetric dilution of 25(OH)D through the greater tissue mass of obese individuals, thereby limiting the 25(OH)D in the blood and indicating a lower vitamin D status. Reduced sun exposure, sun protective behaviours and covering of skin could also impact endogenous vitamin D production [24,30]. Both liver and kidney disease are common in obese populations and can impair metabolism of vitamin D to 25(OH)D and then the hormonally-active form—$1,25(OH)_2D$ [28,31]. Rare alleles for SNPs in the VDR and DBP have been associated with higher body weight and body mass index (BMI), and lower vitamin D status [32–35], suggesting a potential genetic link between body weight and vitamin D status.

As vitamin D deficiency is an important and common issue for obese individuals, we aimed to investigate the relationship between several factors, including BMI, sun exposure, and skin colour, with vitamin D status in a group of morbidly obese individuals. The aim of this paper is to identify factors beyond the standard 25(OH)D measurement that may aid in assessing vitamin D status of morbidly obese individuals.

2. Materials and Methods

2.1. Participants

Participants were recruited as part of a study into vitamin D supplementation post bariatric surgery at the Wesley Hospital, Brisbane, Australia. The data presented here are the pre-surgical information collected. Inclusion criteria included: age ≥ 18 years, and accepted for bariatric surgery by surgical team. The surgical team use the AACE/TOS/ASMBS Clinical Practice Guidelines for the Perioperative Nutritional, Metabolic, and Nonsurgical Support of the Bariatric Surgery Patient to assess patient suitability for surgery [36]. Exclusion criteria included: pregnancy, age <18 years, taking medications that affected vitamin D levels, vitamin D supplement use in the last three months, or having liver or kidney disease. All subjects gave their informed consent for inclusion before they participated in the study. The study was conducted in accordance with the Declaration of Helsinki, and the protocol was approved by the Human Research Ethics Committee of the University of Queensland (#2015000446) and Uniting Care Human Research Ethics Committee (#1502).

2.2. Study Design

In this cross-sectional study, participants were recruited at the time of their initial consultation with the bariatric surgeon. Participant characteristics were collected from study enrolment forms and clinical records. Data collected included pre-surgery 25(OH)D status, age, gender, BMI, season of vitamin D testing, sun exposure behaviours, and assessment of skin colour using spectrophotometry.

2.3. Data Collection

2.3.1. Anthropometry

Weight (kg) and height (m) were measured to the nearest 0.1 kg and 1 cm. Weight and height were measured using digital column scales (SECA 769, Chino, CA, USA). BMI was calculated using weight (kg)/height (m)^2.

2.3.2. Biochemistry

As part of standard care, the surgical team requested the following biochemical parameters from serum: 25(OH)D, parathyroid hormone, calcium, iron studies (iron, ferritin, transferrin), full blood count (red blood cells, white blood cells, platelets), and liver function tests (aspartate aminotransferase, alkaline phosphatase, alanine aminotransferase, albumin, bilirubin). Participants used one of two pathology laboratories available throughout Queensland. Participants' biochemistry results were collected, where available, pre-surgery, 3 months, 6 months, and 12 months post-surgery. Parathyroid hormone was measured by immunoassay (Centaur XP; Siemens, Tarrytown, NY, USA or Cobas 8000 E602; Roche Diagnostics, Mannheim, Germany). Calcium was measured by immunoassay (Architect I2000sr; Abbott, Abbott Park, IL, USA or Advia 2400; Siemens, Tarrytown, NY, USA). Iron studies were measured by immunoassay (Architect I2000sr; Abbott, Abbott Park, IL, USA or Advia 2400; Siemens, Tarrytown, NY, USA). Full blood counts were measured by XN-10 Hematology Analyser (Sysmex, Kobe, Japan). Liver function tests were measured using immunoassay (Advia 2400; Siemens, Tarrytown, NY, USA).

Vitamin D was measured with automated chemiluminescent competitive immunoassay (Liaison XL; DiaSorin, Stillwater, MN, USA or ADVIA Centaur XP; Siemens, Tarrytown, NY, USA). The Liaison XL measurement range is 10–375 nmol/L (4–150 ng/mL). It is reported to demonstrate equimolar cross-reactivity with 25(OH)D$_3$ (100%) and 25(OH)D$_2$ (104%), and cross reactivity of <1% with 3-epi-25(OH)D$_3$ [37]. Precision analysis for Liaison XL have been reported between 12.6 and 10.8% [38]. The Centaur XP measurement range is 10.5–375 nmol/L (4.2–150 ng/mL). It is reported to demonstrate equimolar cross-reactivity with 25(OH)D$_3$ (100.7%) and 25(OH)D$_2$ (104.5%), and cross-reactivity of 1.1% with 3-epi-25(OH)D$_3$ [39]. Precision analysis for Centaur XP have been reported between

4.2 and 11.9% [38]. Both laboratories use the Royal College of Pathologists of Australasia Quality Assurance Program for vitamin D, and one uses the Vitamin D External Quality Assessment Scheme. Vitamin D status was defined using the following ranges: sufficient ≥50 nmol/L, mildly insufficient 49–25 nmol/L, moderately insufficient 24–12.5 nmol/L, and severely insufficient <12.5 nmol/L [10].

2.3.3. Sun Exposure

Participants completed a questionnaire on sun exposure and clothing worn on either workdays or non-workdays in the last three months, based on a previously validated survey [40]. From this data, an average sun exposure time per day was calculated (min/day). Using a modified rule of nines method for estimating percentage of Body Surface Area (%BSA) in individuals with obesity [41], an average daily %BSA exposed to the sun was calculated from information on clothing worn each day.

2.3.4. Skin Colour

Skin colour measurements were taken using a Spectrophotometer CM-2600/D (Konica Minolta, Tokyo, Japan). This instrument measures skin reflectance of light within the wavelength range of 360 nm to 740 nm. The data is reported using the Commission Internationale de L'Eclairage L*a*b* system. Where L* indicates the lightness or brightness of the skin [42]. Readings were taken on the inner arm (natural skin colour) and the outer forearm (tanned skin colour) using the specular component included (SCI) results for L*a*b. Individual typology angles were calculated using the following formula: ITA = (ArcTangent ((L − 50)/b)) × 180/π [43]. Skin colour was then classified using the ITA into the following groups: very light > 55 > light > 41 > intermediate > 28 > tanned > −10 > brown > −30 > dark [43]. ITA calculations were used to create a measure of tan by subtracting the natural skin colour score (ITAC) from the tanned skin colour score (ITAF), i.e., the difference in ITA score between natural and tanned skin.

2.3.5. UV Index

The average UV index in the three months prior to vitamin D testing was recorded for each participant using the data from the Australian Radiation Protection and Nuclear Safety Agency (http://www.arpansa.gov.au). Average UV Index in the three months prior to testing was used as it can take 2–5 months for serum 25(OH)D concentrations to plateau, and it is suggested to not retest for three months [10].

2.3.6. Dietary Vitamin D Intake

Participants completed a diet questionnaire based on a previously validated food frequency questionnaire [44]. Serve sizes were based on the Australia Guide to Healthy Eating [45]. Vitamin D_3 equivalents per serve were calculated based on the NUTTAB 2011-12 Vitamin D food database [46]. The NUTTAB 2011-12 Vitamin D database determined vitamin D_3, 25(OH)D_3, vitamin D_2, and 25(OH)D_2 content using normal phase high-performance liquid chromatography, with ultraviolet detection, on an extract of saponified samples of each food. Vitamin D equivalents were calculated with a factor that takes into account the potentially higher bioavailability of the 25-hydroxy forms of vitamin D. Dietary vitamin D equivalents intake for each participant was calculated for foods containing vitamin D, by calculating the vitamin D equivalents per serve, and multiplying by the minimum number of serves per week indicated by the participant's response (see Table 1).

Table 1. Vitamin D equivalents calculations by response option.

Vitamin D Source	Serve Size	0–1 Serves Per Week (µg/week)	1 to 4 Serves Per Week (µg/week)	5+ Serves Per Week (µg/week)
Beef	65 g cooked	0.0	0.3	1.3
Canned fish, tuna	85 g	0.0	2.0	10.2
Mushrooms	75 g	0.0	1.7	8.6
Eggs, whole	120 g	0.0	2.5	12.6
Milk, whole	250 mL	0.0	0.3	1.5
Salmon	100 g	0.0	20.0	100.0
Diary blend spread	10 g	0.0	1.0	5.0

Based on source: NUTTAB 2010 (Food Standards Australia New Zealand); The University of New South Wales; Professor Heather Greenfield and co-workers at the University of New South Wales; Tables of composition of Australian Aboriginal Foods (J Brand-Miller, KW James and PMA Maggiore).

2.3.7. Single Nucleotide Polymorphisms

DNA was extracted from whole blood samples from 45 participants using QIAamp DNA Blood Mini kit (#51104, Qiagen, Hilden, Germany). Five SNPs were genotyped using a MassARRAY System (Agena Bioscience, San Diego, CA, USA), conducted by the Australian Genomics Research Facility, The University of Queensland, Brisbane, Australia. Participants were identified as either common homozygous, heterozygous, or rare homozygous for each SNP (see Table 2). Global minor allele frequency data was sourced from 1000 Genomes [47].

Table 2. Single nucleotide polymorphisms of interest.

SNP	Gene	MAF	Common Homozygous	Heterozygous	Rare Homozygous
Rs1544410 (*bsm1*)	VDR	0.2959	GG	GA	AA
Rs2228570 (*fok1*)	VDR	0.3285	CC	TC	TT
Rs731236 (*taq1*)	VDR	0.2766	TT	TC	CC
Rs4588	DBP	0.2079	CC	CA	AA
Rs7041	DBP	0.3816	GG	GT	TT

MAF minor allele frequency.

2.4. Statistical Analysis

Statistical analysis was conducted using SPSS 24 (IBM Corp. Released 2015. IBM SPSS Statistics for Macintosh, Version 24.0. Armonk, NY, USA: IBM Corp.). Variables were assessed for normality and transformed where possible. Pearson correlation and Spearman Rank Correlation were used where appropriate. Linear and multiple regression models were used to determine the effect of independent variables on serum 25(OH)D. One-way ANCOVA was used to determine significant differences between mean serum 25(OH)D concentrations while accounting for covariates, and Bonferroni multiple comparisons test was used to identify significant differences between groups. Allelic frequencies were tested against Hardy–Weinburg equilibrium. Significance was set at $p < 0.05$.

3. Results

3.1. Characteristics

See Table 3 for participant characteristics. Fifty participants were recruited (80% female), the age range was 23 to 61 years, 70% were Obese Class III (>40 kg/m^2), 58% were vitamin D sufficient (>50 nmol/L), 35% were vitamin D insufficient (<50 nmol/L), and serum 25(OH)D concentrations ranged from 21 to 103 nmol/L with a normal distribution. The majority (83%) had very light/light constitutive skin colour, and 74% had intermediate/tanned facultative skin colour. Sun exposure times ranged from 0 to 309 min/day, and body surface area exposed to the sun ranged from 0 to 52.5%. Skin colour measurements were not conducted on three participants due to equipment malfunction. Average sun exposure time, body surface exposure and dietary vitamin D intake were not reported in all participants, due to missing or inaccurate data reported in the sun and diet questionnaires.

Table 3. Participant characteristics.

	n	Mean (SD)	95% CI
Weight (kg)	50	126.7 (24.4)	119.8–133.7
BMI (kg/m^2)	50	43.9 (7.3)	41.8–46.0
Plasma 25(OH)D (nmol/L)	48	56.8 (20.3)	50.9–62.7
Natural skin colour (ITAC score)	47	50.2 (8.2)	47.8–52.6
Tanned skin colour (ITAF score)	47	26.6 (11.7)	23.1–30.0
Degree of tan (ITAC–ITAF)	47	23.6 (8.2)	21.2–26.0
Average sun exposure (min/day)	42	65.4 (64.9)	45.2–85.7
Average BSA exposed (%)	41	17.6 (14.9)	12.9–22.3
Dietary Vitamin D (ug/day)	40	1.9 (1.4)	1.4–2.4

BMI body mass index, BSA body surface area, 25(OH)D 25-hydroxyvitamin D, SD standard deviation.

3.2. Correlation Analysis

Pearson's or Spearman's rank correlations were run between all variables (Figure 1). Significant correlations with serum 25(OH)D were found for age and natural skin colour (ITAC). Correlation between serum 25(OH)D and tanned skin colour trended toward significance ($p = 0.074$).

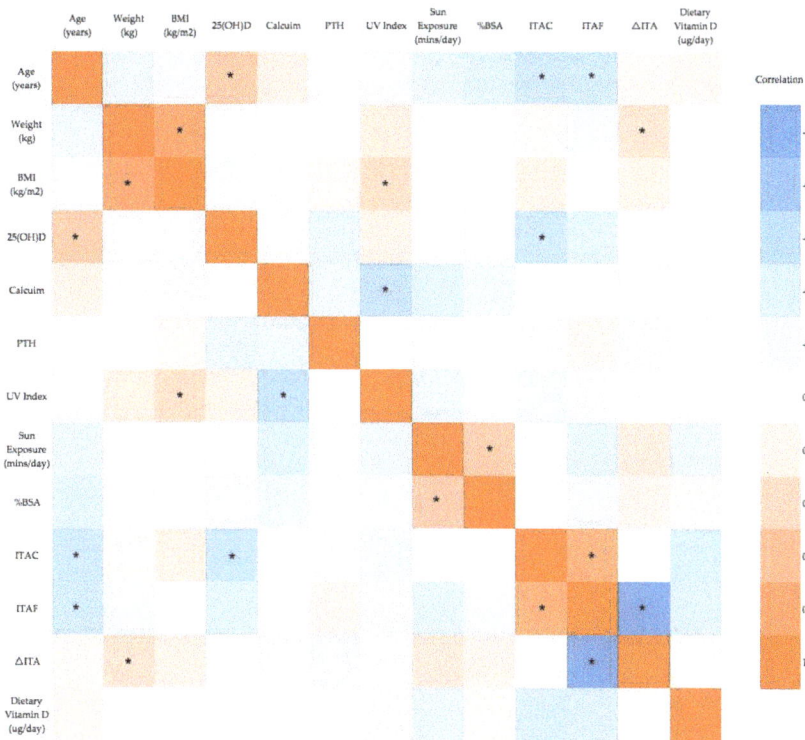

Figure 1. Correlation heat map for all variables. Blue indicates strong negative correlation and Orange indicates strong positive correlation. * $p < 0.05$. BMI body mass index, PTH parathyroid hormone, UV ultraviolet, BSA body surface area, ITA individual typology angle.

3.3. Weight and BMI

No significant correlation was found between weight or BMI, and serum 25(OH)D concentrations. A one-way ANOVA was conducted to determine if serum 25(OH)D concentrations were different between weight or BMI quartiles. There was no significant difference in serum 25(OH)D concentration between weight quartiles, $F(3, 44) = 0.305$, $p = 0.822$, or BMI quartiles, $F(3, 44) = 1.041$, $p = 0.384$ (Table 4).

Table 4. Serum 25(OH)D concentrations by weight and BMI quartile. Serum 25(OH)D is presented as mean $\pm$ standard deviation.

Quartile	Weight (kg)	Serum 25(OH)D (nmol/L)	BMI (kg/m^2)	Serum 25(OH)D (nmol/L)
1	≤107 kg	59.5 ± 21.5	≤39	58.9 ± 22.4
2	108–123 kg	59.8 ± 18.3	40–42.6	64.1 ± 22.3
3	124–141 kg	54.2 ± 23.7	42.7–46.8	50.5 ± 18.2
4	≥142 kg	53.7 ± 18.1	≥42.6	53.8 ± 17.5

3.4. Dietary Vitamin D

Dietary intake of vitamin D is predicted to contribute 5–10% of total vitamin D intake in Australian populations [10]. The Recommended Daily Intakes for vitamin D are 5 µg/day for those aged 19–50 years, and 10 µg for those aged 51–70 years. Average maximum dietary intake prior to surgery was calculated as 1.9 µg/day for this group of individuals, with a range of 0 to 4.7 µg/day. The average Australia adult is estimated to obtain 1.2 to 2.6 µg/day [48] showing this population is within the normal range for Australian adults. There was no significant correlation between dietary vitamin D and serum 25(OH)D concentrations (Figure 1).

3.5. Skin Colour

There was a significant correlation between natural skin colour (ITAC) and serum 25(OH)D concentrations, a trend towards a significant correlation between tanned skin colour (ITAC) ($p = 0.074$) and serum 25(OH)D concentrations, and no significant correlation between degree of tan (ΔITA) and serum 25(OH)D concentrations (Figure 1). ITAC was significantly correlated with age, ($r = -0.315$, $p = 0.015$) and ITAF ($r = 0.716$, $p < 0.01$). ITAF was significantly correlated with age ($r = -0.340$, $p = 0.019$), and change in ITA ($r = 0.719$, $p < 0.01$).

Linear regression analysis was completed to assess the relationship between natural skin colour (ITAC) and serum 25(OH)D concentrations. Natural skin colour accounted for 13.5% of the variation in serum 25(OH)D concentrations, (adj. $R^2 = 11\%$). Natural skin colour significantly predicted serum 25(OH)D concentrations, $F(1, 43) = 6.711$, $p = .013$. For each 10° increase of ITAC score (i.e., lighter natural skin colour), serum 25(OH)D concentrations decrease by 9 nmol/L. Serum 25(OH)D concentrations were predicted using this model for each skin colour group (Table 5).

Linear regression analysis was completed to assess the relationship between tanned skin colour (ITAF) and serum 25(OH)D concentrations. Tanned skin colour accounted for 7.2% of the variation in serum 25(OH)D concentrations, (adj. $R^2 = 5.1\%$). Tanned skin colour was trending toward significance with serum 25(OH)D concentrations, $F(1, 43) = 3.344$, $p = 0.074$. For each 10° decrease in ITAF score (i.e., darker tan) serum 25(OH)D concentrations increase by 5 nmol/L. Serum 25(OH)D concentrations were predicted using this model for each skin colour group (Table 6).

Table 5. Predicted serum 25(OH)D concentrations from linear regression model for ITAC score.

ITAC Score	Serum 25(OH)D Range (nmol/L)
Very light	<53
Light	54–66
Intermediate	67–78
Tanned	79–95
Brown	96–132
Dark	>133

Table 6. Predicted serum 25(OH)D concentrations from linear regression model for ITAF score.

ITAF Score	Serum 25(OH)D Range (nmol/L)
Very light	<44
Light	45–51
Intermediate	52–57
Tanned	58–66
Brown	67–85
Dark	>85

3.6. Sun Exposure

Sun exposure was measured through the sun exposure questionnaire, where participants reported the times spent in direct sunlight, and clothing worn at that time. From this information, an average minutes of sun exposure per day and the %BSA exposed to the sun were calculated. There was no correlation between %BSA or sun exposure minutes and serum 25(OH)D concentrations (Figure 1). Sun exposure minutes and %BSA were significantly positively correlated ($r = 0.486$, $p = 0.001$), suggesting those who spent more time in the sun had more skin exposed.

3.7. Single Nucleotide Polymorphisms

No statistically significant differences in mean serum 25(OH)D concentration were found for any SNP genotype (Table 7); however, lower serum 25(OH)D concentrations were found in the rare genotype compared to the common genotype for all vitamin D SNPs (*bsm1*, *taq1*, *fok1*, rs4588, rs7041). Combinations of two rare genotypes were also examined for any differences in serum 25(OH)D concentrations, weight, or BMI. No significant differences in serum 25(OH)D, weight or BMI were found between those with or without both rare genotypes for *bsm1* and *taq1* ($n = 8$), or rs4588 and rs7041 ($n = 14$), or *fok1* and rs4588 ($n = 10$).

Table 7. Minor allele frequencies for each SNP, and mean serum 25(OH)D concentration, weight, and BMI by genotype for SNPs of interest. *p* values calculated from one-way ANOVAs.

SNP	MAF	Genotype	*n*	Serum 25(OH)D (nmol/L)	*p* Value	Weight (kg)	*p* Value	BMI (kg/m^2)	*p* Value
Rs1544410 (*bsm1*)		GG	18	57.8 (22.9)	0.820	118.4 (23.9)	0.340	42.5 (7.5)	0.426 [a]
		GA	17	54.2 (17.1)		130.7 (27.8)		45.5 (8.8)	
	0.38	AA [b]	8	53.4 (19.0)		126.0 (18.1)		44.9 (6.2)	
Rs2228570 (*fok1*)		CC	18	59.5 (20.6)	0.238	123.4 (31.5)	0.585 [a]	44.0 (9.7)	0.342 [a]
		CT	19	55.6 (20.1)		124.1 (18.4)		43.7 (6.8)	
	0.36	TT [b]	6	43.7 (11.1)		130.5 (22.7)		45.8 (3.6)	
Rs731236 (*taq1*)		TT	19	57.3 (22.4)	0.878	117.7 (23.4)	0.213	42.2 (7.4)	0.238 [a]
		TC	16	54.7 (17.6)		132.4 (27.8)		46.0 (8.7)	
	0.37	CC [b]	8	53.4 (19.0)		126.0 (18.1)		44.9 (6.2)	
Rs4588		CC	23	56.9 (20.4)	0.210	121.0 (25.7)	0.117 [a]	44.0 (7.5)	0.440 [a]
		CA	16	57.8 (19.0)		125.4 (24.8)		42.9 (7.7)	
	0.28	AA [b]	4	39.0 (12.7)		142.7 (8.7)		49.4 (9.8)	
Rs7041		GG	14	59.6 (20.9)	0.601	123.4 (31.6)	0.275 [a]	45.7 (8.7)	0.237 [a]
		GT	23	54.4 (19.1)		122.6 (21.1)		42.0 (6.6)	
	0.41	TT [b]	6	50.7 (20.6)		135.5 (20.5)		48.3 (8.5)	

[a] Kruskal–Wallis H test; [b] homozygous risk genotype, SNP single nucleotide polymorphism, MAF minor allele frequency, BMI body mass index.

3.8. Multiple Regression Model

A multiple regression model was developed to identify the contributions of independent variables to serum 25(OH)D concentrations. Variables were chosen based on their univariate relationship with serum 25(OH)D concentrations, and effect sizes $\geq$ intermediate. Independent variables included in the model were age, ITAC, and UV Index. The multiple regression model statistically significantly predicted serum 25(OH)D concentrations, $F(3, 41) = 7.202$, $p = 0.001$, adj. $R^2 = 29.7\%$, intermediate effect size [49] (Table 8). Age was the only variable that significantly predicted serum 25(OH)D, showing each year increase in age is associated with an increase of 0.9 nmol/L serum 25(OH)D.

Table 8. Multiple regression coefficients.

Model	B	SE$_B$	β	*p* Value
Constant	19.588	28.908		0.502
Age	0.932	0.273	0.467	0.001 *
ITAC	−0.444	0.346	−0.176	0.206
UV Index	3.528	1.965	0.232	0.080

* $p < 0.05$, B unstandardized coefficient, SE$_B$ standard error of unstandardized coefficient, β beta, ITA individual typology angle, UV ultraviolet.

4. Discussion

Determinants of vitamin D status in morbidly obese individuals were examined, and factors considered were dietary vitamin D intake, BMI, skin colour, and sun exposure. The key findings were (i) natural skin colour accounted for 13.5% of the variation in serum 25(OH)D concentrations; (ii) there was a significant positive association between age and serum 25(OH)D; (iii) weight and BMI were not significantly associated with serum 25(OH)D concentrations; (iv) there was relationship between sun exposure time, or amount of skin exposed, with 25(OH)D concentrations in this group.

Natural skin colour (ITAC score) accounted for 13.5% of the variation in serum 25(OH)D concentrations. Results showed that as natural skin colour becomes darker, serum 25(OH)D concentrations increased, suggesting those with darker natural skin colour have higher 25(OH)D concentrations. ITAC score was also used to predict maximal mean serum 25(OH)D concentrations for each skin colour category. It is well documented that those with darker natural skin colour have lower serum 25(OH)D concentrations [21,50]. As this study had only recruited participants with an intermediate skin colour or lighter, it is possible the increase in 25(OH)D concentration with increasing natural skin colour was due to sun protective behaviours from those with lighter skin. For similar reasons, the predictive model became unreliable when dealing with those in the tanned and brown skin colour categories. Although when comparing changes in ITA score i.e., degree of tanning, sun exposure times, and %BSA, there was no correlation between any of these measures and natural skin colour, potentially suggesting no differences in sun protective behaviours regardless of natural skin colour.

A trend towards significance was seen between tanned skin colour (ITAF score) and serum 25(OH)D concentrations. Tanned skin colour accounted for 7.2% of the variation in serum 25(OH)D concentrations in this group. As ITAF score increased (i.e., darker tan), 25(OH)D concentrations increased, suggesting that those with a darker tan (up to intermediate) will have higher 25(OH)D concentrations. Previous research has shown that tanned skin colour is a significant predictor of 25(OH)D [23]. This result came from a larger group but with similar proportions of participants in each skin colour group. Our results confirm those of Rockell et al. [23], showing that for each $10°$ decrease in ITAF score (i.e., darker tan) serum 25(OH)D concentrations increase by 5 nmol/L [23].

The Australian Health Survey (2011–12) showed similar rates of deficiency between genders, and an increase in vitamin D status with age, concurrent with increases in supplement use [12]. Population data in Australia show varying effects of age on serum 25(OH)D, with some showing an increase with age [12,51] and others a decrease with age [19]. There was a significant positive association between age and serum 25(OH)D concentrations in our study. Further investigation of the variables showed that age positively correlated with natural skin colour and tanned skin colour, suggesting that the older participants had darker natural and tanned skin colour. There was no relationship between age and degree of tan, or %BSA exposed to the sun, or sun exposure time.

Weight and BMI were not significantly associated with serum 25(OH)D concentrations. There are several meta-analyses that have shown a significant decrease in serum 25(OH)D concentrations with increasing weight or BMI, although not all included morbidly obese individuals [52–54]. There are several studies in morbidly obese individuals that found a significant [55–61] or borderline significant [62,63] inverse relationship between BMI and 25(OH)D concentrations, with small to large effect sizes. It is possible that once a certain BMI threshold is reached, the dilution effects of obesity on vitamin D status plateau, and the effect becomes minimal, hence the trend of lower serum 25(OH)D in this study, but the lack of a significant difference. Sun exposure, or lack of it, appears to have a major influence on vitamin D status in Australian obese populations. A study into determinants of serum 25(OH)D in Australian Adults reported that the amount of skin exposed to the sun was the single largest contributor to serum 25(OH)D concentrations, followed by location, season, and personal UV radiation exposure [19]. BMI only explained 4% of the variance in their population, which include a wide range of BMI [19].

As the majority of vitamin D_3 is produced endogenously in the skin, it is logical to expect that a relationship would exist between sun exposure times, the %BSA exposed, and vitamin D status. There was no relationship between sun exposure times or %BSA, with serum 25(OH)D concentrations in our study. Previous research into determinants of vitamin D status in Australian adults found a significant association between vitamin D status and time spent outdoors ($r_s = 0.16$, $p < 0.0001$), and vitamin D status and the percentage of clothing cover ($r_s = -0.50$, $p < 0.001$), in a population with a wide range of BMI, including individuals with obesity [19]. There are a few possible reasons why no relationship was identified between these measures and vitamin D status in our study. This study reports behaviours of a specific group of morbidly obese individuals, and so represented only their sun exposure practices, whereas the AusD study included a wide range of BMI and a larger sample size. The data provided on sun exposure times and body surface area exposed was self-reported data, and may not have been accurate. There was a trend toward a positive correlation between change in ITA (degree of tan) and time in the sun. This would be expected, as longer sun exposure would generally lead to an increase in tan, providing some evidence that this measure of sun exposure is accurate. Vitamin D is stored in adipose tissue [64], and there is some evidence that muscle may store 25(OH)D [65], thereby reducing the amount of 25(OH)D available in the circulation for measurement. This may impact the ability to correlate vitamin D status with any measures of skin colour, or sun exposure, especially in those with high amounts of adipose tissue or large muscle mass, as seen in this group of morbidly obese individuals.

Three SNPs for the VDR and two for the DBP were analysed in this group. No significant differences in serum 25(OH)D concentrations were seen between genotypes of any gene. Although all homozygous rare genotypes had lower mean serum 25(OH)D concentrations than the common homozygous genotype. From a clinical perspective, VDR *fok1* and DBP rs4588 both indicated insufficient vitamin D status for those with homozygous rare genotypes compared to homozygous common genotypes. Rare alleles for all four of the main variants for the VDR gene have been associated with lower serum 25(OH)D concentration and vitamin D deficiency in a range of populations [15–17,66–68]. This suggests a possible method of personalised nutrition in this population, by considering specialised treatments for the patients with a genetic predisposition for lower serum 25(OH)D, based on the SNP genotype, particularly for *fok1* and rs4588. This information could contribute to the overall assessment of vitamin D status, and identify those that may achieve more benefit from supplementation.

The VDR *bsm1* rare allele has been associated with higher weight, BMI [32,33], and lower percentage of excess weight loss in bariatric patients [69]. The *taq1* rare allele has also been associated with higher BMI and weight [34]. The *fok1* rare allele has not been associated with weight and BMI previously [70–72]. In this group of morbidly obese individuals, there was no statistically significant difference in weight, BMI or %EWL, between rare or common genotypes for *bsm1*, *taq1*, and *fok1*. Of clinical significance was the difference in mean serum 25(OH)D concentrations between common homozygous and rare homozygous individuals for *fok1* and rs4588, where the common homozygous genotype was vitamin D sufficient, and the rare homozygous genotype was vitamin D deficient.

Both DBP SNP common alleles have been associated with higher BMI in females, but not males [35]. We found no significant differences in weight or BMI between the genotypes for both DBP SNPs. The difference in results could be related to differences in sample populations, this study only included patients with BMI > 30, whereas the previous study included a wide range of BMI (16.93–57.21 kg/m^2) [35]. It is important to note that the SNP analysis from this study was under powered, and so results must be considered with caution. Particularly those that conflict with results from adequately powered studies. Post hoc power analysis using G*Power [73] indicated that power ranged from 6 to 63% for these analyses, and required sample sizes from 69 to 957 for 80% power.

There are several limitations to this study. Serum 25(OH)D concentrations were measured using chemiluminescent competitive immunoassays, on two different platforms. The gold standard in measuring 25(OH)D concentration is liquid chromatography with tandem mass spectrometry. Issues with measuring 25(OH)D arise from the ability of these assays to release 25(OH)D from its binding protein or other carriers like albumin, the hydrophobic properties of 25(OH)D, and the differing antibody specificities to the metabolites [9]. Although both pathology laboratories reported using quality assurance programs, both platforms have potential issues with under or over recovering metabolites, negative biases, and large deviations at lower concentrations of 25(OH)D (~50 nmo/L) [38]. This highlights an issue for clinicians in interpreting results for the 25(OH)D assay. Recruitment did not occur over a full year, this led to lower numbers of participants recruited post summer and autumn. This influences the results of differences in serum 25(OH)D between seasons, and potentially, the range of tanned skin colours. Using a small range of BMI has also minimised the effects of weight and BMI on serum 25(OH)D; use of a wider range, including normal, overweight, and obese individuals may have shown a more pronounced effect. A similar issue is found with the skin colour assessments, as individuals recruited only had natural skin colour from very light to intermediate. This limits the ability of results to be applied to those with darker natural skin colour. Our sample size was also under powered for SNP analysis, and so results should be considered with caution.

5. Conclusions

In this group of morbidly obese individuals lighter natural skin colour and younger age are potential risk factors for vitamin D insufficiency. It appears sun exposure time, the amount of skin exposed to the sun, weight and BMI, do not influence vitamin D status in this population. The vitamin D pathway SNPs investigated showed no statistically significant effects on vitamin D status, although clinically significant differences were found for VDR *fok1* and DBP rs4588. Future research into the determinants of vitamin D status using a larger group of morbidly obese individuals could provide further information on the genetic susceptibility to vitamin D deficiency in this at-risk group. A group with a wider range of natural skin colours could also help to develop an understanding of the contribution of skin colour and tanned skin colour to vitamin D status.

Acknowledgments: This research was supported by The University of Queensland. Open access was funded by PhD funds. The authors would like to acknowledge the valuable support from the Wesley Medical Research (Project No. 2015-03).

Author Contributions: C.F.D. conceived and designed the study, collected and analysed data, and contributed to manuscript preparation. B.D.R. collected data, and contributed to manuscript preparation. I.M. collected data, and contributed to manuscript preparation. S.R. collected data, and contributed to manuscript preparation. J.B.P. conceived and designed the study, and contributed to manuscript preparation. J.D.B. conceived and designed the study, and contributed to manuscript preparation. O.R.L.W. conceived and designed the study, and contributed to manuscript preparation.

Conflicts of Interest: The authors declare no conflict of interest. The funding sponsors had no role in the design of the study; in the collection, analyses, or interpretation of data; in the writing of the manuscript, and in the decision to publish the results.

References

1. Anderson, P.H.; Turner, A.G.; Morris, H.A. Vitamin D actions to regulate calcium and skeletal homeostasis. *Clin. Biochem.* **2012**, *45*, 880–886. [CrossRef] [PubMed]
2. Gorham, E.D.; Holick, M.F.; Garland, C.F.; Garland, F.C.; Grant, W.B.; Mohr, S.B.; Lipkin, M.; Newmark, H.L.; Giovannucci, E.; Wei, M. Optimal vitamin D status for colorectal cancer prevention: A quantitative meta analysis. *Am. J. Prev. Med.* **2007**, *32*, 210–216. [CrossRef] [PubMed]
3. Szodoray, P.; Zeher, M.; Bodolay, E.; Nakken, B.; Gaal, J.; Jonsson, R.; Szegedi, A.; Zold, E.; Szegedi, G.; Brun, J.G.; et al. The complex role of vitamin D in autoimmune diseases. *Scand. J. Immunol.* **2008**, *68*, 261–270. [CrossRef] [PubMed]
4. Bikle, D.D. Extra renal synthesis of 1,25-dihydroxyvitamin D and its health implications. *Clin. Rev. Bone Min. Metab.* **2009**, *7*, 114–125. [CrossRef]
5. Yamamoto, Y.; Yoshizawa, T.; Fukuda, T.; Shirode-Fukuda, Y.; Yu, T.; Sekine, K.; Sato, T.; Kawano, H.; Aihara, K.-I.; Nakamichi, Y.; et al. Vitamin D receptor in osteoblasts is a negative regulator of bone mass control. *Endocrinology* **2013**, *154*, 1008–1020. [CrossRef] [PubMed]
6. Balesaria, S.; Sangha, S.; Julian, R.F.W. Human duodenum responses to vitamin D metabolites of TRPV6 and other genes involved in calcium absorption. *Am. J. Physiol. Gastrointest. Liver Physiol.* **2009**, *297*, 1193–1197. [CrossRef] [PubMed]
7. Kriebitzsch, C.; Verlinden, L.; Eelen, G.; Tan, B.K.; Van Camp, M.; Bouillon, R.; Verstuyf, A. The impact of 1,25(OH)2D3 and its structural analogs on gene expression in cancer cells—A microarray approach. *Anticancer Res.* **2009**, *29*, 3471–3483. [PubMed]
8. Norman, A.W.; Okamura, W.H.; Bishop, J.E.; Henry, H.L. Update on biological actions of 1α,25(OH)2-vitamin D3 (rapid effects) and 24R,25(OH)2-vitamin D3. *Mol. Cell. Endocrinol.* **2002**, *197*, 1–13. [CrossRef]
9. Holick, M.F.; Binkley, N.C.; Bischoff-Ferrari, H.A.; Gordon, C.M.; Hanley, D.A.; Heaney, R.P.; Murad, M.H.; Weaver, C.M.; Endocrine, S. Evaluation, treatment, and prevention of vitamin D deficiency: An Endocrine Society clinical practice guideline. *J. Clin. Endocrinol. Metab.* **2011**, *96*, 1911–1930. [CrossRef] [PubMed]
10. Nowson, C.A.; McGrath, J.J.; Ebeling, P.R.; Haikerwal, A.; Daly, R.M.; Sanders, K.M.; Seibel, M.J.; Mason, R.S. Vitamin D and health in adults in Australia and New Zealand: A position statement. *Med. J. Aust.* **2012**, *196*, 686–687. [CrossRef] [PubMed]
11. Bischoff-Ferrari, H.A.; Henschkowski, J.; Dawson-Hughes, B.; Staehelin, H.B.; Orav, J.E.; Stuck, A.E.; Theiler, R.; Wong, J.B.; Egli, A.; Kiel, D.P. Fall prevention with supplemental and active forms of vitamin D: A meta-analysis of randomised controlled trials. *Br. Med. J.* **2009**, *339*, 843–846. [CrossRef] [PubMed]
12. Australian Bureau of Statistics. *Australian Health Survey: First Results 2011–12*; Australian Bureau of Statistics: Canberra, Australia, 2012.
13. Looker, A.C.; Johnson, C.L.; Lacher, D.A.; Pfeiffer, C.M.; Schleicher, R.L.; Sempos, C.T. Vitamin D status: United States, 2001–2006. *NCHS Data Brief* **2011**, *59*, 1–8.
14. Santos, B.R.; Mascarenhas, L.P.G.; Satler, F.; Boguszewski, M.C.S.; Spritzer, P.M. Vitamin D deficiency in girls from South Brazil: A cross-sectional study on prevalence and association with vitamin D receptor gene variants. *BMC Pediatr.* **2012**, *12*. [CrossRef] [PubMed]
15. Kitanaka, S.; Isojima, T.; Takaki, M.; Numakura, C.; Hayasaka, K.; Igarashi, T. Association of vitamin D-related gene polymorphisms with manifestation of vitamin D deficiency in children. *Endocr. J.* **2012**, *59*, 1007–1014. [CrossRef] [PubMed]
16. Bora, G.; Ozkan, B.; Dayangaç-Erden, D.; Erdem-Yurter, H.; Coşkun, T. Vitamin D receptor gene polymorphisms in Turkish children with vitamin D deficient rickets. *Turk. J. Pediatr.* **2008**, *50*, 30–33. [PubMed]
17. Santos, B.R.; Mascarenhas, L.P.G.; Boguszewski, M.C.S.; Spritzer, P.M. Variations in the Vitamin D-binding protein (DBP) gene are related to lower 25-hydroxyvitamin D levels in healthy girls: A cross-sectional study. *Horm. Res. Paediatr.* **2013**, *79*, 162–168. [CrossRef] [PubMed]
18. Cheung, C.L.; Lau, K.S.; Sham, P.C.; Tan, K.C.; Kung, A.W. Genetic variant in vitamin D binding protein is associated with serum 25-hydroxyvitamin D and vitamin D insufficiency in southern Chinese. *J. Hum. Genet.* **2013**, *58*, 749–751. [CrossRef] [PubMed]

19. Kimlin, M.G.; Lucas, R.M.; Harrison, S.L.; van der Mei, I.; Armstrong, B.K.; Whiteman, D.C.; Kricker, A.; Nowak, M.; Brodie, A.M.; Sun, J. The Contributions of solar ultraviolet radiation exposure and other determinants to serum 25-hydroxyvitamin D concentrations in Australian adults: The AusD study. *Am. J. Epidemiol.* **2014**, *179*, 864–874. [CrossRef] [PubMed]

20. Yu, C.-L.; Li, Y.; Freedman, D.M.; Fears, T.R.; Kwok, R.; Chodick, G.; Alexander, B.; Kimlin, M.G.; Kricker, A.; Armstrong, B.K.; et al. Assessment of lifetime cumulative sun exposure using a self-administered questionnaire: Reliability of two approaches. *Cancer Epidemiol. Biomark. Prev.* **2009**, *18*, 464–471. [CrossRef] [PubMed]

21. Hall, L.M.; Kimlin, M.G.; Aronov, P.A.; Hammock, B.D.; Slusser, J.R.; Woodhouse, L.R.; Stephensen, C.B. Vitamin D intake needed to maintain target serum 25-hydroxyvitamin D concentrations in participants with low sun exposure and dark skin pigmentation is substantially higher than current recommendations. *J. Nutr.* **2010**, *140*, 542–550. [CrossRef] [PubMed]

22. Malvy, D.J.M.; Guinot, C.; Preziosi, P.; Galan, P.; Chapuy, M.C.; Maamer, M.; Arnaud, S.; Meunier, P.J.; Hercberg, S.; Tschachler, E. Relationship between vitamin D status and skin phenotype in general adult population. *Photochem. Photobiol.* **2000**, *71*, 466–469. [CrossRef]

23. Rockell, J.E.P.; Skeaff, C.M.; Williams, S.M.; Green, T.J. Association between quantitative measures of skin color and plasma 25-hydroxyvitamin D. *Osteoporos. Int.* **2008**, *19*, 1639–1642. [CrossRef] [PubMed]

24. Wortsman, J.; Matsuoka, L.Y.; Chen, T.C.; Lu, Z.; Holick, M.F. Decreased bioavailability of vitamin D in obesity. *Am. J. Clin. Nutr.* **2000**, *72*, 690–693. [PubMed]

25. Blum, M.; Dallal, G.E.; Dawson-Hughes, B. Body size and serum 25 hydroxy vitamin D response to oral supplements in healthy older adults. *J. Am. Coll. Nutr.* **2008**, *27*, 274–279. [CrossRef] [PubMed]

26. Calle, E.E.; Thun, M.J. Obesity and cancer. *Oncogene* **2004**, *23*, 6365–6378. [CrossRef] [PubMed]

27. Apovian, C.M.; Gokce, N. Obesity and cardiovascular disease. *Circulation* **2012**, *125*, 1178–1182. [CrossRef] [PubMed]

28. Eliades, M.; Hernaez, R.; Spyrou, E.; Agrawal, N.; Lazo, M.; Brancati, F.L.; Potter, J.J.; Koteish, A.A.; Clark, J.M.; Guallar, E. Meta-analysis: Vitamin D and non-alcoholic fatty liver disease. *Aliment. Pharmacol. Ther.* **2013**, *38*, 246–254. [CrossRef] [PubMed]

29. Holick, M.F. Sunlight and vitamin D for bone health and prevention of autoimmune diseases, cancers, and cardiovascular disease. *Am. J. Clin. Nutr.* **2004**, *80*, 1678–1688.

30. Norval, M.; Wulf, H.C. Does chronic sunscreen use reduce vitamin D production to insufficient levels? *Br. J. Dermatol.* **2009**, *161*, 732–736. [CrossRef] [PubMed]

31. González, E.A.; Sachdeva, A.; Oliver, D.A.; Martin, K.J. Vitamin D insufficiency and deficiency in chronic kidney disease. *Am. J. Nephrol.* **2004**, *24*, 503–510. [CrossRef] [PubMed]

32. Nasser, M.A.-D.; Franca, R.G.; Omar, S.A.-A.; Majed, S.A.; Khalid, M.A.; Hossam, M.D.; Cristina, A.; Andrea, S.C.; Irma, S.; Abdul Khader, M.; et al. Vitamin D receptor gene polymorphisms are associated with obesity and inflammosome activity. *PLoS ONE* **2014**, *9*. [CrossRef]

33. Ye, W.Z.; Reis, A.F.; Dubois-Laforgue, D.; Bellanné-Chantelot, C.; Timsit, J.; Velho, G. Vitamin D receptor gene polymorphisms are associated with obesity in type 2 diabetic subjects with early age of onset. *Eur. J. Endocrinol.* **2001**, *145*, 181–186. [CrossRef] [PubMed]

34. Vasilopoulos, Y.; Sarafidou, T.; Kotsa, K.; Papadimitriou, M.; Goutzelas, Y.; Stamatis, C.; Bagiatis, V.; Tsekmekidou, X.; Yovos, J.G.; Mamuris, Z. VDR TaqI is associated with obesity in the Greek population. *Gene* **2013**, *512*, 237–239. [CrossRef] [PubMed]

35. Almesri, N.; Das, N.S.; Ali, M.E.; Gumaa, K.; Giha, H.A. Independent associations of polymorphisms in vitamin D binding protein (GC) and vitamin D receptor (VDR) genes with obesity and plasma 25OHD3 levels demonstrate sex dimorphism. *Appl. Physiol. Nutr. Metab.* **2016**, *41*, 345. [CrossRef] [PubMed]

36. Mechanick, J.I.; Youdim, A.; Jones, D.B.; Garvey, W.T.; Hurley, D.L.; McMahon, M.M.; Heinberg, L.J.; Kushner, R.; Adams, T.D.; Shikora, S. Clinical practice guidelines for the perioperative nutritional, metabolic, and nonsurgical support of the bariatric surgery patient—2013 update: Cosponsored by American Association of Clinical Endocrinologists, The Obesity Society, and American Society for Metabolic & Bariatric Surgery. *Obesity* **2013**, *21*, S1–S27. [CrossRef] [PubMed]

37. DiaSorin. LIAISON 25 OH Vitamin D TOTAL Assay [directional insert]. DiaSorin: Stillwater, MN, USA, 2012. Available online: http://www.diasorin.com/en/liaisonr-25-oh-vitamin-d-total-assay (accessed on 27 September 2017).

38. Freeman, J.; Wilson, K.; Spears, R.; Shalhoub, V.; Sibley, P. Performance evaluation of four 25-hydroxyvitamin D assays to measure 25-hydroxyvitamin D2. *Clin. Biochem.* **2015**, *48*, 1097–1104. [CrossRef] [PubMed]

39. Siemens Healthineers. ADVIA Centaur Vitamin D Total (VitD) Assay [directional insert 10699279_EN Rev. A, 2013–07]. Siemens Healthcare Diagnostics Inc.: Tarrytown, NY, USA, 2013. Available online: https://www.healthcare.siemens.com/laboratory-diagnostics/assays-by-diseases-conditions/bone-metabolism-assays/advia-centaur-vitamin-d-total-assay (accessed on 27 September 2017).

40. Vu, L.H.; Whiteman, D.C.; van der Pols, J.C.; Kimlin, M.G.; Neale, R.E. Serum Vitamin D Levels in Office Workers in a Subtropical Climate. *Photochem. Photobiol.* **2011**, *87*, 714–720. [CrossRef] [PubMed]

41. Neaman, K.C.; Andres, L.A.; McClure, A.M.; Burton, M.E.; Kemmeter, P.R.; Ford, R.D. A new method for estimation of involved bsas for obese and normal-weight patients with burn injury. *J. Burn Care Res.* **2011**, *32*, 421–428. [CrossRef] [PubMed]

42. Taylor, S.; Westerhof, W.; Im, S.; Lim, J. Noninvasive techniques for the evaluation of skin color. *J. Am. Acad. Dermatol.* **2006**, *54*, S282–S290. [CrossRef] [PubMed]

43. Chardon, A.; Cretois, I.; Hourseau, C. Skin colour typology and suntanning pathways. *Int. J. Cosmet. Sci.* **1991**, *13*, 191–208. [CrossRef] [PubMed]

44. Collins, C.E.; Boggess, M.M.; Watson, J.F.; Guest, M.; Duncanson, K.; Pezdirc, K.; Rollo, M.; Hutchesson, M.J.; Burrows, T.L. Reproducibility and comparative validity of a food frequency questionnaire for Australian adults. *Clin. Nutr.* **2014**, *33*, 906–914. [CrossRef] [PubMed]

45. National Health and Medical Research Council. *Australian Dietary Guidelines*; National Health and Medical Research Council: Canberra, Australia, 2013.

46. Food Standards Australia New Zealand. *NUTTAB 2010—Australian Food Composition Tables*; Food Standards Australia New Zealand: Canberra, Australia, 2010.

47. The 1000 Genomes Project Consortium. A global reference for human genetic variation. *Nature* **2015**, *526*, 68–74. [CrossRef]

48. Nowson, C.A.; Margerison, C. Vitamin D intake and vitamin D status of Australians. *Med. J. Aust.* **2002**, *177*, 149–152. [PubMed]

49. Cohen, J. *Statistical Power Analysis for the Behavioral Sciences*, 2nd ed.; L. Erlbaum Associates: Hillsdale, NJ, USA, 1988.

50. Libon, F.; Cavalier, E.; Nikkels, A.F. Skin color is relevant to vitamin D synthesis. *Dermatology* **2013**, *227*, 250–254. [CrossRef] [PubMed]

51. Gill, T.K.; Hill, C.L.; Shanahan, E.M.; Taylor, A.W.; Appleton, S.L.; Grant, J.F.; Shi, Z.; Dal Grande, E.; Price, K.; Adams, R.J. Vitamin D levels in an Australian population. *BMC Public Health* **2014**, *14*, 1001. [CrossRef] [PubMed]

52. Pereira-Santos, M.; Costa, P.R.F.; Assis, A.M.O.; Santos, C.A.S.T.; Santos, D.B. Obesity and vitamin D deficiency: A systematic review and meta-analysis. *Obes. Rev.* **2015**, *16*, 341–349. [CrossRef] [PubMed]

53. Yao, Y.; Zhu, L.; He, L.; Duan, Y.; Liang, W.; Nie, Z.; Jin, Y.; Wu, X.L.; Fang, Y. A meta-analysis of the relationship between vitamin D deficiency and obesity. *Int. J. Clin. Exp. Med.* **2015**, *8*, 14977–14984. [PubMed]

54. Saneei, P.; Salehi-Abargouei, A.; Esmaillzadeh, A. Serum 25-hydroxy vitamin D levels in relation to body mass index: A systematic review and meta-analysis. *Obes. Rev.* **2013**, *14*, 393–404. [CrossRef] [PubMed]

55. Nguyen, V.T.; Li, X.; Elli, E.F.; Ayloo, S.M.; Castellanos, K.J.; Fantuzzi, G.; Freels, S.; Braunschweig, C.L. Vitamin D, inflammation, and relations to insulin resistance in premenopausal women with morbid obesity. *Obesity* **2015**, *23*, 1591–1597. [CrossRef] [PubMed]

56. Boonchaya-Anant, P.; Holick, M.; Apovian, C. Serum 25-Hydroxyvitamin D Levels and Metabolic Health Status in Extremely Obese Individuals. *Obesity* **2014**, *22*, 2539–2543. [CrossRef] [PubMed]

57. Censani, M.; Stein, E.M.; Shane, E.; Oberfield, S.E.; McMahon, D.J.; Lerner, S.; Fennoy, I. Vitamin D Deficiency Is Prevalent in Morbidly Obese Adolescents Prior to Bariatric Surgery. *ISRN Obesity* **2013**, *2013*. [CrossRef] [PubMed]

58. Fish, E.; Beverstein, G.; Olson, D.; Reinhardt, S.; Garren, M.; Gould, J. Vitamin D Status of Morbidly Obese Bariatric Surgery Patients. *J. Surg. Res.* **2010**, *164*, 198–202. [CrossRef] [PubMed]

59. Mahlay, N.F.; Verka, L.G.; Thomsen, K.; Merugu, S.; Salomone, M. Vitamin D Status Before Roux-en-Y and Efficacy of Prophylactic and Therapeutic Doses of Vitamin D in Patients After Roux-en-Y Gastric Bypass Surgery. *Obes. Surg.* **2009**, *19*, 590–594. [CrossRef] [PubMed]

60. Aasheim, E.T.; Hofsø, D.; Hjelmesæth, J.; Birkeland, K.I.; Bøhmer, T. Vitamin status in morbidly obese patients: A cross-sectional study. *Am. J. Clin. Nutr.* **2008**, *87*, 362–369. [PubMed]

61. Ybarra, J.; Sanchez-Hernandez, J.; Gich, I.; De Leiva, A.; Rius, X.; Rodriguez-Espinosa, J.; Perez, A. Unchanged hypovitaminosis D and secondary hyperparathyroidism in morbid obesity after bariatric surgery. *Obes. Surg.* **2005**, *15*, 330–335. [CrossRef] [PubMed]

62. Grace, C.; Vincent, R.; Aylwin, S.J. High prevalence of vitamin D insufficiency in a United Kingdom urban morbidly obese population: Implications for testing and treatment. *Surg. Obes. Relat. Dis.* **2014**, *10*, 355–360. [CrossRef] [PubMed]

63. Goldner, W.S.; Stoner, J.A.; Thompson, J.; Taylor, K.; Larson, L.; Erickson, J.; McBride, C. Prevalence of vitamin D insufficiency and deficiency in morbidly obese patients: A comparison with non-obese controls. *Obes. Surg.* **2008**, *18*, 145–150. [CrossRef] [PubMed]

64. Mawer, E.B.; Backhouse, J.; Holman, C.A.; Lumb, G.A.; Stanbury, S.W. The distribution and storage of vitamin D and its metabolites in human tissues. *Clin. Sci.* **1972**, *43*, 413–431. [CrossRef] [PubMed]

65. Abboud, M.; Puglisi, D.A.; Davies, B.N.; Rybchyn, M.; Whitehead, N.P.; Brock, K.E.; Cole, L.; Gordon-Thomson, C.; Fraser, D.R.; Mason, R.S. Evidence for a specific uptake and retention mechanism for 25-hydroxyvitamin D (25OHD) in skeletal muscle cells. *Endocrinology* **2013**, *154*, 3022. [CrossRef] [PubMed]

66. Vupputuri, M.R.; Goswami, R.; Gupta, N.; Ray, D.; Tandon, N.; Kumar, N. Prevalence and functional significance of 25-hydroxyvitamin D deficiency and vitamin D receptor gene polymorphisms in Asian Indians. *Am. J. Clin. Nutr.* **2006**, *83*, 1411–1419. [PubMed]

67. Mao, S.; Huang, S. Vitamin D receptor gene polymorphisms and the risk of rickets among Asians: A meta-analysis. *Arch. Dis. Child.* **2014**, *99*, 232–238. [CrossRef] [PubMed]

68. Al-Daghri, N.M.; Al-Attas, O.S.; Alkharfy, K.M.; Khan, N.; Mohammed, A.K.; Vinodson, B.; Ansari, M.G.A.; Alenad, A.; Alokail, M.S. Association of VDR-gene variants with factors related to the metabolic syndrome, type 2 diabetes and vitamin D deficiency. *Gene* **2014**, *542*, 129–133. [CrossRef] [PubMed]

69. Alexandrou, A.; Armeni, E.; Kaparos, G.; Rizos, D.; Tsoka, E.; Deligeoroglou, E.; Creatsa, M.; Augoulea, A.; Diamantis, T.; Lambrinoudaki, I. Bsm1 vitamin D receptor polymorphism and calcium homeostasis following bariatric surgery. *J. Investig. Surg.* **2015**, *28*, 8–17. [CrossRef] [PubMed]

70. Gu, J.; Xiao, W.; He, J.; Zhang, H.; Hu, W.; Hu, Y.; Li, M.; Liu, Y.; Fu, W.; Yu, J. Association between VDR and ESR1 gene polymorphisms with bone and obesity phenotypes in Chinese male nuclear families—Association between VDR and ESR1 gene polymorphisms with bone and obesity phenotypes in Chinese male nuclear families. *Acta Pharmacol. Sin.* **2009**, *30*, 1634–1642. [CrossRef] [PubMed]

71. Ochs-Balcom, H.M.; Chennamaneni, R.; Millen, A.E.; Shields, P.G.; Marian, C.; Trevisan, M.; Freudenheim, J.L. Vitamin D receptor gene polymorphisms are associated with adiposity phenotypes. *Am. J. Clin. Nutr.* **2011**, *93*, 5–10. [CrossRef] [PubMed]

72. Filus, A. Relationship between vitamin D receptor BsmI and FokI polymorphisms and anthropometric and biochemical parameters describing metabolic syndrome. *Aging Male* **2008**, *11*, 134–139. [CrossRef] [PubMed]

73. Faul, F.; Erdfelder, E.; Lang, A.-G.; Buchner, A. G*Power 3: A flexible statistical power analysis program for the social, behavioral, and biomedical sciences. *Behav. Res. Methods* **2007**, *39*, 175–191. [CrossRef] [PubMed]

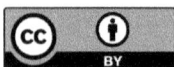

![nutrients logo] *nutrients*

MDPI

Article

Association between Vitamin D Genetic Risk Score and Cancer Risk in a Large Cohort of U.S. Women

Paulette D. Chandler [1,2,*], Deirdre K. Tobias [1,2], Lu Wang [1,2], Stephanie A. Smith-Warner [2,3,4], Daniel I. Chasman [1,2], Lynda Rose [1], Edward L. Giovannucci [2,3,4,5], Julie E. Buring [1,4], Paul M. Ridker [1,2,6], Nancy R. Cook [1,2], JoAnn E. Manson [1,2,4,5,7] and Howard D. Sesso [1,2,4]

[1]   Division of Preventive Medicine, Department of Medicine, Brigham and Women's Hospital, Boston, MA 02115, USA; dtobias@partners.org (D.K.T.); lwang284@its.jnj.com (L.W.); Dchasman@partners.org (D.I.C.); lrose@rics.bwh.harvard.edu (L.R.); jburing@partners.org (J.E.B.); pridker@partners.org (P.M.R.); ncook@partners.org (N.R.C.); jmanson@partners.org (J.E.M.); hsesso@partners.org (H.D.S.)
[2]   Harvard Medical School, Boston, MA 02115, USA; swarner@hsph.harvard.edu (S.A.S.-W.); egiovann@hsph.harvard.edu (E.L.G.)
[3]   Department of Nutrition, Harvard T.H. Chan School of Public Health, Boston, MA 02115, USA
[4]   Department of Epidemiology, Harvard T.H. Chan School of Public Health, Boston, MA 02115, USA
[5]   Channing Division of Network Medicine, Department of Medicine, Brigham and Women's Hospital, Boston, MA 02115, USA
[6]   Cardiovascular Division, Brigham and Women's Hospital, Boston, MA 02115, USA
[7]   Mary Horrigan Connors Center for Women's Health and Gender Biology, Brigham and Women's Hospital, Boston, MA 02115, USA
*   Correspondence: pchandler@partners.org; Tel.: +1-(617)-732-6043; Fax: +1-(617)-632-5370

Received: 29 September 2017; Accepted: 13 December 2017; Published: 9 January 2018

Abstract: Some observational studies suggest an inverse association between circulating 25-hydroxyvitamin D (25OHD) and cancer incidence and mortality. We conducted a Mendelian randomization analysis of the relationship between a vitamin D genetic risk score (GRS, range 0–10), comprised of five single nucleotide polymorphisms (SNPs) of vitamin D status in the DHCR7, CYP2R1 and GC genes and cancer risk among women. Analysis was performed in the Women's Genome Health Study (WGHS), including 23,294 women of European ancestry who were cancer-free at baseline and followed for 20 years for incident cancer. In a subgroup of 1782 WGHS participants with 25OHD measures at baseline, the GRS was associated with circulating 25OHD mean (SD) = 67.8 (26.1) nmol/L, 56.9 (18.7) nmol/L in the lowest versus 73.2 (27.9) nmol/L in the highest quintile of the GRS (p trend < 0.0001 across quintiles). However, in age-adjusted Cox proportional hazards models, higher GRS (reflecting higher 25OHD levels) was not associated (cases; Hazard Ratio (HR) (95% Confidence Interval (CI)), p-value) with incident total cancer: (n = 3985; 1.01 (1.00–1.03), p = 0.17), breast (n = 1560; 1.02 (0.99–1.05), p = 0.21), colorectal (n = 329; 1.06 (1.00–1.13), p = 0.07), lung (n = 330; 1.00 (0.94–1.06), p = 0.89) or total cancer death (n = 770; 1.00 (0.96–1.04), p = 0.90). Results were similar in fully-adjusted models. A GRS for higher circulating 25OHD was not associated with cancer incidence or mortality.

Keywords: vitamin D; cancer; genetic risk score; Mendelian randomization; mortality

---

1. Introduction

Controversy remains whether chronic insufficiency of vitamin D is a causal determinant of incident cancer and mortality [1,2]. Although several observational studies indicate an inverse association between circulating 25-hydroxyvitamin D (25OHD) and cancer incidence and mortality, randomized trials assessing the effect of vitamin D supplementation on cancer incidence have not found clear benefits to date [2,3]. Mendelian randomization studies of single nucleotide polymorphisms (SNPs) influencing plasma level of 25OHD can be used to investigate the effect of lifelong differences in 25OHD and risk of cancer and mortality. If circulating 25-hydroxyvitamin D (25OHD) is causally related to cancer risk, then participants inheriting alleles predictive of low 25OHD concentrations may be at increased cancer risk compared to subjects with alleles predictive of high 25OHD.

Two recent genome-wide association studies (GWAS) [4,5] and other studies identified SNPs significantly associated with circulating 25OHD concentrations and vitamin D metabolism [6–8]. A recent publication reported that genetically low 25OHD concentrations were associated with increased all-cause mortality and cancer mortality in three large Danish cohorts [1]. The 25OHD SNPs used to calculate 25OHD genetically [1] included rs11234027 and rs12794714 in the DHCR7 gene encoding the enzyme that converts 7-dehydrocholesterol to cholesterol rather than vitamin D_3 and rs10741657 and rs7944926 in the CYP2R1 gene, encoding the 25-hydroxylase that converts vitamin D to 25OHD in the liver [9]. Given the association of rs11234027, rs12794714, rs10741657 and rs794492 with genetically low 25OHD and increased all-cause mortality and cancer mortality, we evaluated these same four SNPs in addition to the rs2282679 in the GC gene encoding the vitamin D binding protein, the major transporter of circulating vitamin D compounds [9]. These five SNPs explain about 5% of the between-person variation in concentrations of circulating 25OHD [9]. We leveraged the Women's Genome Health Study (WGHS) [10], a cohort of 23,294 women of European ancestry with genome-wide genotyped data, to derive a genetic risk score (GRS) of these SNPs. This instrumental variable was used to investigate the causal association of vitamin D deficiency and the risk of incident cancer and cancer mortality.

2. Methods

2.1. Women's Genome Health Study

The Women's Health Study (WHS) began in 1992 and is a completed randomized, double-blind, placebo-controlled, 2×2 factorial trial that examined the role of aspirin (100 mg every other day) and vitamin E (600 IU every other day) in the primary prevention of cancer and cardiovascular disease (CVD) among 39,876 United States female health professionals aged 45 years and older. When the trial ended in 2004, 33,682 women (88.6% of those alive) consented to continue with observational follow-up, reporting on their health habits and medical history annually on questionnaires. The cohort continues to be monitored, now with greater than 20 years of follow-up. The WGHS is a majority subset of WHS women who agreed to participate in additional genomics analyses; baseline blood samples were used to extract DNA. The current analysis included 23,294 WGHS women of verified European ancestry free of cancer at baseline and who had provided baseline blood samples with available DNA. Of these, 1782 participants had both previously available 25OHD measurements and genotype data.

All subjects provided written informed consent. The study was conducted in accordance with the Declaration of Helsinki, and the Institutional Review Board of Brigham and Women's Hospital approved the protocol.

2.2. Cancer Endpoint Ascertainment

During follow-up, every 6 months in the first year and almost every year thereafter, participants received questionnaires that assessed their compliance, potential side effects, updated risk factors and outcomes of interest. When the trial ended in 2004, 33,682 women (88.6% of those alive) consented to continue with observational follow-up, reporting their health habits and medical history annually on questionnaires. Morbidity follow-up in the WHS was complete for 97.2% and mortality follow-up for 99.4% of women. For cases of cancer reported during the study period, subjects provided written consent for medical record review. A committee of physicians reviewed medical records. For the current analysis, we included confirmed invasive cancer cases through 2015. With a median follow-up of 20 years, 3985 confirmed cancer cases include 1560 breast, 329 colorectal, 330 lung cancers and 770 cancer deaths and 2973 total deaths. Endpoint review was complete for 95% of reported cancer cases. The confirmation rate among participants with records is 82%. Of all deaths, 60% have a cause confirmed by medical records and 85% are confirmed with death certificates or National Death Index reports.

2.3. Genotyping in the WGHS

Detailed methods of genotyping in the WGHS have been previously reported [10]. In brief, genotyping used the Illumina's Infinium II assay [11] applied to the HumanHap300 Duo + platform (Illumina, San Diego, CA, USA). The final WGHS data included 23,294 participants of self-reported European ancestry confirmed by a multi-dimensional scaling procedure in PLINK10 (http://zzz.bwh.harvard.edu/plink/summary.shtml, PLINK10 is an open-source whole genome association analysis toolset). Genotyping was successful for rs11234027 and rs7944926 in 99.9% of the WGHS participants. The other SNPs, rs10741657, rs12794714, and rs2282679, were 1000G imputed (dosages of the 3 imputed SNPs were converted to genotypes by rounding to the closest genotype value).

2.4. Dietary and Lifestyle Factors

Body mass index (BMI), lifestyle (e.g., physical activity) and dietary data (e.g., vitamin D intake) were derived from the baseline questionnaire. The validity and reproducibility of a semi-quantitative food-frequency questionnaire (FFQ) have been described previously [12–14].

2.5. Laboratory Assessment of 25OHD

We combined samples from1782 women with previously-measured 25OHD in WGHS: a colorectal cancer case-control study [15], hypertension case/control subgroup, breast cancer case-control subgroup and a vitamin D pilot subgroup. Plasma 25OHD was measured at Heartland Assays, Inc. (Ames, IA, USA) with the FDA-approved direct, competitive chemiluminescence immunoassay (CLIA) using the DiaSorin LIAISON 25-OH Vitamin D Total assay (DiaSorin LIAISON 25OHD assay is a chemiluminsecent immunoassay for the quantitiative determination of 25OHD and other hydroxylated vitamin D metabolites). The assay utilizes a specific antibody to 25OHD for coating magnetic particles (solid phase) and a vitamin D analogue, 22-carboxy-23,24,25,26,27-pentanorvitamin D3, linked to an isoluminol derivative. This assay is co-specific for 25-hydroxyvitamin D3 and 25-hydroxyvitamin D2. Samples for plasma 25OHD were shipped in three batches to the reference laboratory, with laboratory personnel blinded to case, control or quality control status. For the colorectal cancer case-control study, the inter- and intra-assay coefficient of variations (CVs) were 5.0% and 9.3%, respectively. For the breast cancer case-control subgroup, the inter- and intra-assay CVs were 5.1% and 6.4%, respectively. For the hypertension case-control subgroup, the inter- and intra-assay CVs were 11.2% and 8.1%, respectively.

3. Statistical Analysis

Genetic Variant Selection

Mendelian randomization (genetic variant as an instrumental variable) assumes that the SNP is associated solely with the exposure of interest. In linear regression models, we estimated the association of the five selected 25OHD SNPs and the GRS with BMI and other variables that may influence circulating 25OHD. A five-SNP polygenic additive GRS was created by summing the number (0, 1 or 2) of higher 25OHD-associated alleles (i.e., "high vitamin D alleles"/risk alleles). Therefore, higher values of the GRS were associated with high levels of 25OHD. The unweighted GRS ranged from 1–10.

We performed Cox proportional-hazard regression models to estimate the association between the individual SNPs and GRS for circulating 25OHD with incident total cancer ($n = 3985$), major site-specific cancers (breast, $n = 1560$; colorectal, $n = 329$; and lung, $n = 330$) and total ($n = 2973$) and cancer ($n = 770$)

mortality. We analyzed the GRS continuously, per one-point increase in score, as well as categorically (0–5 (reference group), 6–7 and 8–10 points). The proportionality assumption was verified for each model. Multiple testing was accounted for by using Bonferroni correction, and thus, associations were considered significant if $p < 0.0008$ (0.05/6; 5 SNPs + GRS). Models were adjusted for baseline age (continuous) with an additional model that adjusted for body mass index (BMI). SAS Version 9.3 (SAS Institute, Cary, NC, USA) was used for the analyses. In a sensitivity analysis excluding rs2282679 (GC, vitamin D binding protein) from the GRS, we estimated the hazard ratio (HR) per 20 nmol/L increase in genetically-determined 25OHD to be able to compare results with a previously-published Mendelian randomization evaluating genetically low vitamin D concentrations and mortality [1]. We multiplied the beta and standard error (SE) for association with cancer by the ratio 20/(slope of association with 25OHD). The computer code used is available upon request.

We calculated Mendelian instrumental variable estimates of genetically determined odds ratios by exponentiation of the Wald-type estimator, which is the ratio of the log hazard ratio of the genetic risk score-disease outcome association (incident total cancer and site-specific cancer, total mortality, and cancer mortality) and the linear regression coefficient of the genetic risk score-25OHD association. Standard errors of the Wald-estimator were determined using the delta method. The adjusted 25OHD allele score coefficient came from 1782 participants who had both genotypic and 25OHD measurements. The Mendelian instrumental variable estimate was scaled to 25OHD 20 nmol/L.

4. Role of the Funding Sources

The funding sources had no role in the design, conduct or analysis of our study or the decision to submit the manuscript for publication.

5. Results

Baseline characteristics are reported in Table 1; all women were of European ancestry with mean (SD) age of 54.7 (7.1) years.

Table 1. Baseline characteristics of Women's Genome Health Study European ancestry participants (*n* = 23,294) *.

Age (Years)	54.7 (7.1)
Randomized aspirin, %	50
Randomized vitamin E, %	50
Season of blood draw, %	
Winter	32.1
Spring or fall	17.2
Summer	50.7
HRT [1] use, never, %	48.3
No oral contraceptive use, %	30.1
Postmenopausal, %	54.5
Body mass index (kg/m^2)	25.9 (5.0)
Exercise (METS-h/week) [2]	14.2 (18.3)
Alcohol (g/day)	4.3 (8.4)
Total vitamin D intake (IU/day)	354.7 (242.8)
Vitamin D without supplement (IU/day)	236.1 (111.2)
Smoking, %	
Current	11.6
Past	37.5
Never	50.9
Family history of colorectal cancer [3], %	10.6

Table 1. *Cont.*

Age (Years)	54.7 (7.1)
Family history of breast cancer, %	6.3
Mammogram screening, %	62.7
Colonoscopy or sigmoidoscopy screening [4], %	8.0
Diabetes, %	2.5

* Values represent the mean and standard deviation (SD) unless otherwise specified; [1] hormone replacement therapy (HRT) use at baseline; [2] metabolic equivalents (METS)-hours per week; [3] family history of colorectal cancer in first degree relative at baseline; [4] history of colonoscopy or sigmoidoscopy screening for screening or symptoms at baseline.

There were 3985 total (total cancer excluding non-melanoma skin cancer), 1560 breast, 329 colorectal and 330 lung cancer cases that developed, along with 770 cancer deaths. Minor allele frequencies ranged from 16–44% (Table S1: Minor allele frequencies of circulating 25OHD SNPs). Selected SNPs explain 2.6% ($F = 48$, $p < 0.0001$) of the variance in circulating 25OHD between individuals in WGHS.

5.1. Candidate SNP Analyses

Except for the correlation of rs11234027 (DHCR7) with age ($p = 0.009$), we did not identify any significant correlations between genetically-determined 25OHD with age, BMI or physical activity. (Table S2: Concentration of 25OHD according to genotypes used as instrumental variables in GRS (DHCR7/CYP2R1/GC) adjusted for potential confounders individually). However, as expected [1,9], each SNP was associated with circulating 25OHD, and the associations were similar with and without adjustment for vitamin D-associated covariates including BMI (Table S3: Concentration of 25OHD according to genotypes used as instrumental variables in GRS (DHCR7/CYP2R1/GC)). For WGHS participants with 25OHD measures at baseline ($n = 1782$), the concentration of 25OHD by genotype copies of risk allele is reported (Table S4: Concentration of 25-hydroxyvitamin D mean (SD) nmol/L by genotype copies of risk allele in WGHS subgroup ($n = 1782$)). The GRS was associated with circulating 25OHD mean (SD) = 67.8 (26.1) nmol/L, 56.9 (18.7) nmol/L in the lowest quintile versus 73.2 (27.9) nmol/L in the highest quintile of the GRS) (p trend < 0.0001 across quintiles).

None of the five SNPs was associated with incident total, breast, colorectal or lung cancer or total mortality after Bonferroni adjustment for multiple comparisons (Table S5: Cox proportional hazards for incident cancer and mortality by circulating vitamin D SNP per allele associated with increase in 25-hydroxyvitamin D). However, for colorectal cancer, two SNPs, rs12794714 (CYP2R1) and rs10741657 (CYP2R1) had nominally significant associations (HR (95% CI), p-values-rs12794714: 1.21 (1.03–1.41), $p = 0.02$ and rs10741657: 1.22 (1.05–1.43), $p = 0.01$). (Table S5: Cox proportional hazards for incident cancer and mortality by circulating vitamin D SNP per allele associated with increase in 25-hydroxyvitamin D) The circulating 25OHD values for the GRS continuous and categorical increased with higher GRS values and categories (Table S6: Mean 25-hydroxyvitamin D level nmol/L for each value of GRS in the case/control cohort ($n = 1782$) and Table S7: Mean 25OHD level nmol/L for each category of GRS in the case/control cohort ($n = 1782$)). The GRS was also not associated with any of the outcomes we evaluated, when analyzed continuously (HR per one unit increase (95% CI), p value incident total cancer: 1.01 (1.00–1.03), $p = 0.17$ and total mortality: 1.00 (0.98–1.01), $p = 0.71$) or in categories (Table 2).

The hazard ratios were similar with the addition of BMI to the age-adjusted models for the outcomes we evaluated (Table S8: Cox proportional hazards for cancer and mortality for genetic risk score of alleles associated with increase in circulating 25-hydroxyvitamin D (continuous and categorical) additionally adjusted for BMI). For site-specific cancers, most GRS hazard ratios centered on 1.0 (Table 2). In a sensitivity analysis, we excluded rs2282679 (GC, vitamin D binding protein) from the GRS (range 0–8) and estimated hazard ratios for our targeted outcomes (Table S9: Cox proportional hazards for cancer and mortality for genetic risk score without vitamin D binding protein (GC) alleles associated with increase in circulating 25OHD (continuous and categorical)). Hazard ratios for GRS without GC (Table S9: Cox proportional Hazards for Cancer and Mortality for Genetic Risk Score without vitamin D binding protein (GC) alleles associated with increase in circulating 25OHD (continuous and categorical)) were similar to estimates using GRS with GC (Table 2) with the exception of an increased risk of colorectal cancer for continuous GRS without GC, HR (95% CI) for colorectal cancer (1.08 (1.01–1.15); *p*-value = 0.03) (Table S9: Cox proportional Hazards for Cancer and Mortality for Genetic Risk Score without vitamin D binding protein (GC) alleles associated with increase in circulating 25OHD (continuous and categorical)). We estimated the HR per 20 nmol/L increase in genetically-determined 25OHD to be able to compare results with a previously-published Mendelian randomization evaluating genetically low vitamin D concentrations and mortality in three large Danish cohorts [1]. We found HR (95% CI) for total mortality (0.99 (0.79–1.19)) and cancer mortality (0.99 (0.59–1.39)).

Table 2. Cox proportional hazards for cancer and mortality for genetic risk score of alleles associated with an increase in circulating 25OHD (continuous and categorical) *.

	Cases/Sample Size	Rate/1000 pyrs [1]	HR (95% CI)
Breast			
Continuous	1560/23,294		1.02 (0.99–1.05)
Reference	417/6477	3.56	1.00
GRS 6–7	626/9619	3.60	1.02 (0.90–1.15)
GRS 8–10	517/7196	4.00	1.13 (0.99–1.28)
Colorectal			
Continuous	329/23,294		1.06 (1.00–1.13)
Reference	83/6477	0.69	1.00
GRS 6–7	136/9621	0.76	1.12 (0.85–1.47)
GRS 8–10	110/7195	0.82	1.21 (0.91–1.61)
Lung			
Continuous	330/23,294		1.00 (0.94–1.06)
Reference	99/6477	0.82	1.00
GRS 6–7	129/9621	0.72	0.89 (0.68–1.15)
GRS 8–10	102/7196	0.76	0.94 (0.71–1.23)
Total			
Continuous	3985/23,294		1.01 (1.00–1.03)
Reference	1091/6468	9.71	1.00
GRS 6–7	1626/9610	9.76	1.01 (0.93–1.09)
GRS 8–10	1268/7183	10.23	1.06 (0.98–1.15)
Total Mortality			
Continuous	2973/23,294		1.00 (0.98–1.02)
Reference	850/6477	6.87	1.00
GRS 6–7	1193/9621	6.49	0.96 (0.88–1.05)
GRS 8–10	930/7196	6.77	1.00 (0.91–1.09)
Cancer mortality			
Continuous	770/23,294		1.00 (0.96–1.04)
Reference	217/6468	1.93	1.00
GRS 6–7	305/9610	1.83	0.95 (0.80–1.13)
GRS 8–10	248/7183	2.00	1.05 (0.87–1.26)

* Adjusted for age; Reference is genetic risk score (GRS) = 0–5. [1] Person-years (pyrs).

5.2. Mendelian Instrumental Variable Estimates

The odds ratio (OR) (95% CI) for a Mendelian genetically determined 20 nmol/L higher plasma 25OHD concentration was 0.97 (0.84–1.13), *p*-value = 0.71, total mortality; 0.98 (0.73–1.32), *p*-value = 0.90, cancer mortality; incident cancer: total, 1.10 (0.96–1.25), *p*-value = 0.17; breast,

1.14 (0.92–1.41), *p*-value = 0.22; colorectal, 1.54 (0.96–2.46), *p*-value = 0.07; lung, 0.96 (0.55–1.68), *p*-value = 0.89.

6. Discussion

We found no significant association between SNPs previously associated with 25OHD and risk of incident total, breast, colorectal and lung cancer or total mortality. There was suggestive evidence for associations of rs12794714 (CYP2R1) and rs10741657 (CYP2R1) with CRC, but these associations did not reach Bonferroni corrected significance. This study had fewer cases than a previous European ancestry Mendelian randomization study [1] that showed an inverse relationship between these vitamin D SNPs and total and cancer mortality. In a sensitivity analysis, we looked at the same allele score, by excluding rs2282679 (GC, vitamin D binding protein), that Afzai et al. [1] evaluated in a Danish population of 95,766 European participants with 10,349 deaths. We estimated the Mendelian OR per 20 nmol/L increase in genetically-determined 25OHD, and the OR (95% CI) for total mortality (0.97 (0.84–1.13)) and cancer mortality (0.98 (0.73–1.32)) were statistically different from the point estimates of the Afzai study [1] (OR (95% CI) per 20 nmol/L lower plasma 25OHD concentration; total mortality: 1.30 (1.05–1.61) and cancer mortality 1.43 (1.02–1.99)). Afzai et al.'s findings correspond to a 30% reduced cancer mortality for a genetically 20 nmol/L increase in 25OHD concentration.

The genetic increment may be modified by the underlying vitamin D status of the population (e.g., limited sun exposure and limited vitamin D in diet); the underlying vitamin D status of the U.S. population may differ from that of the Copenhagen population. Thus, the incremental change in circulating vitamin D by GRS may have different implications for different populations based on their average vitamin D levels. A pooled analysis (2304 participants) of a randomized trial and prospective cohort study reported that women with 25OHD concentrations >100 nmol/L had a 67% lower risk of all invasive cancers combined (excluding skin cancer) than women with concentrations <50 nmol/L [16]. Similarly, a meta-analysis of studies evaluating circulating vitamin D levels, functionally relevant vitamin D receptor genetic variants and variants within vitamin D pathway genes and cancer survival or disease progression showed a benefit of higher vitamin D levels on survival [17]. In contrast, Skaaby et al. prospectively reported no association between vitamin D status and incident total and specific type of cancer [18] or mortality [19] in three cohorts from the general Danish population. The Vitamin D and Omega-3 Trial (VITAL) [20] is expecting a 50 nmol/L increase in 25OHD with vitamin D supplementation, 2000 IU/day, and should be sufficiently powered to detect reduced cancer mortality if the Afzai results are applicable to a randomized vitamin D supplementation clinical trial. Yet, recent meta-analyses of randomized vitamin D intervention trials found little effect of vitamin D supplementation on mortality endpoints [2,3].

Mendelian randomization analyses of genetic variants, which likely reflect lifetime, biologic exposures, represent a complementary approach to testing vitamin D-cancer hypotheses through trials of vitamin D supplementation. Our study agrees with prior studies that suggested that circulating vitamin D genetic markers account for only 2–5% of the variance in 25OHD [4,5,21]. Since the effect sizes of individual alleles are often small, the predictive value of a single variant of a small effect on circulating 25OHD levels is negligible [22]. In one study, four (rs11234027, rs12794714, rs7944926, rs12794714) of the five SNPS used in our study explained more variation in circulating 25OHD (5.2%) than a polygenic score including 9000 SNPs (0.16%) [9]. Our GRS instrumental variable *F* statistic = 40, which is generally considered a strong genetic instrument measurement [23]. Yet, some biostatisticians suggest that even with an *F* statistic >10, the results from Mendelian randomization may lead to wrong inferences [23].

Although family studies have estimated the heritability of circulating 25OHD ranging from 43–80% [24–27], the known SNPs account for only about 5% of the variance in 25OHD and highlight the complex trait of circulating 25OHD. The majority of the genetic effect for circulating 25OHD may be related to rare variants, structural variants other than SNPs or gene-environment interactions [28,29]. It is also possible that other genetic variants affect circulating 25OHD and cancer risk through entirely different mechanisms independent of 25OHD levels. We assumed an additive allelic effect and do not account for potential gene-gene interactions in our Cox proportional models because we did not see a main association of GRS with cancer and mortality.

Our findings do not support an association between vitamin D status, as reflected by 25OHD-related genotypes, and breast cancer risk. Our findings are in agreement with the Women's Health Initiative (WHI) vitamin D and calcium intervention trial, which reported no effect of vitamin D and calcium supplementation on incident invasive postmenopausal breast cancer [30]. Limitations of the WHI trial included compliance, the low vitamin D dose used and duration of the trial (average of seven years) [31]. Our study includes a longer period of follow-up than prior studies and is embedded within a chemoprevention randomized clinical trial of aspirin and vitamin E. Further, the vitamin D genetic score was unrelated to breast cancer risk based on 9500 cases and 11,000 controls in a multicohort analysis that included WGHS participants [32]. Our study is a prospective analysis compared to this retrospective case-control multicohort analysis. In case-control analyses, one cannot predict whether exposure to the risk factor, circulating 25OHD, preceded development of the cancer. We may not have observed an association of our GRS with breast cancer because of the weak association of plasma 25OHD with breast cancer, resulting in an underpowered analysis. In a meta-analysis of prospective studies including nested case-control studies and cohort studies, every 25 nmol/L increase in serum 25OHD concentration significantly reduced breast cancer risk by 3.2% [33].

Our null findings for colorectal cancer are consistent with a pooled analysis of 13 studies (WGHS participants not included) included in the Genetics and Epidemiology of Colorectal Cancer Consortium (GECCO) and Colon Cancer Family Registry (CCFR) with about 10,000 cases and 13,000 controls that demonstrated no association between genetic markers of circulating 25OHD and colorectal cancer [21]. Furthermore, randomized clinical trials of vitamin D supplementation, including the Women's Health Initiative [34] and a British trial [35] showed no effect on total or colorectal cancer incidence or total mortality. In contrast, cohort studies have generally shown an inverse association between high circulating 25OHD and colorectal cancer risk [36]. The Circulating Biomarkers and Breast and Colorectal Cancer Consortium (BBC3), a large international pooling project of 21 cohorts with absolute concentrations of circulating vitamin D measured in prediagnostic samples in approximately 10,000 breast cancer and 6000 colorectal cancer cases and their matched controls, and the VITAL study [20] may offer additional and more conclusive insights for colorectal and breast cancer.

6.1. Strengths

The strengths of our study are the prospective design and homogeneous nature of the WGHS cohort. Our genetic instrumental variable was robustly associated with circulating 25OHD. Genotypes, randomly distributed at birth, are unlikely to be confounded by lifestyle or environmental factors such as poor nutrition or inactivity, which is a noted strength of the Mendelian randomization approach.

6.2. Limitations

Statistically-significant effect estimates for specific cancer sites are difficult to establish unless large magnitudes of association are observed, or large sample sizes are achieved. While we had a large sample size, the HRs close to one suggest there was no overall effect for the vitamin D GRS on cancer endpoints in WGHS. Yet, this study adds to the current literature, because WGHS total mortality and cancer mortality data have not been included in previous vitamin D genetic meta-analyses [16]. A limitation of the current analysis is that we do not evaluate the structural and functional impact of these five SNPs through in silico models that examine coding variants associated with change in protein function and activity.

7. Conclusions

A genetic risk score for higher 25OHD blood levels was not associated with cancer incidence or mortality in this large cohort of U.S. women. Our findings do not provide support for a causal association between vitamin D status, as reflected by 25OHD-related genotypes, and cancer risk. Future research is needed to investigate the efficacy of vitamin D supplementation in reducing cancer risk, as well as the role of vitamin D-related genetic variation in the setting of vitamin D supplementation. VITAL [20] and other ongoing large-scale randomized trials of vitamin D supplementation have the potential to address these important questions, as well as to elucidate some of the relevant biologic mechanisms.

Supplementary Materials: The following are available online at www.mdpi.com/2072-6643/10/1/55/s1, Table S1: Minor allele frequencies of circulating 25OHD SNPs, Table S2: Concentration of 25OHD according to genotypes used as instrumental variables in GRS (DHCR7/CYP2R1/GC) adjusted for potential confounders individually Table S3: Concentration of 25OHD according to genotypes used as instrumental variables in GRS (DHCR7/CYP2R1/GC), Table S4: Concentration of 25-hydrovyvitamin D mean (SD) nmol/L by genotype copies of risk allele in WGHS subgroup (*n* = 1782), Table S5: Cox proportional hazards for incident cancer and mortality by circulating vitamin D SNP per allele associated with increase in 25-hydroxyvitamin D, Table S6: Mean 25-hydroxyvitamin D level nmol/L for each value of GRS in the case/control cohort (*n* = 1782), Table S7: Mean 25OHD level nmol/L for each category of GRS in the case/control cohort (*n* = 1782), Table S8: Cox proportional hazards for cancer and mortality for Genetic Risk Score of alleles associated with increase in circulating 25-hydroxyvitamin D (continuous and categorical) additionally adjusted for BMI, Table S9: Cox proportional Hazards for Cancer and Mortality for Genetic Risk Score without vitamin D binding protein (GC) alleles associated with increase in circulating 25OHD (continuous and categorical).

Acknowledgments: We are indebted to the 39,876 participants in the Women's Health Study for their dedicated and conscientious collaboration; to the staff of the Women's Health Study for their expert and unfailing assistance; and to the programmers for providing assistance with the analyses. The sponsors were not involved in the design, data collection, analysis, interpretation of the study or in writing the manuscript. Sources of funding: The Women's Genome Health Study is supported by HL043851 and HL080467 from the National Heart, Lung and Blood Institute and CA 047988 from the National Cancer Institute and the Donald W. Reynolds Foundation, with collaborative scientific support and funding for genotyping provided by Amgen. The vitamin D assays were conducted in conjunction with the Circulating Biomarkers and Breast and Colorectal Cancer Consortium (BBC3) R01 grant (CA152071). The Women's Health Study is supported by Grants CA-182913, CA-047988, HL-043851, HL-080467 and HL-099355 from the National Institutes of Health, Bethesda, MD. Dr. Chandler received support from Grant U01CA138962 from the National Cancer Institute and Grant 127524-MRSG-15-012-01-CNE from the American Cancer Society.

Author Contributions: P.D.C., D.K.T., D.I.C. and J.E.M. conceived of and designed the analysis. L.R., D.K.T., E.L.G., P.D.C., J.E.M., J.E.B. and D.I.C. analyzed the data. S.S.A.-W., E.L.G., P.D.C., H.E.S., D.K.T., D.I.C. and N.R.C. performed the interpretation of the data. All wrote the paper. All authors read and approved the final manuscript.

Conflicts of Interest: Paul M. Ridker received research support from AstraZeneca, Novartis, Roche and Sanofi-Aventis. No other authors declare any conflict of interest.

References

1. Afzal, S.; Brondum-Jacobsen, P.; Bojesen, S.E.; Nordestgaard, B.G. Genetically low vitamin D concentrations and increased mortality: Mendelian randomisation analysis in three large cohorts. *BMJ* **2014**, *18*, 349. [CrossRef] [PubMed]

2. Chowdhury, R.; Kunutsor, S.; Vitezova, A.; Oliver-Williams, C.; Chowdhury, S.; Kiefte-de-Jong, J.C. Vitamin D and risk of cause specific death: Systematic review and meta-analysis of observational cohort and randomised intervention studies. *BMJ* **2014**, *348*. [CrossRef] [PubMed]

3. Theodoratou, E.; Tzoulaki, I.; Zgaga, L.; Ioannidis, J.P. Vitamin D and multiple health outcomes: Umbrella review of systematic reviews and meta-analyses of observational studies and randomised trials. *BMJ* **2014**, *348*. [CrossRef] [PubMed]

4. Wang, T.J.; Zhang, F.; Richards, J.B.; Kestenbaum, B.; van Meurs, J.B.; Berry, D.; Kiel, D.P.; Streeten, E.A.; Ohlsson, C.; Koller, D.L.; et al. Common genetic determinants of vitamin D insufficiency: A genome-wide association study. *Lancet* **2010**, *376*, 180–188. [CrossRef]

5. Ahn, J.; Yu, K.; Stolzenberg-Solomon, R.; Simon, K.C.; McCullough, M.L.; Gallicchio, L.; Jacobs, E.J.; Ascherio, A.; Helzlsouer, K.; Jacobs, K.B.; et al. Genome-wide association study of circulating vitamin D levels. *Hum. Mol. Genet.* **2010**, *19*, 2739–2745. [CrossRef] [PubMed]

6. Pibiri, F.; Kittles, R.A.; Sandler, R.S.; Keku, T.O.; Kupfer, S.S.; Xicola, R.M.; Llor, X.; Ellis, N.A. Genetic variation in vitamin D-related genes and risk of colorectal cancer in African Americans. *Cancer Causes Control* **2014**, *25*, 561–570. [CrossRef] [PubMed]

7. Jacobs, E.T.; Van Pelt, C.; Forster, R.E.; Zaidi, W.; Hibler, E.A.; Galligan, M.A.; Haussler, M.R.; Jurutka, P.W. CYP24A1 and CYP27B1 polymorphisms modulate vitamin D metabolism in colon cancer cells. *Cancer Res.* **2013**, *73*, 2563–2573. [CrossRef] [PubMed]

8. Dong, L.M.; Ulrich, C.M.; Hsu, L.; Duggan, D.J.; Benitez, D.S.; White, E.; Slattery, M.L.; Farin, F.M.; Makar, K.W.; Carlson, C.S.; et al. Vitamin D related genes, CYP24A1 and CYP27B1, and colon cancer risk. *Cancer Epidemiol. Biomark. Prev.* **2009**, *18*, 2540–2548. [CrossRef] [PubMed]

9. Hiraki, L.T.; Major, J.M.; Chen, C.; Cornelis, M.C.; Hunter, D.J.; Rimm, E.B.; Simon, K.C.; Weinstein, S.J.; Purdue, M.P.; Yu, K.; et al. Exploring the genetic architecture of circulating 25-hydroxyvitamin D. *Genet. Epidemiol.* **2013**, *37*, 92–98. [CrossRef] [PubMed]

10. Ridker, P.M.; Chasman, D.I.; Zee, R.Y.; Parker, A.; Rose, L.; Cook, N.R.; Buring, J.E.; Women's Genome Health Study Working Group. Rationale, design, and methodology of the Women's Genome Health Study: A genome-wide association study of more than 25,000 initially healthy american women. *Clin. Chem.* **2008**, *54*, 249–255. [CrossRef] [PubMed]

11. Gunderson, K.L.; Steemers, F.J.; Ren, H.; Ng, P.; Zhou, L.; Tsan, C.; Chang, W.; Bullis, D.; Musmacker, J.; King, C.; et al. Whole-genome genotyping. *Methods Enzymol.* **2006**, *410*, 359–376. [PubMed]

12. Willett, W.C.; Reynolds, R.D.; Cottrell-Hoehner, S.; Sampson, L.; Browne, M.L. Validation of a semi-quantitative food frequency questionnaire: Comparison with a 1-year diet record. *J. Am. Diet. Assoc.* **1987**, *87*, 43–47. [PubMed]

13. Willett, W.C.; Sampson, L.; Stampfer, M.J.; Rosner, B.; Bain, C.; Witschi, J.; Hennekens, C.H.; Speizer, F.E. Reproducibility and validity of a semiquantitative food frequency questionnaire. *Am. J. Epidemiol.* **1985**, *122*, 51–65. [CrossRef] [PubMed]

14. Salvini, S.; Hunter, D.J.; Sampson, L.; Stampfer, M.J.; Colditz, G.A.; Rosner, B.; Willett, W.C. Food-based validation of a dietary questionnaire: The effects of week-to-week variation in food consumption. *Int. J. Epidemiol.* **1989**, *18*, 858–867. [CrossRef] [PubMed]

15. Chandler, P.D.; Buring, J.E.; Manson, J.E.; Giovannucci, E.L.; Moorthy, M.V.; Zhang, S.; Lee, I.M.; Lin, J.H. Circulating Vitamin D Levels and Risk of Colorectal Cancer in Women. *Cancer Prev. Res.* **2015**, *8*, 675–682. [CrossRef] [PubMed]

16. McDonnell, S.L.; Baggerly, C.; French, C.B.; Baggerly, L.L.; Garland, C.F.; Gorham, E.D.; Lappe, J.M.; Heaney, R.P. Serum 25-Hydroxyvitamin D Concentrations ≥40 ng/mL Are Associated with >65% Lower Cancer Risk: Pooled Analysis of Randomized Trial and Prospective Cohort Study. *PLoS ONE* **2016**, *11*, e0152441. [CrossRef] [PubMed]

17. Vaughan-Shaw, P.G.; O'Sullivan, F.; Farrington, S.M.; Theodoratou, E.; Campbell, H.; Dunlop, M.G.; Zgaga, L. The impact of vitamin D pathway genetic variation and circulating 25-hydroxyvitamin D on cancer outcome: Systematic review and meta-analysis. *Br. J. Cancer* **2017**, *116*, 1092–1110. [CrossRef] [PubMed]

18. Skaaby, T.; Husemoen, L.L.; Thuesen, B.H.; Pisinger, C.; Jørgensen, T.; Roswall, N.; Larsen, S.C.; Linneberg, A. Prospective population-based study of the association between serum 25-hydroxyvitamin-D levels and the incidence of specific types of cancer. *Cancer Epidemiol. Biomark. Prev.* **2014**, *23*, 1220–1229. [CrossRef] [PubMed]

19. Skaaby, T.; Husemoen, L.L.; Pisinger, C.; Jørgensen, T.; Thuesen, B.H.; Fenger, M.; Linneberg, A. Vitamin D status and cause-specific mortality: A general population study. *PLoS ONE* **2012**, *7*, e52423. [CrossRef] [PubMed]

20. Bassuk, S.S.; Manson, J.E.; Lee, I.M.; Cook, N.R.; Christen, W.G.; Bubes, V.Y.; Gordon, D.S.; Copeland, T.; Friedenberg, G.; D'Agostino, D.M.; et al. Baseline characteristics of participants in the VITamin D and OmegA-3 TriaL (VITAL). *Contemp. Clin. Trials* **2016**, *47*, 235–243. [CrossRef] [PubMed]

21. Hiraki, L.T.; Qu, C.; Hutter, C.M.; Baron, J.A.; Berndt, S.I.; Bézieau, S.; Brenner, H.; Caan, B.J.; Casey, G.; Chang-Claude, J.; et al. Genetic predictors of circulating 25-hydroxyvitamin d and risk of colorectal cancer. *Cancer Epidemiol. Biomark. Prev.* **2013**, *22*, 2037–2046. [CrossRef] [PubMed]

22. Evans, D.M.; Visscher, P.M.; Wray, N.R. Harnessing the information contained within genome-wide association studies to improve individual prediction of complex disease risk. *Hum. Mol. Genet.* **2009**, *18*, 3525–3531. [CrossRef] [PubMed]

23. Lawlor, D.A.; Harbord, R.M.; Sterne, J.A.; Timpson, N.; Davey Smith, G. Mendelian randomization: Using genes as instruments for making causal inferences in epidemiology. *Stat. Med.* **2008**, *27*, 1133–1163. [CrossRef] [PubMed]

24. Hunter, D.; De Lange, M.; Snieder, H.; MacGregor, A.J.; Swaminathan, R.; Thakker, R.V.; Spector, T.D. Genetic contribution to bone metabolism, calcium excretion, and vitamin D and parathyroid hormone regulation. *J. Bone Miner. Res.* **2001**, *16*, 371–378. [CrossRef] [PubMed]

25. Orton, S.M.; Morris, A.P.; Herrera, B.M.; Ramagopalan, S.V.; Lincoln, M.R.; Chao, M.J.; Vieth, R.; Sadovnick, A.D.; Ebers, G.C. Evidence for genetic regulation of vitamin D status in twins with multiple sclerosis. *Am. J. Clin. Nutr.* **2008**, *88*, 441–447. [PubMed]

26. Shea, M.K.; Benjamin, E.J.; Dupuis, J.; Massaro, J.M.; Jacques, P.F.; D'Agostino, R.B., Sr.; Ordovas, J.M.; O'Donnell, C.J.; Dawson-Hughes, B.; Vasan, R.S.; et al. Genetic and non-genetic correlates of vitamins K and D. *Eur. J. Clin. Nutr.* **2009**, *63*, 458–464. [CrossRef] [PubMed]

27. Wjst, M.; Altmuller, J.; Braig, C.; Bahnweg, M.; Andre, E. A genome-wide linkage scan for 25-OH-D(3) and 1,25-(OH)2-D3 serum levels in asthma families. *J. Steroid Biochem. Mol. Biol.* **2007**, *103*, 799–802. [CrossRef] [PubMed]

28. Maher, B. Personal genomes: The case of the missing heritability. *Nature* **2008**, *456*, 18–21. [CrossRef] [PubMed]

29. Manolio, T.A.; Collins, F.S.; Cox, N.J.; Goldstein, D.B.; Hindorff, L.A.; Hunter, D.J.; McCarthy, M.I.; Ramos, E.M.; Cardon, L.R.; Chakravarti, A.; et al. Finding the missing heritability of complex diseases. *Nature* **2009**, *461*, 747–753. [CrossRef] [PubMed]

30. Chlebowski, R.T.; Johnson, K.C.; Kooperberg, C.; Pettinger, M.; Wactawski-Wende, J.; Rohan, T.; Rossouw, J.; Lane, D.; O'Sullivan, M.J.; Yasmeen, S.; et al. Calcium plus vitamin D supplementation and the risk of breast cancer. *J. Natl. Cancer Inst.* **2008**, *100*, 1581–1591. [CrossRef] [PubMed]

31. Speers, C.; Brown, P. Breast cancer prevention using calcium and vitamin D: A bright future? *J. Natl. Cancer Inst.* **2008**, *100*, 1562–1564. [CrossRef] [PubMed]

32. Mondul, A.M.; Shui, I.M.; Yu, K.; Weinstein, S.J.; Tsilidis, K.K.; Joshi, A.D.; Agudo, A.; Berg, C.D.; Black, A.; Buring, J.E.; et al. Vitamin D-associated genetic variation and risk of breast cancer in the breast and prostate cancer cohort consortium (BPC3). *Cancer Epidemiol. Biomark. Prev.* **2015**, *24*, 627–630. [CrossRef] [PubMed]

33. Wang, D.; Vélez de-la-Paz, O.I.; Zhai, J.X.; Liu, D.W. Serum 25-hydroxyvitamin D and breast cancer risk: A meta-analysis of prospective studies. *Tumour Biol.* **2013**, *34*, 3509–3517. [CrossRef] [PubMed]

34. Wactawski-Wende, J.; Kotchen, J.M.; Anderson, G.L.; Assaf, A.R.; Brunner, R.L.; O'Sullivan, M.J.; Margolis, K.L.; Ockene, J.K.; Phillips, L.; Pottern, L.; et al. Calcium plus vitamin D supplementation and the risk of colorectal cancer. *N. Engl. J. Med.* **2006**, *354*, 684–696. [CrossRef] [PubMed]

35. Trivedi, D.P.; Doll, R.; Khaw, K.T. Effect of four monthly oral vitamin D3 (cholecalciferol) supplementation on fractures and mortality in men and women living in the community: Randomised double blind controlled trial. *BMJ* **2003**, *326*, 469. [CrossRef] [PubMed]

36. Ekmekcioglu, C.; Haluza, D.; Kundi, M. 25-Hydroxyvitamin D Status and Risk for Colorectal Cancer and Type 2 Diabetes Mellitus: A Systematic Review and Meta-Analysis of Epidemiological Studies. *Int. J. Environ. Res. Public Health* **2017**, *14*, 127. [CrossRef] [PubMed]

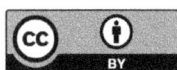

nutrients

MDPI

Review

Iron Supplementation during Pregnancy and Infancy: Uncertainties and Implications for Research and Policy

Patsy M. Brannon [1,2,*] and Christine L. Taylor [2]

1   Division of Nutritional Sciences, Cornell University, Ithaca, NY 14853, USA
2   Office of Dietary Supplements, National Institutes of Health, 6100 Executive Blvd, 3B01,
    Bethesda, MD 20892, USA; TaylorCL3@od.nih.gov
*   Correspondence: pmb22@cornell.edu; Tel.: +1-607-255-3770; Fax: +1-607-255-1033

Received: 12 October 2017; Accepted: 28 November 2017; Published: 6 December 2017

Abstract: Iron is particularly important in pregnancy and infancy to meet the high demands for hematopoiesis, growth and development. Much attention has been given to conditions of iron deficiency (ID) and iron deficient anemia (IDA) because of the high global prevalence estimated in these vulnerable life stages. Emerging and preliminary evidence demonstrates, however, a U-shaped risk at both low and high iron status for birth and infant adverse health outcomes including growth, preterm birth, gestational diabetes, gastrointestinal health, and neurodegenerative diseases during aging. Such evidence raises questions about the effects of high iron intakes through supplementation or food fortification during pregnancy and infancy in iron-replete individuals. This review examines the emerging as well as the current understanding of iron needs and homeostasis during pregnancy and infancy, uncertainties in ascertaining iron status in these populations, and issues surrounding U-shaped risk curves in iron-replete pregnant women and infants. Implications for research and policy are discussed relative to screening and supplementation in these vulnerable populations, especially in developed countries in which the majority of these populations are likely iron-replete.

Keywords: iron supplementation; iron-replete; pregnancy; infancy

1. Introduction

Iron has long been recognized as essential, but its nutritional status is nonetheless characterized by many challenges and unknowns, especially when the focus is pregnancy and infancy. Iron plays key roles in oxygen transport by red blood cells (RBC), energy production, growth and development, functions particularly important during the demands in pregnancy and infancy for hematopoiesis, growth and development. Much attention has been given to conditions of iron deficiency (ID) during these vulnerable life stages, but more recently questions have arisen about the effects of iron supplementation when individuals are iron-replete. Resolving these questions in general as well as in the case of pregnancy and infancy requires better understanding of iron homeostasis, biological adaptations, approaches to determining iron status, and the risk from not only too little but also too much iron.

The highly reactive chemical nature of the iron molecule, particularly its redox chemistry [1] and interaction with oxygen [2], underlie both its essential functions and cytotoxic actions. Its ability to form iron polymers through hydroxide complexes is also important for its storage complexed to the protein, ferritin. In physiologic concentrations, iron functions in both oxygen transport and energy production through its redox potential. In excess, however, iron is a pro-oxidant and produces reactive hydroxyl radicals and other reactive oxygen species (ROS) that damage DNA, proteins, lipids, other cellular molecules and stem cells [2]. Thus, ensuring adequate availability, but not excess, drives iron homeostasis. Iron exhibits a U-shaped nutrient-health relationship because of functional impairment when inadequate and cytotoxicity when excessive. This duality of its effect on health reflects a continuum of iron status from frankly deficient to inadequate stores to replete stores to high stores to toxic levels.

ID, well recognized as a public health concern, results when iron stores are inadequate to meet tissue needs and culminates in iron deficiency anemia (IDA) and fatigue when stores are fully depleted and erythropoiesis is impaired. The risk of ID or IDA increases in physiologic states of high blood loss (reproductive aged women) or increased physiologic need (pregnancy and infancy). ID and IDA receive greater attention than iron excess, both in research and policy, because of their high global prevalence, especially in developing countries.

Globally, over 40% of pregnant women and 47% of preschool children are anemic from all causes [3]. The World Health Organization (WHO) estimates that 50% of these anemias are due to ID and reflect IDA. However, Petry et al. [4] recently suggested based on their systematic review and meta-analysis of nationally representative survey data for preschool children and non-pregnant women that only about 25% of such anemia overall is attributable to ID. Although the global prevalence of IDA has not been measured directly, 10 to 20% of pregnant women and 15 to 24% of school-aged children are likely to have IDA when WHO estimates are reconsidered in light of the recent evidence from Petry et al. The WHO recommends universal iron supplementation [5,6] for pregnant women and young children 6 to 24 months because of this high prevalence of IDA.

However, the environmental and health context for developed countries differs because the prevalence of ID and IDA is lower. The most recent analysis of 1999–2010 National Health and Nutrition Examination Survey (NHANES) data found a prevalence of 2.6% and 2.2% IDA in pregnant women and young children (12–23 months) in the United States [7]. The prevalence of ID was 16.3%and 15.1% in pregant women and young ehildren with a significantly higer prevalence among Non-hispanic black, Mexican American and low-income pregnant women. The prevalence of IDA varies from a low of 3% in Switzerland to 15% in Belgium in European pregnant women [8] and below 5% in Northern and Western Europe in European young children [9]. Despite the lack of established cutpoints for iron-replete status, it appears that the majority of these populations in developed countries are likely to be iron-replete [10] even among ethnic and low socioeconomic individuals in whom the prevalence of ID may be higher than the general population.

Concerns exist and continue to emerge, as discussed in detail below, about the risk of adverse outcomes including growth, gestational length, gestational diabetes mellitus, and gastrointestinal health [11–15] with high intakes and iron status during pregnancy and infancy. Physiologic or developmental adaptation of iron homeostasis appears to occur in pregnancy [11] and infancy [12] to meet the higher physiologic needs for iron during these periods, but these adaptations, along with the lower loss of iron due to the cessation of menses during pregnancy, may potentially enhance the vulnerability to high iron intakes in iron-replete individuals.

This review examines the emerging as well as the current understanding of iron needs and homeostasis during pregnancy and infancy, uncertainties in ascertaining iron status in these populations, and issues surrounding U-shaped risk curves in iron-replete pregnant women and infants. It concludes with a discussion of the implications for research and policy relative to screening and supplementation in these vulnerable populations.

2. Iron Needs: Considerations during Pregnancy and Infancy

The physiologic demand for iron is especially high in pregnancy and infancy with an estimated 1000–1200 mg of iron needed during pregnancy [8,11]. About two thirds of this iron is for maternal needs, and 1/3 is for placental-fetal tissue needs [11]. However, the need varies across gestation with lower need in the first trimester (0.8 mg/day) than the need before pregnancy and much higher need in the third trimester (3.0–7.5 mg/day) [13]. This progressive increase reflects the temporal pattern of hematopoiesis and fetal growth [11]. Maternal hematopoiesis and RBC expansion as well as fetal growth are much higher in the second half of pregnancy. Thus much of the 330–400 mg for fetal growth is, therefore, needed in the last trimester. Some of the total iron need may be met by maternal iron stores in iron-replete women, and approximately 300 mg of this total iron is recycled and again available to the mother as her RBC volume contracts postpartum [16]. About 750 mg of additional iron is needed during pregnancy beyond that mobilized from and then returned to maternal stores in iron-replete women. For women with low or depleted iron stores, 1000 mg or more of additional iron might be required to meet maternal and fetal iron needs during pregnancy.

Despite this progressive physiologic need, established reference intake values for iron in several developed countries average the need for iron across pregnancy rather than varying requirements by trimester. The United States, Canada, Australia and New Zealand recommend 150% higher intakes for pregnant women than for reproductive age women beginning at the initial stages of pregnancy (Table 1). However, the United Kingdom and Europe do not identify a need for an increase during pregnancy, and WHO does not specify intakes for pregnancy. Consequently, the reference intake values vary internationally. Specifically, the Estimated Average Requirement (EAR) or Average Requirement (AR) varies from 7 mg/day to 22 mg/day to meet the needs of 50% of the population, and Recommended Daily Allowance (RDA) or Population Nutrient Intake (PNI) or Recommended Nutrient Intake (RNI) varies from 11.5 mg/day to 27 mg/day, to meet the needs of 97.5% of the population (see Table 1).

Table 1. Dietary iron reference intake values (mg/day) for pregnant women, infants and young children (12–23 months) in the United States, Canada, Europe, Australia, New Zealand and World.

	Women of Reproductive Age	Pregnant Women	Infants 0 to 6 Months 0 to 3	4 to 6	6 to 12 Months	Young Children 12 to 23 Months
United States & Canada (IOM [1])	8.1/18 [2]	22/27 [2]	0.26 [3]		6.9/11 [2]	3/7 [2]
Europe						
EFSA [4]	7/16 [2]	7/16 [2]	Not specified		8/11 [2]	5/7 [2]
UK (SACN [5])	11.4/14.8 [2]	11.4/14.8 [2]	1.3/1.7 [2]	2.3/3.3 [2]	6/7.9 [2]	5.3/6.9 [2]
Australia & New Zealand [6]	8/18 [2]	22/27 [2]	0.2 [3]		7/11 [2]	4/9 [2]
WHO/FAO [7]	19.5/24.5/29.4/58.8 [8]	Not specified	Not specified		6.2/7.7/9.3/18.6 [8]	3.9/4.8/5.8/11.6 [8]

[1] Institute of Medicine (IOM) [17]; [2] Estimated Average Requirement/Recommended Dietary Allowance or Recommended Dietary Intake or Population Reference Intake or Recommended Nutrient Intake; [3] Adequate Intake; [4] European Food Safety Authority (EFSA) [18]; [5] Standing Advisory Committee on Nutrition (SACN) [19]; [6] Nutrient Reference Intakes for Australia and New Zealand [20]; [7] Food and Agricultural Organization (FAO)/World Health Organization (WHO) [21]; [8] Reference Nutrient Intake for 15/12/10/5% bioavailability of dietary iron.

After birth, the need for iron is met primarily from iron stores in the exclusively breastfed full-term infant for the first 4 to 6 months because human milk is low in iron even though this iron is highly bioavailable. These iron stores derive from a portion of the approximate 270–330 mg of iron transferred in utero. Typically, such infants have approximately 80 mg of iron per kg [12,22] and an initially higher hemoglobin (Hb) concentration of about 17.0–19.0 g/dL [23]. Hb concentration steadily declines in the first 12 weeks [23], and iron is scavenged from the degraded Hb. The magnitude of iron stores, however, depends on the iron status of the mother, the gestational age at birth, the delay in cord clamping, and the birth weight of the infant. Thus, preterm or small for gestational age (SGA) infants and infants born to women with IDA are more likely to have lower iron stores that may be depleted earlier than 4 to 6 months [12]. Established reference intake values are low in the first six months when iron needs are met by stores (Table 1). Several developed countries recommend an Adequate Intake of 0.2 to 0.26 mg/day (United States, Canada, Australia and New Zealand), but the United Kingdom recommends a higher RNI (1.7 to 3.3 mg/day for 0–3 and 4–6 months). After iron stores are depleted, dietary iron needs increase to meet the sustained high demands for hematopoiesis, tissue accretion and brain development. Some suggest that during human evolutionary history this additional dietary iron may have come from pre-mastication of meat, a source of highly bioavailable heme iron [24]. Currently, the American Academy of Pediatrics encourages early introduction of pureed meat as a highly bioavailable source of heme iron [25], but intakes of meat by infants are low in the United States [26]. Canadian and Australian health authorities also recommend iron-rich complementary foods including meat (Table 2). Most developed countries (US, Canada, UK, Australia, New Zealand and Europe) recommend an EAR/AR of 6–8 mg/day and an RDA/PNI/RNI of 7.9–11 mg/day for older infants (6 to 12 months) and an EAR/AR of .3–5.3 mg/day and an RDA/PNI/RNI of 6.9–9 mg/day for young children (12 to 23 months).

Recommendations for supplementation vary across developed countries (Table 2) with no routine supplementation recommended for pregnant women and young infants by Canadian and Australian health authorities and for young infants by the European Society Pediatric Gastroenterology, Hepatology and Nutrition but universal supplementation for pregnant women and breast-fed infants four months and older by the United States Center for Disease Control and the American Academy of Pediatrics, respectively. Other authoritative groups in Europe, Britain and New Zealand (Table 2) recommend screening of pregnant women and supplementation if "at risk" or evidence of ID is found. The United States Preventative Services Task Force's recent finding of insufficient evidence for or against universal iron screening and supplementation of pregnant women [27] and screening of young children 6 to 24 months [28] underscores the need for research to inform policy and practice decisions to ensure adequate iron status in these vulnerable populations in developed countries.

Table 2. Recommendations for Iron Screening, Supplementation and Complementary Feeding of Pregnant Women and Infants in the United States, Canada, Europe, Australia, New Zealand and World.

Source	Recommendations	
	Supplement	Supplement and Iron-Rich Complementary Feeding
	Pregnant Women	Infants (0–12 Months)
United States		
UpToDate [1]	15–30 mg/day increase	Supplement 1 mg/kg/day (max. 15 mg/day) breastfed ≥4 months. until consuming sufficient quantities of iron-rich complementary foods
American College of Gynecology [2]	If iron deficiency anemia (IDA) identified	–
Centers for Disease Control [3]	Universal (30 mg/day)	Suggest supplement (1 mg/kg/day) breast-fed infants ≥6 months. consuming insufficient iron from supplementary foods (<1 mg/kg/day)
American Academy of Pediatrics [4]	-	Screen for ID/IDA at 12 months. Supplement (1 mg/kg/day) infants ≥4 months. exclusively breast-fed or consuming >1/2 intake from breast milk until receiving appropriate iron-containing complementary foods
Canada		
Infant Feeding Working Group for Health Canada, Canadian Paedritic Society, Dietitians of Canada & Breastfeeding Committee for Canada [5]		Recommend meat, meat-alternatives & iron-fortified cereals for firs complementary foods at 6 months.
Europe		
European Food Safety Authority [6]	If at risk	-
European Society Pediatric Gastroenteroloy, Hepatoloy & Nutrition [7]	No evidence iron supplementation of European women improves iron status of their infants.	No convincing evidence for iron supplements of exclusively breast-fed term infant <6 months. except on individual basis in high risk groups. Recommend iron rich complementary foods (meat, iron-fortified follow-on formulas & iron-fortified foods)

[1] UpToDate [29]; [2] American College Gynecology [30]; [3] Centers for Disease Control [31]; [4] American Academy of Pediatrics [25]; [5] Infant Feeding Working Group [32]; [6] European Food Safety Authority [18]; [7] European Society Pediatric Gastroenterology, Hepatology & Nutrition [33]; [8] British Committee for Standards on Haematology [34]; [9] Australian Department of Health [35]; [10] Australian Government National Health and Medical Research Council [36]; [11] National Women's Health [37]; [12] World Health Organization (WHO) [6]; [13] WHO [5].

Table 2. *Cont.*

Source	Recommendations	
	Supplement	Supplement and Iron-Rich Complementary Feeding
	Pregnant Women	Infants (0–12 Months)
UK – British		
Committee for Standards in Haematology [8]	Supplement if serum ferritin (SF) <30 µg/L	-
Australia		
Department of Health [9]	Do not routinely supplement	-
National Health and Medical Research Council [10]	-	Introduce first iron-containing nutritious foods (iron-fortified cereals, pureed meat and poultry dishes; care with plant sources such as cooked plain tofu and legumes/beans)
New Zealand		
National Women's Health [11]	Screen SF & Hb mid 26–28 weeks; supplement low dose (65 mg) if iron deficient and high dose (130 mg) if IDA	-
World		
WHO [12,13]	Supplement (30–60 mg/day)	Iron supplementation (10–12.5 mg/day) in young children (6–23 months) for 3 consecutive months/year. in settings ≥40% anemia prevalence

3. Iron Homeostasis: Physiologic and Developmental Adaptations during Pregnancy and Infancy

Iron homeostasis is the coordinated process through which key proteins regulate iron absorption, recycling, transport and storage to ensure iron availability without excess. The hepatic protein, hepcidin, functions as a master regulator in this homeostasis through its down-regulation of intestinal and tissue release of iron. It interacts with the cellular iron exporter, ferroportin (FPN) to reduce iron efflux and, thus, availability. When iron stores and availability are low, hepcidin is low; and more iron is released from that absorbed in the intestine or stored in tissues. In contrast when iron stores and availability are high, hepcidin is elevated; and less iron is released from that absorbed in the intestine or stored in tissues [38]. Hepcidin is also upregulated by inflammation and infection to sequester iron stores and reduce iron absorption as a part of anti-infective responses [39] and downregulated by hypoxia and erythropoiesis to meet iron needs. Mutations in selected key regulatory proteins that interact with hepcidin impair this homeostasis and result in hemochromatosis characterized by iron overload and cytotoxicity [40]. Allelic variants in selected iron regulatory or transport proteins also appear to enhance susceptibility to either high iron stores or ID in some ethnic sub-populations [40].

Adaptations in this iron homeostasis have been suggested both in pregnancy and early infancy, most likely to meet the substantive needs for iron during these periods. In pregnancy, physiologic adaptations appear to increase iron absorption [11]. Although the mechanism of this adaptation is not well understood, iron homeostasis appears to be "reset" through suppression of hepcidin, even though hepcidin still responds to iron availability, erythropoiesis, inflammation and hypoxia albeit at a "blunted" level [11]. Irrespective of maternal or fetal iron status [41], hepcidin concentrations decrease during pregnancy to nearly undetectable levels in the latter half of pregnancy Nemeth has proposed that an as-yet unidentified regulatory factor reduces the regulatory responsiveness of hepcidin to a lower level [11].

Developmental adaptations may also alter the homeostatic regulation of iron absorption by hepcidin in the young infant. Although both hepcidin and its target FPN are present [12], limited preliminary evidence suggests that iron absorption may not be regulated by iron status or supplementation in the infant prior to 6 months [42] or in the suckling-only rat pup prior to day 10 [43,44]. Later in the older human infant and rat pup with complementary feeding or nibbling-suckling transitional feeding, iron absorption does exhibit its usual homeostatic regulation in response to hepcidin. The mechanisms of this attenuated iron homeostatic regulation are largely unknown [12]. One potential consequence of this apparent developmental adaptation is high absorption of the limited amount of iron in human and mammalian milk during the suckling-only period. Conceivably, evolution of infants and other mammals led to unrestrained absorption of limited dietary iron [10].

The relevance of these physiologic and developmental adaptations of iron homeostasis is not understood, but these may serve to facilitate iron availability during peak periods of erythropoiesis. Given the widespread recommendation and use of iron supplements in both pregnant women and infants and iron-fortified formula in developed countries, however, these adaptations may also limit the primary protective mechanisms against excessive iron uptake. What is even less well understood is the extent to which these might, therefore, enhance the risk of high or excess iron status in the context of largely iron-replete populations [38]. Also unknown is how effectively these adapted homeostatic systems respond to key regulators such as iron status and inflammation although in pregnancy some limited evidence suggest that they do. Equally unclear is the extent to which maternal baseline iron status influences the resetting of maternal iron homeostasis [11].

In addition to the physiologic and developmental adaptations of this homeostatic regulation, developing tissues in the fetus and infant differentially acquire iron [45], such that hematopoietic needs are met before the needs of critical tissues such as the brain. In the context of sufficient iron, this does not limit availability to all developing tissues. However, in the context of limited iron availability, the brain can experience ID and permanent damage without impairment of hematopoiesis and hematologic indicators of iron status [45]. The mechanisms of this differential prioritization are also not understood, but clearly have implications for assessing iron status with the common hematologic indicators in the young child through 24 months, the period of rapid and critical brain development and high brain iron needs.

In summary, adaptations in iron homeostasis appear to occur physiologically in pregnancy and developmentally in young infants. They enhance iron absorption, but may limit feedback regulation in response to high iron status. The mechanisms of these adaptations are unknown. Moreover, the extent to which they might also enhance or not susceptibility to excessive absorption with high supplementation or iron-fortification is not understood.

4. Iron Status: Uncertainties in Assessment of Pregnant Women and Infants

4.1. Commonly Used Indicators

Assessing iron status is complex at any life stage, in part because no single indicator is sufficiently specific or sensitive to be used alone; thus, multiple indicators must be measured and integrated to estimate iron status. The most commonly used indicators are presented in Table 3. All are primarily hematologic indicators, but differ where they assess the continuum of iron status from iron stores to tissue depletion to impaired erythropoiesis to anemia resulting from impaired erythropoiesis.

Table 3. Commonly used indicators of iron status in pregnancy and infancy [1].

Indicator	Assesses	Advantages	Limitations
Hemoglobin (Hb)	Anemia	Is commonly available Has low complexity of analytic procedures	Has low specificity and sensitivity Affected by hemodilution in pregnancy and postnatal red blood cell turnover in early infancy May be complicated by certain factors (elevation? age? ethnicity?) Affected by inflammation and obesity
Ferritin (primarily serum, SF)	Size of iron stores	Is commonly available Has World Health Organization (WHO) International Standard Material	Confounded by inflammation
Soluble transferrin receptor (sTfR)	Inadequate tissue availability Iron deficient erythropoiesis	Less affected by inflammation	Has limited availability Exhibits assay differences Lacks a standard reference material (although one is in development)
Ratio of sTfR-to-ferritin (derived using various calculations)	Total body iron stores	Reflects full range of status	Requires two measurements Less affected by inflammation
Transferrin saturation	Iron deficient erythropoiesis	Is commonly available	Varies diurnally and prandially
Erythrocyte protoporphyrin	Iron deficient erythropoiesis		Is reliability infield instrumentation
Hepcidin	Determinant of iron needs and utilization	Is relatively sensitive	Is experimental and under development May possibly be less affected by inflammation

[1] Adapted from Taylor and Brannon [10].

Uncertainties exist in assessing iron status in pregnant women and infants, as well as in other life stages, because of analytic issues including lack of standardization of the assays; confounding especially by inflammation; and lack of established health outcomes relative to cutpoints. Unique to pregnancy are physiologic changes due to plasma volume expansion resulting in hemodilution and a mild inflammatory state [16]. The extent to which this affects common indicators has only been partially assessed for Hb concentration. Collectively, these uncertainties may result in misclassification of ID and IDA, introducing further uncertainties in estimating the prevalence of ID and IDA. In addition, the full continuum of iron status including iron repletion and excess cannot be determined because there are no cutpoints for common iron indicators for repletion and excess. This is true even for Total Body Iron stores (TBI, the log ratio of serum ferritin (SF) to soluble transferrin receptor (sTfR), which theoretically can be used to assess the full continuum of iron status, but in practice is limited by the lack of established cutpoints for repletion and excess. Finally, iron status, especially the level of stores which are essential to assess, change throughout the course of pregnancy as stored iron is mobilized to meet the high demand. Few studies have examined longitudinally the physiologic use of stores in iron-replete women, and none have assessed longitudinally repletion of iron stores postpartum.

4.2. Analytic Challenges

The analytic issues surround the lack of harmonization and standardization of the indicator assays [46]. The available WHO international standard material for SF concentration derives from "consensus" values because no standard reference method exists. This will also be the case for the other WHO international standard material for sTfR in development. The prospect for developing standard reference methods for SF and sTfR is poor because of the size of the proteins involved and technical challenges inherent in doing so [46,47]. In the absence of such standardization, measures may exhibit imprecision and inflated Confidence Intervals [46,48] that can create interpretative challenges and also contribute to misclassification of ID and IDA.

4.3. Confounding

Exacerbating these uncertainties is the documented confounding of SF and to a lesser extent sTfR, as well as indicators based on these two measures such as TBI, by inflammation. The Biomarkers

Reflecting Inflammation and Nutrition Determinants of Anemia (BRINDA) project reports linear regression algorithms to adjust SF based on cross-sectional data from multinational population indicators of acute (C-reactive protein) and chronic (alpha1-acid glycoprotein) inflammation [49–51]. Application of these proposed adjustments to TBI in U.S. women of reproductive age increased slightly by 7 percentage points the prevalence of ID [7]. However, none of these algorithms derive from analysis of data from pregnant women, who experience a mild inflammatory state due to pregnancy itself In addition, hepcidin concentration and inflammation during pregnancy do not appear to correlate [11], but some caution is warranted as this relationship has yet to be evaluated in infection or severe inflammation in pregnant women. Emphasizing the uncertain feasibility of adjusting for inflammation in pregnancy is the lack of correlation of inflammatory and iron status indicators in pregnant adolescents except at delivery [52]. Further, the BRINDA algorithms do not derive from analysis of data for young children (0–24 months). The relationship remains unknown between iron status and inflammatory indicators during pregnancy and young children, but the nature of these relationship needs to be evaluated in order to assess whether there may be ways to adjust for inflammation during pregnancy.

4.4. Linking Measures to Health Outcomes

A major limitation in, and the resulting uncertainty for, current cutpoints stem from the lack of their established relationships to non-hematologic or clinically relevant health outcomes in pregnant women, infants and young children for all common measures of iron status. Currently, cutpoints for pregnancy and young children derive from the lowest percentile distribution of the population, typically below the 5th percentile for Hb concentrations for anemia and, thus, IDA. For pregnant women, the Centers for Disease Control and Prevention (CDC) trimester-specific cutpoints were informed by four small longitudinal studies from 30 years ago [52], These trimester-specific cutpoints do consider hemodilution due to plasma volume expansion, but today's gynecologic population is older and has greater adiposity and incidence of gestational diabetes as well as higher mortality [16]. All of these factors in today's population may affect plasma volume expansion and hemodilution, such that the distribution of common indicators longitudinally in current populations may differ from those upon which these cutpoints were based. Thus, longitudinal studies in today's gynecologic population are needed. Further, cutpoints for SF are the same in pregnant women as those for reproductive age women, ranging from <10 to <15 µg/L and varying among clinical laboratories [8,46,53]. Therefore, the cutpoints for SF do not consider hemodilution due to plasma volume expansion or longitudinal physiologic changes in SF documented in iron-replete pregnant women. Whether TBI, is more independent of plasma volume expansion needs to be evaluated because TBI was only evaluated in a small number of adult males and non-pregnant females [47]. In addition to these limitations in the current population-based cutpoints and lack of evaluation in pregnancy or infancy for SF and TBI, the United States Preventive Services Task Force (USPSTF) noted an additional uncertainty because evidence is lacking on whether changes in these hematologic indicators in pregnant women, infants or young children reflect "meaningful improvements in health outcomes" beyond the hematologic outcome of anemia [54].

Evaluation of these indicators relative to health outcomes, especially non-hematologic outcomes, could inform cutpoints with clinical and public health relevance for the full spectrum of iron status [53]. In particular, TBI may be a useful indicator as it has the potential to be related to the full continuum of iron status. Such evaluation might, in fact, need to use different outcomes for assessing high and low exposure. The relationship of common iron indicators to meaningful outcomes across the full continuum of iron status is also important for developing stronger evidence-based clinical and public health guidelines to ensure adequate iron status and, thus, ensure normal development of critical tissues. Such evaluation based on non-hematologic outcomes is also important for monitoring supplementation, especially during pregnancy, infancy and young childhood when iron is differentially prioritized to erythropoiesis. Indicators that only assess hematologic outcomes fail to identify partially depleted iron stores that could adversely affect critically developing tissues such as the heart brain when hematopoiesis is not yet affected. To improve screening and monitoring, we need indicators that are particularly informative of tissue ID in pregnancy, infancy and young children.

Collectively, the lack of standardization and harmonization of assays, confounding by inflammation, impacts of physiologic changes on the indicators and lack of established relationship with non-hematologic outcomes introduce uncertainty in the measurement and interpretation of iron indicators in pregnant women, infants and young children. These uncertainties increase the risk of misclassification of ID and IDA and also limit interpretation of screening and monitoring of these vulnerable populations.

5. U-Shaped Risk for Iron Status: Concerns for Pregnant Women and Young Infants

Iron exhibits a U-shaped risk, typical of essential nutrients, in which risk of adverse outcomes in pregnant women, infants and young children increases not only with low or inadequate availability but also at higher availability [55,56]. Research and public health programs have focused primarily on the increased risk with low availability, particularly in pregnant women, infants and young children because of the high global prevalence of low iron status, namely ID and IDA. However, emerging evidence calls attention to possible increased risk of adverse outcomes with higher iron status. The 2016 USPSTF finding of insufficient evidence for or against iron screening and supplementation in these populations prompted the National Institutes of Health (NIH) Office of Dietary Supplements to hold a workshop on Iron Screening and Supplementation in Iron-Replete Pregnant Women and Young Children in September 2016 to consider the evidence of risk in iron-replete populations and identify research needs. During the workshop, the clear concern for increased risk of adverse outcome with ID and IDA was evident, but so, too, were the uncertainty and concern for the potential risk for adverse outcomes with high iron status. The physiologic need for iron and apparent adaptations of iron homeostasis as well as common and often routine supplementation of largely iron-replete pregnant and young children in developed countries underlay these concerns as well. The nature of the evidence for this U-shaped risk with iron and the uncertainties of this evidence are worthy of consideration.

5.1. Left-Side of U-Shapes Risk Curve: Low Iron Status

In terms of low iron status during pregnancy, most of the evidence has examined the relationship of Hb concentration or anemia and increased risk of maternal and fetal adverse outcomes without consideration of concomitant inflammation [56]. Low Hb concentrations associate with increased risk of low birthweight (LBW), small for gestational age (SGA), and preterm births [55,56] and maternal mortality [55], but closer examination of the synthesized evidence reveals that this association holds for LBW and preterm birth with low Hb concentrations in the first trimester, but not the second or third trimesters [56]. Although variable cutpoints for anemia and low Hb concentrations were used across the studies, a meta-analysis in 2012 found that the increased risk of SGA associated only with moderate to severe anemia [57] or Hb concentrations <9 g/dL for SGA and preterm births [55]. However, many factors can cause anemia, but only a few studies have examined the relationship of IDA, low SF and high sTfR with adverse pregnancy outcomes and reported less consistent findings than those examining the relationship of low Hb concentrations. Only one of two studies in the first trimester and one of three studies in the second trimester found an association of low SF with SGA or preterm birth and LBW, respectively [56]. Dewey also reported that the higher iron status (lower sTfR or higher SF within normal ranges) early in pregnancy generally associated with better birth outcomes in three cohorts in Ghana, Malawi and Bangladesh, whereas later in pregnancy it did not. Despite the limited evidence and lack of control for confounding by inflammation, the current evidence does suggest s increased risk of maternal and fetal adverse outcomes with anemia and low iron status as assessed by SF and sTfR, particularly early in pregnancy.

ID even more so than IDA is a concern in the infant and young child because of the vulnerable period of brain development in the first 24 months. As discussed earlier, the differential prioritization of iron to erythropoiesis exacerbates the vulnerability of the brain when iron is limiting during this critical period. A limited number of studies find impaired cognitive and brain development with ID [45,58–60]. Nonetheless, the importance of adequate iron is emphasized by this evidence relative to this vulnerable period in the infant's and young child's brain development and likelihood of lasting impairment without adequate iron. Further emphasizing the importance of sufficient iron during this period is a recent systematic review that reports improved psychomotor development in young infants < 6 months exclusively breastfed and supplemented with iron [61] without improvement of ID, IDA, or SF.

Another important evaluation of the risk of low iron status is improvement in outcomes with iron supplementation of pregnant women, infants and young children with low iron status. Although such supplementation generally improves hematologic indicators, which can be viewed as intermediate outcomes for anemia [53,54,62], the benefits and harms of routine iron supplementation on other non-hematologic health outcomes is uncertain. Both the USPSTF and the updated 2011 Cochrane review [63] noted the lack of quality studies reporting on clinical or health outcomes. A meta-analysis in both developed and developing countries, however, reported improved birthweight in a linear dose-response relationship and maternal Hb concentrations in the third trimester with daily iron supplement use in both high, middle and low income countries [64]. In contrast, a recent systematic review of iron supplementation of young children (6–24 months) in developed countries found no clear benefit for growth outcomes (5/6 trials) or infant development in the first 12 months (2 trials), inconsistent findings for improvement of hematologic outcomes and no reports in any of the identified studies related to neurodevelopmental delay or improvement of hematologic indicators and clinical outcomes [65]. As noted previously, the 2017 systematic review [61] found only four randomized clinical trials (RCTs) on iron supplementation of young exclusively breastfed infants <6 months and reported both benefit in terms of psychomotor development and harm in terms of reduced growth without consistent improvement of iron status in terms of IDA, ID, or SF. In spite of the need for more evidence from well-controlled RCTs especially evaluating non-hematologic health outcomes and the relationship of improved iron status with supplementation and health outcomes, all agree that treatment of ID and IDA during pregnancy and young children is important and warranted.

5.2. Right-Side of U-Shaped Risk Curve: High Iron Status

High iron status during pregnancy also associates with increased risk for maternal and fetal adverse outcomes. Across studies, high Hb concentrations, especially in the second trimester, associate with LBW as comprehensively reviewed by Dewey and Oaks [56] and Breymann [55], but has an inconsistent in relationship with preterm birth or SGA [56]. High SF concentrations also associates with increased risk for LBW or preterm birth [56] and SGA [55]. Dewey and Oaks also reported that higher iron status associated with lower birth size in some of the cohorts in Ghana, Malawi and Bangladesh [56]. Again, most of the studies have focused on the relationship of high Hb concentrations and high SF and adverse birth outcomes without consideration of inflammation or impaired plasma volume expansion, which is a major and serious limitation of the evidence to date. Scholl emphasizes the concern that high Hb may reflect impaired plasma volume expansion or inflammation due to infections [66]. Future studies need to consider carefully plasma volume expansion and the presence of inflammation in evaluating the relationship of high iron status assessed by Hb or SF concentrations.

In addition, preliminary evidence also links supplementation or high iron status to emerging adverse outcomes in pregnancy including gestational diabetes mellitus (GDM) in observational case-control and prospective cohort studies and limited RCTs [14]. At present, the evidence for GDM is inconsistent and limited by predominant assessment of high iron status by high Hb or SF concentrations without consideration of concomitant inflammation. Further, GDM itself is associated with inflammation, making it essential to assess acute and chronic inflammation in evaluating the linkage of high iron status with GDM. Although the mechanism is unknown, one possibility may be ROS and damage of pancreatic β cells resulting in diabetes [14]. Further research is needed to clarify the relationship of high iron status and supplementation of iron-replete pregnant women to the risk for GDM.

Iron supplementation of iron-replete infants and young children increased the risk of vomiting and fever in a systematic review of the evidence [67] and altered microbiome profiles in Tanzanian children [15] and impaired linear growth in Swedish infants [68]. In contrast, consumption of iron-fortified formula (9–12 mg/L) by older infants in the United Kingdome from 9 to 18 months did not affect infections, gastrointestinal problems or weight gain, but linear growth was not measured [69]. Although the mechanism whereby iron supplementation of iron-replete young children could adversely impact the gastrointestine and its microbiome are not known, most of the iron in a supplement is not absorbed and could promote a more pathogenic microbiome that depend on iron with resulting diarrhea. However, the environmental context may influence such a response depending on the overall risk for infection. In terms of impaired linear growth, Lonnerdal has proposed that iron supplementation of iron-replete infants might impair such growth through interactions of excess iron with zinc or copper [68]. Nonetheless, further research evaluating the potential adverse effects of iron supplementation of iron-replete young children particularly in developed countries is needed to clarify the risk and its nature to evaluate the risk relative to benefit. Given the observational nature of much of this emerging evidence, strongly designed studies are needed to determine the causality of these relationships.

Another proposed adverse outcome of high neonatal exposure relates to cumulative high brain iron and neurodegeneration in older adults [70]. Supportive evidence in humans includes the association of high iron concentrations in the brain with neurodegenerative diseases such as Parkinson's and Alzheimer's from primarily from case-control studies [2,70]. A systematic review of cross-sectional epidemiologic studies reports inconsistent association of measures of iron status with cognitive impairment [70]. However, preclinical studies of neonatal iron supplementation in rodent models identified in this systematic review report increased brain iron later in life with adverse effects on brain morphology and biochemistry in a variety of areas. Possible mechanisms include ROS damage to brain cells and to stem cells [2], but remain unknown. These preliminary findings and proposed relationship of early high iron exposure and subsequent neurodegenerative disease raise the possibility of Developmental Origins of Adult Disease (DOHaD) in relation to excess early iron.

Overall, current evidence supports a U-shaped risk curve for a variety of adverse birth outcomes in mother and neonate as well as in young children. Emerging evidence also raise concerns about adverse short-term and long-term health outcomes with iron supplementation of iron-replete pregnant women and children. Uncertainties in this evidence, particularly the failure to consider concomitant inflammation and limited evidence for non-hematologic health outcomes, emphasizes the need for well-controlled cohort longitudinal studies and RCT to evaluate the benefits and harms of iron supplementation in iron-replete populations.

6. Implications for Research and Policy

A number of knowledge gaps and research needs were identified at the NIH Workshop on Iron Screening and Supplementation of Iron-Replete Pregnant Women and Young Children in 2016. Four major themes emerged from these gaps and research needs focusing on (1) elucidating adaptations of iron homeostasis in pregnancy and early infancy including their mechanisms, responsiveness to iron status, interaction with genetic and ethnic factors and implication's for the differential prioritization of iron to developing tissues and hematopoiesis; (2) improving the assessment of iron status particularly in these two vulnerable periods including the measurement uncertainties, need for indicators across the full continuum of iron status that are adjustable or independent of inflammation; (3) evaluating iron status relative to maternal and infant health outcomes, especially non-hematologic outcomes; and

(4) determination of short and long term beneficial and adverse health outcomes, especially non-health outcomes such as GDM, LBW, SGA, postnatal growth and DOHaD, with iron supplementation of iron-replete pregnant women and young children [45,48]. In Figure 1, an analytic framework of these knowledge gaps and research needs is depicted along the pathway from screening to supplementation to outcomes. This pathway is based on current evidence (shown in solid lines) with the research needs and gaps of knowledge (shown in dashed lines).

Illustrated from this framework and the discussion above of the limitations of the evidence even from the benefit of improved hematologic outcomes with supplementation is the limited and preliminary nature of the current evidence. Clearly, well-controlled longitudinal cohort studies in iron-replete and generally well-nourished populations in developed countries are needed to understand the dynamic mobilization of iron stores and its impact on clinically-relevant and non-hematologic health outcomes. So too, are well-designed RCTs examining both the benefits and potential harms of iron supplementation on such health outcomes.

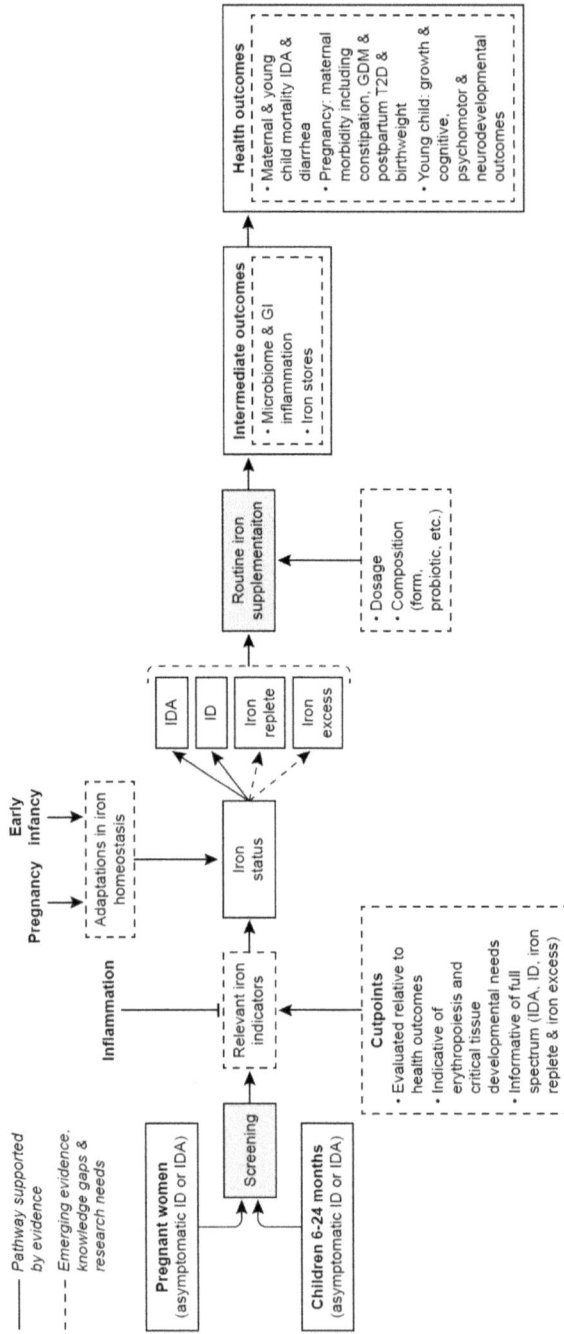

Figure 1. Analytic framework for iron screening and supplementation of pregnant women and young children in developed countries. Solid lines highlight pathways supported by current evidence. Dashed lines highlight emerging evidence, uncertainties and research needs. Abbreviations include ID, iron deficiency; IDA, iron deficient anemia; GI, gastrointestine; GDM, gestational diabetes; T2D, type 2 diabetes. (From Brannon et al. [48] and reprinted with permission by American Journal of Clinical Nutrition: Am. J. Clin. Nutr. 2017; 106(Suppl): 1703S–12S. Printed in USA. © 2017 American Society for Nutrition).

Importantly, little if any research has considered the interaction of baseline iron status (and level of stores) and the beneficial or harmful response to iron supplementation. Critical to understand however regarding this interaction is the determination of who is at risk of adverse outcomes from low iron status and would benefit from iron supplementation. A parallel consideration is the amount and form of iron that is most effective with least adverse effect for either supplementation or food fortification. Based on emerging data, the interaction of the level of iron stores among iron-replete pregnant women and infants with high dietary iron intakes from supplementation or fortified foods may become important to understand relative to the possibility of adverse health outcomes. Until the needed research is available, well-informed public policy will be limited by the insufficiency of the evidence for benefit or harm of routine screening and supplementation. The historical focus on concerns for iron inadequacy remains critical for these vulnerable population groups. But, the concerns should now also begin to encompass the parallel interests in ensuring that those who are iron-replete are not put at risk in the broad-brush efforts to avoid iron deficiency. For many understandable reasons, pregnancy and infancy have been almost universally characterized as "automatically" resulting in ID. The situation, especially in more developed regions of the world, many be more nuanced. Research agendas, and in turn public policy, now need to more fully embrace the competing nature of the concerns and find the best balance. Examples of policy decisions that could be better informed by addressing these knowledge gaps and research needs include, but are not limited to clinical guidelines for screening and supplementation; decisions on supplements and food fortification (formulas and infant cereals) such as the type and amount of iron, dietary guidance both for recommended nutrient and food intakes for these two vulnerable populations. The dilemma at present for policy-decisions in developed countries is the duality both of the U-shaped risk and of the nature of iron status of their pregnant women and young children, most of whom are likely iron, but some of whom have sufficient low iron status to be a concern.

In summary, our knowledge is limited by critical gaps and methodologic challenges that increase the uncertainty in the assessment of iron status across its full continuum in pregnant women and young children whose iron needs are high and in whom adaptations of iron homeostasis may affect their susceptibility to iron excess. Adding to this uncertainty is the lack of cutpoints across the full continuum of iron status that have been related to health outcomes, especially those clinically-relevant and beyond hematologic outcomes. Indicators are also needed that can be appropriated adjusted for or are not affected by inflammation. Advancing our knowledge on the benefits and adverse outcomes of iron supplementation in pregnant women and young children will also inform strong evidence-based policy that ensure sufficiency without excess iron availability in largely iron-replete pregnant women and children in developed countries.

Acknowledgments: P.M.B. and C.L.T. received support from the Office of Dietary Supplements, National Institutes of Health, for this manuscript as a part of the office's iron initiative.

Author Contributions: P.M.B. conceived, developed and drafted the manuscript; C.L.T. conceived and contributed to the interpretation and writing of the manuscript.

Conflicts of Interest: The authors declare no conflict of interest.

References

1. Aisen, P.; Enns, C.; Wessling-Resnick, M. Chemistry and biology of eukaryotic iron metabolism. *Int. J. Biochem. Cell Biol.* **2001**, *33*, 940–959. [CrossRef]
2. Wessling-Resnick, M. Excess iron: Considerations related to development and early growth. *Am. J. Clin. Nutr.* **2017**. [CrossRef]
3. World Health Organization. *World-Wide Prevalence of Anaemia 1993–2005: Who Global Database on Anaemia*; WHO Press: Geneva, Switzerland, 2005.
4. Petry, N.; Olofin, I.; Hurrell, R.F.; Boy, E.; Wirth, J.P.; Moursi, M.; Donahue, A.M.; Rohner, F. The proportion of anemia associated with iron deficiency in low, medium, and high human development index countries: A systematic analysis of national surveys. *Nutrients* **2016**, *8*, 693. [CrossRef] [PubMed]

5. World Health Organization. Daily Iron Supplementation in Children 6–23 Months of Age. Available online: http://www.who.int/elena/titles/guidance_summaries/iron_children/en/ (accessed on 11 July 2017).

6. World Health Organization. Who Recommendations on Antenatal Care for a Positive Pregnancy Experience. Available online: http://www.who.int/reproductivehealth/publications/maternal_perinatal_health/anc-positive-pregnancy-experience/en/ (accessed on 14 September 2017).

7. Gupta, P.M.; Hamner, H.C.; Suchdev, P.S.; Flores-Ayala, R.; Mei, Z. Iron deficiency and adequacy in young children, non-pregnant, and pregnant women in the United States. *Am. J. Clin. Nutr.* **2017**, *106*, 1640S–1646S. [CrossRef] [PubMed]

8. Milman, N.; Taylor, C.; Merkel, J.; Brannon, P. Iron status in pregnant women and women of reproductive age in Europe. *Am. J. Clin. Nutr.* **2017**, *106*, 1655S–1662S. [CrossRef] [PubMed]

9. Van der Merwe, L.F.; Eussen, S.R. Iron status of young children in Europe. *Am. J. Clin. Nutr.* **2017**, *106*, 1663S–1671S. [CrossRef] [PubMed]

10. Taylor, C.L.; Brannon, P.M. Introduction to workshop on iron screening and supplementation in iron-replete pregnant women and young children. *Am. J. Clin. Nutr.* **2017**, *106*, 1547S–1554S. [CrossRef] [PubMed]

11. Fisher, A.L.; Nemeth, E. Iron homeostasis during pregnancy. *Am. J. Clin. Nutr.* **2017**, *106*, 1567S–1574S. [CrossRef] [PubMed]

12. Lönnerdal, B. Development of iron homeostasis in infants and young children. *Am. J. Clin. Nutr.* **2017**, *106*, 1575S–1580S. [CrossRef] [PubMed]

13. Bothwell, T.H. Iron requirements in pregnancy and strategies to meet them. *Am. J. Clin. Nutr.* **2000**, *72*, 257S–264S. [PubMed]

14. Zhang, C.; Rawal, S. Dietary iron intake, iron status and gestational diabetes. *Am. J. Clin. Nutr.* **2017**, *106*, 1672S–1680S. [CrossRef] [PubMed]

15. Paganini, D.; Zimmermann, M.B. The effects of iron fortification and supplementation on the gut microbiome and diarrhea in infants and children: A review. *Am. J. Clin. Nutr.* **2017**, *106*, 1688S–1693S. [CrossRef] [PubMed]

16. Vricella, L.K. Emerging understanding and measurement of plasma volume expansion in pregnancy. *Am. J. Clin. Nutr.* **2017**, *106*, 1620S–1625S. [CrossRef] [PubMed]

17. Institute of Medicine (US) Panel on Micronutrients. *Dietary Reference Intakes for Vitamin A, Vitamin k, Arsenic, Boron, Chromium, Copper, Iodine, Iron, Manganese, Molybdenum, Nickel, Silicon, Vanadium, and Zinc*; National Academies Press: Washington, DC, USA, 2001.

18. EFSA Panel on Dietetic Products Nutrition and Allergies (NDA). Scientific opinion on dietary reference values for iron. *EFSA J.* **2015**, *13*, 115.

19. Scientific Advisory Committee on Nutrition (SACN). *Iron and Health*; The Stationery Office: London, UK, 2010.

20. Australian Ministry of Health. Nutrient Reference Intakes for Australia and New Zealand: Iron. Available online: https://www.nrv.gov.au/nutrients/iron (accessed on 15 September 2017).

21. FAO/WHO. *Human Vitamin and Mineral Requirements*; Iron; FAO: Geneva, Switzerland, 2002; Chapter 13.

22. Rios, E.; Lipschitz, D.A.; Cook, J.D.; Smith, N.J. Relationship of maternal and infant iron stores as assessed by determination of plasma ferritin. *Pediatrics* **1975**, *55*, 694–699. [PubMed]

23. Proytcheva, M.A. Issues in neonatal cellular analysis. *Am. J. Clin. Pathol.* **2009**, *131*, 560–573. [CrossRef] [PubMed]

24. Dewey, K.G. The challenge of meeting nutrient needs of infants and young children during the period of complementary feeding: An evolutionary perspective. *J. Nutr.* **2013**, *143*, 2050–2054. [CrossRef] [PubMed]

25. Baker, R.D.; Greer, F.R. Diagnosis and prevention of iron deficiency and iron-deficiency anemia in infants and young children (0–3 years of age). *Pediatrics* **2010**, *126*, 1040–1050. [CrossRef] [PubMed]

26. Finn, K.; Callen, C.; Bhatia, J.; Reidy, K.; Bechard, L.J.; Carvalho, R. Importance of dietary sources of iron in infants and toddlers: Lessons from the fits study. *Nutrients* **2017**, *9*, 733. [CrossRef] [PubMed]

27. Siu, A.L.; U.S. Preventive Services Task Force. Screening for iron deficiency anemia and iron supplementation in pregnant women to improve maternal health and birth outcomes: U.S. Preventive services task force recommendation statement. *Ann. Intern. Med.* **2015**, *163*, 529–536. [CrossRef] [PubMed]

28. Siu, A.L.; U.S. Preventive Services Task Force. Screening for iron deficiency anemia in young children: Uspstf recommendation statement. *Pediatrics* **2015**, *136*, 746–752. [CrossRef] [PubMed]

29. Garner, C.D. Nutrition in pregnancy. In *Uptodate*; Post, T.W., Ed.; UpToDate: Waltham, MA, USA, 2017.

30. American College of Obstetrics and Gynecology. Acog practice bulletin No. 95: Anemia in pregnancy. *Obstet. Gynecol.* **2008**, *112*, 201–207.

31. Yip, R.; Parvanta, I.; Cogswell, M.E.; McDonnell, S.M.; Bowman, B.A.; Grummer-Strawn, L.M.; Trowbridge, F. Recommendations to prevent and control iron deficiency in the United States. *Morb. Mortal. Wkly. Rep.* **1998**, *47*, 1–29.

32. Infant Feeding Working Group. Nutrition for Healthy Term Infants: Recommendations from Birth to Six Months. Available online: http://www.hc-sc.gc.ca/fn-an/nutrition/infant-nourisson/recom/index-eng.php (accessed on 18 September 2017).

33. Domellöf, M.; Braegger, C.; Campoy, C.; Colomb, V.; Decsi, T.; Fewtrell, M.; Hojsak, I.; Mihatsch, W.; Molgaard, C.; Shamir, R.; et al. Iron requirements of infants and toddlers. *J. Pediatr. Gastroenterol. Nutr.* **2014**, *58*, 119–129. [CrossRef] [PubMed]

34. Pavord, S.; Myers, B.; Robinson, S.; Allard, S.; Strong, J.; Oppenheimer, C.; British Committee for Standards in Haematology. UK guidelines on the management of iron deficiency in pregnancy. *Br. J. Haematol.* **2012**, *156*, 588–600. [CrossRef] [PubMed]

35. Australian Department of Health. Nutritional Supplements, 10.4.4 Iron Supplementation. Available online: http://www.health.gov.au/internet/publications/publishing.nsf/Content/clinical-practice-guidelines-ac-mod1~part-b~lifestyle-considerations~nutritional-supplements (accessed on 18 September 2017).

36. Australian Government National Health and Medical Research Council. Infant Feeding Guidelines: Summary. Available online: https://www.eatforhealth.gov.au/sites/default/files/files/the_guidelines/n56b_infant_feeding_summary_130808.pdf (accessed on 18 September 2017).

37. Auckland District Health Board—National Women's Health. Iron in Pregnancy. Available online: http://nationalwomenshealth.adhb.govt.nz/Portals/0/Documents/Policies/Iron%20in%20Pregnancy_.pdf (accessed on 18 September 2017).

38. Anderson, G.W.; Frazer, D.M. Current understanding of iron homeostasis. *Am. J. Clin. Nutr.* **2017**, *106*, 1547S–1554S. [CrossRef] [PubMed]

39. Ross, A.C. Impact of chronic and acute inflammation on extra- and intracellular iron homeostasis. *Am. J. Clin. Nutr.* **2017**, *106*, 1581S–1587S. [CrossRef] [PubMed]

40. Gordeuk, V.R.; Brannon, P.M. Ethnic and genetic factors of iron status in women of reproductive age. *Am. J. Clin. Nutr.* **2017**, *106*, 1594S–1599S. [CrossRef] [PubMed]

41. Rehu, M.; Punnonen, K.; Ostland, V.; Heinonen, S.; Westerman, M.; Pulkki, K.; Sankilampi, U. Maternal serum hepcidin is low at term and independent of cord blood iron status. *Eur. J. Haematol.* **2010**, *85*, 345–352. [CrossRef] [PubMed]

42. Domellöf, M.; Lönnerdal, B.; Abrams, S.A.; Hernell, O. Iron absorption in breast-fed infants: Effects of age, iron status, iron supplements, and complementary foods. *Am. J. Clin. Nutr.* **2002**, *76*, 198–204. [PubMed]

43. Leong, W.I.; Bowlus, C.L.; Tallkvist, J.; Lönnerdal, B. Iron supplementation during infancy—Effects on expression of iron transporters, iron absorption, and iron utilization in rat pups. *Am. J. Clin. Nutr.* **2003**, *78*, 1203–1211. [PubMed]

44. Leong, W.I.; Bowlus, C.L.; Tallkvist, J.; Lönnerdal, B. DMT1 and FPN1 expression during infancy: Developmental regulation of iron absorption. *Am. J. Physiol. Gastrointest. Liver Physiol.* **2003**, *285*, G1153–G1161. [CrossRef] [PubMed]

45. Georgieff, M.K. Iron assessment to protect the developing brain. *Am. J. Clin. Nutr.* **2017**, *106*, 1588S–1593S. [CrossRef] [PubMed]

46. Hoofnagle, A.N. Bioindicator harmonization in clinical research: Making the hard work matter. *Am. J. Clin. Nutr.* **2017**, *106*, 1615S–1619S. [CrossRef] [PubMed]

47. Pfeiffer, C.M.; Looker, A.C. Laboratory methodologies for indicators of iron status: Strengths, limitations and analytical challenges. *Am. J. Clin. Nutr.* **2017**, *106*, 1606S–1614S. [CrossRef] [PubMed]

48. Brannon, P.M.; Stover, P.J.; Taylor, C.L. Integrating themes, evidence gaps and research needs identified by workshop on iron screening and supplementation in iron-replete pregnant women and young children. *Am. J. Clin. Nutr.* **2017**, *106*, 1703S–1712S. [CrossRef] [PubMed]

49. Namaste, S.M.; Rohner, F.; Huang, J.; Bhushan, N.L.; Flores-Ayala, R.; Kupka, R.; Mei, Z.; Rawat, R.; Williams, A.M.; Raiten, D.J.; et al. Adjusting ferritin concentrations for inflammation: Biomarkers reflecting inflammation and nutritional determinants of anemia (brinda) project. *Am. J. Clin. Nutr.* **2017**, *106*, 359S–371S. [PubMed]

50. Rohner, F.; Namaste, S.; Larson, L.; Addo, Y.; Mei, Z.; Suchdev, P.S.; Ashour, F.; Rawat, R.; Raiten, D.J.; Northrop-Clewes, C. Adjusting soluble transferrin receptor concentrations for inflammation: Brinda project. *Am. J. Clin. Nutr.* **2017**, *106*, 372S–382S. [PubMed]

51. Mei, Z.; Namaste, S.M.; Serdula, M.; Suchdev, P.S.; Rohner, F.; Flores-Ayala, R.; Addo, O.Y.; Raiten, D.J. Adjusting total body iron for inflammation: Biomarkers reflecting inflammation and nutrition determinants of anemia (BRINDA) project. *Am. J. Clin. Nutr.* **2017**, *106*, 383S–389S. [PubMed]

52. O'Brien, K.O. Iron status of north american pregnant women: Other evidence from the united states and canada. *Am. J. Clin. Nutr.* **2017**, *106*, 1647S–1654S. [CrossRef] [PubMed]

53. Daru, J.; Colman, K.; Stanworth, S.J.; De La Salle, B.; Wood, E.M.; Pasricha, S.R. Serum ferritin as an indicator of iron status: What do we need to know? *Am. J. Clin. Nutr.* **2017**, *106*, 1634S–1639S. [CrossRef] [PubMed]

54. Kemper, A.R.; Fan, T.; Grossman, D.C.; Phipps, M.G. Gaps in evidence regarding iron deficiency anemia in pregnant women and young children: Summary of united states preventive services task force recommendations. *Am. J. Clin. Nutr.* **2017**, *106*, 1555S–1558S. [CrossRef] [PubMed]

55. Breymann, C. Iron deficiency anemia in pregnancy. *Semin. Hematol.* **2015**, *52*, 339–347. [CrossRef] [PubMed]

56. Dewey, K.G.; Oaks, B.M. U-shaped curve for risk associated with maternal iron status or supplementation. *Am. J. Clin. Nutr.* **2017**, *106*, 1694S–1702S. [CrossRef] [PubMed]

57. Kozuki, N.; Lee, A.C.; Katz, J. Moderate to severe, but not mild, maternal anemia is associated with increased risk of small-for-gestational-age outcomes. *J. Nutr.* **2012**, *142*, 358–362. [CrossRef] [PubMed]

58. Lozoff, B.; Beard, J.; Connor, J.; Barbara, F.; Georgieff, M.; Schallert, T. Long-lasting neural and behavioral effects of iron deficiency in infancy. *Nutr. Rev.* **2006**, *64*, S34–S43. [CrossRef] [PubMed]

59. Lozoff, B.; Goerogieff, M. Iron deficiency and brain development. *Semin. Pediatr. Neonatol.* **2006**, *13*, 158–165. [CrossRef] [PubMed]

60. Georgieff, M.K. Long-term brain and behavioral consequences of early iron deficiency. *Nutr. Rev.* **2011**, *69*, S43–S48. [CrossRef] [PubMed]

61. Cai, C.; Granger, M.; Eck, P.; Friel, J. Effect of daily iron supplementation in healthy exclusively breastfed infants: A systematic review with meta-analysis. *Breastfeed. Med.* **2017**. [CrossRef] [PubMed]

62. McDonagh, M.S.; Blazina, I.; Dana, T.; Cantor, A.; Bougatsos, C. Screening and routine supplementation for iron deficiency anemia: A systematic review. *Pediatrics* **2015**, *135*, 723–733. [CrossRef] [PubMed]

63. Reveiz, L.; Gyte, G.M.; Cuervo, L.G.; Casasbuenas, A. Treatments for iron-deficiency anaemia in pregnancy. *Cochrane Database Syst. Rev.* **2011**, *10*, CD003094.

64. Haider, B.A.; Olofin, I.; Wang, M.; Spiegelman, D.; Ezzati, M.; Fawzi, W.W.; Nutrition Impact Model Study Group. Anaemia, prenatal iron use, and risk of adverse pregnancy outcomes: Systematic review and meta-analysis. *BMJ* **2013**, *346*, f3443. [CrossRef] [PubMed]

65. McDonagh, M.; Blazina, I.; Dana, T.; Cantor, A.; Bougatsos, C. *Routine Iron Supplementation and Screening for Iron Deficiency Anemia in Children Ages 6 to 24 Months: A Systematic Review to Update the U.S. Preventive Services Task Force Recommendation*; Agency for Healthcare Research and Quality: Rockville, MD, USA, 2015.

66. Scholl, T.O. Iron status during pregnancy: Setting the stage for mother and infant. *Am. J. Clin. Nutr.* **2005**, *81*, 741–748.

67. Pasricha, S.R.; Hayes, E.; Kalumba, K.; Biggs, B.A. Effect of daily iron supplementation on health in children aged 4–23 months: A systematic review and meta-analysis of randomised controlled trials. *Lancet Glob. Health* **2013**, *1*, e77–e86. [CrossRef]

68. Lönnerdal, B. Excess iron intake as a factor in growth, infections and development of infants and young children. *Am. J. Clin. Nutr.* **2017**, *106*, 1681S–1687S. [CrossRef] [PubMed]

69. Singhal, A.; Morley, R.; Abbott, R.; Fairweather-Tait, S.; Stephenson, T.; Lucas, A. Clinical safety of iron-fortified formulas. *Pediatrics* **2000**, *105*, E38. [CrossRef] [PubMed]

70. Agrawal, S.; Berggren, K.L.; Marks, E.; Fox, J.H. Impact of high iron intake on cognition and neurodegeneration in humans and in animal models: A systematic review. *Nutr. Rev.* **2017**, *75*, 456–470. [CrossRef] [PubMed]

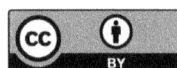

nutrients

MDPI

Review

Protein Hydrolysates as Promoters of Non-Haem Iron Absorption

Yanan Li [1], Han Jiang [1] and Guangrong Huang [1,2,3,*]

1   College of Life Sciences, China Jiliang University, Hangzhou 310018, China;
    dreamforlyn@gmail.com (Y.L.); jianghan@cjlu.edu.cn (H.J.)
2   Key Lab of Marine Food Quality and Hazard Controlling Technology of Zhejiang Province,
    Hangzhou 310018, China
3   National and Local United Engineering Lab of Quality Controlling Technology and Instrument for
    Marine Food, Hangzhou 310018, China
*   Correspondence: grhuang@126.com; Tel.: +86-571-8687-5628

Received: 24 March 2017; Accepted: 13 June 2017; Published: 15 June 2017

Abstract: Iron (Fe) is an essential micronutrient for human growth and health. Organic iron is an excellent iron supplement due to its bioavailability. Both amino acids and peptides improve iron bioavailability and absorption and are therefore valuable components of iron supplements. This review focuses on protein hydrolysates as potential promoters of iron absorption. The ability of protein hydrolysates to chelate iron is thought to be a key attribute for the promotion of iron absorption. Iron-chelatable protein hydrolysates are categorized by their absorption forms: amino acids, di- and tri-peptides and polypeptides. Their structural characteristics, including their size and amino acid sequence, as well as the presence of special amino acids, influence their iron chelation abilities and bioavailabilities. Protein hydrolysates promote iron absorption by keeping iron soluble, reducing ferric iron to ferrous iron, and promoting transport across cell membranes into the gut. We also discuss the use and relative merits of protein hydrolysates as iron supplements.

Keywords: amino acid; di-peptide; tri-peptide; polypeptide; iron chelate; food supplement; bioactive peptides

1. Introduction

Iron (Fe) is an essential micronutrient for human growth and health. Iron affects the health of children, the development of teenagers and the immune system of adults. Iron also plays a role in many cellular metabolic activities, such as carrying oxygen in haemoglobin and myoglobin and transporting electrons in the various cytochrome systems, as well as in ferredoxin for respiration. Anaemia and iron deficiency reduce an individual's well-being, cause fatigue and lethargy, and impair physical capacity and work performance. Maternal anaemia is associated with mortality and morbidity in the mother and baby, including increased risks of miscarriages, stillbirths, prematurity and low birth weight [1]. However, iron deficiency and iron deficiency anaemia (IDA) are classified as the most prevalent nutritional disorders in the world by the WHO; they affect more than 3.5 billion people in the developing world [2]. Almost half of children are anaemic, most of whom live in undeveloped countries [3]. More than 20% of women experience iron deficiency during their reproductive lives [4].

Inadequate iron intake and absorption are the main causes of iron deficiency, which leads to IDA. In these cases, iron supplements or iron fortifiers are needed to overcome the iron deficiency. Commercially available oral iron supplements include ferrous sulfate, ferrous gluconate, ferrous fumarate, iron dextran, and other iron-containing compounds.

Organic iron is thought to have a better bioavailability and have fewer side effects than inorganic iron salts. For example, for a diet containing only 6% of its total iron as haem, 30% of the iron absorbed was acquired from haem to the exclusion of other dietary iron sources [5]. Alternatively, iron can also chelate with a sugar as an iron supplement, such as iron sucrose (Venofer®), iron polysaccharide (Niferex®), iron dextran and iron carboxymaltose (Ferinject®). These iron-sugar complexes have special advantages, such as their minimal side effects. For example, iron-polymaltose complexes have a bioavailability similar to that of ferrous salts, and are preferable in terms of their balance between efficacy and toxicity [6]. The milks fortified by iron sulfate stabilized with maltodextrin covers toddlers' requirements of iron [7].

Proteins and their hydrolysates are important organic substances, and mineral chelating peptides have the ability to enhance the bioavailability of minerals [8]. Some protein hydrolysates have been used in the iron fortification of food for humans and livestock. Thus, the study of protein hydrolysates as promoters of iron absorption is important.

2. Iron-Chelatable Protein Hydrolysates

Protein hydrolysates are protein fragments produced via hydrolysation and include amino acids and peptides of different sizes. Some hydrolysates can be synthesised or produced through bioengineering depending on their structure. Proteins are hydrolysed by enzymes or chemicals to improve their nutritional value or to search for bioactive peptides. Huge proteins, such as collagen, are hydrolysed by enzymes to improve their bioavailability. Many types of fisheries by-products are hydrolysed to change non-edible proteins into edible peptides. Proteins are also hydrolysed by acids or bases to produce amino acids. Protein hydrolysates have various structures and can be produced in large amounts. They serve as important nutrients and food ingredients, as well as playing other roles, and they are an important resource for us to further develop and utilise.

The positive effects of protein hydrolysates on the absorption of minerals, such as iron or other metals, have been reported in vivo and in vitro. The chelation ability of protein hydrolysates is thought to be a key factor in the promotion of iron absorption. Through metal chelation, peptides or amino acids increase the solubility and bioavailability of metals. Therefore, iron-chelatable protein hydrolysates are potential promoters of iron absorption. We will focus on peptides and amino acids, which have the ability to chelate iron.

Proteins are digested into oligopeptides and amino acids in the digestive tract. Amino acids, di-peptides, tri-peptides and polypeptides all have different absorption routes, except for the paracellular route. We therefore classify iron-chelatable protein hydrolysates into the three classes listed in Table 1, which are the absorbable forms of protein hydrolytic products. Some of the reported iron-chelatable protein hydrolysates are listed in Table 1.

Table 1. Iron-chelatable amino acids, peptides and proteins.

Class	Iron-Chelatable Substance	Sequence	Iron Valence	Reference
Amino acids	Arginine	R	II	[9]
	Aspartic acid	D	II	[10]
	Cysteine	C	III	[11]
	Glycine	G	III/II	[12,13]
	Glutamic acid	E	II/III	[14,15]
	Glutamine	Q	III	[16]
	Histidine	H	II/III	[9,11]
	Lysine	K	III	[11]
	Methionine	M	III	[16]
	Serine	S	III	[15]
	Threonine	T	II	[17]
Small peptides	Aspartame		II	[10]
	Arg-Glu-Glu	REE	II	[18]
	Asn-Cys-Ser	NCS	II	[19]
	Carbamyl glycine		II	[20]
	His-Tyr-Asp	HYD	II	[21]
	Isoleucyl-tryptophan	IW	II	[22]

Table 1. *Cont.*

Class	Iron-Chelatable Substance	Sequence	Iron Valence	Reference
	Aspartame		II	[10]
	Leu-Ala-Asn	LAN	II	[19]
	Reduced glutathione	GSH	II	[19]
Small peptides	Ser-Met	SM	II	[19]
	Ser-Cys-His	SCH	II	[23]
	Ser-Ala-Cys	SAC	II	[24]
	Val-Pro-Leu	VPL	II	[25]
	α-lactalbumin and β-lactoglobulin hydrolysate		II	[25]
	β-casein peptide	PGPIPN	III	[26]
	Anchovy peptide	$S(G)_7LGS(G)_2SIR$	II	[27]
	Barley protein hydrolysate	SVNVPLY	II	[25]
	Buffalo α_S-casein		II	[28]
	Caseinophosphopeptide	$(SpSpSpEE)n$	II	[29,30]
	Chickpea protein hydrolysate		II/III	[31]
	Cod skin peptides		II	[32]
	Ferrichrysin/ferrocins		III	[33]
	Hairtail protein hydrolysate		II	[21,34,35]
Poly-peptides	Hydrolysate of Alaskan pollock skin	GPAGPHGPPG/SGSTGH	II	[23,24]
	Mackerel hydrolysate	NPVRGN/NPDRGN	II	[36,37]
	Lactein		II	[38]
	Peptide-hydroxamate	NAPVSIPQ	II/III	[39]
	Plasma hydrolysate	DLGEQYFKG	II	[40]
	Rice protein hydrolysate		II	[41]
	Scad protein hydrolysate		III	[42]
	Seaweed protein hydrolysate		II	[43]
	Sericin hydrolysate		II	[44]
	Shrimp protein hydrolysates	LPTGPKS	II	[45,46]
	Spirulina protein hydrolysate	TDPI(L)AACI(L)	II	[47]
	Soybean protein hydrolysate	DEGEQPRPFPFP	III/II	[48–51]
	Whey peptide		II	[52]
	Ferritin		III	[53]
Protein	Hen egg white lysozyme		III	[54]
	Thiolated human-like collagen		II	[55]
	Whey proteins		II	[56]

2.1. Iron-Chelatable Amino Acids

Amino acids, the building blocks of proteins, are basic nutrients for all forms of life. They are an important form of protein hydrolysate that are absorbed. Amino acids can be absorbed and transported by multiple transporters, which have been identified and classified in the past several decades. As they are important nutrients that can be absorbed by cells directly, amino acids with iron-absorption promoting abilities will be promising candidates for iron supplements.

Many amino acids have been studied to determine their interactions with iron, such as one study of the equilibrium of L-glutamic acid and L-serine with iron(III) in solution [15]. $Fe(His)_2$, $Fe(Gly)_2$, and $Fe(Arg)_2$ have been studied as iron complexes [9]. In addition, the enhanced effect of histidine, cysteine, and lysine on iron absorption is thought to be based on the tridentate chelates then form with iron [11]. Some of the reported iron-chelatable amino acids are listed in Table 1, such as methionine, glutamine, and aspartic acid. Of all the amino acids-iron complexes, iron-glycine is the most reported. The iron-glycine chelate has been proven to have a positive effect on iron absorption in piglets, rats, broilers and humans [13].

2.2. Iron-Chelatable Di-Peptides and Tri-Peptides

Di-peptides and tri-peptides, similar to free amino acids, are also important nutrients and can be transported intact into epithelial cells by the special transporter PEPT1 [57]. Furthermore, small peptides (di-peptides and tri-peptides) are the major forms of protein that are absorbed by cells. The concentration of oligopeptides (di-, tri- and tetra-peptides) in the intestinal lumen is three to four times that of free amino acids [58]. In addition, the transfer efficiency of PEPT1 is higher than that of the amino acid transporters for some substrates [59]. Thus, di- and tri-peptides are more important candidates for iron supplements than amino acids.

Many types of di- and tri-peptides have been reported to chelate iron, and some of them have been isolated from protein hydrolysates. For example, Ser-Met, Leu-Ala-Asn and Asn-Cys-Ser, which were isolated from sesame protein hydrolysates, can chelate iron to a similar degree as reduced glutathione [19]. Two iron-chelatable tri-peptides, Ser-Cys-His and His-Tyr-Asp were isolated from hydrolysates of Alaskan pollock skin collagen [23] and hairtail protein [21], respectively. Some synthesized small peptides that have iron chelation abilities have also been reported. For example, aspartame (*N*-L-α-aspartyl-L-phenylalanine methyl ester) can interact with ferrous iron, and aspartame-ferrous iron complexes have been synthesized [10]. Fe-carbamyl glycine [20] and Arg-Glu-Glu-iron [18] have also been synthesized and studied as iron supplements.

2.3. Iron-Chelatable Polypeptides and Proteins

Polypeptides and proteins, which are polymers of amino acids, are also important for human and animal nutrition. Polypeptides can be absorbed intact except for some forms of small peptides and amino acids, and they can be absorbed via sodium-coupled oligopeptide transporters (SOPT 1 and SOPT2), paracellular passive transport, transcellular passive diffusion and transcytosis [60]. Proteins, similar to polypeptides, can also be absorbed by the paracellular and transcellular pathways. Insulin, for example, can be absorbed by the small intestine at its apical side via endocytosis [61].

Iron-chelatable polypeptides are also important iron supplement candidates; therefore, we will further discuss polypeptides and proteins. The variations are countless for peptides consisting of four or more amino acids, and therefore, iron-chelatable polypeptides are also innumerable. Generally, iron-chelatable polypeptides can be classified into several groups: proteins, protein hydrolysates and other polypeptides.

2.3.1. Iron-Chelatable Proteins

Approximately 30% of proteins and enzymes contain metal or metalloid ions in their structures. Most of these proteins contain an iron or iron-like metal ion because they contain an amino acid motif that can chelate iron. Many proteins, such as thiolated human-like collagen, can chelate iron, as can the iron metabolism-related proteins [55]. In iron-enriched baker's yeast and soybeans, iron also binds proteins [53,62]. Some complexes, such as iron-bound whey proteins, have good stability under different processing conditions [56].

2.3.2. Iron-Chelatable Protein Fragments

The iron-chelating subunits of proteins in food can be released by cooking, digestion and hydrolyzation. These released protein hydrolysates or their fragments are potential iron supplements due to their iron chelation abilities. Proteins that are inexpensive and easy to obtain are major sources for the production of metal-chelatable peptides or other bioactive peptides. Proteins from cereals, aquatic products, milk, and other sources can be hydrolysed by many different types of enzymes to identify iron-chelatable peptides.

For example, a polypeptide from a barley protein, Ser-Val-Asn-Val-Pro-Leu-Tyr, spontaneously forms a complex with an iron ion at physiological pH [25]. Several iron-chelatable peptides were identified from soybean proteins that were hydrolysed by pepsin, trypsin, protease, deamidase and other enzymes [49,51]. Hydrolysates of shrimp, fish and seaweed also have the ability to chelate iron, and several iron-chelatable peptides have been isolated from these sources [32,43,45,46].

In particular, phosphopeptides from casein [28], egg white [63] and other similar sources make up one category of peptides that have the ability to chelate iron. Peptides derived from collagen also have the ability to chelate iron. This category includes peptides from the skin of Alaskan pollock [23,24] and cod [32] and the scales of *Latescalcarifer*, *Mugilcephalus*, *Chanoschanos*, and *Oreochromis* spp. [64].

2.3.3. Other Iron-Chelatable Peptides

In addition to the two categories discussed above, many natural and synthetic peptides have also been studied. Cell-penetrating peptides that can efficiently translocate through the plasma membrane are able to deliver cargos across the membrane both in vitro and in vivo [65]. These cargos range from small to large molecules and can include medicines and proteins. An iron ion can also be cargo. The tri-peptide Arg-Glu-Glu [18] was designed using the rules governing cell-penetrating peptides; the Arg residue improves the penetrability of the peptide and has been proven to promote iron absorption in the form of a chelate. Peptides produced by microorganisms have also been reported to contain iron or to have the ability to chelate iron. Four kinds of ferrocins, which are iron-containing peptides, have been found in one species of gram-negative bacterium [66]. Probiotic bacteria grown in culture media with different nitrogen sources have been shown to produce iron-binding peptides [67]. Iron-binding peptides from *Aspergillus versicolour* [68], *Aspergillus oryzae* [33] and *Lactococcus lactis* [38] are all thought to be promising bioactive peptides that are able to promote iron absorption.

2.4. Structural Characteristics of Iron-Chelatable Protein Hydrolysates

Many protein hydrolysates can chelate iron. However, the protein hydrolysate constituents that are responsible for chelating iron are identified randomly, which is inefficient. Nonetheless, identifying the active components of these protein hydrolysates is necessary to find or synthesize a peptide that has the ability to chelate iron. The chelates of protein hydrolysates and iron ions are complicated because both peptides and amino acids are amphoteric molecules. Protein hydrolysates contain cationic, anionic and zwitterionic forms of peptides at different pH values, and iron ions have different valence states (Fe^{2+} and Fe^{3+}). However, all protein hydrolysates have a similar chemical nature: terminal amino and carboxyl groups with various side-chains. Iron ions have limited differences in their extra-nuclear electron configurations. Therefore, there are rules that can be followed to identify or design peptides. Iron ions acting as a Lewis acid can react with oxygen-rich and nitrogen-rich groups, which are Lewis bases. Fe^{2+} can be classified as a borderline Lewis metal ion, and Fe^{3+} belongs to the hard group of Lewis metal ions. According to this rule, Fe^{3+} prefers oxygen-rich groups, such as the carboxyl groups and phosphate groups (which are hard Lewis bases), and Fe^{2+} has a preference for nitrogen-containing groups [69].

2.4.1. Structural Characteristics of Iron-Chelatable Amino Acids

Every natural amino acid has two effective donor groups (amino and carboxyl) and is capable of forming a stable, five-membered chelate ring with a metal atom [70]. In addition to these two groups, the side-chain of an amino acid (R group), which defines each amino acid, also plays an important role in determining the chelate that is formed. In general, the R group affects the complex by changing the chemical environment of the amino and carboxyl groups. Furthermore, the electron rich R groups of some amino acids, such as the imidazole group of histidine and the sulfhydryl group of cysteine, can also participate in chelation. Additionally, Glu and Asp prefer to form chelates with Fe^{3+} at their oxygen-rich R groups; however, Arg and Asn prefer to form chelates with Fe^{2+} at their oxygen-rich R groups.

2.4.2. Structural Characteristics of Iron-Chelatable Peptides

Peptides have many variants, and their iron chelates are more complicated. There are several factors affecting the stability of these chelates.

Special Amino Acids

Certain special amino acids have strong iron chelation abilities, and peptides containing these amino acids have higher iron chelation abilities than other peptides. The activity of these iron chelates is related to these special amino acids, and those special amino acids can also determine whether they prefer Fe^{3+} or Fe^{2+}. Peptides containing Glu and Asp have higher affinities for Fe^{3+}, and peptides containing Arg and Asn prefer to form chelates with Fe^{2+}.

His has a strong metal chelating ability due to its imidazole group. Peptides that are rich in His have higher iron-chelating activities than other peptides in the hydrolysates of some proteins [31,43,71]. Serine is also an important amino acid that affects the stability of iron-containing peptides, likely due to its hydroxyl group [23]. Peptides containing Ser have higher iron and zinc chelating abilities [19,43]. Similar to serine, cysteine also contributes to iron-chelating activity of a peptide due to its sulfhydryl group. In peptides derived from meat protein, Cys has been recognized as an important amino acid that promotes iron absorption through its chelating activity [58,72]. Peptides containing Cys also show higher activities for iron and zinc chelation than other peptides [19]. Phosphorylated amino acids, especially phosphoserine, make up another category of important amino acids since they can create suitable chelating sites for positively charged iron ions [23]. Caseinophosphopeptides (CPPs) derived from milk proteins contain a high proportion of phosphoserines [73] and can stably chelate iron. Asp and Glu have also been reported to contribute to the chelating ability of peptides due to their carboxyl groups.

Size of the Peptides

Only a single amino or carboxyl group is available at each terminus of a peptide, while other amino and carboxyl groups exist within the peptide bonds that connect the amino acids of the peptide. If the peptides are smaller in size, the proportion of amino and carboxyl groups (the oxygen of the C-terminus and the nitrogen of the N-terminus) will be higher, and the iron chelation activity may be higher as well, and it has been shown that peptides with lower molecular weights have higher iron-chelating activities in protein hydrolysates of *P. columbina* [43]. The iron-binding capacity of sea cucumber (*Stichopus japonicus*) ovum hydrolysates increased significantly, from 55.7% to 92.1%, as their molecular weight decreased and as the proportion of fractions larger than 1000 Da decreased markedly from 58.5% to 36.4% [74]. Conversely, for large peptides, the terminal groups represent a very small proportion of the total peptide mass and can result in these peptides having lower chelation abilities. However, some large peptides contain special amino acids, and they actually have stronger iron chelation abilities due to the greater amount of dentate areas. The proper size of a peptide is determined by both the content of special amino acids and the other aforementioned factors. Thus, peptides with a proper size that offer higher ratios of dentate areas will have higher iron chelation abilities.

Sequences of the Peptides

When peptides, as well as those with more dentate areas, are composed of certain special amino acids, these peptides have low iron-chelating activities, which is inconsistent with the rules stated above. In this situation, the peptides may not be in an appropriate sequence. Chemical substances prefer to form a thermodynamically stable five- or six-member ring. Furthermore, some R groups are large or have strong charges that can affect the stability of the chelate. Thus, the side-chains and their positions or sequences will also affect the chelation ability of a peptide.

In summary, almost all amino acids can chelate iron ions; however, the stabilities of the chelation complexes vary due to the R groups of the amino acids and their chemical environments. The chelates of peptides with iron can be affected by the content of special amino acids and the size and sequence of the peptide. The equilibrium constants of the complexes are very different for different substrates and environments. Only some peptides have high equilibrium constants and can stably chelate with iron. In the future, a model that predicts the equilibrium constant of an iron complex could be designed computationally. Then, with the help of bioinformatic methods, we could choose and produce iron-chelatable peptides from food proteins or synthesize one purposefully. At such a time, our ability to identify and use iron-chelatable protein hydrolysates will progress more efficiently.

3. Mechanisms of Promoting Non-Haem Iron Absorption

3.1. Iron Absorption

In mammalian systems, iron absorption differs significantly with various host- and diet-related variables, including the life-stage and iron status of the organism, as well as the enhancers and inhibitors of iron absorption present in the consumed food. However, dietary iron can be absorbed in the ion and molecular form irrespective of the paracellular route. For the iron ion, Fe^{3+} must be reduced to Fe^{2+} by a reducing substance, such as cytochrome *b* or another reductase on the brush border membrane, or by reductants in our food or gastrointestinal secretions. Then, Fe^{2+} is internalized by enterocytes via the apical transporter divalent metal transporter 1 (DMT1). The iron is stored as ferritin inside the enterocytes and can be transported to the interstitial fluids by the basolateral transporter ferroportin when necessary. The iron is then distributed throughout the body in the form of transferrin-bound iron via the circulatory system [75]. In addition, these iron ions can chelate other molecules and be absorbed in a molecularly bound form, such as polysaccharide-iron complexes [76]. In general, the absorption of molecular iron occurs through either endocytosis or importers. For example, haem-iron is absorbed in the form of haem, and its absorption occurs mainly via receptor-mediated endocytosis that is partially mediated by the proton coupled folate transporter (PCFT) or other unidentified low-affinity haem importers [77]. In intestinal epithelial cells, some internalized iron chelates are catabolized to liberate Fe^{2+}, similar to haem, which then follows the fate of dietary Fe^{2+}. Of course, some iron chelates may be transferred in their unmodified molecular form, just as some haem can be transported intact to the plasma. The mechanisms of iron absorption are shown in Figure 1.

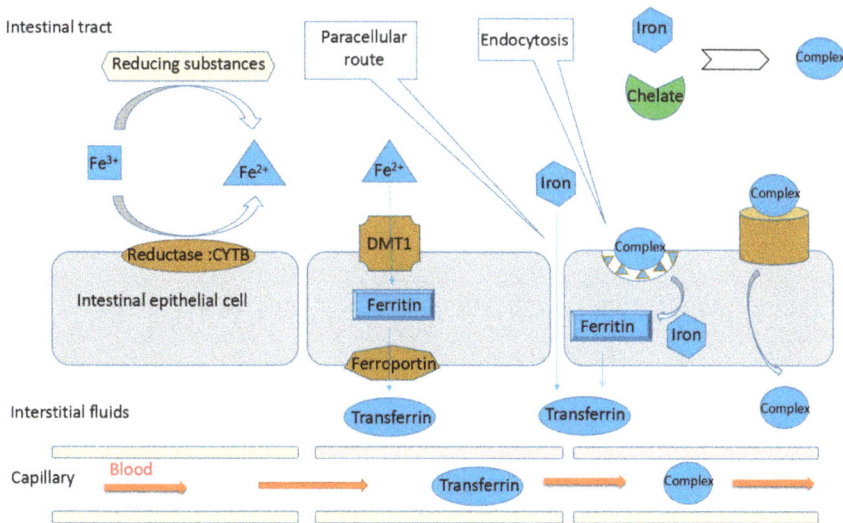

Figure 1. Mechanisms of iron absorption. Iron is absorbed both in ion and complexed forms, as well as via the paracellular route. For iron ions, Fe^{3+} must be reduced to Fe^{2+} by reductases, such as cytochrome *b*, and then be absorbed by the divalent metal transporter 1. The iron is stored in ferritin, transported out of cells by ferroportin and distributed by transferrin. In addition, iron (both Fe^{2+} and Fe^{3+}) can chelate other molecules and be absorbed in the form of complexes via endocytosis and importers, after which their fate includes transformation to iron ions and transfer in their complexed form.

3.2. Mechanisms of Protein Hydrolysates Promoting Non-Haem Iron Absorption

Currently, three theories exist regarding how protein hydrolysates promote iron absorption in mammalian systems. Protein hydrolysates are thought to maintain the solubility of iron, to reduce ferric ion to ferrous ion and keep iron at a low valence state, and/or to promote iron uptake through intestinal cell membranes. The first two theories involve increasing the concentration of soluble iron to promote the entrance of iron into enterocytes through the DMT1 receptor, whereas the latter theory suggests that protein hydrolysates mediate the absorption of bound iron through a peptide or amino acid transporter localized in the brush border membranes.

3.2.1. Maintaining the Solubility of Iron

All nutrients must be absorbed in solution. However, our diet generally contains iron absorption inhibitors, such as phytic acid, tannins, oxalate and polyphenols, which can chelate iron ions and decrease their solubility [78]. In addition, ferric iron becomes insoluble at pH values greater than 3.0, and the pH in the intestinal lumen is basic.

Peptides and amino acids can chelate iron, and their complexes protect iron ions from these inhibitors and the conditions in the fluid of the small intestine, keeping the iron ions in solution. For example, Cys and reduced cysteinylglycine can significantly increase the solubility of iron in a solution containing insoluble iron [58]. Additionally, the hydrolysates of red seaweed (*P. columbina*) protein can maintain iron in a soluble and bioaccessible form after gastrointestinal digestion [43]. CPPs derived from milk proteins with a special sequence of three phosphoseryl residues followed by two glutamic acid residues, Ser(P)-Ser(P)-Ser(P)-Glu-Glu, act as mineral absorption enhancing peptides [8,79,80]. The binding of iron to CPPs increases iron solubility in the alkaline intestinal environment and influence how accessible iron is to apical membranes [81].

3.2.2. Reducing Ferric Ion to Ferrous Ion

As discussed in Section 3.1, most iron ions must be reduced to ferrous ions before being transported by DMT1. Some reductive or antioxidant peptides and amino acids promote iron absorption by reducing ferric iron to ferrous iron, just like ascorbic acid. In addition, Cys and reduced cysteinylglycine enhance ferric iron absorption in Caco-2 cells, but they have no positive effect on ferrous iron [58], suggesting that they may promote iron absorption by reducing ferric iron.

3.2.3. Promoting the Passage of Iron through Intestinal Cell Membranes

Thus far, we have focused on discussing ways to increase the concentration of ferrous iron that arrives at intestinal cell membranes, and we will now consider approaches for promoting the uptake of iron through intestinal cell membranes. Protein hydrolysates have the potential to be excellent iron absorption promoters. Peptides and amino acids have special transporters or pathways in the brush border membranes, and they may carry iron ions when they are absorbed. This absorption of iron is not related to DMT1, but does increase overall iron absorption. For example, Fe-Gly has a special transit system that is different from the absorption system of $FeSO_4$ [5,82,83]. The tri-peptide iron complex Arg-Glu-Glu-Fe, an effective iron supplement for IDA rats, was designed as a cell-penetrating peptide [18]. Some CPP-iron complexes seem to be absorbed via endocytosis in vivo [84].

In conclusion, protein hydrolysates improve iron absorptionin three ways: maintaining the solubility of iron, facilitating the conversion of ferric iron to ferrous iron and promoting the absorption of iron through the intestinal cell membranes. In other words, peptides and amino acids can maintain the solubility of iron through their chelation and reducing abilities. Some complexes can also be absorbed in the form of molecules via PET1, endocytosis, and other modes.

4. Usages, Advantages and Challenges of Protein Hydrolysates as Non-Haem Iron Promoters

4.1. Usagesof Protein Hydrolysates as Non-Haem Iron Promoters

Protein hydrolysates, especially those derived from food protein, are safe when used as iron supplements. Iron chelates of protein hydrolysates have attracted a great amount of attention as a new type of iron supplement [18]. Amino acids [12], small peptides [85] and polypeptides [36] have been confirmed to be able to improve iron bioavailability or absorption. They also have the potential to be used in the food and feed industries, and many of them are already being used. Some of the peptides and amino acids that have been used as iron supplements are listed in Table 2.

Table 2. The use of peptides or amino acids as iron supplements.

Class	Substance	Product Branch	Nation	References
Amino acids	The full spectrum of amino acids	FerrActiv®	America	[86]
	Glycine	Ferbisol®	Spain	[87]
Small peptides	Carbamyl glycine		China	[88]
Polypeptides	Deferrichrysin		Worldwide	[89]
	Donkey-hide gelatine	Dong E®	China	[90]

4.1.1. Amino Acidsas Non-Haem Iron Promoters

Many types of amino acids have been reported to promote iron absorption at the cellular and organismal level, including in humans. Both the full spectrum of amino acids and single amino acids have been shown to promote iron absorption in research and commercial usage.

Aspartic acid, glutamic acid and histidine enhance the uptake and transport of iron by Caco-2 cells [91]. Histidine, cysteine, and lysine enhance in vivo iron uptake in segments of rat duodenum [11]. Iron-amino acid chelates provided faster rates of improvement in haemoglobin levels and were better tolerated by the patients than ferrous-fumarate in a randomized controlled study [92]. Multi-amino acid-iron chelates have been used in premenopausal women and preschool children and have shown positive effects in combating iron deficiency and reducing the number of adverse effects [86,93].

Of all the amino acids, glycine is the most widely used iron chelation ligand. The iron in Fe-Gly can be more easily absorbed than $FeSO_4$ in Caco-2 cells [82]. An addition of Fe-Gly to feed mixtures for broilers contributed to significant changes in the level of biochemical and haematological indicators in their blood [13,94]. Ironbis-glycine chelatesare a suitable compound for food fortification as they prevent the inhibitory effect of phytates [95]. Ferrous bis-glycine chelates can be used for iron fortification in milk as they improve haemoglobin and ferritin serum levels and do not alter milk's organoleptic properties [96]. Furthermore, ferrous bis-glycine can be used in high-phytate foods [12].

4.1.2. Di-Peptides and Tri-Peptidesas Non-Haem Iron Promoters

Di- and tri-peptides can be absorbed quickly. Although there are few reports about the use of di-peptide and tri-peptide iron chelates as iron supplements, it is still a promising direction for us to study. Di-peptides, anserine and carnosine enhanced the uptake and transport of iron by Caco-2 cells [91]. Glutathione also possess iron absorption-enhancing ability [97]. The Arg-Glu-Glu-Fe complex is an effective iron source for IDA rats [18]. Fe-carbamyl glycine is used as an iron fortifier in feed [88].

4.1.3. Polypeptidesas Non-Haem Iron Promoters

Complexes synthesized with low-molecular-mass peptides (<5 kDa) and $FeCl_2$ increased iron uptake by approximately 70% compared with uptake of $FeSO_4$ in a Caco-2 cell model [52]. Caco-2 cellular uptake increased 4-fold for the Fe^{2+}-(Ser-Val-Asn-Val-Pro-Leu-Tyr), a barley-derived peptide complex, after pepsin-pancreatin digestion compared to the uptake of iron sulfate salt [25]. Iron-binding peptides derived from sericin have been shown to improve iron bioavailability and hasten the alleviation of iron deficiency in experimental rats [44]. Ferrichrysin (an iron-chelated cyclic peptide) exhibited the same beneficial effect in improving IDA as ferric citrate, being significantly greater than the effect of haem iron in anaemic Sprague–Dawley (SD) rats [33]. Cysteine-containing peptides derived from meat have apromoting effect on the absorption of non-haem iron in human [72]. Deferrichrysin can be used in food as a food supplement, to prevent colour change and to create iron-fortified foods [89]. A component of traditional Chinese medicine, A 'Jiao (*Collacoriiasini*, donkey-hide gelatine), has been used to enrich the blood for thousands of years in China [90]. Egg white protein is useful for recovery of IDA in SD rats [98]. Soybean sprouts fortified with iron (ferritin) are a good iron supplement with no side effects [53]. Iron-enriched baker's yeast, which contains iron bound to proteins in the yeast cells, is more efficient than inorganic iron in treating anaemic rats [62].

The CPPs derived from casein are important sources of mineral-chelating peptides. The addition of 5–10 g CPPs/100 g soya flour enhanced the level of bioaccessible iron in native and iron-fortified flour to a significant extent [30], and the addition of CPPs in a milk system improved iron binding abilities [99]. Fe uptake compared to that of $FeSO_4$ was significantly increased in tissues (liver, spleen and sacrum) when Fe-β-CN(1–25)4P or $FeSO_4$ was administered once to 10 young females (20–30 years) [100].

Collagen, a major protein constituent of skin, cartilage, and tendons, is also an important source of mineral-chelating peptides. Collagen peptides derived from by-products of *Gadus chalcogrammus*, *Lates calcarifer*, *Mugil cephalus*, *Chanos chanos*, and *Oreochromis* spp. are reported to have iron-chelating ability [24,64]. Collagen peptides derived from deer sinew and fish scales have calcium (calcium is similar to iron) absorption-promoting effects [101,102]. GPAGPHGPPG has been shown to have significant promotional effects on iron transport in Caco-2 cell monolayers [103].

Besides casein and collagen, other proteins, such as soy protein, fish protein, are also hydrolyzed and the resulting hydrolysates have been studied as iron chelation or ironabsorption-promoting peptides.

In conclusion, all of these protein hydrolysates have representative materials that are used in iron supplements, with their structure deciding their properties, but it is hard to compare their promoting effect. However, based on the number of variants, peptides have more advantages for use in iron supplements. Furthermore, di-peptides and tri-peptides have faster absorption rates than amino acids and are more easily absorbed than polypeptides. Therefore, the small peptides, as well as some larger peptides that can be digested down to small peptides, may be more suitable for use in developing new iron supplements.

4.2. Advantagesof Protein Hydrolysates as Non-Haem Iron Promoters

4.2.1. Dual-Purpose Nutrients

Protein hydrolysate iron complexes provide iron for humans and other animals. At the same time, ligands of iron, amino acids and peptides are also important nutrients. A major nutrient, proteins and their hydrolysates can be used to synthesize the basic materials needed by our bodies and can be metabolized to provide energy when they are absorbed. Moreover, peptides and amino acids are safer than other chemical substances in the conditions that they are absorbed and utilized.

4.2.2. Reducing the Side Effects of Iron Ions

Peptides and amino acids with iron-chelating activities can also reduce the production of reactive oxygen species (ROS). ROS are generated in Fenton reactions where iron or other metal ions are involved [31]. ROS are related to the off-flavour of foods [104], as well as a variety of pathologic situations [105]. The reason for this is that ROS promote destructive free-radical reactions in foods or in our bodies. Thus, chelatable protein hydrolysates maintain the quality of foods and reduce the risk of disease while increasing the bioavailability of iron.

Excess iron can be extremely toxic to animals because it catalyses the generation of ROS [106]. Under iron-overload conditions, iron is deposited in organs, such as the liver, heart and pancreas, and damage can then be caused by the production of free radicals. However, protein hydrolysates can reduce the damage caused by iron overload. The compound ferrous gluconate, stabilized with glycine, has a higher liver iron content than ferrous sulfate, and its LD_{50} (median lethal dose) is six times higher than that of ferrous sulfate in SD rats [107]. Glutamylcysteine has been shown to protect the liver against iron overload-induced injury in an iron-overload rat model due to its antioxidant properties and chelation ability [108]. In addition, yeast that is enriched with iron is a less toxic iron source than other iron sources [109].

4.2.3. Bioactivity

Protein hydrolysates and their iron chelates may have some special functions for people and animals, such as acting as an antioxidant and improving immune system activity.

Some peptides or amino acids, such as glutathione, have antioxidant functions and can reduce the production of ROS in vitro and in vivo. Fe-Gly improves the antioxidant status of broiler chickens [110] and protects hypobaric hypoxia-induced tissue injury [111]. S-Allyl cysteine, a sulphur containing amino acid derived from garlic, has a protective effect against alterations to iron metabolism induced by oxidative stress in diabetic rats [112]. Histidine di-peptides, carnosine and *N*-acetyl-carnosine significantly reduce ferritin aggregation and protect against salsolinol-mediated ferritin modification, which is the consequence of free radical scavenging activity [113]. For example, carnosine has antioxidant properties, and it has the ability to react with ROS, reactive nitrogen species and harmful aldehydes [114].

Some protein hydrolysates chelated with iron can improve immune system function. An example is Fe-Gly, which stimulates cellular defence mechanisms by increasing the percentage of Th1 cells and by enhancing the production of cytotoxic CD8+ T cells and IL-2 [115]. The complexing of di-peptide isoleucyl-tryptophan with Fe^{2+} has been studied as an immunomodulatory formulation [22], and hairtail protein hydrolysate-Fe^{2+} complexes increase the growth and non-specific immunity of crayfish [35].

Other functions may also be possessed by protein hydrolysate-iron chelates. For example, ferrous-amino acid chelates can effectively lower blood glucose and improve insulin sensitivity [116], and the collagen peptide-iron complexes may function in promoting skin and bone repair, which is a property possessed by collagen peptides.

In conclusion, complexes of peptides and amino acids with iron are promising iron supplements for three reasons. First, peptides and amino acids are important for nutrition; second, they can decrease the side effects of iron by decreasing the ROS produced by iron ions, as well as the damage caused by iron overload; and third, peptides, amino acids and their iron complexes have special functions and can be used as bioactive ingredients in foods.

4.3. Challenges of Protein Hydrolysates as Non-Haem Iron Promoters

Although many peptides and amino acids have been confirmed to promote iron absorption, some problems still need to be overcome before these iron complexes can be commercialized.

The crucial problem is the stability of the iron complexes. Iron supplements undergo many changes as they are surrounded by many materials during long periods of storage and processing. An iron casein succinylated liquid oral preparation has an unpalatable taste after a long period of storage [117]. Similarly, peptides and amino acids also face the same issues. In addition, the released iron ions undesirably change the colour of water and milk to dark grey. Gastrointestinal stability is also one of the problems that must be overcome. The changes to the chelates that occur during passage through the gastrointestinal tract are still not clear, and we do not know what form of iron arrives at the small intestinal epithelium. A significant proportion of iron in iron bis-glycine chelates is released in the stomach at a low pH [118]. In other words, data concerning the compatibility of peptides, amino acids and hydrolysates with different food matrices, as well as data on their stability during gastrointestinal passage and long-term storage, are needed.

Furthermore, the mechanisms by which protein hydrolysates promote iron absorption remain unclear, and more details are needed. Are there any protein hydrolysate iron complexes that can be absorbed by small intestinal cells via PEPT? Perhaps other transporters and their proportional contributions to total iron absorption should be studied. There are too many iron-chelatable peptides for us to choose from, and new peptides are still being reported. However, we do not know which class of protein hydrolysates or which kind of peptides (amino acids) have better iron promoting effects. It is hard to select the perfect peptide or amino acid for an iron supplement if we do not know its precise mechanism. Furthermore, amino acids and peptides are zwitterions, and they have different dissociated states at different pH values. In addition, they can form one or more rings with iron ions under different conditions. In these cases, their iron complexes will exist in many variations with different equilibrium constants, which is also an issue for their usage. Although most protein hydrolysate iron complexes have been shown to have iron supplementation effects on animals or cells, their use for nutritional or medical purposes are just theoretical and have only been hypothesized. Therefore, there are still additional factors to determine for their use in humans, which need to be tested.

In addition, safety is also a problem. Although protein hydrolysates are relatively safe, some protein hydrolysates may still be allergens, which may cause immunoreactions. Furthermore, the sources of peptides also affect their safety. Non-food proteins and contaminated food proteins, such as venom proteins or proteins from animals with prions, are not safe sources of protein hydrolysates.

5. Conclusions

Protein hydrolysates are promising iron supplements in the form of iron chelates. Iron deficiency is a global issue. The work to find effective and safe iron supplements is never-ending. Much of the literature focuses on protein hydrolysates, which have a promoting effect on iron absorption. Iron chelation ability is thought to be a key factor for the chelating effect of protein hydrolysates. We reviewed the reported iron-chelatable protein hydrolysates and described their structural characteristics. These amino acids and peptides show us that there are abundant sources of iron-chelatable protein hydrolysates. Their relevant characteristics, which include special amino acid compositions, as well as size- and sequence-dependent peptide properties, can guide us to find or synthesize potential iron-chelatable protein hydrolysates.

Protein hydrolysates promote iron absorption in three ways: maintaining the solubility of iron, reducing ferric ions to ferrous ions to keep iron at a low valence state, and promoting the absorption of iron through intestinal cell membranes. Maintaining the solubility of iron, which is related tochelation ability, is of great concern. Reducing ferric ion to ferrous ion with protein hydrolysates or other substrates is also important. However, the method by which iron is carried through the intestinal cell membrane has not been sufficiently studied, and more research should focus on this problem.

Protein hydrolysates can be used in iron supplements as safe food ingredients. Some amino acids, peptides and proteins have been used as iron supplements. Furthermore, protein hydrolysates have some excellent characteristics. First, they can be used as nutrients while promoting iron absorption. Second, their chelation ability can protect individuals from the side effects of iron ions and reduce the damage caused by iron overload. Lastly, they have bioactivities alone and when complexed. Although some protein hydrolysates have been used as iron supplements, many problems still need to be overcome. Their compatibility with different food matrices must be studied systematically. Both their gastrointestinal and long-term storage stabilities also require further investigation. The details of how the complexes are absorbed are still not clear, and we have no rules by which to choose the best peptide or amino acid iron supplement among all of the candidates.

We predict that more and more organic iron supplements will be used and that peptide-iron complexes and amino acids-iron complexes will become popular in the market of iron fortifiers. Similarly, the bioavailability of other minerals, such as zinc, calcium and copper, can also be improved by chelatable peptides or amino acids. Protein hydrolysates have a promising future in the mineral supplement market.

Acknowledgments: This research was supported by the Science and Technology Project of Zhejiang Province, China (Grant No.: 2016C32064). The funding sponsor did not have a role in the design of the study; in the collection, analysis, or interpretation of the data; in the writing of the manuscript; or in the decision to publish the results.

Author Contributions: Yanan Li and Guangrong Huang designed the review. Yanan Li wrote the first draft of the manuscript. Han Jiang and Guangrong Huang revised the manuscript. All authors edited the manuscript and approved the final version.

Conflicts of Interest: The authors declare no conflicts of interest.

References

1. World Health Organization (WHO). *Global Nutrition Targets 2025: Anaemia Policy Brief*; Working Papers; WHO: Geneva, Switzerland, 2016.
2. Baltussen, R.; Knai, C.; Sharan, M. Iron fortification and iron supplementation are cost-effective interventions to reduce iron deficiency in four subregions of the world. *J. Nutr.* **2016**, *134*, 2678–2684.
3. Low, M.; Farrell, A.; Biggs, B.A.; Pasricha, S.R. Effects of daily iron supplementation in primary-school-aged children: Systematic review and meta-analysis of randomized controlled trials. *Can. Med. Assoc. J.* **2013**, *185*, 791–802. [CrossRef] [PubMed]
4. Mfsrh, L.P.; Ffsrh, D.M.; Ffsrh, I.F.D.M. Iron deficiency and iron deficiency anaemia in women. *Best Pract. Res. Clin. Obstet. Gynaecol.* **2017**, *19*, 55–67. [CrossRef]
5. Pineda, O. Iron bis-glycine chelate competes for the non heme-iron absorption pathway. *Am. J. Clin. Nutr.* **2003**, *78*, 495–496. [PubMed]
6. Geisser, P.; Burckhardt, S. The pharmacokinetics and pharmacodynamics of iron preparations. *Pharmaceutics* **2011**, *3*, 12–33. [CrossRef] [PubMed]
7. Pizarro, F.; Olivares, M.; Maciero, E.; Krasnoff, G.; Cócaro, N.; Gaitan, D. Iron Absorption from Two Milk Formulas Fortified with Iron Sulfate Stabilized with Maltodextrin and Citric Acid. *Nutrients* **2015**, *7*, 8952–8959. [CrossRef] [PubMed]
8. Guo, L.; Harnedy, P.A.; Li, B.; Hou, H.; Zhang, Z.; Zhao, X.; Fitzgerald, R.J. Food protein-derived chelating peptides: Biofunctional ingredients for dietary mineral bioavailability enhancement. *Trends Food Sci. Technol.* **2014**, *37*, 92–105. [CrossRef]
9. Ghasemi, S.; Khoshgoftarmanesh, A.H.; Hadadzadeh, H.; Jafari, M. Synthesis of Iron-amino acid chelates and evaluation of their efficacy as iron source and growth stimulator for tomato in nutrient solution culture. *J. Plant Growth Regul.* **2012**, *31*, 498–508. [CrossRef]
10. Zhang, Y.; Yang, Y.; Xue, A.; Li, C. The synthesis of iron chelate with L—Aspartic acid and aspartame. *China Food Ind.* **2009**, *1*, 60–61. (In Chinese)
11. Van Campen, D. Enhancement of iron absorption from ligated segments of rat intestine by histidine, cysteine, and lysine: Effects of removing ionizing groups and of stereoisomerism. *J. Nutr.* **1973**, *103*, 139–142. [PubMed]
12. Bovell-Benjamin, A.C.; Viteri, F.E.; Allen, L.H. Iron absorption from ferrous bisglycinate and ferric trisglycinate in whole maize is regulated by iron status. *Am. J. Clin. Nutr.* **2000**, *71*, 1563–1569. [PubMed]
13. Kwiecien, M.; Samolinska, W.; Bujanowicz-Haras, B. Effects of iron-glycine chelate on growth, carcass characteristic, liver mineral concentrations and haematological and biochemical blood parameters in broilers. *J. Anim. Physiol. Anim. Nutr.* **2015**, *99*, 1184–1196. [CrossRef] [PubMed]
14. Huang, J.; Yu, X.; Diao, L.; Huang, X. Optimization of the preparation process of ferrous glutamate by response surface methodology. *Food Sci.* **2015**, *36*, 81–85. [CrossRef]
15. Djurdjevic, P.; Jelic, R. Solution equilibria in l-glutamic acid and l-serine + iron(III) systems. *Transit. Met. Chem.* **1997**, *22*, 284–293. [CrossRef]

16. Van Campen, D.; Gross, E. Effect of histidine and certain other amino acids on the absorption of iron-59 by rats. *J. Nutr.* **1969**, *99*, 68–74. [PubMed]

17. Tao, J.; Hu, X.; Sun, W.; Nie, S.; Xie, M. Study on antioxidant activity of lipids with iron threonine chelate. *Sci. Technol. Food Ind.* **2012**, *33*, 137–139. [CrossRef]

18. Chen, X.; Lei, X.; Wang, Q.; Du, Z.; Lu, J.; Chen, S.; Zhang, M.; Hao, Z.; Ren, F. Effects of a tripeptide iron on iron-deficiency anemia in rats. *Biol. Trace Elem. Res.* **2015**, *169*, 211–217. [CrossRef]

19. Wang, C.; Li, B.; Jing, A. Separation and identification of zinc-chelating peptides from sesame protein hydrolysate using IMAC-Zn^{2+} and LC-MS/MS. *Food Chem.* **2012**, *134*, 1231–1238. [CrossRef] [PubMed]

20. Zhang, Y.; Sun, X.; Xie, C.; Shu, X.; Oso, A.O.; Ruan, Z.; Deng, Z.Y.; Wu, X.; Yin, Y. Effects of ferrous carbamoyl glycine on iron state and absorption in an iron-deficient rat model. *Genes Nutr.* **2015**, *10*, 1–8. [CrossRef] [PubMed]

21. Lin, H.M.; Deng, S.G.; Zhang, B.; Pang, J. Separation, Structure Identification and Antimicrobial Activity of Ferrous Chelate of Protein Hydrolysate in *Hairtail* (*Hrichiurus haumela*). *J. Sin. Mol. Res.* **2013**, *1*, 2–6. [CrossRef]

22. Kholnazarov, B.M.; Bunyatyan, N.D.; Shakhmatov, A.N.; Bobiev, G.M. Development of an immunotropic drug based on coordination compounds of a synthetic low molecular weight thymus peptide with iron Ions. *Pharm. Chem. J.* **2014**, *48*, 632–634. [CrossRef]

23. Guo, L.; Hou, H.; Li, B.; Zhang, Z.; Wang, S.; Zhao, X. Preparation, isolation and identification of iron-chelating peptides derived from Alaska pollock skin. *Process Biochem.* **2013**, *48*, 988–993. [CrossRef]

24. Guo, L.; Harnedy, P.A.; O'Keeffe, M.B.; Li, Z.; Li, B.; Hu, H.; Fitzgerald, R.J. Fractionation and identification of Alaska pollock skin collagen-derived mineral chelating peptides. *Food Chem.* **2015**, *173*, 536–542. [CrossRef] [PubMed]

25. Eckert, E.; Lu, L.; Unsworth, L.D.; Chen, L.; Xie, J.; Xu, R. Biophysical and in vitro absorption studies of iron chelating peptide from barley proteins. *J. Funct. Foods* **2016**, *25*, 291–301. [CrossRef]

26. Argyri, K.; Miller, D.D.; Glahn, R.P.; Zhu, L.; Kapsokefalou, M. Peptides isolated from in vitro digests of milk enhance iron uptake by Caco-2 cells. *J. Agric. Food Chem.* **2007**, *55*, 10221–10225. [CrossRef] [PubMed]

27. Wu, H.; Liu, Z.; Zhao, Y.; Zeng, M. Enzymatic preparation and characterization of iron-chelating peptides from anchovy (*Engraulis japonicus*) muscle protein. *Food Res. Int.* **2012**, *48*, 435–441. [CrossRef]

28. Jaiswal, A.; Bajaj, R.; Mann, B.; Lata, K. Iron (II)-chelating activity of buffalo α$_S$-casein hydrolysed by corolase PP, alcalase and flavourzyme. *J. Food Sci. Technol.* **2015**, *52*, 3911–3918. [CrossRef] [PubMed]

29. Garcíanebot, M.J.; Alegría, A.; Barberá, R.; Gaboriau, F.; Bouhallab, S. Effect of caseinophosphopeptides from αs- and β-Casein on iron bioavailability in HuH7 cells. *J. Agric. Food Chem.* **2015**, *63*, 6757–6763. [CrossRef] [PubMed]

30. Prakash, D.; Lakshmi, A.J. Preparation of caseinophosphopeptides and assessing their efficacy in enhancing the bioaccessibility of iron and zinc. *J. Food Sci. Technol.* **2015**, *52*, 7493–7499. [CrossRef]

31. Torres-Fuentes, C.; Alaiz, M.; Vioque, J. Iron-chelating activity of chickpea protein hydrolysate peptides. *Food Chem.* **2012**, *134*, 1585–1588. [CrossRef] [PubMed]

32. Cai, B.N.; Chen, X.; Pan, J.Y.; Deng, W.H.; Wan, P.; Chen, D.K.; Sun, H.L. Optimization of preparation process for cod skin collagen peptide-iron (II) Chelate via Response Surface Methodology. *Food Sci.* **2012**, *33*, 48–52. [CrossRef]

33. Suzuki, S.; Fukuda, K.; Irie, M.; Hata, Y. Iron chelated cyclic peptide, ferrichrysin, for oral treatment of iron deficiency: Solution properties and efficacy in anemic rats. *Int. J. Vitam. Nutr. Res.* **2007**, *77*, 13–21. [CrossRef] [PubMed]

34. Lin, H.M.; Deng, S.G.; Huang, S.B.; Li, Y.J.; Song, R. The effect of ferrous-chelating hairtail peptides on iron deficiency and intestinal flora in rats. *J. Sci. Food Agric.* **2015**, *96*, 2839–2844. [CrossRef] [PubMed]

35. Zhang, B.; Shi, Z.R.; Wang, X.L.; Deng, S.G. The effects of hairtail protein hydrolysate-Fe^{2+} complexes on growth and non-specific immune response of red swamp crayfish (*Procambarus clarkii*). *Aquac. Int.* **2016**, *24*, 1039–1048. [CrossRef]

36. Wang, P.F.; Huang, G.R.; Jiang, J.X. Optimization of hydrolysis conditions for the production of iron-binding peptides from mackerel processing byproducts. *Adv. J. Food Sci. Technol.* **2013**, *5*, 921–925.

37. Lin, H.M.; Deng, S.G.; Huang, S.B. Antioxidant activities of ferrous-chelating peptides isolated from five types of low-value fish protein hydrolysates. *J. Food Biochem.* **2014**, *38*, 627–633. [CrossRef]

38. Figueroa-Hernández, C.; Cruz-Guerrero, A.; Rodríguez-Serrano, G.; Gómez-Ruiz, L.; García-Garibay, M.; Jiménez-Guzmán, J. Calcium and iron binding peptides production by *Lactococcus lactis* sp. Cremoris NCFB 712. *Rev. Mex. Ing. Quím.* **2012**, *11*, 259–267.

39. Blat, D.; Weiner, L.; Youdim, M.B.; Fridkin, M. A novel iron-chelating derivative of the neuroprotective peptide NAPVSIPQ shows superior antioxidant and antineurodegenerative capabilities. *J. Med. Chem.* **2008**, *51*, 126–134. [CrossRef] [PubMed]

40. Lee, S.H.; Song, K.B. Purification of an iron-binding nona-peptide from hydrolysates of porcine blood plasma protein. *Process Biochem.* **2009**, *44*, 378–381. [CrossRef]

41. Cao, Y.; Chen, Q.; Xiong, H.; Liang, L. Optimal conditions for preparing iron chelate of enzymic hydrolysis peptides from rice protein. *Food Ferment. Ind.* **2007**, *33*, 61–64. [CrossRef]

42. Zhang, W.; Li, Y.; Zhang, J.; Huang, G. Optimization of hydrolysis conditions for the production of iron-binding peptides from Scad (*Decapterus maruadsi*) processing byproducts. *Am. J. Biochem. Biotechnol.* **2016**. [CrossRef]

43. Cian, R.E.; Garzón, A.G.; Ancona, D.B.; Guerrero, L.C.; Drago, S.R. Chelating properties of peptides from red seaweed *Pyropia columbina* and its effect on iron bio-accessibility. *Plant Foods Hum. Nutr.* **2016**, *71*, 1–6. [CrossRef] [PubMed]

44. Cho, H.J.; Lee, H.-S.; Jung, E.Y.; Park, S.Y.; Lim, W.-T.; Lee, J.-Y.; Yeon, S.-H.; Lee, J.-C.; Suh, H.J. Manufacturing of iron binding peptide using sericin hydrolysate and its bioavailability in iron deficient Rat. *J. Korean Soc. Food Sci. Nutr.* **2010**, *39*, 1446–1451. [CrossRef]

45. Huang, G.; Ren, Z.; Jiang, J.; Chen, W. Purification of a hepta-peptide with iron binding activity from shrimp processing by-products hydrolysates. *Adv. J. Food Sci. Technol.* **2012**, *4*, 207–212. [CrossRef]

46. Huang, G.R.; Ren, Z.Y.; Jiang, J.X. Optimization of hydrolysis conditions for iron binding peptides production from shrimp processing byproducts. *Am. J. Food Technol.* **2014**, *9*, 49–55. [CrossRef]

47. Kim, N.H.; Jung, S.H.; Kim, J.; Kim, S.H.; Ahn, H.J.; Song, K.B. Purification of an iron-chelating peptide from spirulina protein hydrolysates. *J. Korean Soc. Appl. Biol. Chem.* **2014**, *57*, 91–95. [CrossRef]

48. Lv, Y.; Liu, Q.; Bao, X.; Tang, W.; Yang, B.; Guo, S. Identification and characteristics of iron-chelating peptides from soybean protein hydrolysates using IMAC-Fe^{3+}. *J. Agric. Food Chem.* **2009**, *57*, 4593–4597. [CrossRef] [PubMed]

49. Lv, Y.; Bao, X.; Liu, H.; Ren, J.; Guo, S. Purification and characterization of calcium-binding soybean protein hydrolysates by Ca^{2+}/Fe^{3+} immobilized metal affinity chromatography (IMAC). *Food Chem.* **2013**, *141*, 1645–1650. [CrossRef] [PubMed]

50. Wakabayashi, T.; Yamamoto, M.; Hirai, Y. Absorption and availability of iron peptide in pregnant sows. *Bull. Nippon Vet. Zootech. Coll.* **1989**, *38*, 93–105.

51. Zhang, M.N.; Huang, G.R.; Jiang, J.X. Iron binding capacity of dephytinised soy protein isolate hydrolysate as influenced by the degree of hydrolysis and enzyme type. *J. Food Sci. Technol.* **2014**, *51*, 994–999. [CrossRef] [PubMed]

52. Caetano-Silva, M.E.; Cilla, A.; Bertoldo-Pacheco, M.T.; Netto, F.M.; Alegría, A. Evaluation of in vitro iron bioavailability in free form and as whey peptide-iron complexes. *J. Food Compos. Anal.* **2017**. [CrossRef]

53. Małgorzata, K.; Małgorzata, E.; Ewa, I.; Teresa, A.; Hanna, S.; Magdalena, Z.-D.; Dorota, P.-K.; Jadwiga, J.-L. Evaluation of safety of iron-fortified soybean sprouts, a potential component of functional food, in rat. *Plant Foods Hum. Nutr.* **2016**, *71*, 1–6. [CrossRef]

54. And, M.Z.; Hearn, M.T.W. Application of immobilized metal ion chelate complexes as pseudocation exchange adsorbents for protein separation. *Biochemistry* **1996**, *35*, 202–211. [CrossRef]

55. Zhu, C.; Liu, L.; Deng, J.; Ma, X.; Hui, J.; Fan, D. Formation mechanism and biological activity of novel thiolated human-like collagen iron complex. *J. Biomater. Appl.* **2016**, *30*, 1205–1218. [CrossRef] [PubMed]

56. Shilpashree, B.G.; Arora, S.; Sharma, V. Preparation of iron/zinc bound whey protein concentrate complexes and their stability. *Lebensm.-Wiss. Technol.* **2015**, *66*, 514–522. [CrossRef]

57. Freeman, H.J. Clinical relevance of intestinal peptide uptake. *World J. Gastrointest. Pharmacol. Ther.* **2015**, *6*, 22–27. [CrossRef] [PubMed]

58. Glahn, R.P.; Van Campen, D.R. Iron uptake is enhanced in Caco-2 cell monolayers by cysteine and reduced cysteinyl glycine. *J. Nutr.* **1997**, *127*, 642–647. [PubMed]

59. Geissler, S.; Hellwig, M.; Markwardt, F.; Henle, T.; Brandsch, M. Synthesis and intestinal transport of the iron chelator maltosine in free and dipeptide form. *Eur. J. Pharm. Biopharm.* **2011**, *78*, 75–82. [CrossRef] [PubMed]

60. Vij, R.; Reddi, S.; Kapila, S.; Kapila, R. Transepithelial transport of milk derived bioactive peptide VLPVPQK. *Food Chem.* **2016**, *190*, 681–688. [CrossRef] [PubMed]

61. Morishita, M.; Peppas, N.A. Is the oral route possible for peptide and protein drug delivery? *Drug Discov. Today* **2006**, *11*, 905–910. [CrossRef] [PubMed]

62. Kyyaly, M.A.; Powell, C.; Ramadan, E. Preparation of iron-enriched baker's yeast and its efficiency in recovery of rats from dietary iron deficiency. *Nutrition* **2015**, *31*, 1155–1164. [CrossRef] [PubMed]

63. Palika, R.; Mashurabad, P.C.; Nair, M.K.; Reddy, G.B.; Pullakhandam, R. Characterization of iron-binding phosphopeptide released by gastrointestinal digestion of egg white. *Food Res. Int.* **2015**, *67*, 308–314. [CrossRef]

64. Huang, C.Y.; Wu, C.H.; Yang, J.I.; Li, Y.H.; Kuo, J.M. Evaluation of iron-binding activity of collagen peptides prepared from the scales of four cultivated fishes in Taiwan. *J. Food Drug Anal.* **2015**, *23*, 671–678. [CrossRef]

65. Falanga, A.; Galdiero, M.; Galdiero, S. Membranotropic cell penetrating peptides: The outstanding journey. *Int. J. Mol. Sci.* **2015**, *16*, 25323–25337. [CrossRef] [PubMed]

66. Katayama, N.; Nozaki, Y.; Okonogi, K.; Harada, S.; Ono, H. Ferrocins, new iron-containing peptide antibiotics produced by bacteria. Taxonomy, fermentation and biological activity. *J. Antibiot.* **1993**, *46*, 65–70. [CrossRef] [PubMed]

67. ReyesMéndez, A.I.; Figueroa-Hernández, C.; Melgar-Lalanne, G.; Hernández-Sánchez, H.; Dávila-Ortiz, G.; Jiménez-Martínez, C. Production of calcium- and iron-binding peptides by probiotic strains of *Bacillus subtilis*, *B. clausii* and *B. coagulans* GBI-30. *Rev. Mex. Ing. Quím.* **2015**, *14*, 239–245.

68. Barnes, C.L.; Eng-Wilmot, D.L.; Helm, D.V.D. Ferricrocin ($C_{29}H_{44}FeN_9O_{13}.7H_2O$), an iron(III)-binding peptide from *Aspergillus versicolor*. *Acta Crystallogr. Sect. C* **1984**, *40*, 922–926. [CrossRef]

69. Zachariou, M.; Hearn, M.T.W. Protein selectivity in immobilized metal affinity chromatography based on the surface accessibility of aspartic and glutamic acid residues. *J. Protein Chem.* **1995**, *14*, 419–430. [CrossRef] [PubMed]

70. Gurd, F.R.N.; Wilcox, P.E. Complex formation between metallic cations and proteins, peptides, and amino acids. *Adv. Protein Chem.* **1956**, *11*, 311–427. [CrossRef] [PubMed]

71. Amadou, I.; Le, G.W.; Shi, Y.H.; Jin, S. Reducing, Reducing, radical scavenging, and chelation properties of fermented soy protein meal hydrolysate by lactobacillus plantarum lp6. *Int. J. Food Prop.* **2011**, *14*, 654–665. [CrossRef]

72. Taylor, P.G.; Martínez-Torres, C.; Romano, E.L.; Layrisse, M. The effect of cysteine-containing peptides released during meat digestion on iron absorption in humans. *Am. J. Clin. Nutr.* **1986**, *43*, 68–71. [PubMed]

73. García-Nebot, M.J.; Barberá, R.; Alegría, A. Iron and zinc bioavailability in Caco-2 cells: Influence of caseinophosphopeptides. *Food Chem.* **2013**, *138*, 1298–1303. [CrossRef] [PubMed]

74. Na, S.; Cui, P.; Jin, Z.; Wu, H.; Wang, Y.; Lin, S. Contributions of molecular size, charge distribution, and specific amino acids to the iron-binding capacity of sea cucumber (*Stichopus japonicus*) ovum hydrolysates. *Food Chem.* **2017**, *230*, 627–636. [CrossRef]

75. Fillebeen, C.; Gkouvatsos, K.; Fragoso, G.; Calve, A.; Garcia-Santos, D.; Buffler, M.; Becker, C.; Schumann, K.; Ponka, P.; Santos, M.M.; et al. Mice are poor heme absorbers and do not require intestinal Hmox1 for dietary heme iron assimilation. *Haematologica* **2015**, *100*, 334–337. [CrossRef] [PubMed]

76. Taghavi, S.; Amiri, A.; Amin, A.; Ehsani, A.; Maleki, M.; Naderi, N. Oral iron therapy with polysaccharide-iron complex may be useful in increasing the ferritin level for a short time in patients with dilated cardiomyopathy. *Res. Cardiovasc. Med.* **2016**. [CrossRef]

77. Cao, C.; Thomas, C.E.; Insogna, K.L.; O'Brien, K.O. Duodenal absorption and tissue utilization of dietary heme and nonheme iron differ in rats. *J. Nutr.* **2014**, *144*, 1710–1717. [CrossRef] [PubMed]

78. Santos, T.; Connolly, C.; Murphy, R. Trace element inhibition of phytase activity. *Biol. Trace Elem. Res.* **2015**, *163*, 255–265. [CrossRef] [PubMed]

79. Cilla, A.; Perales, S.; Lagarda, M.J.; Barbera, R.; Farre, R. Iron bioavailability in fortified fruit beverages using ferritin synthesis by Caco-2 cells. *J. Agric. Food Chem.* **2008**, *56*, 8699–8703. [CrossRef] [PubMed]

80. Kibangou, I.B.; Bouhallab, S.; Henry, G.; Bureau, F.; Allouche, S.; Blais, A.; Guérin, P.; Arhan, P.; Bouglé, G.L. Milk proteins and iron absorption: Contrasting effects of different caseinophosphopeptides. *Pediatric Res.* **2005**, *58*, 731–734. [CrossRef] [PubMed]

81. Pérès, J.M.; Bouhallab, S.; Bureau, F.; Neuville, D.; Maubois, J.L.; Devroede, G.; Arhan, P.; Bouglé, D. Mechanisms of absorption of caseinophosphopeptide bound iron. *J. Nutr. Biochem.* **1999**, *10*, 215–222. [CrossRef]

82. Ma, W.-Q.; Wu, J.; Zhuo, Z.; Sun, H.; Yue, M.; Feng, J. Comparison of Absorption Characteristics of Iron Glycine Chelate and Ferrous Sulfate in Caco-2 Cells. *Int. J. Agric. Biol.* **2013**, *15*, 372–376.

83. Zhuo, Z.; Fang, S.; Yue, M.; Zhang, Y.; Feng, J. Kinetics absorption characteristics of ferrous glycinate in SD rats and its impact on the relevant transport protein. *Biol. Trace Elem. Res.* **2014**, *158*, 197–202. [CrossRef] [PubMed]

84. Bouhallab, S.; Bouglé, D. Biopeptides of milk: Caseinophosphopeptides and mineral bioavailability. *Reprod. Nutr. Dev.* **2004**, *44*, 493–498. [CrossRef] [PubMed]

85. Hoz, L.D.L.; Silva, V.S.N.D.; Morgano, M.A.; Pacheco, M.T.B. Small peptides from enzymatic whey hydrolyzates increase dialyzable iron. *Int. Dairy J.* **2014**, *38*, 145–147. [CrossRef]

86. Fouad, G.T.; Evans, M.; Sharma, P.; Baisley, J.; Crowley, D.; Guthrie, N. A randomized, double-blind clinical study on the safety and tolerability of an iron multi-amino acid chelate preparation in premenopausal women. *J. Diet. Suppl.* **2013**, *10*, 17–28. [CrossRef] [PubMed]

87. Bisbe, E.; Molto, L.; Arroyo, R.; Muniesa, J.M.; Tejero, M. Randomized trial comparing ferric Carboxymaltose vs oral ferrous glycine sulphate for postoperative anaemia after total knee arthroplasty. *Br. J. Anaesth.* **2014**, *113*, 402–409. [CrossRef] [PubMed]

88. Yin, Y.; Wu, X.; Shu, X. A Kind of Dipeptide-Iron Used for Feed Supplement and Its Preparation Method. CN201010540740.6, 2 November 2011.

89. Galaffu, N.; Habeych Narvaez, E.A.; Ho Dac, T.; Sabatier, M. Food Composition Comprising Desferrichrysin. WO 2014/111532 A1, 24 July 2014.

90. Li, W.L.; Han, H.F.; Zhang, L.; Zhang, Y.; Qu, H.B. Manufacturer identification and storage time determination of "Dong'e Ejiao" using near infrared spectroscopy and chemometrics. *J. Zhejiang Univ.-Sci. B Biomed. Biotechnol.* **2016**, *17*, 382–390. [CrossRef] [PubMed]

91. Kongkachuichai, R.; Yasumoto, K. Effects of amino acids and dipeptides on the uptake and transport of iron by Caco-2 cells cultured in serum-free medium. *Food Sci. Technol. Int.* **1997**, *3*, 279–284. [CrossRef]

92. Abdel Moety, G.A.; Ali, A.M.; Fouad, R.; Ramadan, W.; Belal, D.S.; Haggag, H.M. Amino acid chelated iron versus an iron salt in the treatment of iron deficiency anemia with pregnancy: A randomized controlled study. *Eur. J. Obstet. Gynecol. Reprod. Biol.* **2017**, *210*, 242–246. [CrossRef] [PubMed]

93. Rojas, M.L.; Sanchez, J.; Villada, O.; Montoya, L.; Diaz, A.; Vargas, C.; Chica, J.; Herrera, A.M. Effectiveness of iron amino acid chelate versus ferrous sulfate as part of a food complement in preschool children with iron deficiency, Medellin, 2011. *Biomedica* **2013**, *33*, 350–360. [CrossRef] [PubMed]

94. Shi, R.; Liu, D.; Sun, J.; Jia, Y.; Zhang, P. Effect of replacing dietary FeSO$_4$ with equal Fe-levelled iron glycine chelate on broiler chickens. *Czech J. Anim. Sci.* **2015**, *60*, 233–239. [CrossRef]

95. Layrisse, M.; Garcia-Casal, M.N.; Solano, L.; Baron, M.A.; Arguello, F.; Llovera, D.; Ramirez, J.; Leets, I.; Tropper, E. Iron bioavailability in humans from breakfasts enriched with iron bis-glycine chelate, phytates and polyphenols. *J. Nutr.* **2000**, *130*, 2195–2199. [PubMed]

96. Osman, A.K.; Al-Othaimeen, A. Experience with ferrous bis-glycine chelate as an iron fortificant in milk. *Int. J. Vitam. Nutr. Res.* **2002**, *72*, 257–263. [CrossRef] [PubMed]

97. Layrisse, M.; Martínez-Torres, C.; Leets, I.; Taylor, P.; Ramírez, J. Effect of histidine, cysteine, glutathione or beef on iron absorption in humans. *J. Nutr.* **1984**, *114*, 217–223. [PubMed]

98. Kobayashi, Y.; Wakasugi, E.; Yasui, R.; Kuwahata, M.; Kido, Y. Egg Yolk Protein Delays Recovery while Ovalbumin Is Useful in Recovery from Iron Deficiency Anemia. *Nutrients* **2015**, *7*, 4792–4803. [CrossRef] [PubMed]

99. Smialowska, A.; Matiamerino, L.; Carr, A.J. Assessing the iron chelation capacity of goat casein digest isolates. *J. Dairy Sci.* **2017**, *100*, 2553–2563. [CrossRef] [PubMed]

100. Ait-Oukhatar, N.; Peres, J.M.; Bouhallab, S.; Neuville, D.; Bureau, F.; Bouvard, G.; Arhan, P.; Bougle, D. Bioavailability of caseinophosphopeptide-bound iron. *J. Lab. Clin. Med.* **2002**, *140*, 290–294. [CrossRef] [PubMed]

101. Zhang, H.; Dong, Y.; Qi, B.; Liu, L.; Zhou, G.; Bai, X.; Yang, C.; Zhao, D.; Zhao, Y. Preventive effects of collagen Peptide from deer sinew on bone loss in ovariectomized rats. *Evid. Based Complement. Altern. Med.* **2014**, *2014*, 627285. [CrossRef] [PubMed]

102. Huang, B.-B.; Lin, H.-C.; Chang, Y.-W. Analysis of proteins and potential bioactive peptides from tilapia (*Oreochromis* spp.) processing co-products using proteomic techniques coupled with BIOPEP database. *J. Funct. Foods* **2015**, *19*, 629–640. [CrossRef]

103. Chen, Q.; Guo, L.; Du, F.; Chen, T.; Hou, H.; Li, B. The chelating peptide (GPAGPHGPPG) derived from Alaska pollock skin enhances calcium, zinc and iron transport in Caco-2 cells. *Int. J. Food Sci. Technol.* **2017**, *52*, 1283–1290. [CrossRef]

104. Torresfuentes, C.; Alaiz, M.; Vioque, J. Affinity purification and characterisation of chelating peptides from chickpea protein hydrolysates. *J. Neurochem.* **2011**, *98*, 1746–1762. [CrossRef]

105. Delgado, M.C.O.; Galleano, M.; Añón, M.C.; Tironi, V.A. Amaranth peptides from simulated gastrointestinal digestion: Antioxidant activity against reactive species. *Plant Foods Hum. Nutr.* **2015**, *70*, 27–34. [CrossRef] [PubMed]

106. Wang, L.; Pan, Y.; Yuan, Z.H.; Zhang, H.; Peng, B.Y.; Wang, F.F.; Qian, W. Two-component signaling system VgrRS directly senses extracytoplasmic and intracellular iron to control bacterial adaptation under iron depleted stress. *Pathogens* **2016**. [CrossRef] [PubMed]

107. Lysionek, A.E.; Zubillaga, M.B.; Salgueiro, M.J.; Caro, R.A.; Leonardi, N.M.; Ettlin, E.; Boccio, J.R. Stabilized ferrous gluconate as iron source for food fortification: Bioavailability and toxicity. *Biol. Trace Elem. Res.* **2003**, *94*, 73–77. [CrossRef]

108. Salama, S.A.; Al-Harbi, M.S.; Abdel-Bakky, M.S.; Omar, H.A. Glutamyl cysteine dipeptide suppresses ferritin expression and alleviates liver injury in iron-overload rat model. *Biochimie* **2015**, *115*, 203–211. [CrossRef] [PubMed]

109. Pas, M.; Piskur, B.; Sustaric, M.; Raspor, P. Iron enriched yeast biomass—A promising mineral feed supplement. *Bioresour. Technol.* **2007**, *98*, 1622–1628. [CrossRef] [PubMed]

110. Ma, W.Q.; Sun, H.; Zhou, Y.; Wu, J.; Feng, J. Effects of iron glycine chelate on growth, tissue mineral concentrations, fecal mineral excretion, and liver antioxidant enzyme activities in broilers. *Biol. Trace Elem. Res.* **2012**, *149*, 204–211. [CrossRef] [PubMed]

111. Xu, C.; Chen, D.; Xu, C.; Han, T.; Sheng, B.; Gao, X. Effect of iron supplementation on the expression of hypoxia-Inducible factor and antioxidant status in rats exposed to high-altitude hypoxia environment. *Biol. Trace Elem. Res.* **2014**, *162*, 142–152. [CrossRef] [PubMed]

112. Saravanan, G.; Ponmurugan, P.; Begum, M.S. Effect of S-allylcysteine, a sulphur containing amino acid on iron metabolism in streptozotocin induced diabetic rats. *J. Trace Elem. Med. Biol.* **2013**, *27*, 143–147. [CrossRef] [PubMed]

113. Kang, J.H. Salsolinol, a catechol neurotoxin, induces modification of ferritin: Protection by histidine dipeptide. *Environ. Toxicol. Pharmacol.* **2010**, *29*, 246–251. [CrossRef] [PubMed]

114. Yılmaz, Z.; Kalaz, E.B.; Aydın, A.F.; Soluktekkeşin, M.; Doğruabbasoğlu, S.; Uysal, M.; Koçaktoker, N. The effect of carnosine on methylglyoxal-induced oxidative stress in rats. *Arch. Physiol. Biochem.* **2017**, *123*, 1–7. [CrossRef] [PubMed]

115. Jarosz, L.; Kwiecien, M.; Marek, A.; Gradzki, Z.; Winiarska-Mieczan, A.; Kalinowski, M.; Laskowska, E. Effects of feed supplementation with glycine chelate and iron sulfate on selected parameters of cell-mediated immune response in broiler chickens. *Res. Vet. Sci.* **2016**, *107*, 68–74. [CrossRef] [PubMed]

116. Lin, T.Y.; Jan, H.J.; Fu, C.H.; Chen, T.T.; Chen, M.K.; Lee, H.M. Use of Composition Containing Iron(II) Amino Acid Chelate in Preparation of Drug for Ameliorating Diabetes. U.S. Patent 2017/0007568 A1, 12 January 2017.

117. Min, K.A.; Cho, J.H.; Song, Y.K.; Kim, C.K. Iron casein succinylate-chitosan coacervate for the liquid oral delivery of iron with bioavailability and stability enhancement. *Arch. Pharm. Res.* **2016**, *39*, 94–102. [CrossRef] [PubMed]

118. Pizarro, F.; Olivares, M.; Hertrampf, E.; Mazariegos, D.I.; Arredondo, M.; Letelier, A.; Gidi, V. Iron bis-glycine chelate competes for the nonheme-iron absorption pathway. *Am. J. Clin. Nutr.* **2002**, *76*, 577–581. [PubMed]

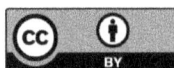

nutrients MDPI

Article

Despite Inflammation, Supplemented Essential Amino Acids May Improve Circulating Levels of Albumin and Haemoglobin in Patients after Hip Fractures

Roberto Aquilani [1], Ginetto Carlo Zuccarelli [2], Anna Maria Condino [3], Michele Catani [2], Carla Rutili [2], Consiglia Del Vecchio [2], Pietro Pisano [2], Manuela Verri [1], Paolo Iadarola [4], Simona Viglio [5] and Federica Boschi [3,*]

[1]   Dipartimento di Biologia e Biotecnologie Università degli Studi di Pavia, Via Ferrata, 1. I-27100 Pavia, Italy; dottore.aquilani@gmail.com (R.A.); manuela.verri@unipv.it (M.V.)
[2]   Istituto Geriatrico P. Redaelli -Reparti di Riabilitazione Geriatrica e di Mantenimento, Via Leopardi, 3. I-20090 Vimodrone, Milano, Italy; zuccarelli1@msn.com (G.C.Z.), m.catani@golgiredaelli.it (M.C.); c.rutili@golgiredaelli.it (C.R.); lidiadelvecchio@libero.it (C.D.V.); p.pisano@golgiredaelli.it (P.P.)
[3]   Dipartimento di Scienze del Farmaco, Università degli Studi di Pavia, Viale Taramelli, 14. I-27100 Pavia, Italy; annamaria.condino@unipv.it
[4]   Dipartimento di Biologia e Biotecnologie Università degli Studi di Pavia, Via Ferrata, 1. I-27100 Pavia, Italy; paolo.iadarola@unipv.it
[5]   Dipartimento di Medicina Molecolare, Università degli Studi di Pavia, Viale Taramelli, 3/B. I-27100 Pavia, Italy; simona.viglio@unipv.it
*   Correspondence: federica.boschi@unipv.it; Tel.: +39-038-298-7398; Fax: +39-038-298-7405

Received: 12 April 2017; Accepted: 15 June 2017; Published: 21 June 2017

Abstract: Essential amino acids (EAAs) are nutritional substrates that promote body protein synthesis; thus we hypothesised that their supplementation may improve circulating albumin (Alb) and haemoglobin (Hb) in rehabilitative elderly patients following hip fractures (HF). Out of the 145 HF patients originally enrolled in our study, 112 completed the protocol. These subjects were divided into two randomised groups, each containing 56 patients. For a period of two months, one group (age 81.4 ± 8.1 years; male/female 27/29) received a placebo, and the other (age 83.1 ± 7.5 years; male/female 25/31) received 4 + 4 g/day oral EAAs. At admission, the prevalence of both hypoAlb (<3.5 g/dL) and hypoHb (<13 g/dL male, <12 g/dL female) was similar in the placebo group (64.3% hypoAlb, 66% hypoHb) and the treated group of patients (73.2% hypoAlb, 67.8% hypoHb). At discharge, however, the prevalence of hypoAlb had reduced more in EAAs than in placebo subjects (31.7% in EAAs vs. 77.8% in placebo; $p < 0.001$). There was a 34.2% reduction of anaemia in hypoHb in EAA subjects and 18.9% in placebo subjects, but the difference was not statistically significant. Oral supplementation of EAAs improves hypoAlb and, to a lesser extent, Hb in elderly rehabilitative subjects with hip fractures. Anaemia was reduced in more than one third of patients, which, despite not being statistically significant, may be clinically relevant.

Keywords: albumin; haemoglobin; essential aminoacids; elderly hip fracture

1. Introduction

Circulating albumin (Alb) and haemoglobin (Hb) proteins are considered to be indicators of the status of general health [1] both in community and clinical settings (acute-, long-term care-, rehabilitation-environments). Low Alb in community-dwelling healthy elderly individuals is independently associated with poorer performance [2] and predicts a greater decline in functional status [2,3]. However, in a clinical setting, low Alb correlates with disease severity and mortality [1,4,5], predicts a prolonged hospital stay, and increases the complication rate and all-cause mortality [5–7]. In institutionalised populations, subjects with hypo-albuminemia (hypoAlb) have increased mortality, which is independent of age, sex, medication use, or protein intake [8]. In the rehabilitation ward, an increase in Alb in elderly patients with hip fractures [9] or ischemic strokes [10] predicts higher functional independence in patients.

With regard to Hb, reduced protein blood levels predispose community-dwelling elderly individuals to the frailty syndrome [11] by inducing alterations in skeletal muscle mass density and strength, which are both responsible for impaired physical performance [12], increased risk of disability [13,14], and impaired quality of life [15]. Moreover, low Hb has been documented to be an independent factor of increased mortality [16,17] in hospitalized medical and surgical patients, and the degree of anaemia is associated with short-term mortality in many studies [18].

One of the patient populations that suffers from anaemia is elderly individuals with hip fractures (HF). The prevalence of anaemia observed in elderly HF at discharge from surgical wards is very high (84%) [19] due to significant blood loss following fractures, surgery, and possible post-operative complications. For the first few days after surgery, anaemia is one of the main factors that delays patient mobilisation [20]. Early mobilisation is the best predictor of both a patient's reduced mortality over one year after trauma and discharge from hospital [21].

Interestingly, Alb and Hb seem to be interrelated and to vary in the same way in older subjects [22]. Alb has been observed to be 1 g/L lower in anaemic individuals compared to normal subjects, and anaemia is associated with a seven-fold higher chance of hypoAlb [22].

Based on all of these studies, we believe that physicians should try to decrease hypoAlb and/or anaemia during a patient's hospital stay. Even though this is also true for Hb, its levels do not seem to negatively influence functional independence either in the acute rehabilitation period [23], or later on after hospital discharge [24]. We believe that Hb improvement should be pursued because anaemia is associated with several adverse outcomes such as the development of cardiovascular and renal diseases [20], death, functional dependence, dementia, and falls [25–28].

As a consequence, improving both hypoAlb and anaemia is of great importance for both individual health and the economic sustainability of the health system. However, improving these circulating proteins in patients with inflammation following trauma and surgery may be difficult, particularly when patients have inadequate protein-energy intakes [29].

In the current study, we aimed to investigate whether supplementation with essential amino acids (EAAs) could improve hypoAlb and anaemia in rehabilitative elderly subjects with HF surgery and mild hypoAlb and anaemia (i.e., not requiring Alb intravenous infusion or transfusion, testosterone, or erythropoietin use). Although a previous study found a negative effect of amino acid supplement on glucose homeostasis, inflammatory markers, and incretins after laparoscopic gastric bypass (Breitman I J Am Coll Surg 2011), we believed there was a strong rationale for using EAAs.

Firstly, these substrates boost protein synthesis [30]. This has even been found to occur during severe inflammation such as that induced by endotoxin [31]; secondly, EAAs have been reported to increase albumin concentrations in sarcopenic patients with chronic obstructive pulmonary disease [32] and in elderly institutionalised individuals [33]; and thirdly, EAAs increase Hb concentrations in haemodialysed subjects [34].

Lastly, EAAs can reduce infection, which negatively impacts albumin and HB syntheses [35].

We therefore studied a cohort of elderly patients admitted to our Geriatric Intensive Rehabilitation Institute after surgery for HF.

2. Subjects and Methods

2.1. Population and Measures

The patients enrolled in this study were consecutively admitted between 1 December 2009 and 30 November 2010. They came straight from the Department of Orthopaedic surgery 20 ± 5 days after undergoing HF surgery. They were all clinically stable and thus received active rehabilitation therapy after surgery for pertrocanteric or sub capital HF. Patients were included independently of their serum levels of Alb because, even within the normal range of values, lower levels of the protein could put the patient at risk of mortality and disease [8]. Furthermore, Alb levels that are higher than the clinical cut-off of 3.8 g/dL are associated with a future loss of skeletal muscle mass (sarcopenia) [2].

The exclusion criteria for patients in our study were as follows: antibiotic therapy on admission, body temperature >36.8 °C, diabetes on insulin treatment, cancer or non-operated cancer, pressure ulcer(s), haematological cancer, acute or advanced chronic renal failure (serum creatinine >2 mg/dL), heart failure, or cognitive alterations (Mini Mental State Examination, <24 scores).

All subjects gave their informed consent for inclusion before they participated in the study. The study was conducted in accordance with the Declaration of Helsinki, and the protocol was approved by the Ethics Committee of the Institute (Direzione Generale/Atti/2008/FF/ R002/13.2.2008).

During the first 48 h after admission, patients underwent the following assessments:

(1) Anthropometric measurements: body weight (kg) was determined using a mechanical weight lifter; height (m) was calculated from knee height [36]; body mass index (BMI) was calculated as kg/m^2; although 70% of patients were able to stand up, we preferred to weigh them by mechanical lifter to avoid instability when they were on the base of the weighing scale.
(2) After overnight fasting, at 7:00 a.m. blood samples were taken from peripheral veins to determine routine variables, which included the measurements of serum/blood protein concentrations (total protein-TP, Alb, prealbumin-preAlb, C-reactive protein (CRP)).

Total serum protein concentrations (normal value 6–8 g/dL) were determined using colorimetric methods (Biurete Colour, Dimention RXL Siemens, Munich, Germany). Alb was measured with capillary electrophoresis (Mini Capillary, Sebia, Cedex, France) and expressed as a percentage of TP (normal value 55.8–66.1%). Serum Alb concentrations were then obtained by multiplying the percentage of Alb by TP (normal value 3.5–5 g/dL). Hypoalbuminemia was indicated as a value <3.5 g/dL. Serum preAlb (normal range 20–40 mg/dL) was measured with an immuno-turbidimetric method (Cobas CCE Roche, Tokyo, Japan). Low preAlb was indicated by a value <20 mg/dL. Serum C-reactive protein (CRP) concentrations were determined with an immuno-turbidimetric method (Dimention RXL Siemens, Munich, Germany). CRP level >0.8 mg/dL was used as a marker of body inflammation. Blood Hb was analysed with a photometric method (Counter XE-2100, Dasit Symex Corporetion, Kobe, Japan). Hb concentrations <13 g/dL in men and <12 g/dL in women indicated the presence of anaemia [19].

2.2. Nutritional Intake

As described elsewhere [35], a three-day food diary was prepared for each patient by nurses who used a diet sheet to keep a record of the type and weight of cooked/uncooked food selected by patients from the hospital catering menu, both before and after their meals. Subsequently, we performed a nutritional analysis to calculate the actual calories and macro/micronutrients that the patients had ingested [35] by using the computer program Food Database DR3 (Dieta ragionata 3. Sintesi Informatica. University of Pavia, Italy). In brief, this program contains all food items and the energy concentrations of macronutrients (kcal/100 g nutrients) and, respectively, of raw and cooked foods. By entering the cooked/uncooked food item that the patient actually ingested into the database, the energy values (É) and macronutrients were calculated by multiplying the weight of the ingested food by its energy density and macro-micronutrient makeup.

2.3. Co-Morbidities

Associated disease(s) with the primary disease (HF) were analysed by the Charlson Index [37].

2.4. Patient Randomisation

After completing all of the above procedures, the patients were assigned a treatment according to a randomised allocation procedure. A randomisation list was generated using Statistical Analysis System SAS software; A and B were the identifiers of the blind treatment. The list was made available to both physicians (G.Z. and C.M.) and the hospital pharmacist. The physicians sequentially allocated patients to treatment A or B according to the randomised list. The first author (R.A.) who interpreted all the results was blinded to patient allocation. The experimental group (EAA group) received an oral nutritional mixture supplement, which provided 8 g of EAAs/day (Aminotrophic, Professional Dietetics, Milan, Italy; 4 g in the morning + 4 g in the afternoon, diluted in half a glass of water) for 60 days.

Each EAA package contained leucine 1250 mg, valine 625 mg, isoleucine 625 mg, lysine 650 mg, threonine 350 mg, cystine 150 mg, histidine 150 mg, phenylalanine 100 mg, methionine 50 mg, tyrosine 30 mg, and tryptophan 20 mg. We chose 8 g EAAs as this dose was found to be effective in several severe chronic diseases to improve insulin resistance [32,33,38] and serum albumin concentrations [32,33].

The calorie content of the single amino acid package was 21.9 kcal (EAA mixture) and 20.2 kcal (casein) (Table 1).

Table 1. Amino acid composition (mg) of a single packet (4 g) of treatment mixture (EAA group) or placebo mixture (casein group).

	EAA Group	Casein Group
	Total amino acid (4 g) of which (mg)	
Leucine	1250	380
Valine	625	272
Isoleucine	625	208
Lysine	650	308
Threonine	350	209
Cysteine	150	16
Histidine	150	104
Phenylalanine	100	192
Methionine	50	96.5
Tyrosine	30	209
Tryptophan	20	32
Serine	-	228
Proline	-	391.5
Glycine	-	52
Glutamic acid	-	801
Aspartic acid	-	268
Arginine	-	128
Alanine	-	105
EAA tot	3820	1801.5
% tot amino acids	95.5%	45%
BCAA	2500	860
% tot	62.5%	21.5%

The placebo group (control group) was given a similar isocaloric, isonitrogenous (casein) product. The nurses assisted each patient during the intake of either the placebo or EAAs in order to be certain of patient compliance.

The duration of the study was 60 days from the randomisation procedure.

All the above procedures were repeated 30 days (T1) and 60 days (T2) after the protocol started (T0).

2.5. A Rehabilitation Protocol

The protocol aimed to restore complete functional recovery of the altered body status, the resumption of a walking pattern that was as normal as possible, and of daily life activities (DLA).

The rehabilitation protocol consisted of two sessions per day, five days per week. Each session lasted 40–50 min and included the following main steps:

- Range of motion (ROM): a passive and assisted active mobilisation of the limb that had been operated on (15 min)
- Muscle strength:

    - isotonic and isometric exercises, neuromuscular facilitation of the sural triceps muscles (three sets of 10 repetitions; 15 min)
    - isotonic exercise and against resistance of: (1) abdominal trunk muscles to contrast the anteversion of the pelvis and (2) Gluteus maximus muscle to restore leg extension movement; (3) Gluteus medius and minimus muscles to keep the pelvis static and to be able to walk without oscillation (3 sets of 10 repetitions; 15 min)

- Assisted gait training with the use of walking sticks (10 min).

2.6. Statistical Analysis

The sample size estimate was determined by performing an appropriate power analysis. More specifically, based on preliminary data, we planned to observe an effect size f(V) (derived from preliminary partial η^2) between treatment groups of about 0.36. Starting from this hypothesis and assuming a type I error of 5% ($\alpha = 0.05$) and a type II error of 10% (power = 0.9), the sample required consisted of 50 patients per group.

Descriptive statistics were performed for all the recorded variables, and data were summarised as mean ± standard deviation (SD). The baseline characteristics between EAA and placebo groups were compared using an independent sample Student's *t* test or chi-square test, as appropriate. Comparisons of trends over time between EAA and placebo groups were performed by applying a repeated measure (times: baseline (T0), day 30 (T1), day 60 (T2)) analysis of variance (ANOVA), with one factor. Specific contrasts were estimated in order to assess differences between the two time points. A repeated measures ANOVA with two factors was used to test the influence on time trends of both treatment supplementation and the presence of infections. The difference in the prevalence of any developed infection between the two groups was tested by performing a chi-square test.

The previous analyses were also carried out to test the variation of the protein concentrations due to the treatment over time in female and male patients.

Linear regression analysis and Pearson's correlation coefficient were estimated to assess the relationship between protein concentrations (as absolute values at admission and discharge and as differences between discharge and admission) and functional tests. Statistical significance was set at $p < 0.05$.

3. Results

A total of 145 patients with hip fractures (HF) were enrolled, 118 of which met the inclusion criteria and were included in the study (Figure 1): 15 patients were excluded because of antibiotic therapy at or up to two days before admission to the Rehabilitation Institute; three for chronic renal failure, six for chronic heart failure, and 3 for diabetes on insulin treatment.

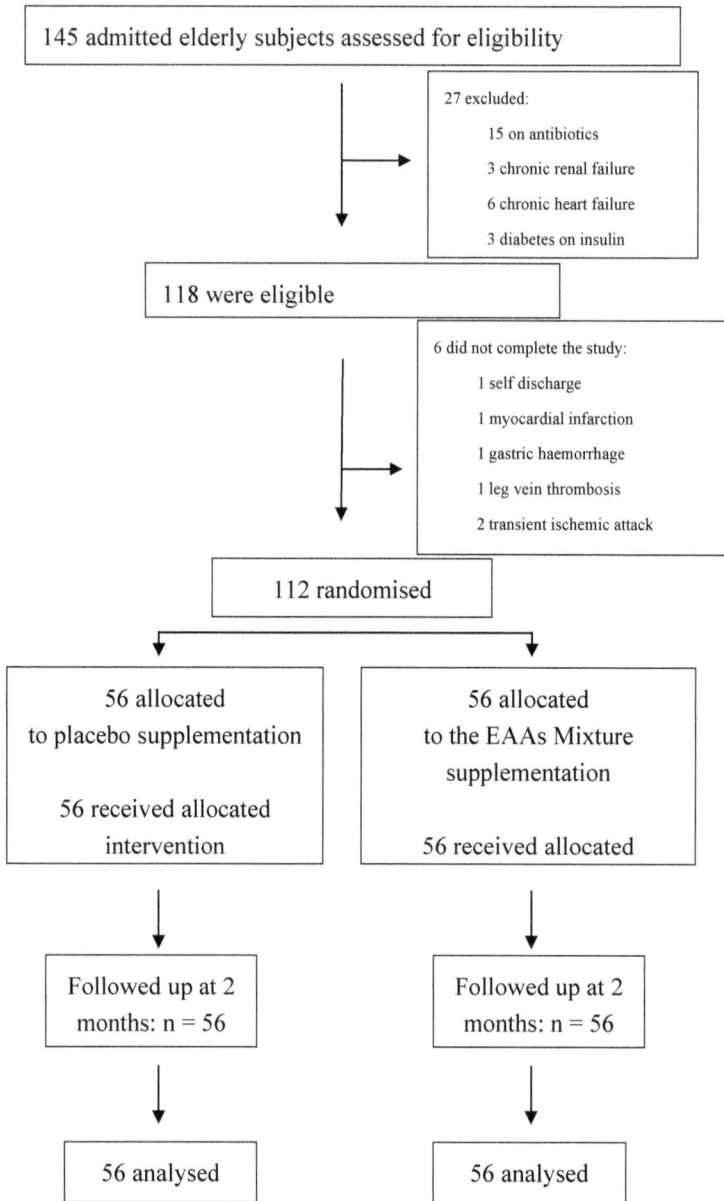

Figure 1. Flow diagram of a trial supplementation with Essential amino acids (EAAs) mixture vs. placebo to treat elderly patients with hip fractures. The diagram includes the number of patients analyzed for the main outcomes (effect on circulating proteins).

A total of 112 out of the 118 patients included in our study completed the study protocol. More specifically, six patients (two in the treated group and four in the placebo group) discontinued the study because of self-discharge (*n* = 1), myocardial infarction (*n* = 1), gastric haemorrhage (*n* = 1), leg deep vein thrombosis (*n* = 1), and transient ischemic attack (*n* = 2). Both the placebo and treated groups included 56 patients. Sixty percent of the placebo group and 65% of the EEA group were given at least one transfusion in the perioperative phase.

3.1. Baseline Characteristics

After randomisation, the treated and placebo groups were similar for co-morbidity (Charlson Index), demographic-anthropometric characteristics, nutritional intake, blood glucose, and urea concentrations. The placebo group was mildly overweight, and the EAA group had a normal body weight (categorisation by using the World Health Organisation WHO database). The daily calorie and protein intakes were slightly lower than recommended for both groups [39] (Table 2). The nutritional analysis conducted on the three-day diaries, showed that in both groups (a) proteins were mainly of animal origin ($77.6 \pm 4.8\%$ in placebo vs. $78.9 \pm 3.6\%$ in treated group; from fresh/cured meats, fish, eggs, milk/dairy products, cheese); (b) EAA dietary intakes were similar; (c) ingested simple sugar (sugar, yoghurt/milk/fruit) comprised 17% of the daily energy intake, which was mildly higher than the recommended amount (<15%); and (d) there was an increased lipid intake with normal ingestion of saturated fats. However, the ingestion of ω3 fatty acids was lower than the recommended amount. A status of systemic body inflammation, indicated by CRP levels (Table 3), was present in and similar for the two patient populations.

Table 2. Demographic-, anthropometric-, co-morbidity index, biohumoral-, and nutritional-variables in two groups of patients after randomisation to either placebo or essential amino acid (EAAs) supplementation.

Variables	nv	Placebo Group (n°56)	EAA Supplemented Group (n°56)	p Value
Demographic				
Male/Female	-	27/29	25/31	0.3
Age (years)	-	81.4 ± 8.1	83.1 ± 7.5	0.15
Anthropometric				
Body weight (kg)	-	63.5 ± 18	62 ± 16.1	0.79
Body Mass Index (BMI) (kg/m²)	-	25.7 ± 7.9	24.9 ± 8.5	0.41
Co-morbidity index (scores)	-	1.8 ± 1.3	1.75 ± 1.2	0.78
Biohumoral				
Glucose (mg/dL)	78–110	98 ± 17	95 ± 8	0.8
Glycated hemoglobin (%)	≤6	6.3 ± 2.7	6.1 ± 1.8	0.71
Urea nitrogen (mg/dL)	4.67–23.3	24.6 ± 6	23 ± 9.1	0.69
Creatinine (mg/dL)	0.5–1.1	1.01 ± 0.6	1 ± 0.9	0.11
Daily nutritional intake	Recommended *			
Energy				
kcal	-	1511 ± 345	1460 ± 319	-
kcal/kg	29.4 M 27 F	23.8 ± 7.2	24.1 ± 6.4	0.9
Proteins				
g	-	58 ± 11	57 ± 13	-
g/kg	≥1.1	0.91 ± 0.2	0.92 ± 0.3	0.89
%E	-	15.3 ± 2.9	15.6 ± 3.5	-
Providing EAAs (mg)				
Lysine	3810 ± 285	4093 ± 457	0.7
Histidine	1669 ± 180	1624 ± 239	0.9
Threonine	2362 ± 341	2258 ± 401	0.8
Valine	3230 ± 454	3347 ± 398	0.8
Isoleucine	2800 ± 375	2899 ± 315	0.9
Leucine	4900 ± 615	4981 ± 585	0.9
Methionine	1342 ± 302	1417 ± 412	0.7
Phenylalanine	2600 ± 299	2757 ± 416	0.5
Tryptophan	650 ± 72	690 ± 122	0.6
Total	23,363 ± 2780	24,066 ± 2954	0.7
% proteins	40.2 ± 4.8	42.2 ± 5.2	0.8
Carbohydrates				
g	-	171.5 ± 41	179.8 ± 51	-
g/kg	2.5–4	2.7 ± 0.55	2.9 ± 0.9	-
%E	-	45.4 ± 10.8	49.3 ± 14	0.78
Simple sugar				
g	-	64.4 ± 4.5	65.1 ± 3.2	-
%E	<15	17 ± 1.2	17.8 ± 0.9	0.9
Lipids				
g	-	66.3 ± 18	60.8 ± 16	-
g/kg	≤1	1.04 ± 0.4	0.98 ± 0.31	0.22
%E	<30	39.5 ± 2.76	40.1 ± 4.9	0.85

Table 2. *Cont.*

Variables	nv	Placebo Group (n°56)	EAA Supplemented Group (n°56)	*p* Value
Saturated				
g		17.5 ± 3.9	12.1 ± 2.6	-
%E	<10	10.4 ± 2.5	7.45 ± 3.7	0.45
Monounsaturated				
g		40 ± 4.3	41.5 ± 6.8	-
%E		23.8 ± 2.5	25.6 ± 4.2	0.75
Polyunsaturated				
g		8.8 ± 2.9	7.2 ± 2.2	-
%E	5–10	5.2 ± 1.7	4.4 ± 1.34	0.8
Omega 6				
g		7.1 ± 2.8	6.1 ± 1.15	-
%E	4–8	4.2 ± 0.45	3.76 ± 0.71	0.65
Omega 3				
g		1.7 ± 0.45	1.2 ± 0.6	-
%E	0.5–2	0.01 ± 0.002	0.007 ± 0.003	0.81
Fibre (g)	>25	14.8 ± 4.3	21.7 ± 9.6	0.4
Calcium (mg)	1200 M; 1200 F	855 ± 184	786 ± 230	0.84
Phosphorous (mg)	700 M; 700 F	1050 ± 351	654 ± 251	0.2
Potassium (mg)	3900 M; 3900 F	2384 ± 146	2185 ± 192	0.85
Sodium (mg)	1200 M; 1200 F	1354 ± 139	1275 ± 235	0.78
Iron (mg)	10 M; 10 F	10.5 ± 3.7	9.8 ± 1.5	0.91
Zinc (mg)	12 M; 9 F	0.7 ± 0.15	0.95 ± 0.21	0.30
Thiamin (mg)	1.2 M; 1.1 F	1.1 ± 0.1	0.99 ± 0.14	0.9
Riboflavin (mg)	1.6 M; 1.3 F	1.25 ± 0.4	1.17 ± 0.15	0.75
Niacin (mg)	18 M; 18 F	14.7 ± 3.6	13.8 ± 2.5	0.85
Vitamin A (µg)	700 M; 600 F	585 ± 128	588 ± 97	0.97
Vitamin C (mg)	105 M; 85 F	75 ± 21	82 ± 32	0.88
Water (mL)	-	854 ± 160	794 ± 89	0.91

Data are expressed as mean ± standard deviation (SD); Statistical analysis: independent sample *t*-test and χ^2-test for placebo group vs. EAA supplemented group; * Livelli di Assunzione di Riferimento di Nutrienti LARN 2014 [39].

Table 3. Changes over time of the study variables. T0 = baseline; T1 = 1 month; T2 = 2 months.

Circulating Proteins	Placebo *n* = 56			EAAs *n* = 56			*p* Interaction
	T0	T1	T2	T0	T1	T2	
Albumin g/dL (n.v. 3.5–5)	3.45 ± 0.34	3.50 ± 0.25	3.51 ± 0.34	3.47 ± 0.41	3.59 ± 0.48	3.7 ± 0.52	=0.038
Haemoglobin g/dL (n.v. ≥12 F; ≥13 M)	11.8 ± 1.7	11.7 ± 1.6	11.7 ± 1.6	11.4 ± 1.7	11.8 ± 1.7	12.2 ± 1.6	=0.008
Prealbumin mg/dL (n.v. 18–38)	15.9 ± 4	15.9 ± 3	16.1 ± 4.1	15.7 ± 5.7	18 ± 7.6	17.6 ± 6.1	=0.3
C-reactive protein mg/dL (n.v. <0.8)	9.3 ± 6.5	16.9 ± 16.1	10.1 ± 9.4	20 ± 17.8	24.5 ± 14.8	13.5 ± 9.3	=0.1

As regards serum proteins (Table 3), Alb was lower than the normal range of values in the entire population. The prevalence of hypoAlb (Figure 2) was similar between treated and placebo subjects (64.3% in placebo and 73.2% in treated patients; ns). The prevalence of anaemia in the entire study population was 67% and was distributed similarly between the two groups (66% in placebo and 67.8% in treated patients; ns).

The results showed that Alb significantly correlated with Hb (r = +0.397; p < 0.001).

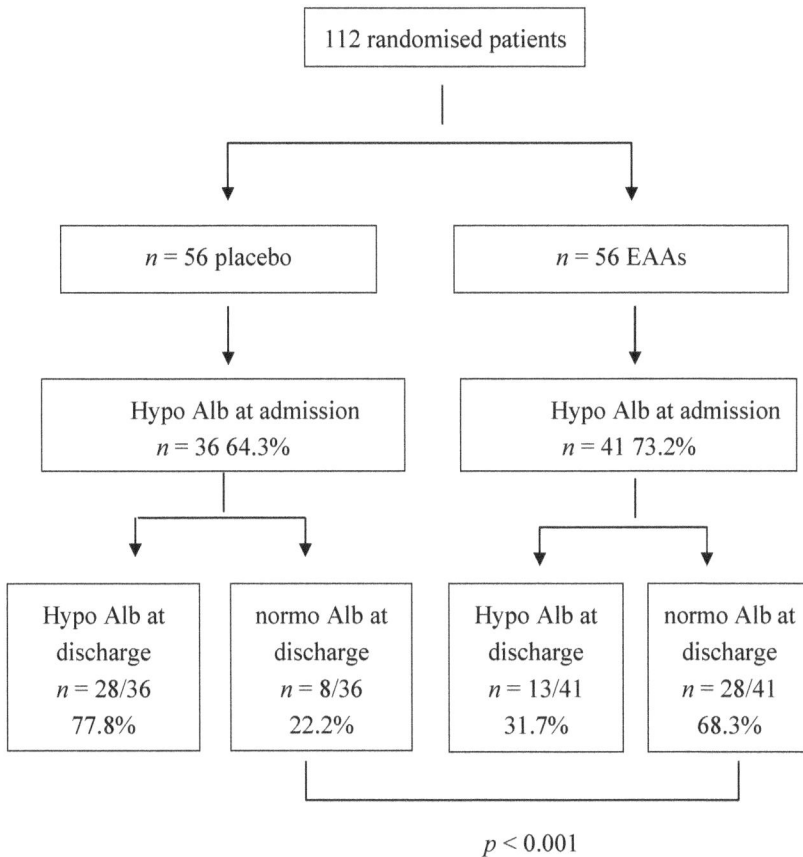

Figure 2. Flow diagram showing the percentage of admitted patients with hypoalbuminemia (Alb < 3.5 g/dL) who did not improve or improved albumin (Alb) during the Rehab period.

3.2. Variable Changes during the Rehabilitation Phase

The results showed significant differences ($p < 0.05$) in the overtime trends of Alb between the two patient populations. In placebo patients, the serum Alb concentrations remained virtually unchanged (Table 3), whereas in treated subjects, the serum Alb concentrations progressively increased over time (Table 3). However, no significant sex-based differences emerged from the model ($p = 0.74$). The normalisation of Alb levels (≥ 3.5 g/dL) occurred in 68.3% of the EAA group and in 22.2% of the placebo group ($p < 0.001$) (Figure 2). The average Alb improvements were +0.46 ± 0.43 g/dL in EAAs and +0.22 ± 0.19 in placebo patients.

At discharge, a status of hypoAlb was still present in 77.8% of placebo patients and in 31.7% of EAAs.

As regards Hb (Table 3), the changes in this protein reflected those of the Alb. Indeed, Hb changed very little in the placebo group, whereas it progressively increased in the treated subjects. This difference was significant ($p = 0.008$). More specifically, in the EAA group, the time course of blood Hb content was different between baseline (T0) and T2 ($p = 0.003$), and between T1 and T2 ($p = 0.002$) and tended to be significant between T0 and T1 ($p = 0.08$). As with Alb concentration, no significant differences of Hb concentration between male and female subjects emerged from the model ($p = 0.5$).

Figure 3 shows that improvements in Hb occurred in 18.9% of placebo subjects and in 34.2% of EAAs. In absolute values, the rates of improved Hb were higher in EAAs than in placebo subjects (+0.75 ± 0.34 g/dL vs. +0.25 ± 0.31 g/dL) (*p* < 0.01).

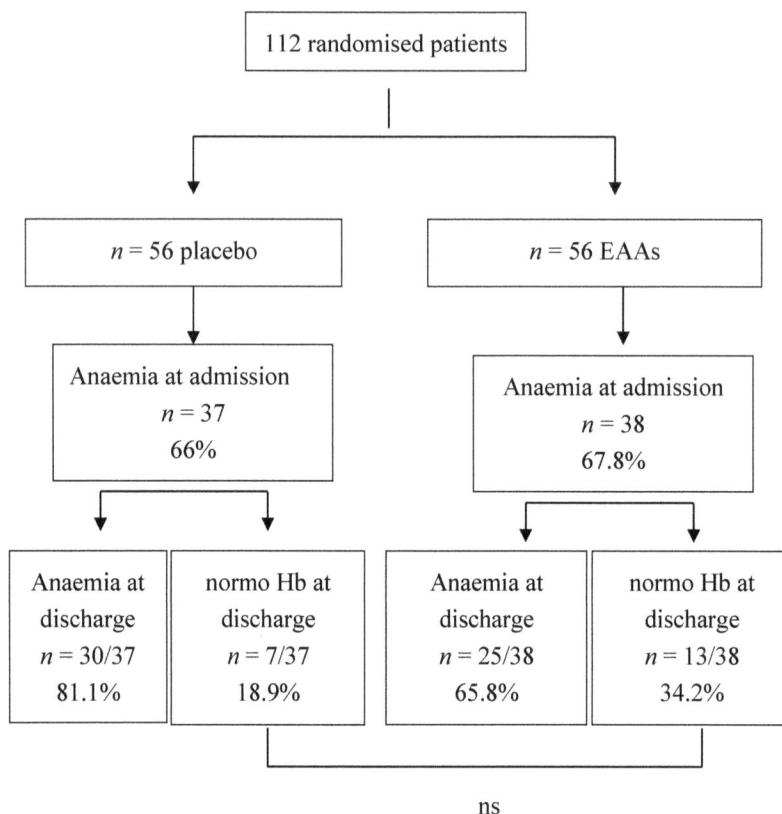

Figure 3. Flow diagram showing the percentage of admitted patients with anaemia (Hb < 13 g/dL male; <12 g/dL female) who did not improve or improved haemoglobin (Hb) during Rehab period.

At discharge, more than 80% of placebo anaemic subjects and more than 65% of treated subjects were still anaemic (Figure 3).

At discharge, Alb and Hb showed a significant correlation (*r* = +0.5, *p* < 0.001).

There were no significant changes of CRP over time either in the placebo or in the EAA group to indicate the persistence of systemic inflammation. No significant changes were observed in either male or female patients (*p* = 0.48). Infections (namely of urinary and lower airway tracts) were higher in placebo (80%) than in treated patients (55%) (*p* < 0.02). Infection did not modify the EAA effects on Alb time courses (*p* = 0.46) or Hb (interaction treatment *p* = 0.73).

After two months of rehabilitation, there was no significant change between baseline body weight or daily nutritional intakes in either patient group or in pre-Alb concentration levels (or in male or female patients) (*p* = 0.8)

To summarise, supplemented EAAs were associated with improvements in Alb and, to a lesser extent, Hb. At about 80 days from the index event, both placebo and EAA subjects were discharged with persistent systemic inflammation.

4. Discussion

This study shows that, despite the presence of systemic inflammation, oral supplementation with EAAs can normalise serum albumin in the majority of hypoAlb patients and reverse anaemia in more than one third of subjects after HF.

4.1. Baseline Circulating Proteins

The hypoalbuminemia observed in both groups of patients at their admission to the Rehabilitation Institute is the result of several mechanisms including systemic inflammation (primed by both trauma and subsequent surgery) [40], the possible inadequacy of patients' calorie-protein intake during their acute orthopaedic hospitalisation, alterations in body tissue composition, or poor nutritional status before the index event.

In catabolic states such as trauma, surgery, and infection, Alb concentrations decrease by approximately 1–1.5 g/dL over a short time (3–7 days) [41]. This reduction in Alb is due to decreased synthesis, accelerated distribution from the intravascular space, and increased catabolism of the protein during metabolic stress [42]. During a catabolic period, low Alb may persist despite nutritional support and the exogenous administration of Alb [1].

Poor nutritional intake during an acute hospital stay is another factor that contributes to impaired circulating Alb levels because low calorie-protein intake reduces synthesis and accelerates the catabolism of Alb [5]. The patients in our study were likely to have had inadequate nutritional intake in the orthopaedic setting [29], as suggested by their low nutrition levels on entry to the Rehabilitation Institute The administered fluid contributed to lower serum albumin concentrations. We believe, however, that this was not important in the study patients as they were admitted to our Institute about 20 days from the index event, while the Extracellular Water ECW is usually lost several days after the acute event because of increased diuresis. In addition, no patient had clinical signs of water retention (edema), and all subjects were clinically and haemodynamically stable.

Both metabolic stress and inadequate nutrition can also explain the low levels of patient preAlb due to the fact that this negative protein of the acute phase response is sensitive to low nutritional intake [38].

The alteration of body tissue composition is another factor that could reduce Alb. Although body composition was not investigated in this study, the patients probably had reduced muscle mass following multiple catabolic factors such as metabolic stress, inflammation, and immobilisation. Even in relatively healthy, well-nourished elderly men and women, low serum Alb has been associated with reduced muscle mass [43].

Lastly, possible malnutrition at the time of fracture may have contributed to a low level of Alb in the patients in our study [44].

At admission to the Rehabilitation Institute, 67% of the entire patient population was anaemic. Reduced Hb levels in subjects with HF is a consequence of several factors including lower Hb on the day before fracture [19], bleeding and fluid shifts before surgery, a drop in Hb levels during surgery, and repeated phlebotomy [19]. Both preoperative Hb concentrations and perioperative bleeding are major determinants of anaemia in post-surgery HF patients. Perioperative transfusions, by inducing immune depression, [45] might have played an important role in favouring infectious complications in the study patients. In this way, transfusion may indirectly have contributed to reducing circulating protein levels. This suggests that it is important to increase presurgery Hb concentrations when needed in order to avoid blood transfusion [46]. Poor nutritional intake is also a co-factor of low Hb.

4.2. EAA-Associated Improvements in Alb and HB

This study provides a positive answer to our investigation into whether EAAs may increase concentrations of serum Alb and Hb. The results show that increases in Alb and Hb were similar in males and females. Indeed, at discharge, the percentage of hypoalbuminemic patients on EAAs dropped to about 31.7% from an initial 73.2%. The treatment group ingested more than double the amount of EAAs (from diet and supplementation) than the placebo group did. In addition, the contribution of EAAs to total amino acid content was higher in the treated group (95.5%) than in the placebo group (45%).

Given that both groups of patients had a similar intake of EAAs in their diet, the difference between the two groups in terms of albumin gain was clearly due to the EAA supplements that were given to the treated group.

Multiple mechanisms may explain the efficacy of EAAs in improving Alb and Hb. EAAs directly promote overall body protein synthesis [47] and inhibit proteolysis, which is particularly relevant to Alb [48]. These activities are present in several tissues including the liver, which is the site of Alb production [49]. Indirectly, EAAs stimulate body protein synthesis by increasing the biological activity of insulin-like growth factor-1 [50].

In addition, the leucine metabolite ß-hydroxy-ß-methylbutyrate (HMB) improves protein synthesis and reduces protein destruction, even in cancer subjects [51,52].

It is interesting to note that the amino acid tryptophan, contained in the mixture used in this study, can promote Alb production as it is the most important amino acid for Alb synthesis [53]. Indeed, in the liver, tryptophan stimulates the ribosomal re-aggregation leading to enhanced Alb production in a fasting state or in conditions of inadequate protein intake [54]. It is unlikely that diet played a role in improving Alb, given that nutritional intake was similar at admission to and discharge from our institute. It was also similar in both placebo and treated patients.

At discharge, patient body weight was similar to baseline values. This indicates that the ingestion of calories, even though it lower than recommended, met the patients' actual body needs, suggesting that inactivity/immobilisation reduced their total body energy requirements.

The lower infection rate that occurred in EAA compared to placebo patients confirms the findings of our previous studies [35,54] and may be due to the fact that EAAs play an important role in improving immunological defences by inducing protein synthesis of immune cells [35]. The proimmunologic EAA activity may explain why infection did not preclude the improvements of Alb and Hb over time.

Lower infection rates probably aid Alb improvement. In this study, the improvement of Alb is in line with two investigations reporting EEA-induced Alb increase in sarcopenic patients with chronic obstructive pulmonary disease [32] and in institutionalized elderly subjects [33]. Conversely, our results are in contrast with a previous investigation, which showed that two-thirds of HF patients failed to increase their serum Alb despite both calorie and protein enrichment of a routine hospital diet [55]. This discrepancy may be reconciled considering the differences in the methodologies adopted. Indeed, ageing is associated with reduced anabolism efficiency in response to a normal protein meal [56], particularly under conditions of insulin resistance frequently found in post-traumatic elderly subjects. On the contrary, ingesting EAAs as free substrates can actually stimulate protein anabolism to a greater degree than amino acids from food proteins [57], even in diabetic subjects [58].

With regards to Hb, the positive influence of EAA supplementation was only partial, given that improvements in Hb, though significant, only occurred in just over a third of the anaemic patients. EAAs probably promote the synthesis rate of globin, the protein group of Hb. Considering the fact that globin consists of four polypeptide chains containing an extraordinarily high percentage of amino acids which are essential for maintaining its helicoidally form [59], supplemented EAAs can stimulate and enhance initiation, prolongation, and termination of the globin chain [59] involving RNA messengers, RNA transfers, and ribosomes [59]. It is interesting that over the first few months of the protocol for subjects on EAA, Hb improvement, unlike Alb, tended to be significant ($p = 0.08$). This difference could reflect the differences in the half-lives of the two proteins, i.e., 19–21 days for Alb and 7 days for Hb [59]. The positive correlation between Alb and Hb confirms the results of another previous study [22]. Notably, after EAA supplementation, this relationship was stronger than that observed under base conditions.

The study cannot explain why EAA failed to improve serum preAlb, which, like Alb, is a negative reactant of the acute phase response. At present, we can only postulate that inflammation may inhibit preAlb production more than Alb and/or that the synthesis of albumin was more sensitive than that of prealbumin to EAA activity.

The main finding of this study is the chance of improving the recovery of hypoalbuminemia and, to a lesser extent, of anaemia, despite the persistence of systemic inflammation. This should not be surprising, however, given that amino acid supplementation can be anabolic even during severe inflammation such as acute endotoxin-induced inflammation in humans [60]. Antinflammatory EAA activity may be partly due to hydroxy-methylbutyrate HMB, the efficacy of which was demonstrated in chronic obstructive pulmonary disease patients. CRP and white blood cells were shown to be significantly lower in patients in the treated group than in the control group [61].

The dose of supplemented EAAs may not have been sufficient for subjects who were still hypoalbuminemic (31.7%) or anemic (65.8%) at the end of the protocol. In addition, for these patients, the amino acid composition of the EAA mixture was not appropriate to exert a sufficient net synthetic activity, particularly when blood amino acid abnormalities coexisted.

Plasma amino acid alterations can be frequent following trauma/surgery or elective Hip arthroplasty [62]. The results of the current investigation are not in agreement with those found in gastric subjects on supplemented amino acids. However, the two studies are very different from both methodological and clinical context standpoints. Methodologically, gastric bypass subjects were provided with a mixture containing a high amount (24 g twice daily) of three amino acids only, not including EAAs, apart from a metabolite of leucine, as in our study. Arginine and glutamine may play a dual role in the intestinal tract, both protective and proinflammatory [63]. Nitric oxide (NO) overproduction from arginine supplementation has been related to greater colonic damage and inflammation [64]. Glutamine supplementation via the glutamic-citrulline-arginine metabolic pathway [65] may indirectly lead to NO formation. Interestingly, a diet providing 12% glutamine produces lower inflammation, and a diet containing 24% glutamine produces higher inflammation [66]. Supplemented EAAs in our patients did not produce inflammation but were compatible with a trend towards reduced CRP. From a clinical point of view, patients after gastric bypass surgery are in a condition of reduced alimentary intake, malabsorption, and a catabolic state. The patients in the present investigation were in a post acute phase of alimentary, functional, progressive recovery.

Our results found that, in the treated group, 31.7% of HF patients remained hypo-albuminemic and 65.8% remained anaemic at discharge from the Rehabilitation Institute. This raises the important issue of how to increase the number of patients with restored Alb and Hb levels.

The differences in Alb and Hb responses to EAA supplementation deserve to be mentioned. We believe that the factors that influence Alb concentrations, including the availability of tryptophan and methionine [50] (both contained in the formula used in the study), protein-energy intake [51], oncotic pressure [42], and hormones [42], may be easier to control than the factors that influence Hb synthesis and degradation, particularly in an inflammatory state such as relative or absolute erythropoietin (EPO) insufficiency [67] and bone marrow response to EPO. Indeed, inflammation may lower EPO levels and/or hamper the response to EPO [68]. Moreover, changes in the circulating levels of testosterone and thyroid hormones may render patients more susceptible to anaemia [69]. In brief, Hb synthesis may not solely depend on adequate provision of EAAs, but also on body status, EPO, and bone marrow response to EPO. For these reasons, we believe that restoring normal Hb levels in more than one third of the elderly patients with HF sequelae in our study by the simple supplementation of EAAs is clinically important.

5. Clinical Implications

oxygen The study suggests that it is beneficial to supplement EAAs to elderly patients with HF and concomitant mild hypoalbuminemia and/or anaemia. In this study, two months of EAA supplementation induced an average Alb increase of 0.22 g/dL, (+6%) compared to the baseline value.

This change is quantitatively similar to that observed (+0.16 g/dL) in institutionalised elderly patients on an EAA mixture that was identical to the one that was used in the present study [33]. The importance of the degree of Alb improvement in this study may be highlighted by four considerations. Firstly, in elderly subjects, serum Alb levels >3.2 g/dL exert a protective effect on mortality 12 months after discharge from the Rehabilitation Institute [70]. Secondly, the physiological decrease in median Alb levels between ages 30 and 80 years is 9–12% for both men and women [22,71]. Thirdly, in clinical practice, the infusion of Alb in a chronic stable disease is an inefficient method to improve circulating protein because the exogenous supply of Alb increases degradation and reduces the synthesis rate of the protein [5]. Lastly, serum Alb is significantly associated with skeletal muscle mass [42], independently of age, dietary intake, frailty, physical activity, or morbidity. Improvement in Alb (and Hb) could reduce the risk of frailty in elderly subjects, particularly in those with skeletal trauma sequelae.

Although anaemia in elderly subjects after HF fracture does not seem to affect the risk of adverse outcomes at three, six, and 12 months after discharge from hospital [24], we believe that long-term improvement of low Hb levels may prevent patients from suffering from muscle alterations that cause an increased risk of frailty and falls [11,72]. Indeed, low Hb, by inducing chronic hypoxia [73] and higher levels of inflammatory markers [74], reduces muscle density, mass [11,75–77], strength [12], and microcirculation [78]. Muscle damage induced by low Hb is therefore in addition to the damage already produced by fracture, surgery, and immobilisation.

An important consideration for clinical practice is that the improvement of Alb and Hb levels in elderly subjects with low circulating proteins prevents decreased circulatory blood volume [79]. In turn, this causes the instability of arterial pressure and rheological alterations of circulation in vital organs.

It is interesting that our patients still had persistent inflammation 70–90 days after the acute event. This may have limited the number of patients who were able to benefit from EAA supplementation. Moreover, persistent inflammation suggests that CRP levels should be checked over time after patients are discharged, because persistent inflammation places subjects with sequelae of HF at an increased risk of delayed reacquisition of adequate motility and physical activity [35], progression of atherosclerosis, and proliferation of cardiovascular events [80]. Indeed, CRP may be involved in all stages of atherosclerosis by influencing processes such as the endothelial function, lipid effect, angiogenesis and apoptosis, thrombosis, complement activation, and monocyte recruitment and activation [81]. Elevated CRP may lead to the rupture of unstable arterial plaques, causing clinical manifestations of cardio-and/or cerebrovascular disease. Moreover, the persistence of inflammation may limit functional recovery after hip fracture surgery. Local and systemic inflammation, as indicated by increased CRP, favour muscle catabolism over anabolic activity. In our study, the Tumor Necrosis Factor (TNFα), which is the main proinflammatory cytokine, was not determined. TNFα induces a resistance to the growth hormone and reduces the levels of the potent anabolic IGF-1 [82]. Interleukin-6 (IL-6) is another important proinflammatory cytokine, which was not determined in this investigation. IL-6 stimulates liver production of CRP as well as hypothalamus-pituitary corticosurrenal axis [83] leading to cortisol overproduction that causes peripheral muscle insulin resistance and catabolic activity. Both TNF and IL-6, by mediating the inflammatory pathway, cause a shift in liver protein synthesis with increased acute phase protein and reduced non reactant proteins, among which is albumin. Thus, inflammation may contribute to patient muscle wasting, sarcopenia, and frailty, particularly when associated with malnutrition and vitamin D deficiency. This may help to explain why most re-admissions after HF surgery are for co-morbidity conditions such as infection or cardiovascular diseases and not for surgical complications [19]. This is relevant because impaired walking performance is permanent in 20% of HF patients [35,70], and there is a high institutionalisation rate (20–25%) [20]. This study points to a reconsideration of our hospital catering and patient education to a more healthy choice of food. Indeed the low amount of ω3 fatty acids ingested daily by the patients in this study could have favoured the persistent inflammation. Together with increased ω3 [84], vitamin E [85] and moderate alcohol consumption [86] have an impact on CRP levels. Thus, the intake of cold water, ocean fish, alcohol (red wine mainly 200 mL/d), and foods containing vitamin E such as nuts, pulses, grains, lentils, chickpeas and oats should be advised to inflamed HF patients.

6. Conclusions

This study indicates that oral supplementation of EAAs may enhance the recovery of hypoalbumenimia and anaemia in more than two thirds and one third, respectively, of inflamed elderly patients after HF surgery. The anabolic activity of EAAs occurs even in the presence of infection.

7. Limitations

This study has several limitations that need more specific research in order to be resolved. Circulating vitamin D levels were not evaluated. Normal vitamin D or its supplementation may be a factor that contributes to reducing inflammation both directly and indirectly. The vitamin directly regulates the immune system [87], thus playing an important role in patient susceptibility to hospital-acquired infections.

By reducing the risk of infection, vitamin D contributes indirectly to a reduced perpetuation of systemic inflammation [88]. A status of hypovitaminosis D is likely in the study patients. Firstly, the prevalence of suboptimal levels of 25-hydroxyvitamin D (25-OHD) has increased in the general population [89]. Secondly, inflammatory changes and intravenous fluid administration lead to a rapid drop (30–40%) in circulating vitamin D levels during acute stress [90]. In addition, inflammation is associated with a decreased vitamin D binding protein [91]. Thus, a vicious circle of vitamin D deficiency-inflammation might occur. Hypovitaminosis D may also reduce the positive effect of rehabilitation of patients with HF as vitamin D improves musculoskeletal function [92] and postural body sway [93] and reduces the number of falls [94]. Interestingly, a recent study has documented that, when sarcopenic elderly patients are supplemented with vitamin D, whey proteins, and essential amino acids, their physical activity decreases inflammation and increases fat-free mass and strength, functionality, and quality of life [95].

Measuring patient body composition and muscle strength would have strengthened the discussion regarding the improvement in circulating proteins and muscle mass/function [11,42]. An overall improvement of visceral and somatic proteins may be more important than the single factor to ensure that patients with HF have better body stability and performance of daily tasks. The quantification of ECW could indicate whether an excess of water retention still existed and could contribute to lower albumin concentrations [96].

It would have been useful to follow up discharged patients to document whether improved circulating Alb and, to a lesser extent Hb, could have actually influenced patients' return to pre-fracture walking capacity [97], with the consequent effect of reducing the risk of physical frailty. Future studies will address HF patients suffering from co-morbidities that were initially excluded in the study (see the Section 2.1). Determining circulating levels of testosterone and thyroid hormones could contribute to finding the EAA mechanisms, which create improvement in proteins. These hormones are often altered in older individuals, and reduced levels render patients more susceptible to anaemia [26]. Knowledge of the blood amino acid profile may be useful to understand which is the best EAA formula composition for a particular patient.

In elderly subjects, the main nutritional factor for developing anaemia is obviously low iron availability, as indicated by low ferritin concentrations. Given that serum concentrations of this protein were not measured, it was not possible to exclude low iron availability as a nutritional factor contributing to anaemia. However, we believe that the persistent body inflammation observed in the study populations would have masked any possible hypoferritinemia from low iron intake.

As EAAs failed to normalise Alb in one third of patients and correct anaemia in about two thirds of patients, a well-planned study is needed to highlight the extent of the impact of infection on circulating proteins and whether this could be limited by increasing the amounts of supplemented EAAs and/or by changing the amino acid composition of the EAA formula.

Another limitation of the study was the fact that we only kept an alimentary diary for three days. We are aware that it would have been preferable to keep them for longer, although this would have been impractical for the nursing staff from an organisational point of view. However, in our Institute, the protocol for checking long-term patient food intake consists in keeping a daily qualitative (i.e., not weighing foods) diary and in frequently determining Blood Urea Nitrogen BUN to estimate the adequacy of protein (EAA) intake and creatinine levels.

Author Contributions: R.A., F.B. and G.C.Z. conceived and designed the study; G.C.Z., C.R. and M.C. recruited the participants; A.M.C., P.I., S.V. and M.V. performed the experiments; R.A. and F.B. analyzed the data; R.A. wrote the paper; and C.D.V. and P.P. edited the paper.

Conflicts of Interest: The authors declare no conflict of interest.

References

1. Doweiko, J.P.; Nompleggi, D.J. The role of albumin in human physiology and pathophysiology, Part III: Albumin and disease states. *JPEN* **1991**, *15*, 476–483. [CrossRef] [PubMed]
2. Visser, M.; Kritchevsky, S.B.; Newman, A.B.; Goodpaster, B.H.; Tylavsky, F.A.; Nevitt, M.C.; Harris, T.B. Lower serum albumin concentration and change in muscle mass: The health, aging and body composition study. *Am. J. Clin. Nutr.* **2005**, *82*, 531–537. [PubMed]
3. Zuliani, G.; Romagnoni, F.; Volpato, S.; Soattin, L.; Leoci, V.; Bollini, M.C.; Buttarello, M.; Lotto, D.; Fellin, R. Nutritional parameters, body composition, and progression of disability in older disabled residents living in nursing homes. *J. Gerontol. A Biol. Sci. Med. Sci.* **2001**, *56*, 212–216. [CrossRef]
4. Corti, M.C.; Guralnik, J.M.; Salive, M.E.; Sorkin, J.D. Serum albumin level and physical disability as predictors of mortality in older persons. *JAMA* **1994**, *272*, 1036–1042. [CrossRef] [PubMed]
5. Mendez, C.M.; McClain, C.J.; Marsano, L.S. Albumin therapy in clinical practice. *Nutr. Clin. Pract.* **2005**, *20*, 314–320. [CrossRef] [PubMed]
6. Anderson, C.F.; Moxness, K.; Meister, J.; Burritt, M.F. The sensitivity and specificity of nutrition-related variables in relationship to the duration of hospital stay and the rate of complications. *Mayo Clin. Proc.* **1984**, *59*, 477–483. [CrossRef]
7. Rich, M.W.; Keller, A.J.; Schechtman, K.B.; Marshall, W.G.; Kouchoukos, N.T. Increased complications and prolonged hospital stay in elderly cardiac surgical patients with low serum albumin. *Am. J. Cardiol.* **1989**, *63*, 714–718. [CrossRef]
8. Sahyoun, N.R.; Jacques, P.F.; Dallal, G.; Russell, R.M. Use of albumin as a predictor of mortality in community dwelling and institutionalized elderly populations. *J. Clin. Epidemiol.* **1996**, *49*, 981–988. [CrossRef]
9. Mizrahi, E.H.; Fleissig, Y.; Arad, M.; Blumstein, T.; Adunsky, A. Admission albumin levels and functional outcome of elderly hip fracture patients: Is it that important? *Aging Clin. Exp. Res.* **2007**, *19*, 284–289. [CrossRef] [PubMed]
10. Aquilani, R.; Boselli, M.; Baiardi, P.; Pasini, E.; Iadarola, P.; Verri, M.; Viglio, S.; Condini, A.; Boschi, F. Is stroke rehabilitation a metabolic problem? *Brain Inj.* **2014**, *28*, 161–173. [CrossRef] [PubMed]
11. Cesari, M.; Penninx, B.W.; Lauretani, F.; Russo, C.R.; Carter, C.; Bandinelli, S.; Atkinson, H.; Onder, G.; Pahor, M.; Ferrucci, L. Hemoglobin levels and skeletal muscle: Results from the InCHIANTI study. *J. Gerontol. A Biol. Sci. Med. Sci.* **2004**, *59*, 249–254. [CrossRef] [PubMed]
12. Penninx, B.W.; Guralnik, J.M.; Onder, G.; Ferrucci, L.; Wallace, R.B.; Pahor, M. Anemia and decline in physical performance among older persons. *Am. J. Med.* **2003**, *115*, 104–110. [CrossRef]
13. Fuchs, Z.; Blumstein, T.; Novikov, I.; Walter-Ginzburg, A.; Lyanders, M.; Gindin, J.; Habot, B.; Modan, B. Morbidity, comorbidity, and their association with disability among community-dwelling oldest-old in Israel. *J. Gerontol. A Biol. Sci. Med. Sci.* **1998**, *53*, 447–455. [CrossRef]
14. Penninx, B.W.; Pahor, M.; Cesari, M.; Corsi, A.M.; Woodman, R.C.; Bandinelli, S.; Guralnik, J.M.; Ferrucci, L. Anemia is associated with disability and decreased physical performance and muscle strength in the elderly. *J. Am. Geriatr. Soc.* **2004**, *52*, 719–724. [CrossRef] [PubMed]
15. Boogaerts, M.; Coiffier, B.; Kainz, C.; Epoetin Beta QOL Working Group. Impact of epoetin beta on quality of life in patients with malignant disease. *Br. J. Cancer* **2003**, *88*, 988–995. [CrossRef] [PubMed]

16. Izaks, G.J.; Westendorp, R.G.; Knook, D.L. The definition of anemia in older persons. *JAMA* **1999**, *281*, 1714–1717. [CrossRef] [PubMed]

17. Makipour, S.; Kanapuru, B.; Ershler, W.B. Unexplained anemia in the elderly. *Semin. Hematol.* **2008**, *45*, 250–254. [CrossRef] [PubMed]

18. Gruson, K.I.; Aharonoff, G.B.; Egol, K.A.; Zuckerman, J.D.; Koval, K.J. The relationship between admission hemoglobin level and outcome after hip fracture. *J. Orthop. Trauma* **2002**, *16*, 39–44. [CrossRef] [PubMed]

19. Halm, E.A.; Wang, J.J.; Boockvar, K.; Penrod, J.; Silberzweig, S.B.; Magaziner, J.; Koval, K.J.; Siu, A.L. The effect of perioperative anemia on clinical and functional outcomes in patients with hip fracture. *J. Orthop. Trauma* **2004**, *18*, 369–374. [CrossRef] [PubMed]

20. Foss, N.B.; Kristensen, M.T.; Kehlet, H. Anaemia impedes functional mobility after hip fracture surgery. *Age Ageing* **2008**, *37*, 173–178. [CrossRef] [PubMed]

21. Foss, N.B.; Kristensen, M.T.; Kehlet, H. Prediction of postoperative morbidity, mortality and rehabilitation in hip fracture patients: The cumulated ambulation score. *Clin. Rehabil.* **2006**, *20*, 701–708. [CrossRef] [PubMed]

22. Salive, M.E.; Cornoni-Huntley, J.; Phillips, C.L.; Guralnik, J.M.; Cohen, H.J.; Ostfeld, A.M.; Wallace, R.B. Serum albumin in older persons: Relationship with age and health status. *J. Clin. Epidemiol.* **1992**, *45*, 213–221. [CrossRef]

23. Adunsky, A.; Arad, M.; Blumstein, T.; Weitzman, A.; Mizrahi, E.H. Discharge hemoglobin and functional outcome of elderly hip fractured patients undergoing rehabilitation. *Eur. J. Phys. Rehabil. Med.* **2008**, 417–422.

24. Su, H.; Aharonoff, G.B.; Zuckerman, J.D.; Egol, K.A.; Koval, K.J. The relation between discharge hemoglobin and outcome after hip fracture. *Am. J. Orthop.* **2004**, *33*, 576–580. [PubMed]

25. Culleton, B.F.; Manns, B.J.; Zhang, J.; Tonelli, M.; Klarenbach, S.; Hemmelgarn, B.R. Impact of anemia on hospitalization and mortality in older adults. *Blood* **2006**, *107*, 3841–3846. [CrossRef] [PubMed]

26. Ferrucci, L.; Balducci, L. Anemia of aging: The role of chronic inflammation and cancer. *Semin. Hematol.* **2008**, *45*, 242–249. [CrossRef] [PubMed]

27. Atti, A.R.; Palmer, K.; Volpato, S.; Zuliani, G.; Winblad, B.; Fratiglioni, L. Anaemia increases the risk of dementia in cognitively intact elderly. *Neurobiol. Aging* **2006**, *27*, 278–284. [CrossRef] [PubMed]

28. Penninx, B.W.; Pluijm, S.M.; Lips, P.; Woodman, R.; Miedema, K.; Guralnik, J.M.; Deeg, D.J. Late-life anemia is associated with increased risk of recurrent falls. *J. Am. Geriatr. Soc.* **2005**, *53*, 2106–2111. [CrossRef] [PubMed]

29. Patterson, B.M.; Cornell, C.N.; Carbone, B.; Levine, B.; Chapman, D. Protein depletion and metabolic stress in elderly patients who have a fracture of the hip. *J. Bone Jt. Surg. Am.* **1992**, *74*, 251–260. [CrossRef]

30. Liu, Z.; Long, W.; Fryburg, D.A.; Barrett, E.J. The regulation of body and skeletal muscle protein metabolism by hormones and amino acids. *J. Nutr.* **2006**, *136*, 212S–217S. [PubMed]

31. Rittig, N.; Thomsen, H.H.; Bach, E.; Jørgensen, J.O.; Møller, N. Hormone and cytokine responses to repeated endotoxin exposures-no evidence of endotoxin tolerance after 5 weeks in humans. *Shock* **2015**, *44*, 32–35. [CrossRef] [PubMed]

32. Dal Negro, R.W.; Aquilani, R.; Bertacco, S.; Boschi, F.; Micheletto, C.; Tognella, S. Comprehensive effects of supplemented essential amino acids in patients with severe COPD and sarcopenia. *Monaldi Arch. Chest Dis.* **2010**, *73*, 25–33. [CrossRef] [PubMed]

33. Rondanelli, M.; Opizzi, A.; Antoniello, N.; Boschi, F.; Iadarola, P.; Pasini, E.; Aquilani, R.; Dioguardi, F.S. Effect of essential amino acid supplementation on quality of life, amino acid profile and strength in institutionalized elderly patients. *Clin. Nutr.* **2011**, *30*, 571–577. [CrossRef] [PubMed]

34. Bolasco, P.; Cupisti, A.; Locatelli, F.; Caria, S.; Kalantar-Zadeh, K. Dietary management of incremental transition to dialysis therapy: Once-weekly hemodialysis combined with low-protein diet. *J. Ren. Nutr.* **2016**, *26*, 352–359. [CrossRef] [PubMed]

35. Aquilani, R.; Zuccarelli, G.C.; Dioguardi, F.S.; Baiardi, P.; Frustaglia, A.; Rutili, C.; Comi, E.; Catani, M.; Iadarola, P.; Viglio, S.; et al. Effects of oral amino acid supplementation on long-term-care-acquired infections in elderly patients. *Arch. Gerontol. Geriatr.* **2011**, *52*, 123–128. [CrossRef] [PubMed]

36. Chumlea, W.C.; Roche, A.F.; Steinbaugh, M.L. Estimating stature from knee height for persons 60 to 90 years of age. *J. Am. Geriatr. Soc.* **1985**, *33*, 116–120. [CrossRef] [PubMed]

37. Charlson, M.E.; Pompei, P.; Ales, K.L.; MacKenzie, C.R. A new method of classifying prognostic comorbidity in longitudinal studies: Development and validation. *J. Chronic Dis.* **1987**, *40*, 373–383. [CrossRef]

38. Aquilani, R.; Opasich, C.; Gualco, A.; Verri, M.; Testa, A.; Pasini, E.; Viglio, S.; Iadarola, P.; Pastoris, O.; Dossena, M.; et al. Adequate energy-protein intake is not enough to improve nutritional and metabolic status in muscle-depleted patients with chronic heart failure. *Eur. J. Heart Fail.* **2008**, *10*, 1127–1135. [CrossRef] [PubMed]

39. Quarta Revisione dei livelli di Assunzione di Riferimento di Nutrienti (LARN) e di Energia per la popolazione italiana, 2014.

40. Soeters, P.B.; Grimble, R.F. Dangers, and benefits of the cytokine mediated response to injury and infection. *Clin. Nutr.* **2009**, *28*, 583–596. [CrossRef] [PubMed]

41. Margarson, M.P.; Soni, N. Serum albumin: Touchstone or totem? *Anaesthesia* **1998**, *53*, 789–803. [CrossRef] [PubMed]

42. Rothschild, M.A.; Oratz, M.; Schreiber, S.S. Serum albumin. *Hepatology* **1988**, *8*, 385–401. [CrossRef] [PubMed]

43. Baumgartner, R.N.; Koehler, K.M.; Romero, L.; Garry, P.J. Serum albumin is associated with skeletal muscle in elderly men and women. *Am. J. Clin. Nutr.* **1996**, *64*, 552–558. [PubMed]

44. Bastow, M.D.; Rawlings, J.; Allison, S.P. Benefits of supplementary tube feeding after fractured neck of femur: A randomised controlled trial. *Br. Med. J. Clin. Res. Ed.* **1983**, *287*, 1589–1592. [CrossRef] [PubMed]

45. Kendall, S.J.; Weir, J.; Aspinall, R.; Henderson, D.; Rosson, J. Erythrocyte transfusion causes immunosuppression after total hip replacement. *Clin. Orthop. Relat. Res.* **2000**, *381*, 145–155. [CrossRef]

46. Theusinger, O.M.; Spahn, D.R. Perioperative blood conservation strategies for major spine surgery. *Best Pract. Res. Clin. Anaesthesiol.* **2016**, *30*, 41–52. [CrossRef] [PubMed]

47. Kimball, S.R.; Fabian, J.R.; Pavitt, G.D.; Hinnebusch, A.G.; Jefferson, L.S. Regulation of guanine nucleotide exchange through phosphorylation of eukaryotic initiation factor eIF2alpha. Role of the alpha and delta-subunits of eiF2b. *J. Biol. Chem.* **1998**, *273*, 12841–12845. [PubMed]

48. Wang, X.; Campbell, L.E.; Miller, C.M.; Proud, C.G. Amino acid availability regulates p70S$_6$ kinase and multiple translation factors. *Biochem. J.* **1998**, *334*, 261–267. [CrossRef] [PubMed]

49. Fafournoux, P.; Bruhat, A.; Jousse, C. Amino acid regulation of gene expression. *Biochem. J.* **2000**, *351*, 1–12. [CrossRef] [PubMed]

50. Dillon, E.L.; Sheffield-Moore, M.; Paddon-Jones, D.; Gilkison, C.; Sanford, A.P.; Casperson, S.L.; Jiang, J.; Chinkes, D.L.; Urban, R.J. Amino acid supplementation increases lean body mass, basal muscle protein synthesis, and insulin-like growth factor-I expression in older women. *J. Clin. Endocrinol. Metab.* **2009**, *94*, 1630–1637. [CrossRef] [PubMed]

51. May, P.E.; Barber, A.; D'Olimpio, J.T.; Hourihane, A.; Abumrad, N.N. Reversal of cancer-related wasting using oral supplementation with a combination of beta-hydroxy-beta-methylbutyrate, arginine, and glutamine. *Am. J. Surg.* **2002**, *183*, 471–479. [CrossRef]

52. Smith, H.J.; Mukerji, P.; Tisdale, M.J. Attenuation of proteasome-induced proteolysis in skeletal muscle by {beta}-hydroxy-{beta}-methylbutyrate in cancer-induced muscle loss. *Cancer Res.* **2005**, *65*, 277–283. [PubMed]

53. Rothschild, M.A.; Oratz, M.; Mongelli, J.; Fishman, L.; Schreiber, S.S. Amino acid regulation of albumin synthesis. *J. Nutr.* **1969**, *98*, 395–403. [PubMed]

54. Boselli, M.; Aquilani, R.; Baiardi, P.; Dioguardi, F.S.; Guarnaschelli, C.; Achilli, M.P.; Arrigoni, N.; Iadarola, P.; Verri, M.; Viglio, S.; et al. Supplementation of essential amino acids may reduce the occurrence of infections in rehabilitation patients with brain injury. *Nutr. Clin. Pract.* **2012**, *27*, 99–113. [CrossRef] [PubMed]

55. Mizrahi, E.H.; Fleissig, Y.; Arad, M.; Blumstein, T.; Adunsky, A. Rehabilitation outcome of hip fracture patients: The importance of a positive albumin gain. *Arch. Gerontol. Geriatr.* **2008**, *47*, 318–326. [CrossRef] [PubMed]

56. Paddon-Jones, D.; Short, K.R.; Campbell, W.W.; Volpi, E.; Wolfe, R.R. Role of dietary protein in the sarcopenia of aging. *Am. J. Clin. Nutr.* **2008**, *87*, 1562S–1566S. [PubMed]

57. Paddon-Jones, D.; Wolfe, R.R.; Ferrando, A.A. Amino acid supplementation for reversing bed rest and steroid myopathies. *J. Nutr.* **2005**, *135*, 1809–1812.

58. Solerte, S.B.; Gazzaruso, C.; Bonacasa, R.; Rondanelli, M.; Zamboni, M.; Basso, C.; Locatelli, E.; Schifino, N.; Giustina, A.; Fioravanti, M. Nutritional supplements with oral amino acid mixtures increases whole-body lean mass and insulin sensitivity in elderly subjects with sarcopenia. *Am. J. Cardiol.* **2008**, *101*, 69E–77E. [CrossRef] [PubMed]

59. Gaskill, P.; Kabat, D. Unexpectedly large size of globin messenger ribonucleic acid. *Proc. Natl. Acad. Sci. USA* **1971**, *68*, 72–75. [CrossRef] [PubMed]

60. Rittig, N.; Bach, E.; Thomsen, H.H.; Johannsen, M.; Jørgensen, J.O.; Richelsen, B.; Jessen, N.; Møller, N. Amino acid supplementation is anabolic during the acute phase of endotoxin-induced inflammation: A human randomized crossover trial. *Clin. Nutr.* **2016**, *35*, 322–330. [CrossRef] [PubMed]

61. Hsieh, L.C.; Chien, S.L.; Huang, M.S.; Tseng, H.F.; Chang, C.K. Anti-inflammatory and anticatabolic effects of short-term beta-hydroxy-beta-methylbutyrate supplementation on chronic obstructive pulmonary disease patients in intensive care unit. *Asia Pac. J. Clin. Nutr.* **2006**, *15*, 544–550. [PubMed]

62. Baldissarro, E.; Aquilani, R.; Boschi, F.; Baiardi, P.; Iadarola, P.; Fumagalli, M.; Pasini, E.; Verri, M.; Dossena, M.; Gambino, A.; et al. The hip functional retrieval after elective surgery may be enhanced by supplemented essential amino acids. *Biomed. Res. Int.* **2016**, *2016*, 931–952. [CrossRef] [PubMed]

63. Vidal-Casariego, A.; Calleja-Fernández, A.; de Urbina-González, J.J.; Cano-Rodríguez, I.; Cordido, F.; Ballesteros-Pomar, M.D. Efficacy of glutamine in the prevention of acute radiation enteritis: A randomized controlled trial. *JPEN* **2014**, *38*, 205–213. [CrossRef] [PubMed]

64. Klimberg, V.S.; Souba, W.W.; Dolson, D.J.; Salloum, R.M.; Hautamaki, R.D.; Plumley, D.A.; Mendenhall, W.M.; Bova, F.J.; Khan, S.R.; Hackett, R.L. Prophylactic glutamine protects the intestinal mucosa from radiation injury. *Cancer* **1990**, *66*, 62–68. [CrossRef]

65. Bellows, C.F.; Jaffe, B.M. Glutamine is essential for nitric oxide synthesis by murine macrophages. *J. Surg. Res.* **1999**, *86*, 213–219. [CrossRef] [PubMed]

66. Shinozaki, M.; Saito, H.; Muto, T. Excess glutamine exacerbates trinitrobenzenesulfonic acid-induced colitis in rats. *Dis. Colon Rectum* **1997**, *40*, 59–63. [CrossRef]

67. Ferrucci, L.; Guralnik, J.M.; Bandinelli, S.; Semba, R.D.; Lauretani, F.; Corsi, A.; Ruggiero, C.; Ershler, W.B.; Longo, D.L. Unexplained anaemia in older persons is characterised by low erythropoietin and low levels of pro-inflammatory markers. *Br. J. Haematol.* **2007**, *136*, 849–855. [CrossRef] [PubMed]

68. Ferrucci, L.; Guralnik, J.M.; Woodman, R.C.; Bandinelli, S.; Lauretani, F.; Corsi, A.M.; Chaves, P.H.; Ershler, W.B.; Longo, D.L. Proinflammatory state and circulating erythropoietin in persons with and without anemia. *Am. J. Med.* **2005**, *118*, 1288. [CrossRef] [PubMed]

69. Chahal, H.S.; Drake, W.M. The endocrine system and ageing. *J. Pathol.* **2007**, *211*, 173–180. [CrossRef] [PubMed]

70. Bellelli, G.; Magnifico, F.; Trabucchi, M. Outcomes at 12 months in a population of elderly patients discharged from a rehabilitation unit. *J. Am. Med. Dir. Assoc.* **2008**, *9*, 55–64. [CrossRef] [PubMed]

71. Dybkaer, R.; Lauritzen, M.; Krakauer, R. Relative reference values for clinical chemical and haematological quantities in 'healthy' elderly people. *Acta Med. Scand.* **1981**, *209*, 1–9. [CrossRef] [PubMed]

72. Smith, D.L. Anemia in the elderly. *Am. Fam. Physician* **2000**, *62*, 1565–1572. [PubMed]

73. Dodd, S.L.; Powers, S.K.; Brooks, E.; Crawford, M.P. Effects of reduced O_2 delivery with anemia, hypoxia, or ischemia on peak VO_2 and force in skeletal muscle. *J. Appl. Physiol.* **1993**, *74*, 186–191. [PubMed]

74. Olivares, M.; Hertrampf, E.; Capurro, M.T.; Wegner, D. Prevalence of anemia in elderly subjects living at home: Role of micronutrient deficiency and inflammation. *Eur. J. Clin. Nutr.* **2000**, *54*, 834–839. [CrossRef] [PubMed]

75. Hepple, R.T. Skeletal muscle: Microcirculatory adaptation to metabolic demand. *Med. Sci. Sports Exerc.* **2000**, *32*, 117–123. [CrossRef] [PubMed]

76. Anker, S.D.; Ponikowski, P.P.; Clark, A.L.; Leyva, F.; Rauchhaus, M.; Kemp, M.; Teixeira, M.M.; Hellewell, P.G.; Hooper, J.; Poole-Wilson, P.A.; et al. Cytokines and neurohormones relating to body composition alterations in the wasting syndrome of chronic heart failure. *Eur. Heart J.* **1999**, *20*, 683–693. [CrossRef] [PubMed]

77. García-Martínez, C.; López-Soriano, F.J.; Argilés, J.M. Acute treatment with tumour necrosis factor-alpha induces changes in protein metabolism in rat skeletal muscle. *Mol. Cell. Biochem.* **1993**, *125*, 11–18. [CrossRef] [PubMed]

78. Deveci, D.; Marshall, J.M.; Egginton, S. Relationship between capillary angiogenesis, fiber type, and fiber size in chronic systemic hypoxia. *Am. J. Physiol. Heart Circ. Physiol.* **2001**, *281*, 241–252.

79. Kasuya, H.; Kawashima, A.; Namiki, K.; Shimizu, T.; Takakura, K. Metabolic profiles of patients with subarachnoid hemorrhage treated by early surgery. *Neurosurgery* **1998**, *42*, 1268–1274. [CrossRef] [PubMed]

80. Li, J.J.; Fang, C.H. C-reactive protein is not only an inflammatory marker but also a direct cause of cardiovascular diseases. *Med. Hypotheses.* **2004**, *62*, 499–506. [CrossRef] [PubMed]

81. De Maat, M.P.; Trion, A. C-reactive protein as a risk factor versus risk marker. *Curr. Opin. Lipidol.* **2004**, *15*, 651–657.
82. Von Haehling, S.; Steinbeck, L.; Doehner, W.; Springer, J.; Anker, S.D. Muscle wasting in heart failure: An overview. *Int. J. Biochem. Cell Biol.* **2013**, *45*, 2257–2265. [CrossRef] [PubMed]
83. Mastorakos, G.; Chrousos, G.P.; Weber, J.S. Recombinant interleukin-6 activates the hypothalamic-pituitary-adrenal axis in humans. *J. Clin. Endocrinol. Metab.* **1993**, *77*, 1690–1694. [PubMed]
84. Madsen, T.; Skou, H.A.; Hansen, V.E.; Fog, L.; Christensen, J.H.; Toft, E.; Schmidt, E.B. C-reactive protein, dietary *n*-3 fatty acids, and the extent of coronary artery disease. *Am. J. Cardiol.* **2001**, *88*, 1139–1142. [CrossRef]
85. Devaraj, S.; Jialal, I. Alpha tocopherol supplementation decreases serum C-reactive protein and monocyte interleukin-6 levels in normal volunteers and type 2 diabetic patients. *Free Radic. Biol. Med.* **2000**, *29*, 790–792. [CrossRef]
86. Sierksma, A.; van der Gaag, M.S.; Kluft, C.; Hendriks, H.F. Moderate alcohol consumption reduces plasma C-reactive protein and fibrinogen levels; a randomized, diet-controlled intervention study. *Eur. J. Clin. Nutr.* **2002**, *56*, 1130–1136. [CrossRef] [PubMed]
87. Adams, J.S.; Hewison, M. Unexpected actions of vitamin D: New perspectives on the regulation of innate and adaptive immunity. *Nat. Clin. Pract. Endocrinol. Metab.* **2008**, *4*, 80–90. [CrossRef] [PubMed]
88. Pinheiro da Silva, F.; Machado, M.C. Antimicrobial peptides: Clinical relevance and therapeutic implications. *Peptides* **2012**, *36*, 308–314. [CrossRef] [PubMed]
89. Pellicane, A.J.; Wysocki, N.M.; Schnitzer, T.J. Prevalence of 25-hydroxyvitamin D deficiency in the outpatient rehabilitation population. *Am. J. Phys. Med. Rehabil.* **2010**, *89*, 899–904. [CrossRef] [PubMed]
90. Quraishi, S.A.; Camargo, C.A. Vitamin D in acute stress and critical illness. *Curr. Opin. Clin. Nutr. Metab. Care* **2012**, *15*, 625–634. [CrossRef] [PubMed]
91. Jeng, L.; Yamshchikov, A.V.; Judd, S.E.; Blumberg, H.M.; Martin, G.S.; Ziegler, T.R.; Tangpricha, V. Alterations in vitamin D status and anti-microbial peptide levels in patients in the intensive care unit with sepsis. *J. Transl. Med.* **2009**, *7*, 28. [CrossRef] [PubMed]
92. Venning, G. Recent developments in vitamin D deficiency and muscle weakness among elderly people. *BMJ* **2005**, *330*, 524–526. [CrossRef] [PubMed]
93. Pfeifer, M.; Begerow, B.; Minne, H.W.; Schlotthauer, T.; Pospeschill, M.; Scholz, M.; Lazarescu, A.D.; Pollähne, W. Vitamin D status, trunk muscle strength, body sway, falls, and fractures among 237 postmenopausal women with osteoporosis. *Exp. Clin. Endocrinol. Diabetes* **2001**, *109*, 87–92. [CrossRef] [PubMed]
94. Simpson, J.L.; Bischoff, F. Cell-free fetal DNA in maternal blood: Evolving clinical applications. *JAMA* **2004**, *291*, 1135–1137. [CrossRef] [PubMed]
95. Rondanelli, M.; Klersy, C.; Terracol, G.; Talluri, J.; Maugeri, R.; Guido, D.; Faliva, M.A.M.; Solerte, B.S.; Fioravanti, M.; Lukaski, H.; et al. Whey protein, amino acids, and vitamin D supplementation with physical activity increases fat-free mass and strength, functionality, and quality of life and decreases inflammation in sarcopenic elderly. *Am. J. Clin. Nutr.* **2016**, *103*, 830–840. [CrossRef] [PubMed]
96. Hedström, M.; Ljungqvist, O.; Cederholm, T. Metabolism and catabolism in hip fracture patients: Nutritional and anabolic intervention-a review. *Acta Orthop.* **2006**, *77*, 741–747. [CrossRef] [PubMed]
97. Magaziner, J.; Simonsick, E.M.; Kashner, T.M.; Hebel, J.R.; Kenzora, J.E. Predictors of functional recovery one year following hospital discharge for hip fracture: A prospective study. *J. Gerontol.* **1990**, *45*, 101–107. [CrossRef]

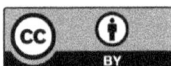

nutrients

MDPI

Article

Iron Absorption from Three Commercially Available Supplements in Gastrointestinal Cell Lines

Francesca Uberti [1],*, Vera Morsanuto [1], Sabrina Ghirlanda [2] and Claudio Molinari [1]

[1] Laboratory of Physiology, Department of Translational Medicine, University of Eastern Piedmont, via Solaroli 17, 28100 Novara, Italy; vera.morsanuto@med.uniupo.it (V.M.); claudio.molinari@med.uniupo.it (C.M.)

[2] noiVita s.r.l.s. Spin-Off of University of Eastern Piedmont, via A. Canobio 4/6, 28100 Novara, Italy; info@noivita.it

* Correspondence: francesca.uberti@med.uniupo.it; Tel.: +39-0321-660-653

Received: 17 July 2017; Accepted: 9 September 2017; Published: 13 September 2017

Abstract: This study compares the absorption characteristics of two iron-based dietary supplements and their biocompatibility to bisglycinate iron, a common chelated iron form. The Caco-2 cell line—a model of human intestinal absorption—and GTL-16 cell line—a model of gastric epithelial cells—were used to perform the experiments; in the first experiments, the kinetics of absorption have been evaluated analyzing the divalent metal transporter 1 (DMT1) expression. Three different iron combinations containing 50 μM iron (named Fisioeme®, Sideral® and bisglycinate) were used for different stimulation times (1–24 h). After this, the effects of the three iron formulations were assessed in both a short and a long time, in order to understand the extrusion mechanisms. The effects of the three different formulations were also analyzed at the end of stimulation period immediately after iron removal, and after some time in order to clarify whether the mechanisms were irreversibly activated. Findings obtained in this study demonstrate that Fisioeme® was able to maintain a significant beneficial effect on cell viability compared to control, to Sideral®, and to iron bisglycinate. This observation indicates that Fisioeme® formulation is the most suitable for gastric and intestinal epithelial cells.

Keywords: iron metabolism; iron mechanisms; Caco-2 permeability; GTL-16 permeability; DMT1 receptor

1. Introduction

Iron deficiency anaemia is the most common nutritional disorder in the world. This condition affects a large number of children as well as women in reproductive age both in developing countries and in industrialized ones. Moreover, iron deficiency affects hemodialysis patients receiving erythropoietic stimulators as well. The numbers are impressive; 2 billion people, over 30% of the world's population, are anaemic, over 50% due to iron deficiency, and, in poorer areas, this is frequently exacerbated by infectious diseases [1]. Several factors can contribute to iron deficiency, but low bioavailability of iron in the diet is one of the most important [2]. Iron in the diet is present both in its non-heme and heme forms, and the two of them are absorbed in duodenum. Non-heme iron accounts for more than 85% of the total iron in the diet, but it features a low bioavailability (2–7%) since several dietary factors strongly interfere with it [3]. Presently, iron supplements are the best options for maintaining iron stores in the body. However, not only the iron content, but also the bioavailability of iron for absorption largely depends on the dietary components [4]. For example, iron in its heme form is highly bioavailable, and meat-containing diets show beneficial effects as well [5]. Recently, the attention of the researchers has focused on the absorption mechanisms in the gut. Inorganic iron absorption, indeed, requires multiple mechanisms for entry and exit from duodenal and jejunal epithelial cells. If inorganic iron from the diet or supplements is not presented in a highly absorbable formulation, it will not be optimally absorbed by the intestine and subsequently transferred into the bloodstream. The part of iron trapped in the intestinal epithelial cells is then eliminated through the stools after the end of the life cycle of the enterocyte [6]. Therefore, several approaches have been attempted to improve the availability and absorption of iron through the gastrointestinal barrier. Most iron supplements are made up of ferrous salts, which is positively charged iron associated with its negatively charged counter-ions. Most common counter-ions are glycinate, sulfate, gluconate, and fumarate. Once ingested, the acidic juice within the stomach acts to dissolve the iron salt. Unfortunately, iron dietary supplementation is associated with potentially dangerous side effects and overload risk. It is well known that iron overdose can cause severe corrosive lesions to the upper gastrointestinal tract, including necrosis of the mucous membrane, ulcer and ischemia. However, epithelial gastrointestinal lesions in patients receiving iron therapy have received little attention despite its extensive use.

The aim of this study was to analyze the differences between different iron supplements in order to understand how to plan better food supplementation.

2. Materials and Methods

2.1. Cell Culture

The human intestinal Caco-2 cell line, purchased from American Type Culture Collection (ATCC, Manassas, VA, USA), was used as an experimental model [7] to predict the features of intestinal absorption following oral intake [8]. This is a widely accepted cellular model to study absorption, metabolism, and bioavailability of drugs and xenobiotics. Furthermore, this cell line has been used in other studies on iron bioavailability [9]. These cells were grown in Dulbecco's Modified Eagle's Medium/Nutrient F-12 Ham (DMEM-F12, Sigma-Aldrich, Milan, Italy) containing 10% fetal bovine serum (FBS, Sigma-Aldrich), 2 mM L-glutamine (Sigma-Aldrich), and 1% penicillin-streptomycin (Sigma-Aldrich) at 37 °C in incubator at 5% CO_2. Cells were used from passages 46 to 49 to perform different experiments, such as 3-(4,5-Dimethylthiazol-2-yl)-2,5-Diphenyltetrazolium Bromide (MTT), plating 1×10^4 cells in 96-well plates, Western blot and interleukin 8 (IL-8) plating 1×10^6 cells in 6-well plates, plating 1×10^6 cells in 6-well plates, 0.5×10^4 cells were placed in Culture Slide (BD Biosciences, Bedford, MA, USA) with 4 chambers to perform iron histochemistry studies, absorption study plating 2×10^4 cells on 6.5 mm transwell with 0.4 µm pore polycarbonate membrane insert (Sigma-Aldrich) in a 24-well plate. Before the experiments, cells were washed and incubated for 8 h in DMEM without red phenol and supplemented with 0.5% FBS, 2 mM L-glutamine, and 1% penicillin-streptomycin at 37 °C in an incubator and then stimulated. Cells plated on transwell insert were maintained in complete medium changed every other day, first basolaterally and then apically for 21 days before the stimulations.

GTL-16 cell line, donated by the Laboratory of Histology of the University of Eastern Piedmont, is a clonal line derived from a poorly differentiated gastric carcinoma cell line [10] widely used as a model of gastric epithelial cells. Cells were cultured in Dulbecco's Modified Eagle Medium (DMEM) supplemented with 10% foetal bovine serum (FBS), 1% penicillin-streptomycin in incubator at 37 °C, 5% CO_2 [11]. This cell line was plated at different densities, 1×10^4 cells were plated on 96-well plates to study cell viability (MTT test); 2×10^4 cells were seeded onto 6.5 mm translucent polyethylene terephthalate (PET) transwell insert 0.4 µm in a 24 well to study absorption; 0.5×10^4 cells were placed in Culture Slide (BD Biosciences, Bedford, MA, USA) with 4 chambers to perform immunohistochemistry tests. Moreover, the cells were plated on 60 mm dishes until confluence to analyze the intracellular pathways through Western blot analysis and IL-8. The cells plated on transwell insert were maintained in complete medium changed every other day, first basolaterally and then apically for 7 days before the stimulations. Before stimulations, cells were synchronized by incubation in DMEM without red phenol and FBS and supplemented with 1% penicillin/streptomycin,

2 mM L-glutamine and 1 mM sodium pyruvate in an incubator at 37 °C, 5% CO_2, and 95% humidity for 18 h [11].

2.2. Experimental Protocol

These cell lines were used to evaluate the absorption of iron through stomach and intestinal epithelial cells, in order to clarify the effects after oral intake. In addition, the role of oxidative stress as a consequence of treatment was investigated both during and further to the removal treatment. Finally, since the effectiveness of iron after oral intake depends on its composition, three different formulations of iron were analyzed.

The study was divided into three parts: in the first part, the kinetics of absorption, by DMT1 expression analysis, were evaluated. Both cell lines were treated with the same iron concentration (50 µM) [12] prepared in 3 different ways (named Fisioeme®, Sideral® and bisglycinate) for different times (ranging from 1 h to 24 h). In the second part, the effects of iron prepared in the same 3 formulations in a short (3 h) and long time (24 h) were assessed, in order to understand the extrusion mechanisms. Finally, in the third part, the effects of iron, prepared in the same 3 formulations, were analyzed at the end of stimulation period and after its removal, at short (3 h plus 3 h) and long time (24 h plus 24 h) in order to clarify whether the mechanisms were irreversibly activated.

2.3. Agent Preparations

Fisioeme® (FIS) and Sideral® (SID) are dietary supplements. FIS combines the properties of iron bysglicinate, folic acid and vitamin C to improve iron absorption while avoiding such negative gastric effects such as hyperacidity. Each tablet is composed of 30 mg iron, 80 mg vitamin C, and 400 µg folic acid. On the other hand, SID is composed of iron encapsulated in a membrane. In detail, iron is associated with vitamin C and B12. Each capsule is composed of 14 mg iron, 60 mg vitamin C and 370 µg vitamin B12. FIS and SID were grinded and dissolved directly in the DMEM without red phenol and FBS but supplemented with 1% penicillin/streptomycin, 2 mM L-glutamine and 1 mM sodium pyruvate to make a 20× concentration and then diluted in the same medium to obtain 1× (50 µM iron). Finally, iron bisglycinate (BIS) formulated in pure powder was prepared directly in DMEM without red phenol and FBS but supplemented with 1% penicillin/streptomycin, 2 mM L-glutamine and 1 mM sodium pyruvate according to the solubility to obtain a concentration of 20× and then diluted in the same medium to use 1× (50 µM iron).

2.4. MTT Test

MTT-based In Vitro Toxicology Assay Kit (Sigma-Aldrich) was performed as described in literature [11] to determine cell viability after stimulations. Briefly, at the end of treatments, Caco-2 and GTL-16 cells were incubated with 1% MTT dye in DMEM without red phenol 0% FBS for 2 h at 37 °C in incubator [13] and cell viability was determined measuring absorbance at 570 nm with correction at 690 nm through a spectrometer (VICTORX4 multilabel plate reader, PerkinElmer, Waltham, MA, USA). Cell viability was obtained comparing the results to control cells (baseline 0).

2.5. Caco-2 Permeability Assay

After 21 days, the three different iron formulations were added to culture medium under different pH conditions, as reported in literature [14,15]; pH 6.5 preparations were added to the apical side, whereas pH 7.4 to the basolateral side. The slightly acidic pH (pH 6.5) in the apical side represents the average pH in the lumen of the small intestine, whereas the neutral pH (pH 7.4) in the basolateral side mimics the pH of the blood. During treatments the cells were maintained in incubator at 5% CO_2 and, at the end of stimulations, the iron quantity was measured by a specific kit.

2.6. GTL-16 Permeability Assay

After 7 days, to study the effects on iron absorption of apical-to-basolateral (Ap–Bl) pH gradients, the medium was changed on both the apical (donor compartment) and basolateral (receiver compartment) sides adding HCl to the medium to obtain pH 3 at apical side for 60 min, as reported in literature [16,17]. At the end, the stimulations were performed in the same manner and conditions as previously described and then iron quantity was measured by kit.

2.7. Apparent Permeability Coefficient (Papp)

The presence of iron was assessed in the apical and basolateral compartments converting the amount of total volume in relationship with the surface area of the transwell ($\mu g/cm^2$), following a classic method [18]. Briefly, the Papp (cm/s) was calculated as:

$$P_{app} = dQ/dt \times 1/m_0 \times 1/A \times V_{Donor}$$

dQ: amount of substance transported (nmol or μg);
dt: incubation time (sec);
m0: amount of substrate applied to donor compartment (nmol or μg);
A: surface area of transwell membrane (cm^2);
V_{Donor}: volume of the donor compartment (cm^3).
Negative controls without cells were tested to exclude transwell membranes influence.

2.8. Iron Quantification Assay

Iron Assay Kit (Sigma-Aldrich) measures ferrous iron (Fe^{2+}), ferric iron (Fe^{3+}), and total iron (total iron – ferrous iron) in samples following the manufacturer's instructions. Briefly, Caco-2 and GTL-16 cells at apical side were lysed in 4 volumes of cold Iron Assay Buffer, centrifuged at 13,000 rpm for 10 min at 4 °C and supernatants were measured. The medium at the basolateral side was directly centrifuged at 13,000 rpm for 10 min at 4 °C and supernatants were measured. To measure total iron, 5 μL of Iron Reducer to each of the sample wells to reduce Fe^{3+} to Fe^{2+} were added. All reactions were incubated for 30 min at room temperature (RT), protected from light and then 100 μL of Iron Probe were added to each well containing standard or test samples and incubated for 60 min at RT and protected from light. The absorbance at 593 nm (A593) was measured by spectrometer (Victor). Total iron ($Fe^{2+} + Fe^{3+}$) concentrations can be determined from the standard curve. Fe^{3+} is equal to total iron (sample plus iron reducer) $-Fe^{2+}$ (sample plus assay buffer). The iron concentration was expressed as ng/μL.

2.9. Iron Histochemistry

Perls' and Turnbull's stains were used to visualize ferric iron (Fe^{3+}) and ferrous iron (Fe^{2+}), respectively [19,20] (see Appendix A).

2.10. IL-8 Assay Kit

Human IL-8 Quantikine ELISA Kits (R&D Systems, Abingdon, UK) [21] were used for sandwich ELISA experiments. Each condition was tested in triplicates according to the manufacturer's specifications, and the output was measured using a microplate reader (Victor) at 450 nm within 30 min with correction to 540 nm. Concentrations (ng/mL) were obtained by fitting data to a standard curve and results expressed as a mean $\pm$ standard deviation (SD) (% vs. control).

2.11. Western Blot of Cell Lysates

Caco-2 and GTL-16 cells were lysed in ice Complete Tablet Buffer (Roche, Milan, Italy) supplemented with 2 mM sodium orthovanadate, 1 mM phenylmethanesulfonyl fluoride (PMSF; Sigma-Aldrich), 1:50 mix

Phosphatase Inhibitor Cocktail (Sigma-Aldrich) and 1:200 mix Protease Inhibitor Cocktail (Calbiochem, San Diego, CA, USA) and 35 µg of proteins of each sample were resolved on 8% and 15% SDS-PAGE gels. Polyvinylidene difluoride membranes (PVDF, GE, Healthcare Europe GmbH, Milan, Italy) were incubated overnight at 4 °C with specific primary antibody: anti-annexin V (1:2000; Sigma-Aldrich), anti-p53 (1:250, Santa Cruz Biotechnology, Heidelberg Germany), anti-ferroportin (1:250, Santa Cruz Biotechnology), anti-ferritin (1:250, Santa Cruz Biotechnology) and anti-DMT1 (1:250, Santa Cruz Biotechnology). Protein expression was normalized and verified through β-actin detection (1:5000; Sigma-Aldrich) and expressed as mean ± SD (% vs. control).

2.12. Statistical Analysis

For each experimental protocol, at least four independent experiments were run; the results are expressed as means ± SD of independent experiments performed on four technical replicates. One-way ANOVA followed by Bonferroni post hoc test were used for statistical analysis, and pairwise differences compared by Mann–Whitney U tests. p-values < 0.05 were considered statistically significant.

3. Results

3.1. Time-Course Study on DMT1 Expression

The effects on DMT1 expression of 50 µM iron were analyzed by the stimulation of Caco-2 and GTL-16 cultures with SID and BIS for different times (ranging from 1 h to 24 h). Since iron formulated in FIS is a combination of BIS with other substances, in these experiments, BIS was used as a control substance. As reported in a time course study (Figure 1), the effect on DMT1 expression on both cell types showed a time dependent increase that was similar using SID to when BIS was used. The effects on DMT1 expression were significantly increased ($p < 0.05$) starting from 3 h after treatments with SID and BIS on both cell types and the maximum effects were observed at 24 h. For this reason, 3 h and 24 h were used for all successive experiments.

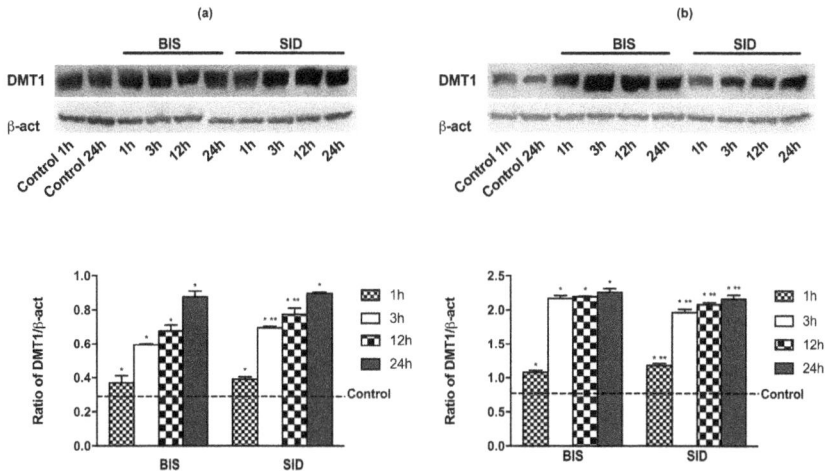

Figure 1. Time-course study (from 1 h to 24 h) of divalent metal transporter 1 (DMT1) receptor in GTL-16 (**a**) and Caco-2 cells (**b**) treated with different iron formulations. Western blot (upper) and densitometric analysis (down) normalized through β-act are reported. The results are expressed as means ± standard deviation (SD) of four independent experiments for each cell type. The control line shows the average of all control measures recorded at different times. BIS = iron bisglycinate; SID = Sideral®. * $p < 0.05$ vs. control (reported as line); ** $p < 0.05$ vs. correspondent column at different times.

3.2. Cell Viability and Cell Regulation

In order to demonstrate the safety of iron supplementation, we evaluated if the levels of the investigated compounds (50 µM iron) were toxic to Caco-2 and GTL-16 cells by conducting cell viability experiments. Iron showed a formulation-dependent effect on cell viability (Figure 2A,B) on both cell types in a time-dependent manner. FIS and SID at 3 h were able to increase ($p < 0.05$) cell viability in GTL-16 cells compared to control and to BIS, confirming their beneficial properties regarding its metabolization, but, at 24 h, only FIS was able to maintain a significant beneficial effect on cell viability compared to control, to SID, and to BIS. This observation indicates that FIS formulation was more suitable for stomach epithelial cells. Moreover, in Caco-2 cells, these effects were more evident, and the differences between 3 h and 24 h obtained from each iron formulation were higher. BIS did not induce any significant change independently from stimulation time ($p > 0.05$), whereas FIS showed the maximum effect on cell viability at 3 h and maintained a minimal effect at 24 h. Finally, SID induced a significant effect at 3 h, but, at 24 h, its effect was decreased and resulted similar to the control ($p > 0.05$). These data confirm the best biocompatibility of iron formulated in FIS during transit time in the intestinal tract. In addition, as reported in Figure 2C,D, the inflammatory marker IL-8 was also investigated to verify the effectiveness of the treatments on both cell types; indeed, the concentration of IL-8 was time-dependent. In particular, in GTL-16 cells, only the sample treated with SID showed a significant increase in IL-8 concentration already at 3 h ($p < 0.05$ versus control), and this effect appeared amplified at 24 h. Similarly, SID formulation increased IL-8 concentration in Caco-2 cells as well. These data confirm the effectiveness and tolerability of FIS compared to SID on both cell types over time. SID induces the inflammatory mediator IL-8 but FIS does not, and, therefore, it may be more suitable as an iron supplement.

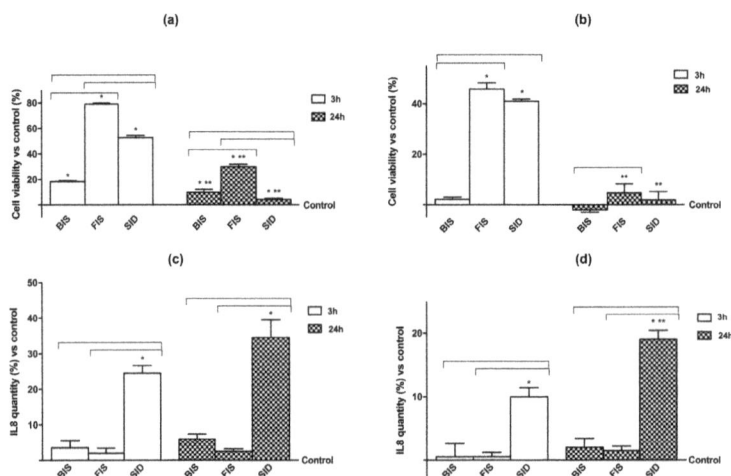

Figure 2. Cell viability (**a,b**) and interleukin 8 (IL-8) concentration (**c,d**) at 3 h and 24 h measured on GTL-16 and Caco-2 cells treated with different iron formulations. In A and B cell viability, measured by 3-(4,5-Dimethylthiazol-2-yl)-2,5-Diphenyltetrazolium Bromide (MTT) assay, and in C and D IL-8 concentration, measured by ELISA kit, on both cell types were reported. Data are expressed as means ± SD (% vs. control) of four independent experiments for each cell type. FIS = Fisioeme[®]. * $p < 0.05$ vs. control (reported as line); ** $p < 0.05$ vs. correspondent column at different time; bars $p < 0.05$ among different treatments at the same time.

In order to confirm this hypothesis, activation of p53 and Annexin V was also investigated in both cell types at 3 h and 24 h after treatment with different iron formulations (Figure 3). In GTL-16 cells at

3 h and 24 h, BIS did not induce any significant change on p53 and Annexin V activation compared to control. On the contrary, FIS and SID were able to reduce p53 and Annexin V levels compared to control ($p < 0.05$) at 3 h; however, only FIS at 24 h was able to maintain the activation at a basal level on both proteins. Indeed, at 24 h, SID significantly ($p < 0.05$) increased the activation of p53 and Annexin V. Similarly, in Caco-2 cells, both BIS and FIS were able to maintain both proteins at low level ($p > 0.05$) at 3 h and 24 h compared to control. On the contrary, SID induced activation of p53 already at 3 h ($p < 0.05$ compared to control); at 24 h, both levels of protein were augmented ($p < 0.05$ compared to control).

All of these data confirm a better influence on cell integrity exerted by the iron formulation contained in FIS compared to the other tested formulations.

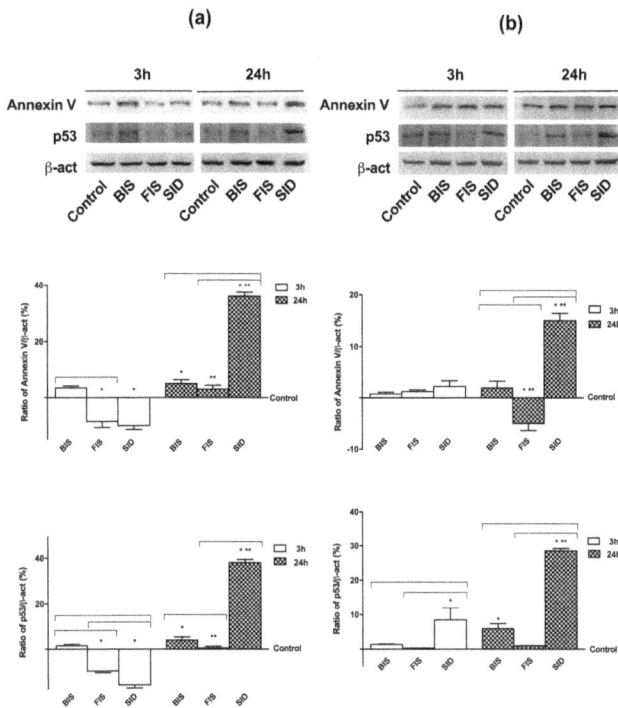

Figure 3. Western blot and densitometric analysis of Annexin V and p53 on GTL-16 (**a**) and Caco-2 cells (**b**) treated with different iron formulations at 3 h and 24 h. Western blot (upper) and densitometric analysis (down) are reported. The results after normalization through β-act and control, are expressed as means ± SD (% vs. control) of four independent experiments for each cell type. * $p < 0.05$ vs. control (reported as line); ** $p < 0.05$ vs. correspondent column at different time; bars $p < 0.05$ among different treatments at the same time.

3.3. Iron Deposition and Quantification

To clarify the beneficial effects of iron supplements, some experiments were performed to evaluate the balance between Fe^{2+} and Fe^{3+} (Appendix B: Figures A1 and A2) in order to verify whether Fe^{3+} was not accumulated into gastric and intestinal epithelia. Control cultures not treated with iron showed a small amount of background staining whose intensity was not different from washing solution. The slides of untreated (control) samples stained with Perls' and Turnbull's methods demonstrated that cells in the control condition appeared to be healthy. The intensity of staining (positive cells) for Fe^{2+} and Fe^{3+} was relatively similar regardless of time and treatments applied on both cell types; the maximum intensity was observed on both cell types at 3 h and 24 h in the presence of BIS and SID, but the differences between the two staining methods were not significant ($p > 0.05$). For this reason, on both cell types, the intracellular and extracellular iron quantity (total Fe) was also investigated (Figure 4). In GTL-16 cells, the intracellular quantity of iron (ng/μL) further to administration of BIS and FIS showed a time-dependent effect (greater at 24 h) and BIS was more present compared to FIS ($p < 0.05$). SID revealed no significant difference in time at the intracellular level. The study of the extracellular environment (iron crossing the membrane in gastric cells and in intestinal cells respectively) showed that the amount of iron was higher with FIS treatment and this effect was maintained over time. These data were confirmed by analysis of transepithelial resistance (Table 1) in which FIS exhibited a moderately higher permeability than SID and BIS both at 3 h and at 24 h. Finally, studying Caco-2 cells (Figure 4) intracellular environment, no significant changes were observed among the different iron formulations at 3 h. On the other hand, at 24 h, BIS and SID were present in greater amounts than FIS. Evaluating the extracellular environment (basolateral side, corresponding to plasma) at 3 h, no significant changes were observed. However, at 24 h, permanence time of FIS was quantitatively present longer ($p < 0.05$) compared to the other formulations. Similar data were obtained by analysis of transepithelial resistance (Table 1). Indeed, the permeability of FIS was higher than BIS and SID in both stimulation times. However, only the apical to basolateral transport was evaluated, which would not indicate whether P-gp was active against the absorption of a particular compound. In both cell types, the cell monolayers used exhibited tight junctions and this allowed the rapid permeation of the highly absorbed compound.

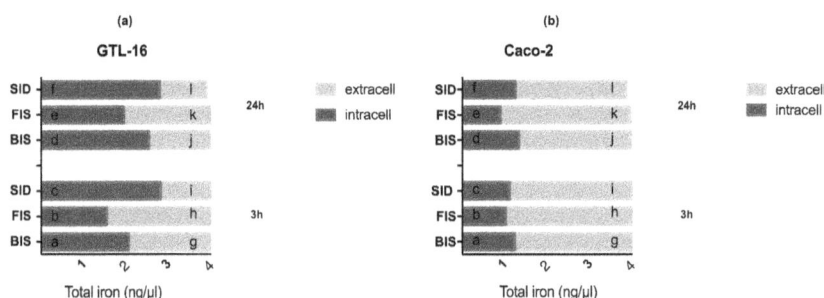

Figure 4. Total iron quantification on intracellular and extracellular environments of GTL-16 (**a**) and Caco-2 (**b**) cells treated with different iron formulations at 3 h and 24 h. The graphics report the iron movements quantified. The results are expressed as means ± SD of four independent experiments for each cell type. In (**a**) a $p < 0.05$ vs. b, c; b $p < 0.05$ vs. c; e $p < 0.05$ vs. d, f; g $p < 0.05$ vs. h, i; h $p < 0.05$ vs. i, k; g $p < 0.05$ vs. j; j $p < 0.05$ vs. k; k $p < 0.05$ vs. l. In (**b**) $p < 0.05$ vs. b, c; e $p < 0.05$ vs. d, f; b $p < 0.05$ vs. e; c $p < 0.05$ vs. f; h $p < 0.05$ vs. g, i; k $p < 0.05$ vs. j, l; g $p < 0.05$ vs. j; h $p < 0.05$ vs. k; i $p < 0.05$ vs. l.

Table 1. Apical to basolateral permeability. Apparent permeability values (Papp) represent mean data ± standard deviation (SD) from three separate measurements of each compound tested in one experiment, each with four independently analyzed.

Iron Formulation	P_{app} (10^{-6} cm/s) at 3 h		P_{app} (10^{-6} cm/s) at 24 h	
	GTL-16	Caco-2	GTL-16	Caco-2
SID	5.02 ± 1.1 **	15.07 ± 1.9 **	0.63 ± 0.035	1.57 ± 0.41
FIS	12.56 ± 1.43 *,**	16.08 ± 2 **	1.38 ± 0.4	1.88 ± 0.43
BIS	10.35 ± 1.82 *,**	13.56 ± 1.8 **	0.94 ± 0.6	1.44 ± 0.35

SID = Sideral®; FIS = Fisioeme®; BIS = iron bisglycinate. * $p < 0.05$ vs. SID; ** $p < 0.05$ between the same treatment at different time.

3.4. Iron Mechanisms

Since iron metabolism is influenced by various conditions, the importance of the different iron formulations on iron uptake (DMT1 analysis) and on transfer across the cell monolayer (ferritin light chain for transportation and ferroportin to extrude) was investigated as well (Figure 5). In GTL-16 cells, BIS was able to induce the expression of DMT1 in a time-dependent manner with a maximum effect at 24 h, but it was mainly embedded inside the cells, as shown by ferritin and ferroportin levels ($p < 0.05$ compared to control). FIS and SID were able to induce the expression of DMT1 in a similar time-dependent manner with a maximum of effectiveness at 24 h, but only FIS was able to effectively pass across the cell at 24 h ($p < 0.05$), indicating the beneficial effect of the composition in the gastric cells metabolism and into the intestinal tract. In Caco-2 cells, a similar effect on DMT1 expression among the treatments can be observed, but the formulations showed a different time-dependent extrusion mechanism with a maximum effect at 24 h. In particular, a greater transfer across the cell with FIS treatment was observed as shown by ferroportin involvement. These data demonstrate the ability of FIS to carry out its effects in a better way, compared to other iron formulations.

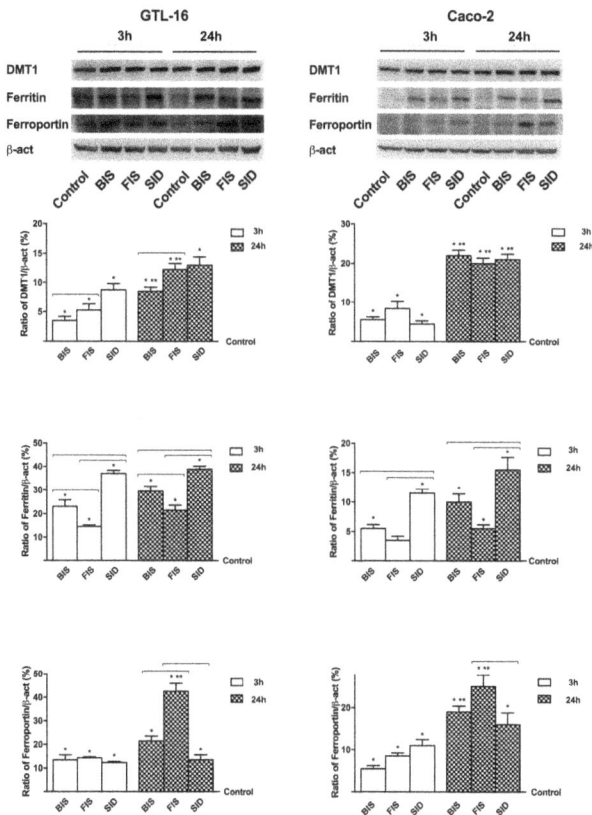

Figure 5. Western blot (upper) and densitometric analysis (down) of DMT1, ferritin light chain and ferroportin expressed on GTL-16 and Caco-2 cells treated with different iron formulations at 3 h and 24 h. The images are an example of four independent experiments for each cell type. The results obtained after normalization through β-act and then through control values are expressed as means ± SD of four independent experiments for each cell types. * $p < 0.05$ vs. control; ** $p < 0.05$ vs. correspondent column at different times; bars $p < 0.05$ among different treatments at the same time

3.5. Irreversible Effects of Iron

Since the effects of iron could be negative for cells following its intracellular accumulation, some additional experiments were carried out maintaining both cell types in absence of the iron formulations for a supplementary time (3 h iron plus 3 h without iron and 24 h with iron plus 24 h without iron).

As shown in Figure 6A, cell viability was time-dependent on both cell lines with a maximum effect at 24 h plus 24 h; in particular, in GTL-16 cells, BIS and FIS were able to maintain a significant cell viability ($p < 0.05$) over time, whereas SID was less effective to maintain viability. Similarly, BIS and FIS in Caco-2 cells were able to maintain viability with a maximum effect at 24 h plus 24 h ($p < 0.05$). On the other hand, SID caused a reduction of viability, thus supporting the hypothesis that iron formulated with SID could be trapped in the intestinal tract. The inflammatory framework (Figure 6B) was associated with the viability and supported the accumulation hypothesis of iron formulated with SID. Indeed, both GTL-16 and Caco-2 cells showed a significant increase in IL-8 concentration compared to control ($p < 0.05$) and to the other treatments ($p < 0.05$) already at 3 h plus 3 h.

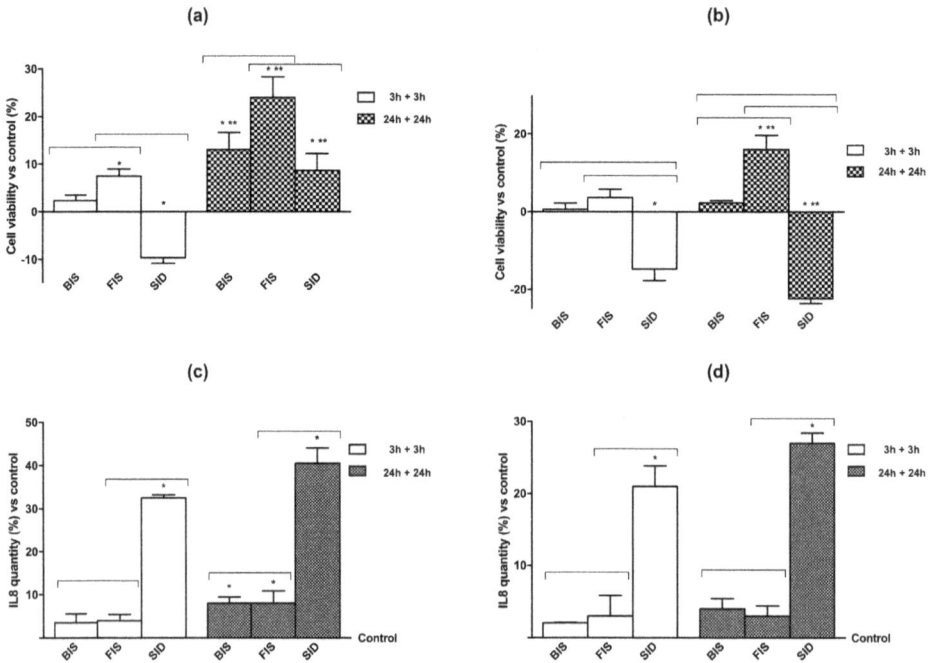

Figure 6. Cell viability and IL-8 concentration measured on GTL-16 and Caco-2 cells maintained for equal time (3 h plus 3 h; 24 h plus 24 h) without iron treatments. In (**a**) and (**b**) cell viability, measured by MTT assay, and in (**c**) and (**d**) IL-8 concentration, measured by ELISA kit, on both cell types are reported. Data are expressed as means ± SD (% vs. control) of four independent experiments for each cell type. * $p < 0.05$ vs. control; ** $p < 0.05$ vs. correspondent column at different time; bars $p < 0.05$ among different treatments at the same time.

In addition, the activation of p53 and annexin V (Figure 7) supported the hypothesis of the accumulation of iron associated with SID treatment on both cell types; indeed, p53 and annexin V already showed an increase at 3 h plus 3 h ($p < 0.05$).

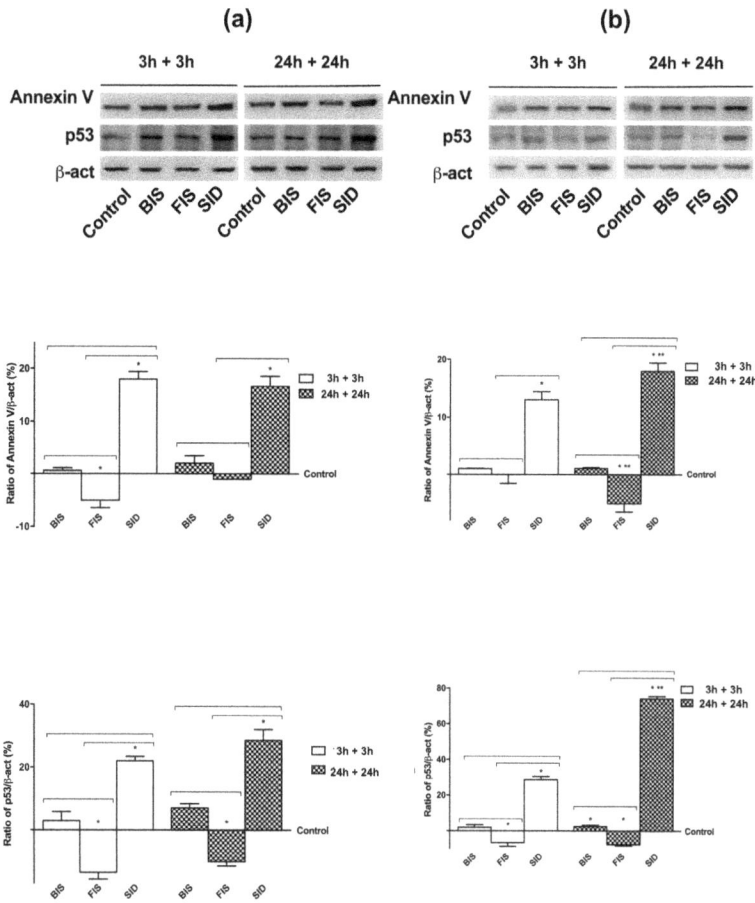

Figure 7. Western blot and densitometric analysis of p53 and Annexin V on GTL-16 (**a**) and Caco-2 cells (**b**) maintained for equal time (3 h plus 3 h; 24 h plus 24 h) without iron treatments. Western blot (upper) and densitometric analysis (down) are reported. The results after normalization through β-act and control, are expressed as a means ± SD (% vs. control) of four independent experiments for each cell type. * $p < 0.05$ vs. control; ** $p < 0.05$ vs. correspondent column at different time; bars $p < 0.05$ among different treatments at the same time.

3.6. Iron Metabolism

Since the different effectiveness of iron formulations on both cell types was demonstrated, the deposition mechanisms and the output of iron were also investigated to evaluate ferritin light chain and ferroportin in the absence of iron treatment (Figure 8).

On both cell lines, the activation of ferritin light chain was significantly reduced in the samples treated with FIS and significantly increased ($p < 0.05$) in the samples treated with SID in a time-dependent manner with maximum effects at 24 h plus 24 h. On the contrary, the output receptor ferroportin, in GTL-16 cells was increased in a time-dependent manner in samples treated with BIS and FIS with maximum effectiveness at 24 h plus 24 h, whereas SID treatment showed a significant reduction ($p < 0.05$) on ferroportin expression. Similar mechanisms have been observed in Caco-2 cells as well, with a greater inhibition of ferroportin at 24 h plus 24 h compared to control ($p < 0.05$). These data demonstrate that iron in all formulations was partially accumulated and slowly released over time; however, this effect did not appear after SID treatment because iron was trapped within the cells. In additon, further experiments were carried out to evaluate the production of reactive oxygen species (ROS) induced both in GTL-16 and Caco-2 cells by the administration of BIS, FIS and SID (Appendix B: Figure A3). The results are comparable to those observed in viability and inflammatory framework experiments. FIS showed the lowest ROS increase in both cell cultures compared to BIS and SID, and this increase in ROS production is always not significant compared to control regardless of exposure time. Finally, in total iron quantification experiments, FIS has always shown to induce a better balance between intracellular and extracellular compartment compared to BIS and SID (Appendix B: Figure A4); indeed, the extracellular amount, which is the one that has passed through the barrier, is higher or equals the intracellular amount. Thus, FIS is better than BIS and SID in regards to this effect. This result was also observed in long exposure time and even without stimulus. Moreover, iron stores are lower in Caco-2 than in GTL-16.

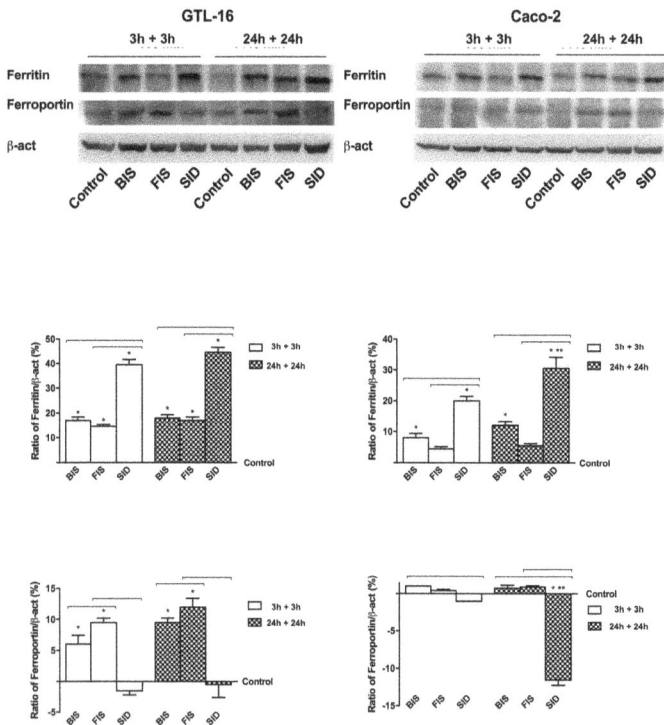

Figure 8. Western blot and densitometric analysis of ferritin light chain and ferroportin expressed on GTL-16 and Caco-2 cells maintained for equal time (3 h plus 3 h; 24 h plus 24 h) without iron treatments. Western blot (upper) and densitometric analysis (down) are reported. The results obtained after normalization through β-act and then through control values, are expressed as a means $\pm$ SD (% vs. control) of four independent experiments for each cell type. * $p < 0.05$ vs. control; ** $p < 0.05$ vs. correspondent column at different times; bars $p < 0.05$ among different treatments at the same time.

4. Discussion

Current strategies about iron deficiency treatment are based on oral ferrous iron supplements; however, these may be poorly tolerated by patients due to gastrointestinal side effects [12,22], which interfere with the efficiency of the treatment itself. The biocompatibility of iron dietary supplements is a common issue in treatment of iron deficiency anaemia. Moreover, the iron formulation can be very important in determining such side effects as severe corrosive injury to the epithelial gastrointestinal cells, including mucosal necrosis, ulceration, and ischemia.

In this study, we compared the biocompatibility and biological activity of a range of commercially available iron supplements using a well-characterized in vitro model of digestive system [23]. Cell lines used in the present work are widely accepted as an experimental model of gastrointestinal system.

The Caco-2 human intestinal cell model is among the most widely used for drug development, toxicology and intestinal physiology studies. Caco-2 cells differ in a monolayer of polarized cells coupled by junctions that express many morpho-functional characteristics of the absorbent epithelium of the small intestine. For this reason, Caco-2 cells have been extensively used for iron uptake studies [24]. On the other hand, the GTL-16 cell line is a clonal line derived from a poorly differentiated gastric carcinoma cell line [10] and is widely used as a model of gastric epithelial cells. Findings obtained in this study demonstrate that FIS was able to maintain a significant beneficial effect on cell viability and integrity compared to control, to SID, and to BIS. Furthermore, the inflammatory framework was maintained at a more basal level by treatments with FIS and BIS than that observed after SID treatment. Similar data were observed after removal of iron. These observations indicate that FIS formulation is more suitable for gastric and intestinal epithelial cells.

It is noteworthy that tests on intracellular iron, total iron quantification, and molecular mechanisms demonstrate that FIS is able to physiologically regulate iron metabolism, whereas iron in SID appears to be trapped within cells. The epithelium of the intestinal mucosa is one of the major barriers in terms of extension between the intestine and the internal organs. As such, it is a dual target of any toxic insult from drugs or substances in the diet: in fact, mucosal alterations are not only a damage to the tissue itself but can cause uncontrolled passage of potentially toxic substances from the intestinal lumen to blood. The physiological role of FIS is further demonstrated by the small and not significant increase in ROS production. Details are reported in Appendix B. In addition, the permeability resistance observed in both cell types showed a mutual relationship between measured iron concentration and cellular permeability, which accounts for the better absorption and solubility of iron bysglicinate compared to iron pyrophosphate. In the future, additional experiments will be performed in vivo to explore the effects of these iron formulations in an anaemic mouse experimental model.

5. Conclusions

In conclusion, FIS that contains iron bisglycinate has a better bioavailability than compound BIS and SID, which we have investigated. For this reason, FIS is a good choice of iron preparation as a food supplement.

Acknowledgments: Laborest Italia S.p.a (Lorenzo Secondini) contributed to preparing and donating compounds. The authors wish to thank Mariangela P. Fortunato for her precious help with the language. This study was partially funded by the "DiMeT-UPO 2016" grant.

Author Contributions: F.U. and C.M. conceived and designed the experiments. F.U., V.M. and S.G. performed the experiments and F.U. analyzed the data, and F.U. and C.M. wrote the paper. All authors critically reviewed and contributed to the final draft.

Conflicts of Interest: The authors declare no conflict of interest.

Appendix A

Appendix A.1. Method: Iron Histochemistry

The cells cultured on chamber slides at the end of stimulations were washed three times with cold PBS 1× supplemented with 2 mM sodium orthovanadate, and fixed using a cold fixative solution (3.7% formaldehyde, 3% sucrose in PBS 1×) for 20 min at RT. Then, the chamber slides were incubated in a sufficient amount of Prussian Blue cell staining reagent composed of an equal amount of potassium ferrocyanide and HCl or of Turnbull staining reagent composed of 5:1 potassium ferrocyanide and HCl for 10 min at RT. Then, the slides were counterstained with Safranin-O for 5 min at RT and mounted with Bio Mount (Bio-Optika, Milan, Italy). The number of positive cells was calculated as described elsewhere [25]. Briefly, 12 different areas (1 mm^2) randomly selected from each section were taken, and the number of signals was determined using ImagePro 3 software (NIH, Bethesda, MD, USA). The results were expressed as means $\pm$ SD (% vs. control).

Appendix A.2. Method: Radical Oxygen Species (ROS) Analysis

ROS production was determined as a superoxide dismutase-inhibitable reduction of cytochrome C, following a standard technique [13,20]. In all samples (both treated and control), 100 μL of cytochrome C (Sigma-Aldrich) and in another one 100 μL of superoxide dismutase (Sigma-Aldrich) were added for 30 min in an incubator. The absorbance was measured at 550 nm by spectrometer (VICTORX3 Multilabel Plate Reader, Perkin Elmer, Waltham, MA, USA) and the O$_2$ was expressed as nanomoles per reduced cytochrome C per microgram of protein and reported as a mean $\pm$ SD (%).

Appendix B

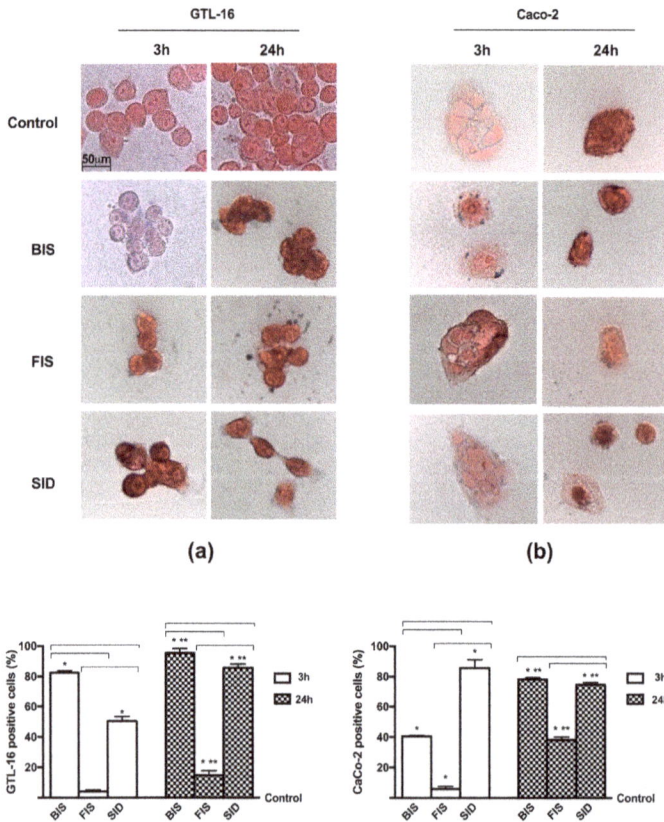

Figure A1. Perl's staining on GTL-16 (**a**) and Caco-2 (**b**) cells treated with different iron formulations at 3 h and 24 h. (**top**) the images show an example of four independent experiments taken at original magnification 40×. The scale bar in the first image can be used for all others; (**bottom**) the positive cells counted were obtained from four independent experiments and expressed as means $\pm$ SD (% vs. control). * $p < 0.05$ vs. control; ** $p < 0.05$ vs. correspondent column at different times; bars $p < 0.05$ among different treatments at the same time.

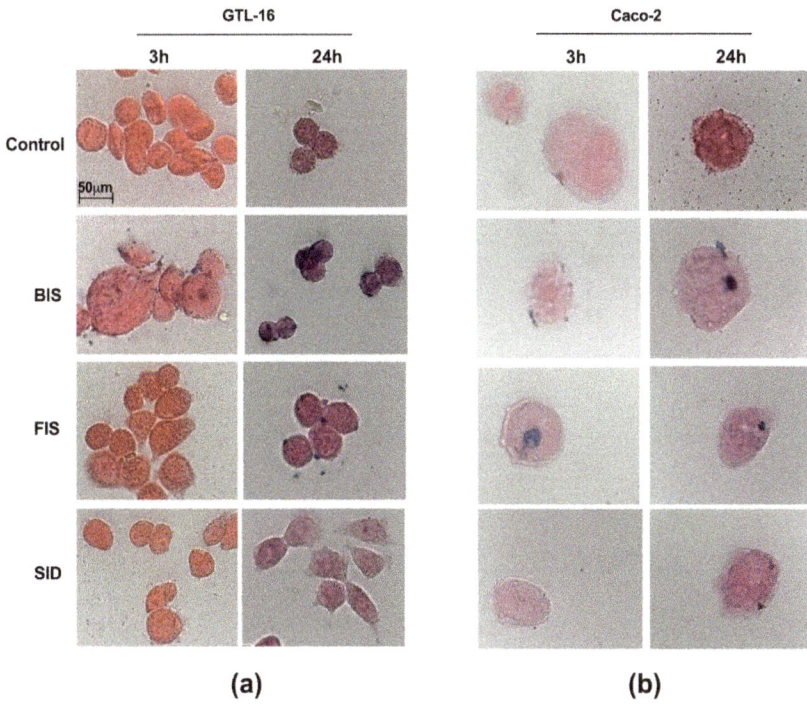

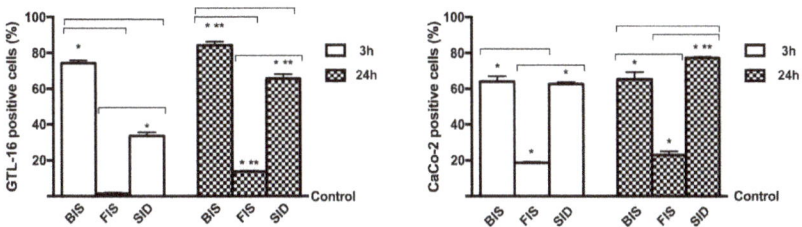

Figure A2. Turnbull staining on GTL-16 (**a**) and Caco-2 cells (**b**) treated with different iron formulations at 3 h and 24 h. (**top**) the images reported are an example of four independent experiments taken at original magnification 40×. The scale bar in the first image can be used for all others; (**bottom**) the positive cells counted were obtained from four independent experiments and expressed as means ± SD (% vs. control). * $p < 0.05$ vs. control; ** $p < 0.05$ vs. correspondent column at different times; bars $p < 0.05$ among different treatments at the same time.

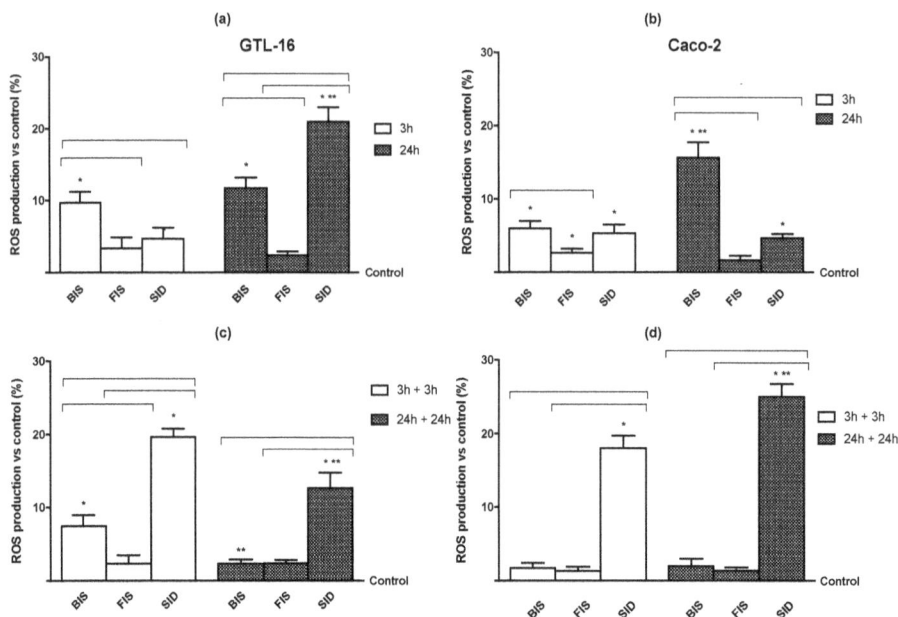

Figure A3. Radical oxygen species (ROS) measurements on GTL-16 (**a,c**) and Caco-2 (**b,d**) cells treated with different iron formulations at 3 h and 3 h plus 3 h or 24 h and 24 h plus 24 h. The results are expressed as means ± SD of four independent experiments for each cell type. * $p < 0.05$ vs. control; ** $p < 0.05$ vs. correspondent column at different time; bars $p < 0.05$ among different treatment at the same time.

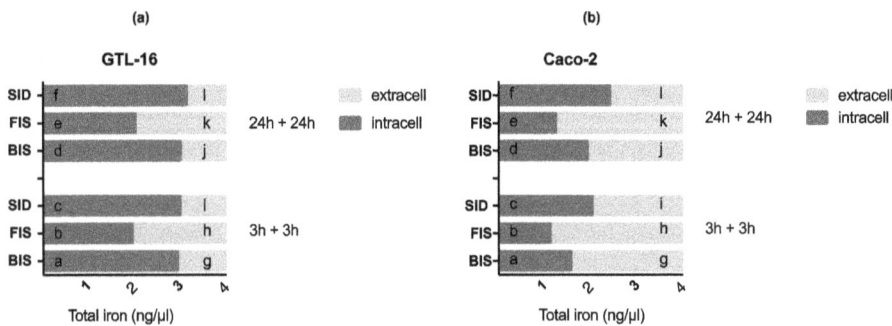

Figure A4. Total iron quantification in GTL-16 (**a**) and Caco-2 (**b**) cells treated with different iron formulations at 3 h plus 3 h and 24 h plus 24 h. The graphs show the iron movements quantified. Results are expressed as mean ± SD of four independent experiments for each cell type. In (**a**) a $p < 0.05$ vs. b, c, d; b $p < 0.05$ vs. c; d $p < 0.05$ vs. e; c, e $p < 0.05$ vs. f; g $p < 0.05$ vs. h, i; h $p < 0.05$ vs. i; j $p < 0.05$ vs. k; i, k $p < 0.05$ vs. l. In (**b**), a $p < 0.05$ vs. b, c, d; b $p < 0.05$ vs. c; d $p < 0.05$ vs. e, f; c, e $p < 0.05$ vs. f; g $p < 0.05$ vs. h, i, j; h $p < 0.05$ vs. i; j $p < 0.05$ vs. k, l; i $p < 0.05$ vs. l.

References

1. Miller, J.L. Iron deficiency anemia: A common and curable disease. *Cold Spring Harb. Perspect. Med.* **2013**, *1*, a011866. [CrossRef] [PubMed]
2. Scheers, N.M.; Almgren, A.B.; Sandberg, A.S. Proposing a caco-2/hepG2 cell model for in vitro iron absorption studies. *J. Nutr. Biochem.* **2014**, *25*, 710–715. [CrossRef] [PubMed]
3. Miret, S.; Tascoglu, S.; Van der Burg, M.; Frenken, L.; Klaffke, W. In vitro bioavailability of iron from the heme analogue sodium iron chlorophyllin. *J. Agric. Food Chem.* **2010**, *58*, 1327–1332. [CrossRef] [PubMed]
4. Sharp, P.A. Intestinal iron absorption: Regulation by dietary & systemic factors. *Int. J. Vitam. Nutr. Res.* **2010**, *80*, 231–242. [CrossRef]
5. López, M.A.; Martos, F.C. Iron availability: An updated review. *Int. J. Food Sci. Nutr.* **2004**, *55*, 597–606. [CrossRef] [PubMed]
6. Fuqua, B.K.; Vulpe, C.D.; Anderson, G.J. Intestinal iron absorption. *J. Trace Elem. Med. Biol.* **2012**, *26*, 115–119. [CrossRef] [PubMed]
7. Fossati, L.; Dechaume, R.; Hardillier, E.; Chevillon, D.; Prevost, C.; Bolze, S.; Maubon, N. Use of simulated intestinal fluid for Caco-2 permeability assay of lipophilic drugs. *Int. J. Pharm.* **2008**, *360*, 148–155. [CrossRef] [PubMed]
8. DiMarco, R.L.; Hunt, D.R.; Dewi, R.E.; Heilshorn, S.C. Improvement of paracellular transport in the Caco-2 drug screening model using protein-engineered substrates. *Biomaterials* **2017**, *129*, 152–162. [CrossRef] [PubMed]
9. Christides, T.; Ganis, J.C.; Sharp, P.A. In vitro assessment of iron availability from commercial Young Child Formulae supplemented with prebiotics. *Eur. J. Nut.* **2016**, *9*, 1–10. [CrossRef] [PubMed]
10. Giordano, S.; Di Renzo, M.F.; Ferracini, R.; Chiadò-Piat, L.; Comoglio, P.M. A protein with associated tyrosine kinase activity in a human gastric carcinoma cell line. *Mol. Cell Biol.* **1988**, *8*, 3510–3517. [CrossRef] [PubMed]
11. Uberti, F.; Bardelli, C.; Morsanuto, V.; Ghirlanda, S.; Molinari, C. Role of vitamin D3 combined to alginates in preventing acid and oxidative injury in cultured gastric epithelial cells. *BMC Gastroenterol.* **2016**, *16*, 127. [CrossRef] [PubMed]
12. Christides, T.; Wray, D.; McBride, R.; Fairweather, R.; Sharp, P. Iron bioavailability from commercially available iron supplements. *Eur. J. Nutr.* **2015**, *54*, 1345–1352. [CrossRef] [PubMed]
13. Uberti, F.; Lattuada, D.; Morsanuto, V.; Nava, U.; Bolis, G.; Vacca, G.; Squarzanti, D.F.; Cisari, C.; Molinari, C. Vitamin D protects human endothelial cells from oxidative stress through the autophagic and survival pathways. *J. Clin. Endocrinol. Metab.* **2014**, *99*, 1367–1374. [CrossRef] [PubMed]
14. Natoli, M.; Leoni, B.D.; D'Agnano, I.; D'Onofrio, M.; Brandi, R.; Arisi, I.; Zucco, F.; Felsani, A. Cell growing density affects the structural and functional properties of Caco-2 differentiated monolayer. *J. Cell Physiol.* **2011**, *226*, 1531–1543. [CrossRef] [PubMed]
15. Obringer, C.; Manwaring, J.; Goebel, C.; Hewitt, N.J.; Rothe, H. Suitability of the in vitro Caco-2 assay to predict the oral absorption of aromatic amine hair dyes. *Toxicol. In Vitro* **2016**, *32*, 1–7. [CrossRef] [PubMed]
16. Fernandes, I.; de Freitas, V.; Reis, C.; Mateus, N. A new approach on the gastric absorption of anthocyanins. *Food Funct.* **2012**, *3*, 508–516. [CrossRef] [PubMed]
17. Lemieux, M.; Bouchard, F.; Gosselin, P.; Paquin, J.; Mateescu, M.A. The NCI-N87 cell line as a gastric epithelial barrier model for drug permeability assay. *Biochem. Biophys. Res. Commun.* **2011**, *412*, 429–434. [CrossRef] [PubMed]
18. Pardridge, W.M.; Triguero, D.; Yang, J.; Cancilla, P.A. Comparison of in vitro and in vivo models of drug transcytosis through the blood–brain barrier. *J. Pharmacol. Exp. Ther.* **1990**, *253*, 884–891. [PubMed]
19. Owen, J.E.; Bishop, G.M.; Robinson, S.R. Uptake and Toxicity of Hemin and Iron in Cultured Mouse Astrocytes. *Neurochem. Res.* **2016**, *41*, 298–306. [CrossRef] [PubMed]
20. Uberti, F.; Morsanuto, V.; Bardelli, C.; Molinari, C. Protective effects of 1α,25-Dihydroxyvitamin D3 on cultured neural cells exposed to catalytic iron. *Physiol. Rep.* **2016**, *4*, e12769. [CrossRef] [PubMed]
21. Uberti, F.; Morsanuto, V.; Lattuada, D.; Colciaghi, B.; Cochis, A.; Bulfoni, A.; Colombo, P.; Bolis, G.; Molinari, C. Protective effects of vitamin D3 on fimbrial cells exposed to catalytic iron damage. *J. Ovarian Res.* **2016**, *9*, 34. [CrossRef] [PubMed]

22. Hyder, S.M.; Persson, L.A.; Chowdhury, A.M.; Ekstrom, E.C. Do side-effects reduced compliance to iron supplementation? A study of daily- and weekly- dose regimens in pregnancy. *J. Health Popul. Nutr.* **2002**, *20*, 175–179. [PubMed]

23. Yun, S.; Habicht, J.P.; Miller, D.D.; Glahn, R.P. An in vitro digestion Caco-2 cell culture system accurately predicts the effects of ascorbic acid and polyphenolic compounds on iron bioavailability in humans. *J. Nutr.* **2004**, *134*, 2717–2721. [PubMed]

24. Garcia, M.N.; Flowers, C.; Cook, J.D. The Caco-2 cell culture system can be used as a model to study food iron availability. *J. Nutr.* **1996**, *126*, 251–258. [PubMed]

25. Chana, K.; Fenwick, P.; Nicholson, A.; Barnes, P.; Donnelly, L. Identification of a distinct glucocorticosteroid-insensitive pulmonary macrophage phenotype in patients with chronic obstructive pulmonary disease. *J. Allergy Clin. Immunol.* **2014**, *133*, 207–216. [CrossRef] [PubMed]

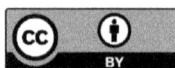

nutrients

MDPI

Review

Development of Databases on Iodine in Foods and Dietary Supplements

Abby G. Ershow [1],*, Sheila A. Skeaff [2], Joyce M. Merkel [1] and Pamela R. Pehrsson [3]

[1] Office of Dietary Supplements, National Institutes of Health, Bethesda, MD 20892, USA; merkelj@od.nih.gov
[2] Department of Human Nutrition, University of Otago, Dunedin 9010, New Zealand; sheila.skeaff@otago.ac.nz
[3] Nutrient Data Laboratory, US Department of Agriculture, Beltsville, MD 20705, USA; pamela.pehrsson@ars.usda.gov
* Correspondence: ershowa@od.nih.gov; Tel.: +1-301-435-2920

Received: 16 November 2017; Accepted: 10 January 2018; Published: 17 January 2018

Abstract: Iodine is an essential micronutrient required for normal growth and neurodevelopment; thus, an adequate intake of iodine is particularly important for pregnant and lactating women, and throughout childhood. Low levels of iodine in the soil and groundwater are common in many parts of the world, often leading to diets that are low in iodine. Widespread salt iodization has eradicated severe iodine deficiency, but mild-to-moderate deficiency is still prevalent even in many developed countries. To understand patterns of iodine intake and to develop strategies for improving intake, it is important to characterize all sources of dietary iodine, and national databases on the iodine content of major dietary contributors (including foods, beverages, water, salts, and supplements) provide a key information resource. This paper discusses the importance of well-constructed databases on the iodine content of foods, beverages, and dietary supplements; the availability of iodine databases worldwide; and factors related to variability in iodine content that should be considered when developing such databases. We also describe current efforts in iodine database development in the United States, the use of iodine composition data to develop food fortification policies in New Zealand, and how iodine content databases might be used when considering the iodine intake and status of individuals and populations.

Keywords: iodine; database; food; dietary supplements; food composition

1. Introduction

Low levels of iodine in the soil and groundwater are common in many parts of the world, often leading to diets that are low in iodine. Severe iodine deficiency is now rare due to widespread salt iodization, but mild-to-moderate deficiency is still prevalent even in many developed countries [1]. Knowledge about all sources of dietary iodine, including foods, beverages, water, salts, and supplements, is important for understanding patterns of iodine intake and for planning interventions. Robust food composition tables specific to individual countries are a key practical resource in providing population-level and individual-level guidance for better iodine nutrition. This article will discuss the importance of well-constructed databases on the iodine content of foods and dietary supplements, the primary causes of variability in iodine content, the desirable characteristics of these databases, and their current availability worldwide. We also describe recent progress in iodine database development and use in the United States (US) and New Zealand, and consider database applications relevant to the assessment of iodine intake of populations and individuals.

2. Background

Iodine is essential for the synthesis of thyroid hormone and thus is required for normal physical, neurological, and intellectual growth of infants and children, and for normal metabolism and function in adults. On a body weight basis, infancy and early childhood are the times of highest iodine requirements. Pregnant and lactating women also have increased requirements to meet their heightened physiologic needs. It is critical that women who are likely to conceive, or are pregnant or lactating, have iodine reserves sufficient for their own health and also sufficient to provide the fetus and infant with the necessary iodine supply [2,3]. The most serious consequences of iodine deficiency are well characterized and include hypothyroidism, neuro-cognitive impairment, and, in cases of severe deficiency in pregnancy, cretinism in the infant. In contrast, the consequences of mild-to-moderate iodine deficiency are less well understood and are an important priority for research and public health practice. In particular, concerns center on the impact of mild-to-moderate iodine deficiency in pregnancy, which has a high prevalence worldwide [1], on child development. Two observational studies found an association between inadequate iodine status in pregnancy and poorer academic performance in their children [4,5], although a recent randomized controlled trial reported no difference in cognitive scores of children born to mildly iodine deficient mothers supplemented with iodine or placebo in pregnancy [6].

Satisfactory iodine nutrition can be achieved in most circumstances through intake of adequately iodized salt in sufficient quantities and/or intake of other iodine-rich foods that are commonly consumed within a country [7]. In the early 1920s, iodized table salt was introduced in many countries, a practice that since then has spread to include the majority of countries with about 86% of the world's population recently estimated as having access to iodized salt [8]. World Health Organization (WHO) recommends Universal Salt Iodization, whereby all salt for human and animal consumption is iodized including salt used in the food industry [9]. Some countries add iodized salt to only a few foods, for example in New Zealand and Australia, where the mandatory use of iodized salt in commercial bread production was implemented in 2009. However, in other countries iodized salt may be available but not used in commercially prepared food [10,11], or the salt may be iodized but at a very low level [10].

Iodine deficiency has re-emerged in countries such as Australia [12] and New Zealand [13]. A drop in iodine intake may reflect recent changes in food consumption patterns in which home-prepared foods, traditionally made with iodized salt, have been replaced with commercially prepared foods made with non-iodized salt. For example, in the case of the US, this point is reinforced by surveys documenting that retail sales of iodized salt have declined [11] and that less time is now spent preparing foods at home [14]. This situation has raised concerns about potentially inadequate intakes of iodine despite high intakes of salt from commercially prepared foods [15]. Likewise, individuals or ethnic groups whose diets exclude or restrict iodine-rich food sources for health, religious, or other reasons (such as vegan/vegetarian diet patterns, lactose intolerance, or low salt diets) may be at risk for inadequate iodine intake [16]. Knowing the iodine content of available foods thus becomes a key component in understanding which foods are the most important contributors to iodine intake for populations as well as individuals.

The need for improved data on the iodine content of foods and beverages has been noted by several expert committees [17,18] and has recently been reviewed in detail [19]. Also, iodine derived from dietary supplements must be included along with foods in order to accurately assess total intake; therefore, data are needed on the iodine content of supplements [20]. Robust approaches to developing databases will include choosing appropriate analytical methodology (including use of standard reference materials [21,22]); designing and implementing sampling plans with good coverage of major country-specific contributors (from foods, beverages, dietary supplements, and salt); and publishing the results in database formats or tables that allow linkage with population surveys and individual intake records (such as food frequency questionnaires and 24-h recalls).

3. The Availability of Databases Including Iodine Content

Many countries have developed national databases that include information on the iodine content of foods, beverages, and salts, and other food components. To identify food and nutrient composition databases for individual countries and to determine if these databases included values for iodine, and also to identify information on national iodization programs for salt or other foods, we conducted an extensive Internet search using resources from FAO INFOODS [23], the recently released ILSI interactive tool [24], and other sites including Google and Google Scholar. In most cases the keywords used were "food composition", "food composition database", "iodine composition", "iodine in foods", and the name of the country using countries listed by the US Department of State. (https://www.state. gov/misc/list/). We did not specify any particular language in our search, although many databases were available in English either in their original form or in translation.

Over 124 countries have known salt iodization programs, either mandatory or voluntary [25], but for many of these countries it was not possible to determine if the country had a national food composition database, and if so, to ascertain the presence or absence of iodine data. Table 1 presents information on the availability of national food composition databases, by country, that have iodine content data, and it also describes national iodization practices. Most databases provide for all kinds of foods with a few exceptions, such as Turkey's database, which contains iodine values only for table salt, fish, and shellfish. However, as shown in Table 2, national iodine databases are not currently available for many countries that do have national food composition databases containing information on other nutrients. In some cases, limited iodine datasets have been published as part of scholarly or other journal publications [26–31]. (NOTE: The compilation presented in Tables 1 and 2 is not exhaustive, nor is it equivalent to a systematic literature review. The information is dynamic, meaning that at the time of this publication, links to databases were verified to be active; however, links may change or become inactive over time.)

Table 1. National food composition databases that include iodine.

Country	Year of Salt Iodization	URL	Database Name
Armenia	2004 [32]	pdf.usaid.gov/pdf_docs/Pdach758.pdf	Armenian Food Composition Table 2010
Australia	1953/54 [1] [33]	www.foodstandards.gov.au/science/ monitoringnutrients/ausnut/foodnutrient/	AUSNUT 2011-13 Food Nutrient Database
Austria	1963 [34]	www.oenwt.at/content/naehrwert-suche/	OENWT Österreichische Nährwerttabelle
Bahrain	Not found [2]	www.fao.org/fileadmin/templates/food_ composition/documents/pdf/ FOODCOMPOSITONTABLESFORBAHRAIN.pdf	Food Composition Tables for the Kingdome of Bahrain
Czech Republic	1950 [34]	www.nutridatabaze.cz/en/	Czech Food Composition Database
Denmark	1998 [34]	frida.fooddata.dk/AlpList.php	Danish Food Composition Databank
Finland	1949 [34]	fineli.fi/fineli/en/index	Fineli, National Food Composition Database in Finland
France	1952 [34]	pro.anses.fr/TableCIQUAL/	CIQUAL French Food Composition Table
Italy	1972 [35]	www.bda-ieo.it/wordpress/en/	Food Composition Database for Epidemiological Studies in Italy (Banca Dati di Composizione degli Alimenti per Studi Epidemiologici in Italia—BDA
Japan	No program	www.mext.go.jp/en/policy/science_technology/ policy/title01/detail01/sdetail01/sdetail01/ 1385122.htm	Tables of Food Composition in Japan-2015-(7th Revised Ed)
Malaysia	2000 [36]	myfcd.moh.gov.my/	Malaysian Food Composition Database (MYFCD)
New Zealand [3]	1924 [37]	www.foodcomposition.co.nz/concise-tables	Concise New Zealand Food Composition Tables 12th Ed
The Netherlands	1942 [34]	nevo-online.rivm.nl/ProductenZoeken.aspx	Dutch Nutrient Material File (NEVO)
Norway	1920 [34]	www.matvaretabellen.no/	Norwegian Food Composition Table
Poland	1997 [34]	www.izz.waw.pl/index.php?lang=en	Poland Food Composition Tables Database

Table 1. *Cont.*

Country	Year of Salt Iodization	URL	Database Name
Slovakia	1953 [34]	www.pbd-online.sk/	Slovak Food Composition Database Online
Slovenia [4]	1964 [34]	opkp.si/en_GB/cms/vstopna-stran	OPKP (Open Platform for Clinical Nutrition)
Spain	1982 [35]	www.bedca.net/bdpub/index_en.php	Spanish Food Composition Database
Sweden	1936 [35]	www.livsmedelsverket.se/en/food-and-content/ naringsamnen/livsmedelsdatabasen	Livsmedelsdatabasen—Swedish Food Composition Database
Switzerland	1922 [34]	www.naehrwertdaten.ch/	Swiss Food Composition Database
Tanzania	1990s [38]	www.hsph.harvard.edu/nutritionsource/food-tables/	Tanzania Food Composition Tables
Tunisia	1990s [39]	www.mpl.ird.fr/tahina/home/doc/sommaire_ table_composition.pdf	Table de Composistion des Aliments Tunisiens
Turkey [5]	1968 [34]	www.turkomp.gov.tr/?locale=en	Turkish Food Composition Database, TürKomp [2]
UK	No program	www.gov.uk/government/publications/ composition-of-foods-integrated-dataset-cofid	Composition of Foods Integrated Dataset (CoFID)

[1] Iodized salt was only added to bread in 1953/1954 but was discontinued in the 1980s; iodized salt was available in Australia from this time. A 2009 iodization program applied to salt added to most bread [33,40]. [2] Search was conducted and salt iodization details were not located, but this does not confirm the absence of a program. [3] Database does not have updated iodine values for all fortified breads. [4] Database lacks some milk/dairy and beverage products. [5] Database iodine content is limited to table salt, fish, and shellfish.

Table 2. National food composition databases that do not include iodine.

Country	Year of Salt Iodization	URL	Source Name
Belgium	1990 [34]	www.nubel.com/fr/table-de-composition-des-aliments.html	Belgian Table of Food Composition
Brazil	No program	www.fcf.usp.br/tbca/	Brazilian Food Composition Table (TBCA)
Cameroon	Not found [1]	www.academia.edu/5451699/A_review_of_ composition_studies_of_Cameroon_traditional_ dishes_Macronutrients_and_minerals	Journal Publication
Canada	1949 [41]	food-nutrition.canada.ca/cnf-fce/index-eng.jsp	Canadian Nutrient File (CNF)
Chile	1979 [42]	web.minsal.cl/composicion-de-alimentos/	Chilean Table of Chemical Composition of Foods, Update 2010
China	1995 [43]	www.neasiafoods.org/dataCenter.do?level=yycfk& language=us	Food and Nutrient Database, Food Nutrition Library
Costa Rica	1970 [44]	www.inciensa.sa.cr/actualidad/Tabla% 20Composicion%20Alimentos.aspx	Tablas de Composición de Alimentos
Cuba	Not found [1]	www.inha.sld.cu/	Tabla de Composición de Alimentos Utilizados en Cuba
Gambia	Not found [1]	ilsirf.org/wp-content/uploads/sites/5/2017/03/ Gambia2011FCT.pdf	Food Composition Table for Use in The Gambia
Germany	1959 [34]	www.blsdb.de/	German Nutrient Database—Bundeslebensmittelschlüssel
Greece	No program	www.hhf-greece.gr/tables/Home.aspx?l=en	Composition Tables of Foods and Greek Dishes
Iceland	No program	old.matis.is/english/service/product-development-and-entrepreneurship/nutrition/ isgem-the-icelandic-food-composition-database/	ISGEM (The Icelandic Food Composition Database)
India	1983 [45]	ifct2017.com/wp-content/uploads/2017/05/ifct-doc.pdf	Indian Food Composition Tables
Ireland	No program	www.ucc.ie/archive/ifcdb/	Irish Food Composition Database
Israel	No program	www.health.gov.il/Subjects/FoodAndNutrition/ Nutrition/professionals/Pages/Tzameret.aspx	Tzameret
Korea	No program	koreanfood.rda.go.kr/eng/fctFoodSrchEng/ engMain	Korean Standard Food Composition Table

Table 2. *Cont.*

Country	Year of Salt Iodization	URL	Source Name
Lesotho	2000 [46]	ilsirf.org/wp-content/uploads/sites/5/2017/03/Lesotho2006FCT.pdf	Lesotho Food Composition Tables
Mexico	Not found [1]	www.innsz.mx/2017/Tablas/index.html#page=8	Tablas de Composicion de Alimentos y Productos Alimenticios Mexicanos (Version condensada 2015)
Mozambique	2000 [47]	ilsirf.org/wp-content/uploads/sites/5/2017/03/Mozambique2011FCT.pdf	Food Composition Tables for Mozambique, Version 2
Nepal	1973 [48]	www.fao.org/fileadmin/templates/food_composition/documents/regional/Nepal_Food_Composition_table_2012.pdf	Food Composition Table for Nepal 2012
Papua New Guinea	1995 [49]	www.fao.org/docrep/007/y5432e/y5432e00.htm	The Pacific Islands Food Composition Tables
Portugal	No program	portfir.insa.pt/foodcomp/search	Portuguese Food Composition Table
Serbia	1937 [50]	www.serbianfood.info/lozinka1.php	Serbian Food & Nutrition Database
Singapore	1988 [51]	focos.hpb.gov.sg/eservices/ENCF/	Energy and Nutrient Composition of Food
South African	1995 [52]	safoods-apps.mrc.ac.za/foodcomposition/	South African Food Database System (SAFOODS)
Sweden	1936 [34]	www.livsmedelsverket.se/en/food-and-content/naringsamnen/livsmedelsdatabasen	Livsmedelsdatabasen—Swedish Food Composition Database
Thailand	1994 [53]	www.inmu.mahidol.ac.th/aseanfoods/download/books/dl1.php?file=A1	ASEAN Food Composition Tables
Togo	Not found [1]	ilsirf.org/wp-content/uploads/sites/5/2017/03/TogoTable_de_Composition_des_Aliments.pdf	Table de Composition des Aliments du Togo
Uganda	1990s [54]	www.harvestplus.org/category/resource-type/technical-monographs	A Food Composition Table for Central and Eastern Uganda
Vietnam	1999 [55]	www.fao.org/fileadmin/templates/food_composition/documents/pdf/VTN_FCT_2007.pdf	Bảng Thành Phần Thực Phẩm Việt Nam Vietnamese Food Composition Table
United States	1924 [56]	ndb.nal.usda.gov/ndb/	USDA Food Composition Database

[1] Search was conducted and salt iodization details were not located, but this does not confirm the absence of a program.

4. Sources of Variability in Food Iodine Content

The amount of iodine in foods can be highly variable, and the nature and degree of this variability can have implications for the complexity and cost of developing databases of iodine content. For example, high variability may affect sampling plans such that more samples may need to be collected over a wider range of geographic areas and a larger number of sales or distribution venues [57]. Also, different chemical assay approaches (i.e., methods and reference materials) may be needed, depending on the anticipated range of iodine concentrations. (Note: see Section 5, below, for further discussion of these methodological issues). Highly variable and non-normal (skewed) distributions of iodine content may be best served by presentations of descriptive statistics that include multiple indicators of central tendency and range [58]. Some of the factors affecting between-country and within-country variability in iodine content of foods are described below.

4.1. Water

Drinking water is particularly variable in its iodine content between and within countries, especially if they are geographically diverse. Levels of iodine in drinking water supplies are reflective of factors such as iodine in the soil and water table, proximity to sea water, and agricultural runoff [59]. Therefore, assessment of iodine intake from drinking water may require data at the regional or local level. For example, the iodine content of water in some regions of China is sufficiently high to lead to excessive intake and potential thyroid hypertrophy in school children [60]. Conversely, the desalinated water used in many parts of Israel has been noted to have very low, essentially zero, iodine levels [61]. In many countries, there is very little information available on the iodine content of drinking water supplies, nor on the iodine content of bottled waters. Food composition databases should include a range of values or a default average value for the iodine content of drinking water.

4.2. Salt

Salt is the preferred vehicle for iodine fortification, and salt iodization has been implemented in 124 countries [62]. Salt can be produced from underground rock salt deposits, natural brine, or by evaporated seawater, with the latter containing <1 mg iodine (I)/kg of salt. This relatively low level of iodine in un-fortified sea salt may not always be appreciated by consumers. Most food-grade salt requires the addition of iodine, usually as potassium iodate or potassium iodide. WHO suggests that the amount of iodine added to salt should be based on the estimated salt consumed by the population; this ranges from 14 mg I/kg when estimated salt intake is high (i.e., 14 g/day) to 65 mg I/kg when salt intake is low (i.e., 3 g/day) [63]. In many countries, the iodine content of iodized salt is legislated and specified by a food standards code. However, the actual iodine content of iodized salt may differ from the reported content, particularly when iodized salt is kept in open containers and exposed to high humidity; the iodine content of salt can vary by 8% to 49% under such conditions [64]. Database developers must consider whether the country practices Universal Salt Iodization, in which case all salt for human use must be iodized, and therefore iodized salt will be used for commercial food products [9]. Alternatively, databases might include paired iodine values for some food products that have been prepared with iodized or non-iodized salt.

4.3. Agricultural Practices—Soils and Crops

Iodine occurs naturally in the earth's crust and is present everywhere in the environment. Soils, shales, and coal rich in organic matter are generally higher in iodine than hard rock [65,66]. Also the iodine content of the soil can be influenced by the proximity of the growing area to ocean water (through which atmospheric iodine is incorporated into rainfall, and thereby raises the iodine content of the soil), the iodine content of ground waters and irrigation waters, and the use of iodine-containing fertilizers [67]. The iodine content of plant crops is affected by the content of iodine in the soil (i.e., plants grown on high iodine soils will contain more iodine than those grown on low iodine soils), but in general, plant-based foods such as vegetables and fruits are relatively poor sources of iodine [59]. The exceptions are seaweeds, which have a great capacity to concentrate iodine [68–70].

4.4. Agricultural Practices—Animal Husbandry

Dairy products and eggs may contain significant but variable amounts of iodine, influenced, to some degree, by the iodine content of supplements in animal feeds and salt licks. These supplements are often provided as part of animal husbandry practice to ensure good health and reproductive outcomes in dairy and beef cattle, sheep, goats, and poultry. Dairy products also have contained adventitious iodine from iodophors, iodine-containing disinfectants used at various points in the production of milk. Iodophors can be used to clean udders, but if the cleansing has not been performed properly some of the iodine from the teat dips can be absorbed and transferred to milk and meat. A recent US Department of Agriculture (USDA) report found that 55% of dairy operations were using iodophor teat dips [71], suggesting that the practice is still relatively common in the US. Iodophors were also used in the cleaning of industrial equipment for processing milk in dairies; a decline in this practice in New Zealand by the mid-1980s is suggested to be responsible for a drop in the iodine content of milk and dairy products [13].

4.5. Food Processing

Commercial baked goods are another source of iodine when iodates are used in the commercial baking industry as dough conditioners. Iodates were introduced in the US 40 years ago and in Tasmania, Australia, over 50 years ago, but now other dough conditioners are being used. Also, some commercial baked goods contain erythrosine (Red No. 3/E127), a common food coloring that contains iodine; however, the iodine from erythrosine is only partially bioavailable [72].

5. Developing an Iodine Database for US Foods—Recent Progress

In 2014, the National Institutes of Health's Office of Dietary Supplements (ODS), Bethesda MD, convened several working groups to consider clinical and population research relevant to human iodine nutrition, particularly in the US [73]. Key areas of applied and clinical research that were reviewed and identified as needing greater effort included: assessing the iodine concentration of US foods and drinking water supplies; evaluating iodine intakes of various US population subgroups; and having a sufficient scientific knowledge base to determine iodine requirements at different lifecycle stages [73]. A database on the iodine content of US foods was considered to be a critical tool for conducting research on all of the identified gap areas. This priority has been operationalized through an interagency agreement (NIH IAA-AOD-17002) between ODS and the USDA to develop the USDA Food Iodine Database. Other federal partners involved in this project include the US Food and Drug Administration and the National Institute of Standards and Technology (NIST).

In this section, as summarized in Table 3, we will describe the main features of the project plan for the nascent USDA Food Iodine Database. A similar scientific and technical approach has been used to develop other databases, including those for choline and flavonoids [74,75]. We note that the scientific and technical approach used by the USDA is, of course, most suitable for the US; however, the concepts and operational components driving the design and execution of the project plan can serve as a prototype for development of iodine databases in other countries.

Table 3. Project Components for Developing the USDA Food Iodine Database.

Design phase (Completed)
• *Define research needs*
• *Review existing data*
• *Assess iodine distribution in the food supply*
• *Develop sampling design and calculate sample sizes*
Preliminary study phase (Completed)
• *Conduct stability studies*
• *Develop sample handling protocols*
• *Identify appropriate analytical methods and quality control materials*
Research implementation phase (Ongoing)
• *Conduct analyses and data quality control reviews*
• *Conduct ancillary studies*
• *Disseminate data and documentation*

5.1. The Design Phase

For any research initiative designed to provide foundational data to explore the connection between food and health, the researcher must address what and why it needs to be done, and how to achieve the answers. Put another way, when developing a new database or dataset, it is important to define the research needs and potential impact at the outset of the project. In the case of iodine, sufficient iodine composition data on food and dietary supplements are needed to estimate intakes and to assess the consequences of deficiency or excess.

Preliminary planning activities include: identifying the "population of interest" of foods and supplements; designing the sampling plan; developing a defensible analytical process (methods and quality control); planning for statistical analysis of the results; and considering a means of data dissemination. In the case of iodine, although the USDA has developed special databases for other nutrient-focused datasets, it was important to identify unique characteristics of iodine-contributing foods and dietary supplements. Other specific challenges related to database development included the need for methods for effective sampling and analysis of foods [19], and for statistical approaches that can accommodate variability in the iodine content of foods [58].

Since resources for composition analyses are rarely sufficient to analyze all potential contributors to iodine intake, it is essential to identify existing useable data of adequate scientific quality. The USDA has long sought to take advantage of published and other available data when data quality criteria have been met to satisfaction [76]. Also, for this same reason of efficiency, when possible, the USDA seeks to harmonize its data with other data generated by complementary activities, most notably, the US Food and Drug Administration (FDA) Total Diet Study (TDS). The FDA TDS is an ongoing program that obtains about 290 foods of various matrices, four times a year, each in a different US location, sampled in order to monitor an array of nutrients and other constituents of the US food supply [77]. For iodine analysis of TDS foods, the FDA has recently synchronized their laboratory assay method, inductively coupled-mass spectrometry (ICP-MS), to that used by the USDA; in addition, the possibility of coordinating selected efforts is under discussion. This approach allows inter-agency exchange of data on iodine. Also, enhanced quality control is achieved through close collaboration to utilize NIST standard reference materials and methods. Thus, existing data from the TDS will be used to enhance the national iodine dataset and also to set priorities for planned new or repeat analyses [19]. When planning the sampling of specific foods, it is critical to identify and acquire other relevant data that clarifies the distribution of iodine in the food supply (e.g., industry uses, agricultural production, sales, and other sources). Another step involves preparing country-specific proportional weighting factors for different versions of the food; an example would the use of industry data on relative amounts sold or used of different types of iodized and non-iodized salt (e.g., conventional, sea, Kosher, etc.).

In developing the sampling plan, it is necessary to determine an appropriate sample size. The acquired food samples must be nationally representative, and the number of samples must be sufficiently large to develop statistically defensible variability estimates. The approach to this plan must be suitable for the country whose food supply is being analyzed; countries with a highly structured and nationally distributed food supply will need an approach different from that in countries where foods are acquired (grown, hunted, or foraged) and consumed within multiple smaller localities. An example of necessary adaptations is that of acquiring food samples from American Indian reservations and Alaska Native villages [78]. In the US, the sampling plan includes identification and procurement of US-representative food samples; many of these samples are selected for analysis under the NIH-USDA National Food and Nutrient Analysis Program (NFNAP) [79]. The USDA typically acquires its food samples in a minimum of 12 geographically diverse locations selected according to current population density data, retail sales data, and other national-level information. NFNAP foods under evaluation for iodine analysis include finfish and other seafood products; seaweeds/seaweed extracts; iodine-containing commercial ingredients and additives; highly-consumed dairy and egg products, commercially processed mixed dishes; retail salts; and other foods containing significant amounts of iodine.

5.2. Preliminary Study Phase

It is necessary to confirm the stability of the analytes in both new and archived analytical samples, particularly when samples are shared from other studies or have been stored for some time. This is a particularly important step when analyzing for iodine in salt and other food substrates. To investigate the possible loss of iodine during sample storage, the USDA reanalyzed a set of samples that had been initially analyzed 5 years previously and was able to confirm that the iodine content of archived NFNAP foods stored at −60 °C had not changed [78,80]. The USDA also plans to evaluate salt industry data regarding iodine volatilization under varying storage, humidity, and temperature conditions.

Sample handling protocols must be developed prior to sample collection to ensure sample integrity during shipping and storage. Pilot testing of protocols including chain-of-custody plans may be warranted to ensure that sample integrity can be maintained from the point of purchase all the way through to analysis. The USDA has developed sample handling protocols for NFNAP that can serve as examples for others who are undertaking collection and eventual assay of foods [76]. An important precaution when utilizing samples of varying provenance (such as from a multicenter study) is to ensure that there has not been inadvertent contamination during the collection or storage process; sources of contamination may include leaching from storage containers that can release iodine into the sample over time and use of iodine-containing preservatives or disinfectants.

For the chemical analysis of foods, it is important to identify appropriate analytical methods and to select a capable laboratory through precertification testing with blinded samples [75]. In terms of analytical methodology, the ICP-MS method [76] is suitable for the analysis of iodine in a variety of foods, as well as dietary supplements, and is known to have good precision and accuracy. Using the ICP-MS method, the USDA contract laboratory has shown that it can generate accurate iodine values that compare well with the iodine values of several NIST-certified reference materials (CRM), notably NIST 1849a Infant/Adult Nutritional Formula and 1548a Typical Diet [21,78,80]. For quality control during analysis of samples, the USDA is using these CRM reference materials, as well as in-house control materials cross-validated to the NIST materials. Other NIST CRM materials with available iodine values (such as iodized salt, egg powder, whole milk powder, and kelp) will be used as warranted as the analytical plan progresses.

5.3. Research Implementation Phase

The USDA's experience with other database development projects has revealed that the greatest effort and cost are incurred when acquiring food products according to the statistical design, conducting direct assays of the prepared samples and quality control materials, and assembling the data in an orderly format. This phase of the USDA Food Iodine Database project is now in progress. To date, over 135 unique foods have been sampled; some of these are newly acquired and others are existing frozen samples that were archived as part of previously completed projects. About 350 prepared samples representing these foods have been analyzed to date, along with quality control materials comprising about 10% of total assays. The predominant food groups analyzed so far are multi-ingredient commercial foods (e.g., restaurant hamburgers and macaroni and cheese, retail frozen pizza, milks and yogurt) and several types of fish (shellfish, crustaceans, mollusks, and finfish).

Following data quality review, data dissemination in the form of accessible databases and professional and peer-reviewed publications will allow transparency of the data and related information. Additional ancillary studies can enhance the value and usefulness of database resources; for example, the USDA is considering a sub-study to utilize direct chemical assay followed by statistical modeling to evaluate the iodine content of home-prepared recipes in comparison with commercial food equivalents. In addition, the USDA will use ancillary studies to explore other factors that that may affect total dietary iodine such as geographic origin of foodstuffs (as reflecting iodine content of soils), the iodine content of water supplies used for drinking and reconstituting foods, and the iodine content of dietary supplements.

6. Iodine Content of Supplements

Nutrient-containing supplements may contribute substantially to total nutrient intake [27,81,82], and therefore should be included along with foods when estimating total dietary intake of iodine. Supplements are used worldwide but are regulated very differently among countries [83], sometimes as foods (as in the US and Europe) [84,85], and sometimes as a form of herbal medicines (as in Germany) [86,87], and product registration or licensing may be required under certain circumstances [88]. Databases describing the content, ingredients, and other information on supplements may be assembled by government entities, manufacturers, or researchers. The information content, definitions, terminology, data formats, and sources of data can vary considerably, and this lack of uniformity and consistency has been noted as a limitation in making between-country comparisons for research and other purposes [85].

Identifying and then accessing dietary supplement databases from different countries can be challenging as there are few readily available and comprehensive compilations [85]. Nevertheless, the task may be approached on a country-by-country basis. For example, the Netherlands provides a database on the composition of supplements that is linked to the national food composition tables [89]; this database has been used as part of an iodine intake assessment study in children and adults [90]. Similarly, dietary supplement databases have been developed and then used for iodine intake assessment in pregnant and lactating women in Norway [26–28] and in pregnant women [29] and adults [30] in Denmark. The Australian dietary supplement database (AUSNUT 2011–2013) contains 35 nutrient values, including iodine, for 2163 dietary supplements consumed during several national nutrition and physical activity surveys conducted from 2011–2013 [91]. The method for constructing a dietary supplement database for adult participants in one of the United Kingdom sub-projects of a multi-country European cohort study has been described in detail [92].

In the US, the Dietary Supplement Label Database (DSLD), sponsored by ODS in collaboration with other US federal agencies, is presently the most comprehensive listing of label information (www.dsld.nlm.nih.gov/dsld-mobile/) [93,94]. The DSLD evolved from earlier questionnaire-based efforts to understand the magnitude of the contribution of supplements to population nutrient intake in the US, starting with the 1999 cycle of the National Health and Nutrition Examination Survey (NHANES) [93,95]. Other currently available databases with label information for US products include DailyMed (dailymed.nlm.nih.gov/dailymed/) and the industry-sponsored Supplement Online Wellness Library (OWL) database (www.supplementowl.org).

Iodine content (per serving) and source (ingredients) are provided for US supplement products as listed on the product label and the Supplement Facts Panel [96]. For example, the label may indicate that the iodine in the supplement product may come from diverse sources such as iodine salts (e.g., potassium iodide) or botanical ingredients (e.g., kelp). When using label information, whether by direct inspection of the product container or through the label databases mentioned above, an important caveat is that results from direct analysis of individual supplement products usually are not publicly available.

To estimate typical nutrient content values—including for iodine—for certain grouped classes of sampled supplement products (e.g., adult multivitamin/multiminerals (MVMs), pediatric MVMs, and non-prescription prenatal MVMs), direct chemical analysis has been conducted on sampled products and standard reference materials [97]; the analysis results have been made available through the Dietary Supplements Ingredient Database (DSID) [20,98]. The DSID assay results suggest that the actual iodine content for adult MVMs, pediatric MVMs, and non-prescription prenatal MVMs may typically exceed the labeled amount by 20–26%. Furthermore, comparisons of labeled iodine contents of prescription and non-prescription prenatal supplements sold in the US have found that, per tablet, non-prescription prenatals contain approximately 10% more iodine than prescription prenatals [99,100].

Given the concerns about the adequacy of iodine intake by pregnant women, data from the US National Health and Nutrition Examination Survey (NHANES) program has provided a means of understanding the contribution of dietary supplements to iodine intake. Use of supplements (multi-vitamins or MVMs) was found to be widespread (~75%) among US pregnant women surveyed in 1999–2006; however, use of iodine-containing supplements was relatively low (~22%) [95]. Since that time, various professional organizations including the American Academy of Pediatrics [101], the Endocrine Society [102], the Teratology Association [103], and the American Thyroid Association [104], as well as the Australian National Health and Medical Research Council [105] and the New Zealand Ministry of Health [106], have recommended that pregnant and lactating women take a daily prenatal MVM supplement that contains 150 µg of iodine. Data on time trends in usage of iodine-containing supplements by pregnant and lactating women will help in understanding whether usage is changing in response to professional recommendations. A recent study undertaken in New Zealand reported that 52% of pregnant and lactating women followed the recommendation for a 150 µg of iodine per day [107].

7. New Zealand: A Case Study Illustrating the Need for a Database with Iodine Content

New Zealand has low levels of iodine in the soil, predisposing the population to iodine deficiency. New Zealand was the first country after Switzerland to introduce iodized salt to address widespread iodine deficiency, albeit at an initial low concentration of 5 mg I/kg; this was increased to 50 mg I/kg in 1939 [37]. Domestic household use of iodized salt, both at the table and in home cooking, successfully eradicated iodine deficiency in New Zealand by the early 1950s. Additional iodine was derived from dairy products when iodophors were used by the dairy industry from the 1960s to the 1980s. However, changes in food habits, including a reduction in the consumption of iodized salt in the home and a drop in the iodine content of dairy products when detergent-based sanitizers replaced iodophors, are factors believed to have contributed to the re-emergence of mild iodine deficiency in the 1990s [13]. Given the widespread nature of the deficiency, which was reported in all population groups, the most effective strategy identified by the government was mandatory fortification [41].

Dietary modeling was used to identify the best dietary approach to increase iodine intake without exceeding the upper limit of intake, with a particular focus on reducing the prevalence of iodine deficiency in pregnant women and children. In order to undertake this process, it was imperative that the iodine content of foods be included in the New Zealand Food Composition Database [108]. Because the most commonly eaten staple foods in the New Zealand diet are low in iodine, and the foods highest in iodine content are consumed in small quantities, a preliminary proposal was put forward to mandate the replacement of non-iodized salt with iodized salt in breads, breakfast cereals, and sweet biscuits (i.e., cookies). Because New Zealand imports and exports biscuits, a requirement to fortify biscuits with iodine would require separate production lines for both overseas and New Zealand biscuit producers. Furthermore, cereal manufacturers suggested that the application of a brine spray to breakfast cereals would produce inconsistent amounts of iodine in breakfast cereals. Thus, concerns about trade regulations for biscuits and technological concerns for breakfast cereal meant that bread, a staple food consumed by 87% of the New Zealand population, was chosen as the sole food for fortification; it was acknowledged that bread would not provide pregnant women with enough iodine to meet their higher requirements. A change to the Food Standards Code came into effect in September 2009 mandating the use of iodized salt in yeast-leavened bread; organic bread was exempt from this requirement [33]. The New Zealand Food Composition Database has included a revised iodine content for some breads, although more information on the iodine content of New Zealand breads can be found in a separate government report [109].

8. Discussion

Iodine has emerged as a nutrient of concern in many developed countries, in part because retail sales (and home use) of non-iodized salts may be increasing [11,110–112] and iodized salt is not always used in the commercially prepared foods that make up an ever-increasing component of the food supply yet whose consumption often leads to excessive sodium intake [11,110–112]. Also, some countries have not yet implemented mandatory salt iodization programs [51,112,113]. Pregnant women and young children are at highest risk of inadequate intake but other groups within populations may also be at risk. At present there is no simple or reliable way to assess the iodine status of an individual. Although other causes cannot be ruled out, altered thyroid function can suggest the presence of iodine deficiency. In the future, validated biomarkers of individual status (such as thyroglobulin levels) may become available [114]. In the meantime, despite the difficulty of directly assessing iodine status of individuals, practical diet-based approaches may prove useful.

Individuals should be asked about the voluntary and involuntary factors that can affect iodine intake and status. This information can provide a basis for assessing risk and providing counseling. For example, interview methodology can be used to gather information on use of iodine-containing dietary supplements, and on intake of food sources of iodine such as dairy products and seafood, including fresh and saltwater fish and seaweeds. A growing concern in many countries is the adoption of dietary patterns that specifically exclude major sources of iodine, including low-salt [115], vegan [116–118], and Paleo diets [119]. Questionnaires must be attuned to phrasing; for example, it is important to enquire about use of dairy vs non-dairy milks, as the iodine content of milk alternatives often is very low [120]. In some situations, it may even be desirable to develop individualized advice regarding type of salt; for example, researchers in China are attempting to develop an online screening tool that informs consumers if they should consume iodized or non-iodized salt [121].

An additional topic that needs appropriate interview methodology includes the type of salt used in the home for cooking and at the table. For example, interviewers should ask how often new iodized salt is purchased, as the iodine content may decline over long periods of storage. Interviewers should also ascertain use of sea salt, which, if not fortified, may have a surprisingly low iodine content. Determining the amount of iodine coming from iodized cooking and table salt can be difficult to quantify for a number of reasons. Firstly, the interpretation of a sprinkle or pinch of salt will vary from person to person. Secondly, if food intake is being weighed, the weighing scales may not be sensitive enough to measure salt added at the table and weight recorded as null (i.e., 0) grams. Thirdly, when iodized salt is used for cooking vegetables or pasta, the amount of iodine in water that is discarded and the amount that becomes incorporated into the cooked food is unknown. Thus, iodine intakes determined using diet records or 24-h recalls are likely to underestimate actual iodine intake, particularly in individuals who regularly and generously add iodized salt to their food. A simpler approach is to add a set amount of iodine to anyone who reports use of iodized discretionary salt; in New Zealand, an additional 48 μg of iodine, representing the consumption of 1 g of salt (48 mg I/kg) per day, is included in the total daily iodine intake to account for discretionary use of iodized salt [109].

Data on the iodine content of foods can also be useful in research settings. Although seldom considered, an estimate of the iodine content of the diet determined using a validated iodine-specific food frequency questionnaire should be included as a variable in studies investigating thyroid function on disease and child development. The iodine content of the diet could also be used to stratify participants in randomized controlled trials of iodine supplementation.

Another use of iodine databases is in the treatment of thyroid disease. Patients undergoing radioablation treatment for thyroid cancer are prescribed a several-week course of a low iodine diet, in order to enhance uptake of radioactive iodine [122,123]. The degree of success in reducing iodine intake usually is estimated using urinary iodine excretion [124]. Some patients find it difficult to adhere to these diets. Also, there is debate about the necessary degree of dietary restriction, as well as about the optimal time frame for dietary modification, both of which may depend, in part, on the background iodine content of the patient's usual diet [125,126]. In some circumstances, iodine data from other countries has been used to develop dietary prescriptions for patients living in a different country [127]. Improved national-level databases will be useful in clinical practice and in research on low iodine diets.

Goitrogens are a chemically diverse group of compounds that have the capacity to interfere with uptake or utilization of iodine by the thyroid gland, and thus pose an additional source of dietary complexity important for understanding issues of adequacy of iodine intake [18]. The impact on thyroid status of eating these foods may depend on the quantity eaten and the background iodine content of the diet. High goitrogen intake may render marginal iodine intakes inadequate for physiologic demands and under some circumstances may actually contribute to goiter endemics and related disorders [128]. Dietary goitrogens often are inherent botanical constituents of foods; examples include cassava (cyanogenic glucosides), cruciferous vegetables (glucosinolates), and soy products (flavonoids). Dietary assessments should include information on intake of goitrogen-source foods, which can be very specific to geographic region, including cultural practices and economic issues related to the cost of foods. Special purpose databases or data tables with information on some of the goitrogenic constituents of foods (e.g., the USDA Flavonoid Database [74,129]) can provide useful corollaries for iodine composition tables and would have potential application for research and for counseling individuals at risk for thyroid disease. Environmental goitrogens also may present dietary exposures of concern in some situations and include perchlorates, nitrates, and disulfides. These compounds may derive from industrial contamination but may also occur naturally in soils and can subsequently leach into the water supply and thereby into foods [130]. Tobacco smoke presents another important goitrogenic exposure due to its thiocyanate content. As individuals are unlikely to be aware of ingestion of most environmental goitrogens, it may be useful to consider estimating exposure through the use of biomarkers [131,132].

In the US, the USDA Food Iodine Database project described in this paper complements the ODS-supported DSID and DSLD resources that provide data on the iodine content of supplements, necessary to determine total iodine intake. Once the USDA Food Iodine Database is complete, it will be possible to generate more complete estimates of iodine intake and iodine sources through linkage to dietary intake tools and to the data generated by surveys such as the NHANES, which heretofore has based its estimates of iodine intake on urinary iodine levels [133]. Also, the eventual availability of iodine values for a large number of foods with descriptive statistics that include multiple measures of variability (e.g., percentile cutoffs, coefficients of variation, and standard deviation) and central tendency (e.g., means and medians) will allow modeling of intakes that account for the spread of iodine levels in many types of foods, thus helping to develop appropriate methods for estimating intake of individuals and populations [58].

Another US concern, which also may be the case in other countries, is that information is available about the iodine content of infant formula but not breast milk. Databases on the typical iodine content of human milk would be desirable. Estimating the likely iodine intake of breast-fed infants is an additional key aspect of understanding adequacy of population level iodine status.

9. Conclusions

Information about the iodine content of national food supplies is essential for understanding the state of human iodine nutrition around the world, with important applications in nutrition research, dietary counseling, treatment of thyroid disease, and public health practice. Collection and evaluation of dietary data are essential components of this work because there is no simple way at present to estimate iodine status of individuals. When possible, iodine composition databases for foods should be complemented by databases for dietary supplements in countries where supplements make a significant contribution to the total intake of iodine. Regularly updated composition data that reflect current food supplies are needed to support nutrition surveys, which generate critical data resources for understanding national-level concerns and identifying sub-populations at risk due to typical dietary patterns or increased physiological need. In future surveys, characterizing the relationship between iodine intake and thyroid function across populations and within population subgroups will require information on total intake, from all sources.

Acknowledgments: We would like to acknowledge the assistance of Amanda Moran, University of Maryland. This paper was supported by the NIH Office of Dietary Supplements.

Author Contributions: A.G.E., S.A.S. and P.R.P. developed the concept for the manuscript. A.G.E., S.A.S., J.M.M. and P.R.P. wrote the manuscript.

Conflicts of Interest: The authors declare no conflicts of interest.

References

1. Iodine Global Network. Global Scorecard of Iodine Nutrition in 2017 in the General Population and in Pregnant Women (PW). Available online: http://www.ign.org/cm_data/IGN_Global_Scorecard_AllPop_and_PW_May2017.pdf (accessed on 20 September 2017).
2. Boyages, S.C. Clinical review 49: Iodine deficiency disorders. *J. Clin. Endocrinol. Metab.* **1993**, *77*, 587–591. [PubMed]

3. Abel, M.H.; Caspersen, I.H.; Meltzer, H.M.; Haugen, M.; Brandlistuen, R.E.; Aase, H.; Alexander, J.; Torheim, L.E.; Brantsaeter, A.L. Suboptimal maternal iodine intake is associated with impaired child neurodevelopment at 3 years of age in the Norwegian mother and child cohort study. *J. Nutr.* **2017**, *147*, 1314–1324. [CrossRef] [PubMed]

4. Bath, S.C.; Steer, C.D.; Golding, J.; Emmett, P.; Rayman, M.P. Effect of inadequate iodine status in UK pregnant women on cognitive outcomes in their children: Results from the Avon Longitudinal Study of Parents and Children (ALSPAC). *Lancet* **2013**, *382*, 331–337. [CrossRef]

5. Hynes, K.L.; Otahal, P.; Hay, I.; Burgess, J.R. Mild iodine deficiency during pregnancy is associated with reduced educational outcomes in the offspring: 9-Year follow-up of the gestational iodine cohort. *J. Clin. Endocrinol. Metab.* **2013**, *98*, 1954–1962. [CrossRef] [PubMed]

6. Gowachirapant, S.; Jaiswal, N.; Melse-Boonstra, A.; Galetti, V.; Stinca, S.; Mackenzie, I.; Thomas, S.; Thomas, T.; Winichagoon, P.; Srinivasan, K.; et al. Effect of iodine supplementation in pregnant women on child neurodevelopment: A randomised, double-blind, placebo-controlled trial. *Lancet Diabetes Endocrinol.* **2017**, *5*, 853–863. [CrossRef]

7. Zimmermann, M.B. Iodine deficiency. *Endocr. Rev.* **2009**, *30*, 376–408. [CrossRef] [PubMed]

8. United Nations International Children's Emergency Fund (UNICEF). Household Consumption of Iodized Salt: Global Database 2017. Available online: https://data.unicef.org/topic/nutrition/iodine-deficiency/ (accessed on 18 December 2017).

9. Venkatesh Mannar, M.G.; Dunn, J.T.; International Council for Control of Iodine Deficiency Disorders. Salt Iodization for the Elimination of Iodine Deficiency. Available online: http://www.ceecis.org/iodine/08_production/00_mp/SI_elim_IDD_1994venkatesh.pdf (accessed on 21 December 2017).

10. Dahl, L.; Johansson, L.; Julshamn, K.; Meltzer, H.M. The iodine content of Norwegian foods and diets. *Public Health Nutr.* **2004**, *7*, 569–576. [CrossRef] [PubMed]

11. Maalouf, J.; Barron, J.; Gunn, J.P.; Yuan, K.; Perrine, C.G.; Cogswell, M.E. Iodized salt sales in the United States. *Nutrients* **2015**, *7*, 1691–1695. [CrossRef] [PubMed]

12. Li, M.; Eastman, C.J.; Waite, K.V.; Ma, G.; Zacharin, M.R.; Topliss, D.J.; Harding, P.E.; Walsh, J.P.; Ward, L.C.; Mortimer, R.H.; et al. Are Australian children iodine deficient? Results of the Australian National Iodine Nutrition Study. *Med. J. Aust.* **2006**, *184*, 165–169. [PubMed]

13. Mann, J.I.; Aitken, E. The re-emergence of iodine deficiency in New Zealand? *N. Z. Med. J.* **2003**, *116*, U351. [PubMed]

14. Smith, L.P.; Ng, S.W.; Popkin, B.M. Trends in US home food preparation and consumption: Analysis of national nutrition surveys and time use studies from 1965–1966 to 2007–2008. *Nutr. J.* **2013**, *12*, 45. [CrossRef] [PubMed]

15. Institute of Medicine Committee on Strategies to Reduce Sodium Intake. The National Academies Collection: Reports funded by National Institutes of Health. In *Strategies to Reduce Sodium Intake in the United States*; Henney, J.E., Taylor, C.L., Boon, C.S., Eds.; National Academies Press: Washington, DC, USA, 2010.

16. Booms, S.; Hill, E.; Kulhanek, L.; Vredeveld, J.; Gregg, B. Iodine deficiency and hypothyroidism from voluntary diet restrictions in the US: Case reports. *Pediatrics* **2016**, *137*, e20154003. [CrossRef] [PubMed]

17. Swanson, C.A.; Zimmermann, M.B.; Skeaff, S.; Pearce, E.N.; Dwyer, J.T.; Trumbo, P.R.; Zehaluk, C.; Andrews, K.W.; Carriquiry, A.; Caldwell, K.L.; et al. Summary of an NIH workshop to identify research needs to improve the monitoring of iodine status in the United States and to inform the DRI. *J. Nutr.* **2012**, *142*, 1175s–1185s. [CrossRef] [PubMed]

18. Rohner, F.; Zimmermann, M.; Jooste, P.; Pandav, C.; Caldwell, K.; Raghavan, R.; Raiten, D.J. Biomarkers of nutrition for development—Iodine review. *J. Nutr.* **2014**, *144*, 1322s–1342s. [CrossRef] [PubMed]

19. Pehrsson, P.R.; Patterson, K.Y.; Spungen, J.H.; Wirtz, M.S.; Andrews, K.W.; Dwyer, J.T.; Swanson, C.A. Iodine in food- and dietary supplement-composition databases. *Am. J. Clin. Nutr.* **2016**, *104* (Suppl. S3), 868s–876s. [CrossRef] [PubMed]

20. Andrews, K.W.; Roseland, J.M.; Gusev, P.A.; Palachuvattil, J.; Dang, P.T.; Savarala, S.; Han, F.; Pehrsson, P.R.; Douglass, L.W.; Dwyer, J.T.; et al. Analytical ingredient content and variability of adult multivitamin/mineral products: National estimates for the Dietary Supplement Ingredient Database. *Am. J. Clin. Nutr.* **2017**, *105*, 526–539. [CrossRef] [PubMed]

21. Long, S.E.; Catron, B.L.; Boggs, A.S.; Tai, S.S.; Wise, S.A. Development of Standard Reference Materials to support assessment of iodine status for nutritional and public health purposes. *Am. J. Clin. Nutr.* **2016**, *104* (Suppl. S3), 902s–906s. [CrossRef] [PubMed]

22. Sharpless, K.E.; Lippa, K.A.; Duewer, D.L.; Rukhin, A.L. *The ABCs of Using Standard Reference Materials in the Analysis of Foods and Dietary Supplements: A Practical Guide*; National Institute of Standards and Technology: Gaithersburg, MD, USA, 2014.

23. Food and Agriculture Organization of the United Nations. International Network of Food Data Systems (INFOODS)—International Food Composition Table/Database Directory. Available online: http://www.fao.org/infoods/infoods/tables-and-databases/en/ (accessed on 7 November 2017).

24. International Life Sciences Institute Research Foundation (ILSI). World Nutrient Databases for Dietary Studies. Available online: http://ilsirf.org/resources/databases/wndds/ (accessed on 20 September 2017).

25. Global Fortification Data Exchange. Map: Count of Nutrients In Fortification Standards. Available online: https://www.fortificationdata.org/map-number-of-nutrients/ (accessed on 19 December 2017).

26. Brantsæter, A.L.; Abel, M.H.; Haugen, M.; Meltzer, H.M. Risk of suboptimal iodine intake in pregnant Norwegian women. *Nutrients* **2013**, *5*, 424–440. [CrossRef] [PubMed]

27. Haugen, M.; Brantsaeter, A.L.; Alexander, J.; Meltzer, H.M. Dietary supplements contribute substantially to the total nutrient intake in pregnant Norwegian women. *Ann. Nutr. Metab.* **2008**, *52*, 272–280. [CrossRef] [PubMed]

28. Henjum, S.; Lilleengen, A.M.; Aakre, I.; Dudareva, A.; Gjengedal, E.L.F.; Meltzer, H.M.; Brantsaeter, A.L. Suboptimal iodine concentration in breastmilk and inadequate iodine intake among lactating women in Norway. *Nutrients* **2017**, *9*, 643. [CrossRef] [PubMed]

29. Andersen, S.L.; Sorensen, L.K.; Krejbjerg, A.; Moller, M.; Laurberg, P. Challenges in the evaluation of urinary iodine status in pregnancy: The importance of iodine supplement intake and time of sampling. *Eur. Thyroid J.* **2014**, *3*, 179–188. [CrossRef] [PubMed]

30. Tetens, I.; Biltoft-Jensen, A.; Spagner, C.; Christensen, T.; Gille, M.B.; Bugel, S.; Banke Rasmussen, L. Intake of micronutrients among Danish adult users and non-users of dietary supplements. *Food Nutr. Res.* **2011**, *55*. [CrossRef] [PubMed]

31. Katagiri, R.; Yuan, X.; Kobayashi, S.; Sasaki, S. Effect of excess iodine intake on thyroid diseases in different populations: A systematic review and meta-analyses including observational studies. *PLoS ONE* **2017**, *12*, e0173722. [CrossRef] [PubMed]

32. United Nations International Children's Emergency Fund (UNICEF). ARMENIA Prevention of Iodine Deficiencies Disorders 2005 Annual Progress Report. Available online: http://pdf.usaid.gov/pdf_docs/Pdach758.pdf (accessed on 6 November 2017).

33. Food Standards Australia New Zealand. Australian User Guide Mandatory Iodine Fortification Implementing the Requirements of Mandatory Fortification with Iodised Salt under Standard 2.1.1—Cereals and Cereal Products. Available online: https://www.foodstandards.gov.au/code/userguide/documents/Rewrite%20Mandatory%20Iodine%20Fortification%20User%20Guide%20_Formated%20Master_.pdf (accessed on 29 September 2017).

34. World Health Organization (WHO). *Comparative Analysis of Progress on the Elimination of Iodine Deficiency Disorders*; WHO: Copenhagan, Denmark, 2000.

35. World Health Organization (WHO). *Iodine Deficiency in Europe: A Continuing Public Health Problem*; WHO: Geneva, Switzerland, 2007.

36. Parman, S.; Ministry of Health Malaysia. Malayia. Available online: http://www.wpro.who.int/nutrition/documents/docs/maa.pdf (accessed on 6 November 2017).

37. Purves, H.D. The aetiology and prophylaxis of endemic goitre and cretinism. The New Zealand experience. *N. Z. Med. J.* **1974**, *80*, 477–479. [PubMed]

38. Assey, V.D.; Peterson, S.; Kimboka, S.; Ngemera, D.; Mgoba, C.; Ruhiye, D.M.; Ndossi, G.D.; Greiner, T.; Tylleskar, T. Tanzania national survey on iodine deficiency: Impact after twelve years of salt iodation. *BMC Public Health* **2009**, *9*, 319. [CrossRef] [PubMed]

39. Doggui, R.; El Ati-Hellal, M.; Traissac, P.; Lahmar, L.; El Ati, J. Adequacy assessment of a universal salt iodization program two decades after its implementation: A national cross-sectional study of iodine status among school-age children in Tunisia. *Nutrients* **2017**, *9*, 6. [CrossRef] [PubMed]

40. Food Standards Australia New Zealand. Proposal P1003 Mandatory Iodine Fortification for Australia Assessment Report. Available online: https://www.foodstandards.gov.au/code/proposals/documents/P1003%20Mandatory%20Iodine%20fortification%20Aust%20AR%20FINAL.pdf (accessed on 30 October 2017).

41. Food Standards Australia New Zealand. Final Assessment Report, Proposal P230, Consideration of Mandatory Fortification with Iodine for New Zealand. Available online: http://www.foodstandards.gov.au/code/proposals/documents/P230_FAR_Attach_1_6___12_13.pdf (accessed on 7 November 2017).

42. Muzzo, S.; Pretell, E. IDD Newsletter—Iodine Excess in Chile. Available online: http://www.ign.org/newsletter/idd_nl_feb09_chile.pdf (accessed on 6 November 2017).

43. Sun, D.; Codling, K.; Chang, S.; Zhang, S.; Shen, H.; Su, X.; Chen, Z.; Scherpbier, R.W.; Yan, J. Eliminating iodine deficiency in China: Achievements, challenges and global implications. *Nutrients* **2017**, *9*, 361. [CrossRef] [PubMed]

44. Ministry of Health Republic of Costa Rica; United Nations Children's Fund (UNICEF). *Iodizing Salt A Health Policy, The Costa Rican Experience*; UNICEF: San José, Costa Rica, 2013.

45. National Iodine Deficiency Disorders Control Program (NIDDCP). Salt Iodiasation Program in INDIA. Available online: http://saltcomindia.gov.in/NIDCCP_Iodised_Program.html (accessed on 30 October 2017).

46. Sebotsa, M.L.; Dannhauser, A.; Jooste, P.L.; Joubert, G. Assessment of the sustainability of the iodine-deficiency disorders control program in Lesotho. *Food Nutr. Bull.* **2007**, *28*, 337–347. [CrossRef] [PubMed]

47. Jooste, P. IDD Newsletter—Mozambique Redoubles Its Salt Iodization Efforts. Available online: http://www.ign.org/newsletter/idd_may14_mozambique.pdf (accessed on 7 November 2017).

48. Gelal, B.; Baral, N. Moving Toward the Sustainable Ellimination of IDD in Nepal. Available online: http://www.ign.org/newsletter/idd_nl_may10_nepal.pdf (accessed on 7 November 2017).

49. Temple, V.J. IDD Newsletter—Progress Towards Elimination of IDD in Papua New Guinea. Available online: http://www.ign.org/cm_data/idd_nl_nov06_papua_new_guinea.pdf (accessed on 7 November 2017).

50. Kazakh Academy of Nutrition (KAN). Serbia Vignette. Available online: http://kan-kaz.org/english/files/serbia_vignette.pdf (accessed on 2 October 2017).

51. Codling, K.; Rudert, C.; Begin, F.; Pena-Rosas, J.P. The legislative framework for salt iodization in Asia and the Pacific and its impact on programme implementation. *Public Health Nutr.* **2017**, *20*, 3008–3018. [CrossRef] [PubMed]

52. Jooste, P.L.; Weight, M.J.; Lombard, C.J. Iodine concentration in household salt in South Africa. *Bull. World Health Organ.* **2001**, *79*, 534–540. [PubMed]

53. Ministry of Public Health Thailand. Notification of Ministry of Public Health No. 153 [B.E. 2537(1994)] Re: Iodized Salt. Available online: http://food.fda.moph.go.th/law/data/announ_moph/V.English/No.%20333%20Edible%20Salt.pdf (accessed on 3 October 2017).

54. Uganda National Bureau of Standards. Revision of the Salt Iodisation Regulations and Standards for Iodised Salt in Uganda. Final Report. Available online: http://library.health.go.ug/download/file/fid/1466 (accessed on 30 October 2017).

55. United Nations International Children's Emergency Fund (UNICEF). Salt Iodisation in Viet Nam: Learning from the Past and Building Back Better. Available online: https://www.unicef.org/vietnam/Final_IDD_Eng_E-mail_version.pdf (accessed on 30 October 2017).

56. Leung, A.M.; Braverman, L.E.; Pearce, E.N. History of U.S. iodine fortification and supplementation. *Nutrients* **2012**, *4*, 1740–1746. [CrossRef] [PubMed]

57. Greenfield, H.; Southgate, D.A.T. *Food Composition Data: Production, Management and Use*, 2nd ed.; Food and Agriculture Organization of the United Nations: Rome, Italy, 2003.

58. Carriquiry, A.L.; Spungen, J.H.; Murphy, S.P.; Pehrsson, P.R.; Dwyer, J.T.; Juan, W.; Wirtz, M.S. Variation in the iodine concentrations of foods: Considerations for dietary assessment. *Am. J. Clin. Nutr.* **2016**, *104* (Suppl. S3), 877s–887s. [CrossRef] [PubMed]

59. Fuge, R.; Johnson, C.C. Iodine and human health, the role of environmental geochemistry and diet: A review. *Appl. Geochem.* **2015**, *63*, 282–302. [CrossRef]

60. Chen, W.; Li, X.; Wu, Y.; Bian, J.; Shen, J.; Jiang, W.; Tan, L.; Wang, X.; Wang, W.; Pearce, E.N.; et al. Associations between iodine intake, thyroid volume, and goiter rate in school-aged Chinese children from areas with high iodine drinking water concentrations. *Am. J. Clin. Nutr.* **2017**, *105*, 228–233. [CrossRef] [PubMed]

61. Ovadia, Y.S.; Gefel, D.; Aharoni, D.; Turkot, S.; Fytlovich, S.; Troen, A.M. Can desalinated seawater contribute to iodine-deficiency disorders? An observation and hypothesis. *Public Health Nutr.* **2016**, *19*, 2808–2817. [CrossRef] [PubMed]

62. United Nations Children's Fund. Sustainable Elimination of Iodine Deficiency: Progress Since the 1990 World Summit for Children. Available online: https://www.unicef.org/publications/files/Sustainable_Elimination_of_Iodine_Deficiency.pdf (accessed on 10 October 2017).

63. World Health Organization (WHO). Fortification of Food-grade Salt with Iodine for the Prevention and Control of Iodine Deficiency Disorders—Guideline. Available online: http://www.who.int/nutrition/publications/guidelines/fortification_foodgrade_saltwithiodine/en/ (accessed on 10 October 2017).

64. Dasgupta, P.K.; Liu, Y.; Dyke, J.V. Iodine nutrition: Iodine content of iodized salt in the United States. *Environ. Sci. Technol.* **2008**, *42*, 1315–1323. [CrossRef] [PubMed]

65. National Academy of Science. The relation of selected trace elements to health and disease. In *Geochemistry and the Environment*; National Academy of Science: Washington, DC, USA, 1974; Volume 1.

66. US DHHS Agency for Toxic Substances and Disease Registry (ATSDR). *Toxicological Profile for Iodine*; ATSDR: Atlanta, GA, USA, 2004.

67. United States Nuclear Regulatory Commission Division of Safeguards. *A Dynamic Model of the Global Iodine Cycle for the Estimation of Dose to the World Population from Releases of Iodine-129 to the Environment*; USNRC: Rockville, MD, USA, 1979.

68. Katagiri, R.; Asakura, K.; Sasaki, S.; Hirota, N.; Notsu, A.; Miura, A.; Todoriki, H.; Fukui, M.; Date, C. Estimation of habitual iodine intake in Japanese adults using 16 d diet records over four seasons with a newly developed food composition database for iodine. *Br. J. Nutr.* **2015**, *114*, 624–634. [CrossRef] [PubMed]

69. Bouga, M.; Combet, E. Emergence of seaweed and seaweed-containing foods in the UK: Focus on labeling, iodine content, toxicity and nutrition. *Foods* **2015**, *4*, 240–253. [CrossRef] [PubMed]

70. Sisasou, E.; Willey, N. Inter-taxa differences in iodine uptake by plants: Implications for food quality and contamination. *Agronomy* **2015**, *5*, 537–554. [CrossRef]

71. USDA APHIS National Animal Health Monitoring System. Dairy 2014 Milk Quality, Milking Procedures, and Mastitis on U.S. Dairies, 2014. Available online: https://www.aphis.usda.gov/animal_health/nahms/dairy/downloads/dairy14/Dairy14_dr_Mastitis.pdf (accessed on 24 October 2017).

72. Wenlock, R.W.; Buss, D.H.; Moxon, R.E.; Bunton, N.G. Trace nutrients. 4. Iodine in British food. *Br. J. Nutr.* **1982**, *47*, 381–390. [CrossRef] [PubMed]

73. Ershow, A.G.; Goodman, G.; Coates, P.M.; Swanson, C.A. Research needs for assessing iodine intake, iodine status, and the effects of maternal iodine supplementation. *Am. J. Clin. Nutr.* **2016**, *104* (Suppl. S3), 941s–949s. [CrossRef] [PubMed]

74. USDA Agricultural Research Service Nutrient Data Laboratory. USDA Special Interest Databases on Flavonoids. Available online: https://www.ars.usda.gov/northeast-area/beltsville-md/beltsville-human-nutrition-research-center/nutrient-data-laboratory/docs/usda-special-interest-databases-on-flavonoids/ (accessed on 30 October 2017).

75. Patterson, K.Y.; Bhagwat, S.A.; Williams, J.R.; Howe, J.C.; Holden, J.M. USDA Database for the Choline Content of Common Foods Release Two. Available online: https://www.ars.usda.gov/ARSUserFiles/80400525/Data/Choline/Choln02.pdf (accessed on 6 November 2017).

76. Haytowitz, D.B.; Lemar, L.E.; Pehrsson, P.R. USDA's Nutrient Databank System—A tool for handling data from diverse sources. *J. Food Compost. Anal.* **2009**, *22*, 433–441. [CrossRef]

77. US Food and Drug Administration. Total Diet Study. Available online: https://www.fda.gov/Food/FoodScienceResearch/TotalDietStudy/default.htm (accessed on 9 November 2017).

78. Trainer, D.; Pehrsson, P.R.; Haytowitz, D.B.; Holden, J.M.; Phillips, K.M.; Rasor, A.S.; Conley, N.A. Development of sample handling procedures for foods under USDA's National Food and Nutrient Analysis Program. *J. Food Compost. Anal.* **2010**, *23*, 843–851. [CrossRef] [PubMed]

79. Haytowitz, D.B.; Pehrsson, P.R. USDA's National Food and Nutrient Analysis Program (NFNAP) produces high-quality data for USDA food composition databases: Two decades of collaboration. *Food Chem.* **2018**, *238*, 134–138. [CrossRef] [PubMed]

80. Patterson, K.Y.; Pehrsson, P.R.; USDA-ARS Beltsville Human Nutrition Research Center, Nutrient Data Laboratory, Beltsville, MD, USA. Personal communication, 2017.

81. Fulgoni, V.L., III; Keast, D.R.; Bailey, R.L.; Dwyer, J. Foods, fortificants, and supplements: Where do Americans get their nutrients? *J. Nutr.* **2011**, *141*, 1847–1854. [CrossRef] [PubMed]

82. Kang, M.; Kim, D.W.; Lee, H.; Lee, Y.J.; Jung, H.J.; Paik, H.Y.; Song, Y.J. The nutrition contribution of dietary supplements on total nutrient intake in children and adolescents. *Eur. J. Clin. Nutr.* **2016**, *70*, 257–261. [CrossRef] [PubMed]

83. Matulka, R.A. Dietary Supplements in the U.S. and Abroad: Similarities and Differences. Available online: http://burdockgroup.com/dietary-supplements-in-the-u-s-and-abroad-similarities-and-differences/ (accessed on 2 October 2017).

84. US Food and Drug Administration. What Is a Dietary Supplement? Available online: https://www.fda.gov/aboutfda/transparency/basics/ucm195635.htm (accessed on 29 September 2017).

85. Skeie, G.; Braaten, T.; Hjartaker, A.; Lentjes, M.; Amiano, P.; Jakszyn, P.; Pala, V.; Palanca, A.; Niekerk, E.M.; Verhagen, H.; et al. Use of dietary supplements in the European Prospective Investigation into Cancer and Nutrition calibration study. *Eur. J. Clin. Nutr.* **2009**, *63* (Suppl. S4), 226s–238s. [CrossRef] [PubMed]

86. Liu, F.X.; Salmon, J. Comparison of herbal medicines regulation between China, Germany, and the United States. *Integr. Med.* **2010**, *9*, 42–49.

87. World Health Organization (WHO). National Policy on Traditional Medicine and Regulation of Herbal Medicines—Report of a WHO Global Survey. Available online: http://apps.who.int/medicinedocs/en/d/Js7916e/9.4.html (accessed on 1 October 2017).

88. Health Canada. About Natural Health Product Regulation in Canada. Available online: https://www.canada.ca/en/health-canada/services/drugs-health-products/natural-non-prescription/regulation.html (accessed on 1 October 2017).

89. National Institute for Public Health and the Environment (RIVM). Dutch Dietary Supplement Database (NES). Available online: http://www.rivm.nl/en/Topics/D/Dutch_Food_Composition_Database/Organisation/Dutch_Dietary_Supplement_Database (accessed on 29 September 2017).

90. Verkaik-Kloosterman, J.; Buurma-Rethans, E.J.M.; Dekkers, A.L.M.; van Rossum, C.T.M. Decreased, but still sufficient, iodine intake of children and adults in the Netherlands. *Br. J.Nutr.* **2017**, *117*, 1020–1031. [CrossRef] [PubMed]

91. Food Standards Australia New Zealand. Dietary Supplement Nutrient Database. Available online: http://www.foodstandards.gov.au/science/monitoringnutrients/ausnut/dietarysupps/ (accessed on 1 October 2017).

92. Lentjes, M.A.; Bhaniani, A.; Mulligan, A.A.; Khaw, K.T.; Welch, A.A. Developing a database of vitamin and mineral supplements (ViMiS) for the Norfolk arm of the European Prospective Investigation into Cancer (EPIC-Norfolk). *Public Health Nutr.* **2011**, *14*, 459–471. [CrossRef] [PubMed]

93. Dwyer, J.T.; Picciano, M.F.; Betz, J.M.; Fisher, K.D.; Saldanha, L.G.; Yetley, E.A.; Coates, P.M.; Milner, J.A.; Whitted, J.; Burt, V.; et al. Progress in developing analytical and label-based dietary supplement databases at the NIH Office of Dietary Supplements. *J. Food Compost. Anal.* **2008**, *21*, S83–S93. [CrossRef] [PubMed]

94. Dwyer, J.T.; Coates, P.M.; Smith, M. Challenges and resources in dietary supplement research. *Nutrients* **2018**, *10*, 41. [CrossRef] [PubMed]

95. Gahche, J.J.; Bailey, R.L.; Mirel, L.B.; Dwyer, J.T. The prevalence of using iodine-containing supplements is low among reproductive-age women, NHANES 1999–2006. *J. Nutr.* **2013**, *143*, 872–877. [CrossRef] [PubMed]

96. US Food and Drug Administration. Nutrition Labeling of Dietary Supplements. e-CFR. 21CFR101.36. Available online: http://www.ecfr.gov/cgi-bin/text-idx?SID=fdb14fc1ad4c9125549a45f13ed6eecb&mc=true&node=se21.2.101_136&rgn=div8 (accessed on 29 September 2017).

97. Turk, G.C.; Sharpless, K.E.; Cleveland, D.; Jongsma, C.; Mackey, E.A.; Marlow, A.F.; Oflaz, R.; Paul, R.L.; Sieber, J.R.; Thompson, R.Q.; et al. Certification of elements in and use of standard reference material 3280 multivitamin/multielement tablets. *J. AOAC Int.* **2013**, *96*, 1281–1287. [CrossRef] [PubMed]

98. USDA Agricultural Research Service; US DHHS NIH Office of Dietary Supplements. Dietary Supplement Ingredient Database (DSID); Release 4.0. Available online: https://dietarysupplementdatabase.usda.nih.gov/ (accessed on 23 October 2017).

99. Saldanha, L.G.; Dwyer, J.T.; Andrews, K.W.; Brown, L.L.; Costello, R.B.; Ershow, A.G.; Gusev, P.A.; Hardy, C.J.; Pehrsson, P.R. Is nutrient content and other label information for prescription prenatal supplements different from nonprescription products? *J. Acad. Nutr. Diet.* **2017**, *117*, 1429–1436. [CrossRef] [PubMed]

100. Lee, K.W.; Shin, D.; Cho, M.S.; Song, W.O. Food group intakes as determinants of iodine status among US adult population. *Nutrients* **2016**, *8*, 325. [CrossRef] [PubMed]

101. Rogan, W.J.; Paulson, J.A.; Baum, C.; Brock-Utne, A.C.; Brumberg, H.L.; Campbell, C.C.; Lanphear, B.P.; Lowry, J.A.; Osterhoudt, K.C.; Sandel, M.T.; et al. Iodine deficiency, pollutant chemicals, and the thyroid: New information on an old problem. *Pediatrics* **2014**, *133*, 1163–1166. [PubMed]

102. De Groot, L.; Abalovich, M.; Alexander, E.K.; Amino, N.; Barbour, L.; Cobin, R.H.; Eastman, C.J.; Lazarus, J.H.; Luton, D.; Mandel, S.J.; et al. Management of thyroid dysfunction during pregnancy and postpartum: An Endocrine Society clinical practice guideline. *J. Clin. Endocrinol. Metab.* **2012**, *97*, 2543–2565. [CrossRef] [PubMed]

103. Obican, S.G.; Jahnke, G.D.; Soldin, O.P.; Scialli, A.R. Teratology public affairs committee position paper: Iodine deficiency in pregnancy. *Birth Defects Res. A Clin. Mol. Teratol.* **2012**, *94*, 677–682. [CrossRef] [PubMed]

104. Alexander, E.K.; Pearce, E.N.; Brent, G.A.; Brown, R.S.; Chen, H.; Dosiou, C.; Grobman, W.A.; Laurberg, P.; Lazarus, J.H.; Mandel, S.J.; et al. 2017 Guidelines of the American Thyroid Association for the Diagnosis and Management of Thyroid Disease During Pregnancy and the Postpartum. *Thyroid* **2017**, *27*, 315–389. [CrossRef] [PubMed]

105. Australian National Health and Medical Research Council (NHMRC). NHMRC Public Statement: Iodine Supplementation for Pregnant and Breastfeeding Women. Available online: https://www.nhmrc.gov.au/_files_nhmrc/publications/attachments/new45_statement.pdf (accessed on 6 November 2017).

106. New Zealand Ministry of Health. Iodine. Available online: http://www.health.govt.nz/our-work/preventative-health-wellness/nutrition/iodine (accessed on 10 October 2017).

107. Reynolds, A.N.; Skeaff, S.A. Maternal adherence with recommendations for folic acid and iodine supplements: A cross-sectional survey. *Aust. N. Z. J. Obstet. Gynaecol.* **2017**. [CrossRef] [PubMed]

108. New Zealand Institute for Plant & Food Research Limited; Ministry of Health (New Zealand). *The Concise New Zealand Food Composition Tables*, 12th ed.; New Zealand Institute for Plant & Food Research Limited; Ministry of Health (New Zealand): Auckland, New Zealand, 2016. Available online: http://www.foodcomposition.co.nz/concise-tables (accessed on 10 October 2017).

109. Ministry for Primary Industries. Update Report on the Dietary Iodine Intake of New Zealand Children Following Fortification of Bread with Iodine. Available online: https://www.mpi.govt.nz/food-safety/food-safety-and-suitability-research/food-science-research/food-composition-research/nutrient-research/ (accessed on 20 December 2017).

110. Zmitek, K.; Pravst, I. Iodisation of salt in Slovenia: Increased availability of non-iodised salt in the food supply. *Nutrients* **2016**, *8*, 434. [CrossRef] [PubMed]

111. Limbert, E.; Prazares, S.; Sao Pedro, M.; Madureira, D.; Miranda, A.; Ribeiro, M.; Jacome de Castro, J.; Carrilho, F.; Oliveira, M.J.; Reguengo, H.; et al. Iodine intake in Portuguese pregnant women: Results of a countrywide study. *Eur. J. Endocrinol.* **2010**, *163*, 631–635. [CrossRef] [PubMed]

112. Ovadia, Y.S.; Arbelle, J.E.; Gefel, D.; Brik, H.; Wolf, T.; Nadler, V.; Hunziker, S.; Zimmermann, M.B.; Troen, A.M. First Israeli national iodine survey demonstrates iodine deficiency among school-aged children and pregnant women. *Thyroid* **2017**, *27*, 1083–1091. [CrossRef] [PubMed]

113. Costa Leite, J.; Keating, E.; Pestana, D.; Cruz Fernandes, V.; Maia, M.L.; Norberto, S.; Pinto, E.; Moreira-Rosario, A.; Sintra, D.; Moreira, B.; et al. Iodine status and iodised salt consumption in Portuguese school-aged children: The Iogeneration Study. *Nutrients* **2017**, *9*, 458. [CrossRef] [PubMed]

114. Pearce, E.N.; Caldwell, K.L. Urinary iodine, thyroid function, and thyroglobulin as biomarkers of iodine status. *Am. J. Clin. Nutr.* **2016**, *104* (Suppl. S3), 898s–901s. [CrossRef] [PubMed]

115. Tayie, F.A.; Jourdan, K. Hypertension, dietary salt restriction, and iodine deficiency among adults. *Am. J. Hypertens.* **2010**, *23*, 1095–1102. [CrossRef] [PubMed]

116. Appleby, P.N.; Thorogood, M.; Mann, J.I.; Key, T.J. The Oxford Vegetarian Study: An overview. *Am. J. Clin. Nutr.* **1999**, *70*, 525S–531S. [PubMed]

117. Leung, A.M.; Lamar, A.; He, X.; Braverman, L.E.; Pearce, E.N. Iodine status and thyroid function of Boston-area vegetarians and vegans. *J. Clin. Endocrinol. Metab.* **2011**, *96*, E1303–E1307. [CrossRef] [PubMed]
118. Schupbach, R.; Wegmuller, R.; Berguerand, C.; Bui, M.; Herter-Aeberli, I. Micronutrient status and intake in omnivores, vegetarians and vegans in Switzerland. *Eur. J. Nutr.* **2017**, *56*, 283–293. [CrossRef] [PubMed]
119. Manousou, S.; Stal, M.; Larsson, C.; Mellberg, C.; Lindahl, B.; Eggertsen, R.; Hulthen, L.; Olsson, T.; Ryberg, M.; Sandberg, S.; et al. A Paleolithic-type diet results in iodine deficiency: A 2-year randomized trial in postmenopausal obese women. *Eur. J. Clin. Nutr.* **2017**. [CrossRef] [PubMed]
120. Bath, S.C.; Hill, S.; Infante, H.G.; Elghul, S.; Nezianya, C.J.; Rayman, M.P. Iodine concentration of milk-alternative drinks available in the UK in comparison with cows' milk. *Br. J. Nutr.* **2017**, *118*, 525–532. [CrossRef] [PubMed]
121. Skalnaya, M.G.; Skalny, A.V.; Tinkov, A.A. TEMA-16 Abstracts. *J. Trace Elem. Med. Biol.* **2017**, *41* (Suppl. S1), 1s–88s.
122. Sawka, A.M.; Ibrahim-Zada, I.; Galacgac, P.; Tsang, R.W.; Brierley, J.D.; Ezzat, S.; Goldstein, D.P. Dietary iodine restriction in preparation for radioactive iodine treatment or scanning in well-differentiated thyroid cancer: A systematic review. *Thyroid* **2010**, *20*, 1129–1138. [CrossRef] [PubMed]
123. Morris, L.F.; Wilder, M.S.; Waxman, A.D.; Braunstein, G.D. Reevaluation of the impact of a stringent low-iodine diet on ablation rates in radioiodine treatment of thyroid carcinoma. *Thyroid* **2001**, *11*, 749–755. [CrossRef] [PubMed]
124. Kim, H.K.; Lee, S.Y.; Lee, J.I.; Jang, H.W.; Kim, S.K.; Chung, H.S.; Tan, A.H.; Hur, K.Y.; Kim, J.H.; Chung, J.H.; et al. Usefulness of iodine/creatinine ratio from spot-urine samples to evaluate the effectiveness of low-iodine diet preparation for radioiodine therapy. *Clin. Endocrinol.* **2010**, *73*, 114–118. [CrossRef] [PubMed]
125. Kim, H.K.; Lee, S.Y.; Lee, J.I.; Jang, H.W.; Kim, S.K.; Chung, H.S.; Tan, A.H.; Hur, K.Y.; Kim, J.H.; Chung, J.H.; et al. Daily urine iodine excretion while consuming a low-iodine diet in preparation for radioactive iodine therapy in a high iodine intake area. *Clin. Endocrinol.* **2011**, *75*, 851–856. [CrossRef] [PubMed]
126. Li, J.H.; He, Z.H.; Bansal, V.; Hennessey, J.V. Low iodine diet in differentiated thyroid cancer: A review. *Clin. Endocrinol.* **2016**, *84*, 3–12. [CrossRef] [PubMed]
127. Morsch, E.P.; Vanacor, R.; Furlanetto, T.W.; Schmid, H. Two weeks of a low-iodine diet are equivalent to 3 weeks for lowering urinary iodine and increasing thyroid radioactive iodine uptake. *Thyroid* **2011**, *21*, 61–67. [CrossRef] [PubMed]
128. Gaitan, E. Goitrogens in food and water. *Annu. Rev. Nutr.* **1990**, *10*, 21–39. [CrossRef] [PubMed]
129. Bhagwat, S.; Haytowitz, D.B.; Holden, J.M. USDA Database for the Flavonoid Content of Selected Foods, Release 3.1. Available online: https://www.ars.usda.gov/ARSUserFiles/80400525/Data/Flav/Flav3.2.pdf (accessed on 30 October 2017).
130. Abt, E.; Spungen, J.; Pouillot, R.; Gamalo-Siebers, M.; Wirtz, M. Update on dietary intake of perchlorate and iodine from U.S. food and drug administration's total diet study: 2008–2012. *J. Expo. Sci. Environ. Epidemiol.* **2018**, *28*, 21–30. [CrossRef] [PubMed]
131. Mortensen, M.E.; Birch, R.; Wong, L.Y.; Valentin-Blasini, L.; Boyle, E.B.; Caldwell, K.L.; Merrill, L.S.; Moye, J., Jr.; Blount, B.C. Thyroid antagonists and thyroid indicators in U.S. pregnant women in the Vanguard Study of the National Children's Study. *Environ. Res.* **2016**, *149*, 179–188. [CrossRef] [PubMed]
132. Corey, L.M.; Bell, G.P.; Pleus, R.C. Exposure of the US population to nitrate, thiocyanate, perchlorate, and iodine based on NHANES 2005–2014. *Bull. Environ. Contam. Toxicol.* **2017**, *99*, 83–88. [CrossRef] [PubMed]
133. Lee, K.W.; Cho, M.S.; Shin, D.; Song, W.O. Changes in iodine status among US adults, 2001–2012. *Int. J. Food Sci. Nutr.* **2016**, *67*, 184–194. [CrossRef] [PubMed]

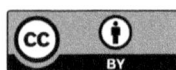

nutrients

MDPI

Review

Efficacy and Effectiveness of Carnitine Supplementation for Cancer-Related Fatigue: A Systematic Literature Review and Meta-Analysis

Wolfgang Marx [1,2,*], Laisa Teleni [2], Rachelle S. Opie [1], Jaimon Kelly [2], Skye Marshall [2], Catherine Itsiopoulos [1] and Elizabeth Isenring [2]

[1]   School of Allied Health, College of Science, Health and Engineering, La Trobe University, Melbourne, VIC 3086, Australia; R.Opie@latrobe.edu.au (R.S.O.); C.Itsiopoulos@latrobe.edu.au (C.I.)

[2]   Faculty of Health Sciences & Medicine, Bond University, Gold Coast, QLD 4226, Australia; laisa.teleni@student.bond.edu.au (L.T.); jkelly@bond.edu.au (J.K.); smarshal@bond.edu.au (S.M.); lisenrin@bond.edu.au (E.I.)

*   Correspondence: w.marx@latrobe.edu.au; Tel.: +61-3-9479-3069

Received: 29 September 2017; Accepted: 3 November 2017; Published: 7 November 2017

Abstract: Background: Carnitine deficiency has been implicated as a potential pathway for cancer-related fatigue that could be treated with carnitine supplementation. The aim of this systematic literature review and meta-analysis was to evaluate the literature regarding the use of supplemental carnitine as a treatment for cancer-related fatigue. Methods: Using the PRISMA guidelines, an electronic search of the Cochrane Library, MEDLINE, Embase, CINAHL and reference lists was conducted. Data were extracted and independently assessed for quality using the Academy of Nutrition and Dietetics evidence analysis by two reviewers. In studies with positive quality ratings, a meta-analysis was performed using the random-effects model on Carnitine and cancer-related fatigue. Results: Twelve studies were included for review with eight reporting improvement in measures of fatigue, while four reported no benefit. However, many studies were non-randomized, open-label and/or used inappropriate dose or comparators. Meta-analysis was performed in three studies with sufficient data. Carnitine did not significantly reduce cancer-related fatigue with a standardized mean difference (SMD) of 0.06 points ((95% CI −0.09, 0.21); $p = 0.45$). Conclusion: Results from studies with lower risk of bias do not support the use of carnitine supplementation for cancer-related fatigue.

Keywords: carnitine; fatigue; cancer; dietary supplement; systematic review

1. Introduction

Cancer-related fatigue (CRF) is one of the most common side-effects of cancer treatment, affecting up to 91% of patients and is now considered one of the most distressing symptoms of cancer [1,2]. CRF is associated with worsened quality of life, depression and anxiety, inability to perform activities of daily living and can have significant financial costs to both patients and their caregivers [3,4]. Furthermore, CRF can persist for months or years after the completion of cancer treatment and is associated with reduced recurrence-free and overall survival [5–8].

Despite its high prevalence, the aetiology of CRF remains unclear. Mechanisms implicated in the development of CRF include inflammation, anaemia and altered neuroendocrine pathways [9]. In addition, most observational studies report that decreased serum carnitine has been associated with fatigue [10–13]. Carnitine is pivotal to energy production; facilitating the uptake of fatty acids into the mitochondria for beta-oxidation. Chemotherapy regimens including cisplatin and ifosfomide disrupt carnitine metabolism by increasing the renal excretion of carnitine [14,15]. Furthermore, muscle wasting, as seen in cancer cachexia, can further exacerbate fatigue. Carnitine may have multiple properties that can prevent or reduce muscle wasting including modulation of protein synthesis and degradation, as well as anti-apoptotic, antioxidant and anti-inflammatory properties [16]. Therefore, it is plausible that the restoration of serum carnitine levels via supplemental carnitine could ameliorate CRF.

Several trials have investigated the effectiveness of supplemental carnitine for the management of CRF. The aim of this review was to systematically evaluate intervention trials regarding the use of supplemental carnitine as a treatment for cancer-related fatigue to inform the clinical management of CRF.

2. Methods

This study was prepared in accordance with the Preferred Reporting Items for Systematic Reviews and Meta-Analyses (PRISMA) guidelines [17].

2.1. Eligibility Criteria

Eligible studies included those evaluating CRF as a primary or secondary outcome in patients of any cancer diagnosis and age, supplemented with carnitine as either a stand-alone intervention or in combination with other agents. Studies were limited to those published in English. Randomized and pseudo-randomized controlled trials were preferred; however, if there were less than five randomized studies, non-randomized and single arm studies were included.

2.2. Data Collection and Extraction

The CINAHL, Cochrane Library (i.e., Cochrane CENTRAL and Cochrane Database of Systematic Reviews), Embase and MEDLINE databases were searched from database inception to December 2016. Two reviewers (Wolfgang Marx and Laisa Teleni) independently screened the titles and abstracts for relevance. Relevant articles were retrieved and two review authors (Wolfgang Marx and Laisa Teleni) independently screened the full text for eligibility. The reference lists of eligible articles were screened for relevant publications. Data extraction was performed in duplicate (Wolfgang Marx and Rachelle S Opie) and a third author (Liz Isenring) was designated as referee.

Extracted data included the study design, inclusion and exclusion criteria, patient demographics (e.g., age, gender), dosing schedule (including dose and frequency), sample size (including dropout rates and reasons), method used to assess fatigue, study outcomes (including self-reported measures of fatigue and adverse events), funding details and potential conflict of interest. We extracted the mean (change from baseline or end-of-study value) and appropriate variance data (standard deviation, standard error or 95% confidence intervals) to perform the meta-analysis.

2.3. Assessment of Study Quality

The quality of the included studies was assessed independently by two authors (Wolfgang Marx and Rachelle S Opie) using the Academy of Nutrition and Dietetics Quality Criteria Checklist which assesses studies for selection, allocation, reporting and attrition bias as well as the level of external validity. Using this checklist, each study was assigned a positive (low risk of bias), negative (high risk of bias) or neutral (moderate risk of bias) rating.

2.4. Data Synthesis

Studies that were rated as positive quality were pooled into Revman for meta-analysis using the DerSimonian and Laird random-effects model [18,19]. Based on the quality rating of the included studies, meta-analysis was deemed inappropriate in 9 of the 12 studies and therefore, findings are presented in narrative form. Treatment effect was calculated as the standardized mean difference (SMD) due to the variability in fatigue measurement scales. One study was standardized to a negative score by multiplying the mean and standard deviation by −1 to reflect a directional score consistent with the other studies [20,21]. A statistically significant ($p < 0.05$) result was considered evidence of an effect.

3. Results

3.1. Study Characteristics

Of the 1727 articles screened, 12 met the eligibility criteria (Figure 1). Population groups included eight advanced cancer, seven mixed diagnoses, two breast cancer only and the remaining studies included pancreatic, gynaecological cancer or multiple myeloma patients only. Three studies included patients with carnitine deficiency only (as confirmed by blood test), five studies included patients with self-reported fatigue and six had no restriction on carnitine deficiency or fatigue in their eligibility criteria.

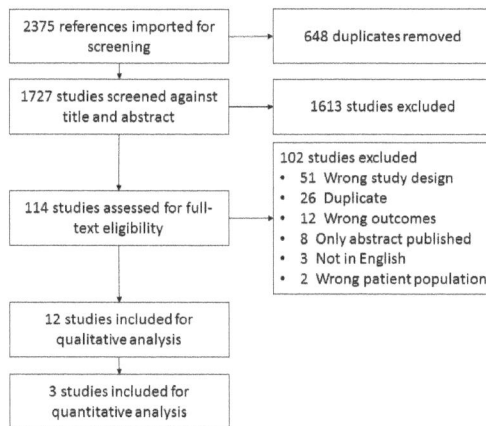

Figure 1. Systematic review flow diagram.

The included studies used a variety of study designs. Three studies were single-arm trials and eight studies used a comparator arm, four of which used a placebo control while five used either standard care or various active ingredients (see Table 1). Eight studies were open-label, two studies were double-blinded throughout the intervention [20,22] and two studies incorporated both a double-blinded and an open-label phase [23,24]. Intervention characteristics and key findings are summarized in Table 1.

There was a large range of sample sizes with eight studies having a total sample size below 100 participants. However, four studies had moderate-to-large sample sizes that ranged from 144 to 409 participants [20,24–26].

3.2. Carnitine Regimens

All studies used an oral dose of carnitine, delivered in a range of forms including liquid ($n = 5$) [22–24,27,28] capsule ($n = 1$) and jelly ($n = 1$) formulations [29]. Nine studies used a dose between 2 to 6 g per day and three studies used <2 g/day, taken once or up to three divided doses per day, with Iwase et al. [29] using the smallest dose of 50 mg [23,27]. Most studies used carnitine as a stand-alone intervention—however, three studies used carnitine as a co-intervention with antioxidant supplements (e.g., coenzyme Q10, alpha lipoic acid), nonsteroidal anti-inflammatories (e.g., celecoxib) and steroids (e.g., megestrol acetate and medroxyprogesterone acetate) [25,29,30]. The intervention period varied from one week up to 24 weeks.

Table 1. Study Design, Population and Quality of Included Studies.

Study & Design	Study Design and Quality	Population and Attrition	Sample Size and Attrition
• Graziano et al. 2002 [31]	• Single arm intervention study • Study quality: Negative • COI: none stated • Funding: none reported	• Advanced cancer. Undergoing first line, palliative chemotherapy. Mixed cancer diagnoses • Mean age: 61 (range: 45–70) years • Female: 40%	• N = 50 • Attrition: 0% • Withdrawal reasons: N/A
• Gramignano et al. 2006 [28]	• Open-label, single-arm intervention study • Study quality: Negative • COI: none stated • Funding: none reported	• Advanced cancer. Mixed cancer diagnoses • Mean age: 60 ± 9 years • Female: 83%	• N = 12 • Attrition: 0% • Withdrawal reasons: N/A
• Cruciani et al. 2006 [27]	• Open-label, Single-arm intervention study • Study quality: Negative • COI: none stated • Funding: none reported	• Carnitine deficient. Advanced cancer. Mixed cancer diagnoses • Mean age: 60 ± 14 years • Female: 37%	• N = 27 (n = 3 to 6 per dosage group) • Attrition: 22% (n = 3 per 7 dosage groups) • Withdrawal reasons: hospitalization (n = 2), severe deterioration (n = 3) and protocol violation (n = 1)
• Callander et al. 2014 [32]	• Open-label, non-randomised controlled trial • Study quality: Negative • COI: none stated • Funding: Partially funded by an unrestricted grant from Millennium	• Relapsed and/or refractory multiple myeloma • Mean age: 65 ± 12 years • Female: 34%	• N = 32 (n = 13 IG; n = 19 CG) • Attrition: 16% (n = 13 IG; n = 14 CG) • IG: withdrawal reasons: unclear. CG withdrawal reasons: LFT abnormality (n = 1); deterioration (n = 4)

Table 1. *Cont.*

Study & Design	Study Design and Quality	Population and Attrition	Sample Size and Attrition
• Cruciani et al. 2009 [30]	• Double-blind, placebo-controlled randomized trial; with control-group open-label cross-over • Study quality: Negative • COI: none stated • Funding: none reported	• Carnitine deficient. Advanced cancer. Mixed cancer diagnoses • Mean age: 66–70 ± 13 years • Female: 55%	• $N = 33$ ($n = 27$ IG including $n = 10$ from CG cross-over; $n = 12$ CG) • Attrition: 36% ($n = 10$ IG; $n = 7$ CG) • IG withdrawal reasons: died ($n = 2$), deterioration ($n = 3$), diarrhoea ($n = 1$), missed follow-up ($n = 1$) • CG withdrawal reasons: died ($n = 1$), deterioration ($n = 2$), fatigue ($n = 2$)
• Kraft et al. 2012 [22]	• Double-blind, placebo-controlled randomized trial • Study quality: Positive • COI: none stated • Funding: unrestricted educational grants from Medinal GmbH, Greven, Germany, Fresenius Kabi Germany GmbH Bad Homburg, Germany and Nutricia GmbH, Erlangen, Germany	• Stage IV Pancreatic cancer • Mean age: 64 ± 2 years • Female: 40%	• $N = 72$ ($n = 38$ IG; $n = 34$ CG) • Attrition: 64% ($n = 14$ IG; $n = 12$ CG) • Withdrawal reasons (groups reported together, no significant difference: died ($n = 2$), deterioration ($n = 3$), diarrhoea ($n = 1$), missed follow-up ($n = 1$)
• Iwase et al. 2016 [29]	• Open-label RCT • Study quality: Negative • COI: none stated • Funding: Otsuka Pharmaceutical Factory Incorporated	• Women with diagnosed breast cancer • Median age: 49–52 (range: 22–70) years • Female: 100%	• $N = 59$ ($n = 28$ IG; $n = 31$ CG) • Attrition: 3% ($n = 59$ IG; $n = 29$ CG) • IG: withdrawal reasons: N/A • CG withdrawal reasons: declined ($n = 1$); deterioration ($n = 1$)

Table 1. *Cont.*

Study & Design	Study Design and Quality	Population and Attrition	Sample Size and Attrition
• Cruciani et al. 2012 [24]	• Double-blind placebo-controlled randomized trial with control-group cross-over • Study quality: Positive • COI: none stated • Funding: Financial support contributed by Ricardo A. Cruciani (lead author)	• Mixed cancer diagnoses • Age not reported • Female: 58%	• $N = 376$ ($n = 198$ IG; $n = 187$ CG) • Attrition: 44% ($n = 104$ IG; $n = 105$ CG) • IG: Withdrawal reasons: died ($n = 8$), refused treatment ($n = 37$), deterioration ($n = 7$), became ineligible ($n = 24$), adverse events ($n = 2$), others ($n = 7$) • CG withdrawal reasons: died ($n = 8$), refused treatment ($n = 30$), deterioration ($n = 5$), adverse events ($n = 29$), others ($n = 9$)
• Hershman et al. 2013 [20]	• Double-blind placebo-controlled randomized trial • Study quality: Positive • COI: none stated • Funding: Financial support by Dawn L. Hershman	• Women with diagnosed breast cancer undergoing taxane-based adjuvant chemotherapy • Median age: 50–52 (range: 26–80) years • Female: 100%	• $N = 409$ ($n = 208$ IG; $n = 201$ CG) • Attrition: 3% ($n = 201$ IG; $n = 194$ CG) • Withdrawal reasons: not described
• Mantovani et al. 2010 [26]	• Open-label, five-arm randomized non-controlled trial • Study quality: Neutral • COI: none stated • Funding: provided by lead author	• Advanced cancer. Cancer-related anorexia/cachexia. Mixed cancer diagnoses • Mean age: 63 ± 12 years • Female: 47%	• $N = 332$ ($n = 88$ IG-a (L-carnitine alone); $n = 88$ IG-b (L-carnitine + other therapies); $n = 156$ other groups) • Attrition: 3% ($n = 85$ IG-a; $n = 86$ IG-b) • IG-a withdrawal reasons: died ($n = 3$) • IG-b withdrawal reasons: died ($n = 2$)

Table 1. *Cont.*

Study & Design	Study Design and Quality	Population and Attrition	Sample Size and Attrition
• Macciò et al. 2012 [25]	• Open-label, two-arm randomized non-controlled trial • Study quality: Neutral • COI: none stated • Funding: none stated	• Gynaecological cancer only. Advanced cancer. • Cancer-related anorexia/cachexia • Mean age: 61 ± 13 years • Female: 100%	• $N = 144$ ($n = 72$ IG-a (L-carnitine + other therapies); $n = 72$ IG-b (MA alone)) • Attrition: 14% ($n = 61$ IG-a; $n = 63$ IG-b)IG-a withdrawal reasons: died ($n = 8$), poor compliance ($n = 3$) • IG-b withdrawal reasons: died ($n = 7$), poor adherence ($n = 2$)
• Madeddu et al. 2012 [30]	• Open-label, two-arm randomized non-controlled trial • Study quality: Negative • COI: not reported • Funding: none stated	• Advanced cancer. • Cancer-related anorexia/cachexia. Mixed cancer diagnoses • Mean age: 65 ± 9 years • Female: 30%	• $N = 60$ ($n = 31$ IG-a (L-carnitine + celecoxib); $n = 29$ IG-b (L-carnitine + celecoxib + MA)) • Attrition: 7% ($n = 29$ IG-a; $n = 27$ IG-b) • IG-a withdrawal reasons: died ($n = 2$) • IG-b withdrawal reasons: died ($n = 2$)

CG, control group; COI, conflict of interest; IG, intervention group; MA, N/A, not applicable.

3.3. Outcome Measures

All studies used a self-reported measure to assess fatigue with most studies using the following validated questionnaires: The Multidimensional Fatigue Symptom Inventory—Short Form, Functional Assessment of Chronic Illness Therapy-Fatigue Scale, or the Brief Fatigue Index (BFI). Three studies calculated sample sizes *a priori* based on fatigue with one study, Cruciani et al. [24], achieving the required sample size [23,24,29]. Five studies did not report on fatigue as their primary outcome but provided powered calculations based on other outcomes (e.g., lean body mass, peripheral neuropathy and inflammation) and four provided no sample size calculation.

Other secondary outcomes included quality of life, anthropometric measures (e.g., lean body mass, grip strength, DEXA), pathology (e.g., reactive oxygen species, glutathione peroxidase, superoxide dismutase, pro-inflammatory cytokines and C-reactive protein), physical function, depression and mood scales, measures of peripheral neuropathy and treatment response (e.g., complete remission, partial response, minimal response).

3.4. Compliance Measures

Five studies reported on compliance with Hershman et al. [20] (pill count) and Kraft et al. [22] (serum carnitine) providing sufficient detail on the method of measuring compliance [25,26,30].

3.5. Quality Rating

Three studies included in this review received a positive quality rating with two receiving a neutral rating and seven receiving a negative rating (Table 1). The primary reasons for the neutral or negative rating were a lack of blinding, lack of inclusion of a placebo/control group, lack of adjustment of potential confounders and randomization, failure to conduct an intention-to-treat analysis.

3.6. Intervention Results on Cancer-Related Fatigue

Four studies reported no improvement in measures of CRF in response to carnitine supplementation and eight studies reported significant improvement in CRF (Table 2). Four single arm studies reported significant improvements when compared to baseline [27,28,30,31]. Iwase et al. [29] reported a significant improvement in worst level of and mean change in fatigue compared to the control group but not average fatigue. Maccio et al. [25] reported that a combination therapy that included carnitine (as well as celecoxib, alpha lipoic acid, carboxycysteine and megestrol acetate) resulted in a significantly improved CRF compared to the control group. Similarly, Mantovani et al. [26] reported a significant improvement in fatigue when using a combination intervention but not when participants received carnitine and an antioxidant supplement only. Cruciani et al. [23] found no significant difference between the intervention and placebo group during a blinded phase; however, after a second, open-label phase whereby all participants received the carnitine supplement, the participants who were originally allocated to the blinded intervention group reported significantly improved levels of fatigue.

All studies with a low risk of bias reported no significant difference in measures of fatigue while most studies with a moderate to high risk of bias reported significant improvements in fatigue.

3.7. Adverse Events

Eight studies provided data on adverse events. Commonly reported adverse events included diarrhoea ($n = 7$ studies) [20,23–26,29,32] and haematological toxicities ($n = 3$ studies) [24,29,32] with both symptoms reported in approximately less than five patients in each study reporting $\geq$grade 3 symptoms. Of the studies that included a control group, no significant increase in adverse events in the intervention group was reported.

Table 2. Intervention and Results of Included Studies.

Study & Design	Intervention	Results
• Graziano et al. 2002 [31]	• Intervention: Levocarnitine supplement, not further described • Comparator: None • Dose: 2 g × 2 per day (4 g total per day) • Duration: 1-week	**Fatigue:** At 3-weeks post-baseline: *FACT-Fatigue* (scored 0–65; lower scores indicate more severe symptoms) • μ 36.5 ± 5.1; mean change from baseline 1.6 ($P > 0.05$ since baseline)
• Gramignano et al. 2006 [28]	• Intervention: Levocarnitine solution • Comparator: none • Dose: 2 g × 3 per day (6 g total per day) • Duration: 4-weeks	**Fatigue:** At 4-weeks post-baseline: *MFSI-SF* (scored 0–150; higher scores indicate more severe symptoms) • μ 12.1 ± 12.6; mean change from baseline −13.3 (**$P < 0.001$ since baseline**) **Quality of Life:** At 4-weeks post-baseline: *QoL–OS* (scored 0–73; higher scores indicate more severe symptoms) • μ 36.8 ± 15.7; mean change from baseline −17.5 (**$P < 0.05$ since baseline**) *EQ-5D Visual Analogue Scale* (scored 0–100; lower scores indicate more severe symptoms) • μ 73.3 ± 12.4; mean change from baseline 22.7 ($P < 0.001$ since baseline) **Anthropometry:** At 4-weeks post-baseline: *Lean body mass via BIA* • μ 40.4 ± 8.6kg; mean change from baseline 2.4 kg (**$P < 0.05$ since baseline**) **Appetite:** At 4-weeks post-baseline: *Numerical scale* (scored 0–10; lower scores indicate more severe symptoms) • μ 6.8 ± 1.9; mean change from baseline 2 (**$P = 0.001$ since baseline**) **Muscle strength:** At 4-weeks post-baseline: *Grip strength* via dynamometer data not reported ($P > 0.05$ since baseline) **Pathology:** At 4-weeks post-baseline: *ROS* • μ 415.2 ± 126.0 FORT units; mean change from baseline −60.6 ($P > 0.05$ since baseline) *GPx* • μ 9890 ± 3004 U/L; mean change from baseline 682 U/L ($P > 0.05$ since baseline) *Pro-inflammatory cytokines IL-1β; IL-6; TNF-α* • data not reported ($P > 0.05$ since baseline)

Table 2. *Cont.*

Study & Design	Intervention	Results
• Cruciani et al. 2006 [27]	• Intervention: Levocarnitine solution (1 g carnitine per mL) • Comparator: None • Dose: 250 mg, 750 mg, 1250 mg, 1750 mg, 2250 mg, 2750 mg or 3000 mg. Given in two doses/day to meet total reported dosage • Duration: 1-week	**CRP** • µ 0.59 ± 0.51 ng/mL; mean change from baseline −0.38 ($P = 0.05$ since baseline) *Haemoglobin* • µ 11.0 ± 1.2 g/dL; mean change from baseline −0.1 ($P > 0.05$ since baseline) For all patients ($n = 27$): **Fatigue:** At 1-week post-baseline: *Brief Fatigue Inventory* (scored 0–90; higher scores indicate more severe symptoms) • µ 39.7 ± 26.0; mean change from baseline −26.4 (**$P < 0.001$ since baseline**) **Mood:** At 1-week post-baseline: *Centre for Epidemiologic Studies Depression Scale* (scored 0–60; higher scores indicate more severe symptoms) • µ 19.0 ± 12.0; mean change from baseline −10.2 (**$P < 0.001$ since baseline**) **Sleep:** At 1-week post-baseline: *Epworth Sleeplessness Scale* (scored 0–24; higher scores indicate more severe symptoms) • µ 9.0 ± 6.0; mean change from baseline −3.9 (**$P = 0.001$ since baseline**) **Pathology:** At 1-week post-baseline: *Haemoglobin* • µ 12.0 ± 2.0 g/dL; mean change from baseline −0.02 g/dL. (**$P = 0.03$ since baseline**) **Adverse events:** • $n = 2$ mild nausea
• Callander et al. 2014 [32]	• Intervention: Acetyl-l-carnitine (not further described) • Dose: 2 × 1.5 g (3 g per day total) • Comparator: IV bortezomib, doxorubicin and oral low-dose dexamethasone (median 3-months) • Duration: variable depending on cycles of therapy needed (median 10-months) • All patients received IV bortezomib, doxorubicin and oral low-dose dexamethasone	**Fatigue:** At end of treatment: *FACT-Fatigue* (scored 0–65; lower scores indicate more severe symptoms) • IG; µ 22.4 ± 11.2; mean change from baseline 7.5 ($P = 0.114$ since baseline) vs. CG: data not reported. Groups not compared

Table 2. *Cont.*

Study & Design	Intervention	Results
• Iwase et al. 2016 [29]	• Supplement: Jelly with BCAA, Co-Q10, L-carnitine • Dose: Unclear. Either BCAA 1250 mg; Co-Q10 15 mg; L-carnitine 25 mg per day or double that dosage • Comparator: Usual care, with recommendations for adequate exercise and relaxation • Duration: 3-weeks	**Fatigue:** At 3-weeks post-baseline: *Brief Fatigue Inventory global fatigue score* (scored 0–10; higher scores indicate more severe symptoms) • IG: outcome data not reported; mean change from baseline −1.50 ± 2.2 vs. CG: outcome data not reported; mean change from baseline −0.2 ± 2.2 • *P* = 0.025 in change between groups **Quality of life:** At 3-months post-baseline: *EORTC-QLQ-C30 global health status sub-group* (scoring unclear; lower scores indicate more severe symptoms) • IG: outcome data not reported; mean change from baseline −3.4 ± 20.4 vs. CG: outcome data not reported; mean change from baseline 2.7 ± 24.0 • *P* = 0.303 change between groups **Mood:** At 3-weeks post-baseline: *Hospital Anxiety and Depression Scale—Anxiety* (scored 0–21; lower scores indicate more severe symptoms) • IG: outcome data not reported; mean change from baseline −0.6 ± 1.9 vs. CG: outcome data not reported; mean change from baseline 0.3 ± 1.5 • *P* = 0.053 in change between groups *Hospital Anxiety and Depression Scale—Depression* (scored 0–21; lower scores indicate more severe symptoms) • IG: outcome data not reported; mean change from baseline 0.6 ± 2.1 vs. CG: outcome data not reported; mean change from baseline −0.1 ± 1.6 • *P* = 0.154 change between groups **Adverse events:** Most common severe adverse events were leukopenia and neutropenia. Detailed list of adverse events included in Iwase et al.

Table 2. *Cont.*

Study & Design	Intervention	Results
• Cruciani et al. 2009 [30]	• Supplement: L-carnitine syrup (1 g carnitine per 10 mL) • Dose: 4-days to progress to 2 × 1 g L-carnitine (2 g carnitine; 10 mL syrup total per day) • Comparator: matching placebo • Duration: 4-weeks including dose-escalation phase (2 weeks for the CG cross-over participants)	**Fatigue:** At 4-weeks post-baseline: *FACT-Anaemia fatigue sub-scale* (scoring unclear; lower scores indicate more severe symptoms) • IG: μ 22.4 ± 10.7; mean change from baseline 6.4 vs. CG: μ 15.1 ± 4.8; mean change from baseline 3.3 • **P = 0.03 between groups** (adjusted) **Quality of life:** At 4-weeks post-baseline: *FACT-Anaemia physical sub-scale* (scoring unclear; lower scores indicate more severe symptoms) • IG: μ 16.5 ± 6.7; mean change from baseline 1.3 vs. CG: μ 14.9 ± 4.0; mean change from baseline 0.9 • P = 0.12 between groups (adjusted) *FACT-Anaemia social/family sub-scale* (scoring unclear; lower scores indicate more severe symptoms) • IG: μ 23.4 ± 6.3; mean change from baseline −0.6 vs. CG: μ 21.3 ± 12.9; mean change from baseline −2.6 • P = 0.21 between groups (adjusted) *FACT-Anaemia emotional sub-scale* (scoring unclear; lower scores indicate more severe symptoms) • IG: μ 14.5 ± 5.8; mean change from baseline 0.3 vs. CG: μ 17.2 ± 4.9 ^{0}; mean change from baseline 5.6 • P = 0.35 between groups (adjusted) *FACT-Anaemia function sub-scale* (scoring unclear; lower scores indicate more severe symptoms) • IG: μ 11.0 ± 3.2; mean change from baseline −0.4 vs. CG: μ 9.2 ± 3.8; mean change from baseline −1.6 • **P = 0.002 between groups** (adjusted) *Linear Analogue Scale Assessments* (scoring unclear; lower scores indicate more severe symptoms) • IG: μ 37.5 ± 18.3; mean change from baseline 8.6 vs. CG: μ 27.5 ± 19.1; mean change from baseline 6.5 • P = 0.11 between groups **Physical function:** At 4-weeks post-baseline: *KPS* (scoring 0–100; lower scores indicate more severe symptoms) • IG: μ 64.2 ± 9.0; mean change from baseline 6 vs. CG: μ 50.0 ± 15.5; mean change from baseline −7 • **P = 0.002 between groups** (adjusted) **Adverse events:** • *n* = 1 constipation • *n* = 1 diarrhoea

Table 2. *Cont.*

Study & Design	Intervention	Results
• Kraft et al. 2012 [22]	• Supplement: L-carnitine liquid formulation (not further described) • Dose: 4 g/day • Comparator: matching placebo • Duration: 3-months	**Fatigue:** At 3-months post-baseline: *Brief Fatigue Inventory* (scored 0–90; higher scores indicate more severe symptoms) • IG: 28.6% had score >4 vs. CG: 41.7% had score >4 • *P* > 0.05 between groups **Anthropometry:** At 6-weeks post-baseline: *Body mass index via BIA* • IG: data not reported; mean change from baseline 3.4% ± 1.5% vs. CG: data not reported; mean change from baseline 1.5% ± 1.4% • **P < 0.018 between groups** **Quality of life:** At 3-months post-baseline: *EORTC-QLQ-C30 global health status sub-group* (scoring unclear; lower scores indicate more severe symptoms) • IG: data not reported; mean change from baseline 0.8 vs. CG: data not reported; mean change from baseline −0.3 • **P < 0.041 between groups** *At 6-weeks post-baseline:* *EORTC-QLQ-C30 cognitive function sub-group* (scoring unclear; lower scores indicate more severe symptoms) • IG: data not reported; mean change from baseline 0.3 vs. CG: data not reported; mean change from baseline −0.1 • **P < 0.034 between groups**
• Cruciani et al. 2012 [24]	• Supplement: 10 g Levocarnitine inert salt in 100 mL solution • Dose: 2 × 1 g L-carnitine per day • Comparator: matching placebo • Duration: 2-months (1-month for CG cross-over participants)	**Fatigue:** At 4-weeks post-baseline: *Brief Fatigue Inventory* (scored 0–90; higher scores indicate more severe symptoms) • IG: data not reported; mean change from baseline −1.0 **(95% CI: −1.3 to −0.6)** vs. CG: data not reported; mean change from baseline −1.1 **(95% CI: −1.4 to 0.8)** • *P* = 0.57 between groups *FACT-Fatigue* (scored 0–65; lower scores indicate more severe symptoms) • Data not reported. • *P* = 0.64 between groups **Mood:** At 4-weeks post-baseline: *Centre for Epidemiologic Studies Depression Scale* (scored 0–60; higher scores indicate more severe symptoms) • Data not reported • *P* = 0.93 between groups **Physical function:** At 8-weeks post-baseline *ECOG PS* (scoring 0–5; higher scores indicate more severe symptoms) • IG: 18% improved and 18% remained stable vs. CG: 64% improved and 20% remained stable • *P* = 0.63 between groups

Table 2. *Cont.*

Study & Design	Intervention	Results
• Hershman et al. 2013 [20]	• Supplement: Acetyl-l-carnitine capsules • Dose: 6 × 500 mg Acetyl-l-carnitine (3 g per day total) • Comparator: matching placebo • Duration: 6-months	**Fatigue:** At 6-months post-baseline: *FACT-Fatigue* (scored 0–65; lower scores indicate more severe symptoms) • IG: mean change from baseline 1.7 vs. CG: mean change from baseline 2.2 • $P = 0.51$ between groups **Functional status:** At 12-weeks post-baseline: *FACT-Taxane Trial Outcome Index* (scoring unclear; lower scores indicate more severe symptoms) • IG: μ 91.9; mean change from baseline −7.4 vs. CG: data not reported; mean change from baseline −7.4 • At 6-months pose-baseline: IG was 3.5 points lower than CG **$P = 0.03$ between groups** **Adverse events:** • IG: grade 3 toxicity ($n = 3$), vomiting ($n = 1$); CG: insomnia ($n = 1$)
• Mantovani et al. 2010 [26]	• Supplement: l-carnitine (not further described) • Dose: 4 g/day • Duration: 4-months • Comparator: MPA (500 mg/day) or MA (320 mg/day) + eicosapentaenoic acid (EPA) enriched supplement (2.2 g/day) + thalidomide (200 mg/day) + l-carnitine (4 g/day) • Other groups (not reported here) were (1) MPA or MA; (2) EPA enriched supplement; (3) thalidomide • All patients given: polyphenols 300 mg/day; lipoic acid 300 mg/day; carbocysteine 2.7 g/day; vitamin E 400 mg/day; vitamin A 30,000 IU/day; and vitamin C 500 mg/day	**Fatigue:** At 4-months post-baseline: *MFSI-SF* (scored 0–150; higher scores indicate more severe symptoms) • IG-a: μ 26.1 ± 25; mean change from baseline 0.85 ± 19.5 ($P = 0.801$ since baseline) vs. IG-b: μ 20 ± 23.1; mean change from baseline −7.5 ± 12.8 (**$P = 0.047$ since baseline**) **$P = 0.004$ between groups (mean change)** **Quality of life:** At 4-months post-baseline: *EORTC-QLQ-C30* (scored 0–100; lower scores indicate more severe symptoms) • IG-a: μ 57.1 ± 21; mean change from baseline 1.9 ($P = 0.832$ since baseline) vs. IG-b: μ 65.8 ± 18; mean change from baseline 9.8 ($P = 0.145$ since baseline). Groups not compared *EQ-5D index* (scoring unclear) • IG-a: μ 0.4 ± 0.5; mean change from baseline −0.1 ($P = 0.151$ since baseline) vs. IG-b: μ 0.6 ± 0.4; mean change from baseline 0.1 ($P = 0.092$ since baseline). Groups not compared *EQ-5D visual analogue scale* (scored 0–100; lower scores indicate more severe symptoms) • IG-a: μ 50.0 ± 26.8; mean change from baseline 4.7 ($P = 0.593$ since baseline) vs. IG-b: μ 49.2 ± 18.0; mean change from baseline −2.5 ($P = 0.950$ since baseline) **Physical function:** At 4-months post-baseline: *ECOG PS* (scoring 0–5; higher scores indicate more severe symptoms) • IG-a: μ 1.5 ± 0.9; mean change from baseline −0.4 (**$P = 0.0001$ since baseline**) vs. IG-b: μ 1.5 ± 0.8; mean change from baseline −0.5 (**$P < 0.0001$ since baseline**). Groups not compared

Table 2. *Cont.*

Study & Design	Intervention	Results
		Anthropometry: At 4-months post-baseline:
		Lean body mass via BIA
		• IG-a: μ 44.6 ± 8.7 kg; mean change from baseline −0.52 ± 3.14 kg ($P = 0.952$ since baseline) vs. IG-b: μ 44.0 ± 7.2 kg; mean change from baseline 0.44 ± 3.1 kg ($P = 0.609$ since baseline)
		$P = 0.144$ between groups
		Lean body mass via DEXA
		• IG-a: μ 45.2 ± 16.7 kg; mean change from baseline −0.7 ± 2.2 kg ($P = 0.980$ since baseline) vs. IG-b: μ 44.9 ± 7.7 kg; mean change from baseline 2.1 ± 2.1 kg (**$P = 0.0148$ since baseline**)
		• **$P < 0.001$ between groups**
		Lean body mass via CT at L3
		• IG-a: μ 43.5 ± 29.4 kg; mean change from baseline 1.2 kg ($P = 0.058$ since baseline) vs. IG-b: μ 45.4 ± 23.9 kg; mean change from baseline 2.6 kg (**$P = 0.001$ since baseline**). Groups not compared
		Muscle strength: At 4-months post-baseline:
		Grip strength via dynamometer
		• IG-a: μ 25.1 ± 11.9; mean change from baseline −0.8 ($P = 0.104$ since baseline) vs. IG-b: μ 24.2 ± 7.2; mean change from baseline −3 ($P = 0.399$ since baseline). Groups not compared
		Appetite: At 4-months post-baseline:
		Visual analogue scale (scoring unclear; lower scores indicate more severe symptoms)
		• IG-a: μ 5.3 ± 3.1; mean change from baseline 0.2 ($P = 0.607$ since baseline) vs. IG-b: μ 6.1 ± 1.5; mean change from baseline 1.0 (**$P = 0.00037$ since baseline**). Groups not compared
		Pathology: At 4-months post-baseline:
		IL-6
		• IG-a: μ 31.6 ± 27.9 pg/mL; mean change from baseline −12.2 pg/mL ($P = 0.663$ since baseline) vs. IG-b: μ 24.7 ± 23.4 pg/mL; mean change from baseline −16.7 pg/mL (**$P = 0.0187$ since baseline**). Groups not compared.
		TFN-α
		• IG-a: μ 37.5 ± 40.7 pg/mL; mean change from baseline 5.3 pg/mL ($P = 0.240$ since baseline) vs. IG-b: μ 22.5 ± 21.8 pg/mL; mean change from baseline −14.8 pg/mL ($P = 0.053$ since baseline). Groups not compared
		ROS
		• IG-a: μ 458 ± 138 FORT U; mean change from baseline 9 FORT U ($P = 0.736$ since baseline) vs. IG-b: μ 445 ± 115 FORT U; mean change from baseline −52 FORT U ($P = 0.262$ since baseline). Groups not compared

Table 2. *Cont.*

Study & Design	Intervention	Results
		GPx
		• IG-a: μ 7107 ± 3398 IU/mL; mean change from baseline 666 IU/mL (*P* = 0.383 since baseline) vs. IG-b: μ 6676 ± 2542 IU/mL; mean change from baseline −758 IU/mL (*P* = 0.816 since baseline). Groups not compared
		Adverse events:
		• IG-a *n* = 1 diarrhoea; IG-b *n* = 1 diarrhoea
		Fatigue: At 4-months post-baseline: *MFSI-SF* (scored 0–150; higher scores indicate more severe symptoms)
		• IG-a: μ 19.9 ± 20.5; mean change from baseline −6.4 (*P* = **0.045 since baseline**) vs. IG-b: μ 23.5 ± 18.2; mean change from baseline 0.9 (*P* = 0.483 since baseline)
		• ***P* = 0.049 between groups**
		Quality of life: At 4-months post-baseline: *EORTC-QLQ-C30* (scored 0–100; lower scores indicate more severe symptoms)
		• IG-a: μ 61.3 ± 20.9; mean change from baseline 7.5 (*P* = **0.029 since baseline**) vs. IG-b: μ 61.1 ± 15.5; mean change from baseline 4.1 (*P* = **0.042 since baseline**)
		• ***P* = 0.042 between groups**
		Anthropometry: At 4-months post-baseline: *Lean body mass* via DEXA
		• IG-a: μ 45.4 ± 10.2 kg; mean change from baseline 2.4 kg (*P* = **0.002 since baseline**) vs. IG-b: μ 45.7 ± 8.2 kg; mean change from baseline 1.3 kg (*P* = 0.584 since baseline)
Maccìo et al. 2012 [25]	• Supplement/treatments: MA + L-carnitine + celecoxib + antioxidants (alpha lipoic acid and carbocysteine) • Dose: MA 320 mg/day; L-carnitine 4 g/day; alpha lipoic acid 600 mg/day; carbocysteine 2.7 g/day; celecoxib 300 mg/day • Comparator: MA (320 mg/day) • Duration: 4-months	• ***P* = 0.032 between groups**
		Appetite: At 4-months post-baseline: *Visual analogue scale* (scoring unclear; lower scores indicate more severe symptoms)
		• IG-a: μ 6.0 ± 1.0; mean change from baseline 1.5 (*P* = **0.019 since baseline**) vs. IG-b: μ 6.3 ± 1.5; mean change from baseline 1.2 (*P* = **0.040 since baseline**)
		• *P* = 0.774 between groups
		Muscle strength: At 4-months post-baseline: *Grip strength* via dynamometer
		• IG-a: μ 27.2 ± 13.9 kg; mean change from baseline 3 (*P* = 0.399 since baseline) vs. IG-b: μ 24.3 ± 8.9; mean change from baseline −1.1 kg (*P* = 0.140 since baseline)
		• *P* = 0.302 between groups
		Physical function: At 4-months post-baseline: *ECOG PS* (scoring 0–5; higher scores indicate more severe symptoms)
		• IG-a: μ 1.1 ± 0.8; mean change from baseline −0.7 (*P* = **0.001 since baseline**) vs. IG-b: μ 1.1 ± 1.2; mean change from baseline −0.5 (*P* = **0.035 since baseline**)
		• *P* = 0.231 between groups

Table 2. *Cont.*

Study & Design	Intervention	Results
		Pathology: At 4-months post-baseline:
		CRP
		• IG-a: μ 15.3 ± 6.7 mg/L; mean change from baseline −9.2 mg/L (**P = 0.038 since baseline**) vs. IG-b: μ 21.2 ± 19.7 mg/L; mean change from baseline −7.4 mg/L (P = 0.292 since baseline)
		• P = 0.056 between groups
		SOD
		• IG-a: μ 96 ± 12; mean change from baseline 11 (P = 0.185 since baseline) vs. IG-b: μ 94 ± 15; mean change from baseline 3 (P = 0.345 since baseline)
		• P = 0.345 between groups
		IL-6
		• IG-a: μ 12.9 ± 10.5 pg/mL; mean change from baseline −9.4 pg/mL (**P = 0.05 since baseline**) vs. IG-b: μ 28.2 ± 23.8 pg/mL; mean change from baseline 1.0 pg/mL (P = 0.622 since baseline)
		• **P = 0.003 between groups**
		TFN-α
		• IG-a: μ 21.4 ± 22.6 pg/mL; mean change from baseline −22 pg/mL (**P = 0.036 since baseline**) vs. IG-b: μ 54.0 ± 25.3 pg/mL; mean change from baseline 13 pg/mL (P = 0.829 since baseline)
		• **P = 0.04 between groups**
		ROS
		• IG-a: μ 444 ± 71.9 FORT U; mean change from baseline −84 FORT U (**P = 0.006 since baseline**) vs. IG-b: μ 427 ± 102 FORT U; mean change from baseline −33 FORT U (P = 0.092 since baseline)
		• **P = 0.037 between groups**
		GPx
		• IG-a: μ 7458 ± 3554 U/L; mean change from baseline 1451 U/L (P = 0.233 since baseline) vs. IG-b: μ 7304 ± 5521; mean change from baseline 683 U/L (P = 0.320 since baseline)
		• P = 0.185 between groups
		Adverse events:
		IG-a *n* = 2 diarrhoea and *n* = 1 epigastria; IG-b *n* = 1 epigastria

Table 2. *Cont.*

Study & Design	Intervention	Results
• Madeddu et al. 2012 [30]	• Supplement/ treatments: L-carnitine + celecoxib • Dose: L-carnitine 4 g/day; celecoxib dose not specified • Comparator: Dose: MA (320 mg/day); L-carnitine (4 g/day); celecoxib dose not specified • Duration: 4-months • All patients also had antioxidants polyphenols 300 mg/day; lipoic acid 300 mg/day; carbocysteine 2.7 g/day; vitamin E 400 mg/day; Vitamin A 30,000 IU/day, vitamin C 500 mg/day	**Fatigue:** At 4-months post-baseline: *MFSI-SF* (scored 0–150; higher scores indicate more severe symptoms) • IG-a: μ 19.9 ± 16.6; mean change from baseline −7.4 (**P = 0.036 since baseline**) vs. IG-b: μ 13.5 ± 11.8; mean change from baseline −8.8 (**P = 0.025 since baseline**) • P = 0.981 between groups **Quality of life:** At 4-months post-baseline: *EORTC-QLQ-C30* (scored 0–100; lower scores indicate more severe symptoms) • IG-a: μ 61.9 ± 16.6; mean change from baseline 1.3 (P = 0.333 since baseline) vs. IG-b: μ 70.5 ± 16.2; mean change from baseline 6.6 (P = 0.258 since baseline) • P = 0.514 between groups *ECOG PS* (scoring 0–5; higher scores indicate more severe symptoms) • IG-a: μ 1.4 ± 0.7; mean change from baseline −0.4 (**P = 0.009 since baseline**) vs. IG-b: μ 1.4 ± 0.8; mean change from baseline −0.3 (**P = 0.030 since baseline**) • P = 0.796 between groups **Appetite:** At 4-months post-baseline: *Visual analogue scale* (scoring unclear; lower scores indicate more severe symptoms) • IG-a: μ 7.6 ± 2.8; mean change from baseline 1.4 (**P = 0.046 since baseline**) vs. IG-b: μ 7.3 ± 2.3; mean change from baseline 1.4 (**P = 0.016 since baseline**) • P = 0.250 between groups **Anthropometry:** At 4-months post-baseline: *Lean body mass via DEXA* • IG-a: μ 41.0 ± 9.2 kg; mean change from baseline 2.4 kg (**P = 0.026 since baseline**) vs. IG-b: μ 43.8 ± 6.4 kg; mean change from baseline 2.5 kg (**P = 0.036 since baseline**) • P = 0.333 between groups *Lean body mass via BIA* • IG-a: μ 40.9 ± 8.7 kg; mean change from baseline 1.1 kg (P = 0.316 since baseline) vs. IG-b: μ 44.6 ± 5.9 kg; mean change from baseline 3.6 kg (P = 0.676 since baseline) • P = 0.407 between groups *Lean body mass via CT at L3* • IG-a: μ 32.4 ± 10.9 kg; mean change from baseline 0.5 kg (**P = 0.048 since baseline**) vs. IG-b: μ 41.8 ± 8.5 kg; mean change from baseline 1.3 kg (**P = 0.041 since baseline**) • P = 0.656 between groups

Table 2. *Cont.*

Study & Design	Intervention	Results
		Muscle strength: At 4-months post-baseline:
		Grip strength via dynamometer
		• IG-a: μ 29.9 ± 7.8 kg; mean change from baseline 3.8 kg (P = 0.140 since baseline) vs. IG-b: μ 29.2 ± 9.1 kg; mean change from baseline 1.7 kg (P = 0.380 since baseline)
		• P = 0.338 between groups
		Physical function: At 4-months post-baseline:
		6-min walk test
		• IG-a: μ 474 ± 79 m; mean change from baseline 45 m (**P = 0.015 since baseline**) vs. IG-b: μ 464 ± 97 m; mean change from baseline 53 m (**P = 0.038 since baseline**)
		• P = 0.626 between groups
		Pathology: At 4-months post-baseline:
		CRP
		• IG-a: μ 21.2 ± 19.7 mg/L; mean change from baseline −7.8 mg/L (P = 0.291 since baseline) vs. IG-b: μ 10.3 ± 11.6 mg/L; mean change from baseline −11.5 mg/L (P = 0.239 since baseline)
		• P = 0.840 between groups
		IL-6
		• IG-a: μ 20.6 ± 17.8 pg/mL; mean change from baseline −4.1 pg/mL (P = 0.543 since baseline) vs. IG-b: μ 19.4 ± 29.2 pg/mL; mean change from baseline −3 pg/mL (P = 0.781 since baseline)
		• P = 0.877 between groups
		TFN-α
		• IG-a: μ 26.4 ± 5.2 pg/mL; mean change from baseline −0.6 pg/mL (P = 0.829 since baseline) vs. IG-b: μ 26.5 ± 6.7 pg/mL; mean change from baseline −1.1 pg/mL (P = 0.475 since baseline)
		• P = 0.548 between groups
		Adverse events
		• IG-a: diarrhoea (n = 1), epigastria (n = 1); IG-b: diarrhoea (n = 1), epigastria (n = 1)

μm, micrometre; BCAA, branched chain amino acid; BIA, bioelectrical impedance analysis; CG, control group; CG, control group; Co-Q10, coenzyme Q10; COI, conflict of interest; CRP, c-reactive protein; CT, computed tomography; DEXA, dual-energy X-ray absorptiometry; ECOG PS, decilitre; Eastern Cooperative Oncology Group performance status; dL, decilitre; FACT, Functional Assessment of Cancer Therapy; g, gram; GPx, Glutathione peroxidase; IG, intervention group; IL, interleukin; kcal, kilocalorie; IU, international unit; IV, intravenous; kg, kilogram; KPS, Karnofsky Performance Status; L, litre; L3, third lumbar vertebrae; m, meter; megestrol acetate; MPA, medroxyprogesterone acetate; MFSI-SF, Multidimensional Fatigue Symptoms Inventory-Short Form; mg, milligrams; MPA, medroxyprogesterone acetate; N/A, not applicable; pg, picogram; QoL, quality of life; ROS, Reactive oxygen species; SOD, superoxide dismutase; TNF, tumour necrosis factor. $^\Omega$ Data reported in Cruciani et al. 2009 [23] was a mean of 117.2 ± 4.9; however, due to the scoring of the assessment tool sub-scale and other data points reported in using this tool the review authors believe this to be an error and that the mean was 17.2.

3.8. Meta-Analysis

In three studies involving a total of 659 participants [20,22,24], carnitine did not significantly reduce CRF (SMD of 0.06 points (95% CI −0.09, 0.21); *p* = 0.45; Figure 2). There was no evidence of statistical heterogeneity (I^2 = 0%). Clinical heterogeneity was evident from the three studies in regards to the dose (2–4 g of carnitine per day), patient demographics (40–100% females included) and carnitine status. However, there were not enough studies to conduct sensitivity analyses to isolate these potential sources of heterogeneity and test the robustness of findings.

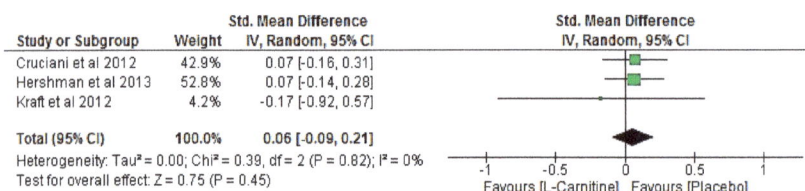

Study or Subgroup	Weight	Std. Mean Difference IV, Random, 95% CI	Std. Mean Difference IV, Random, 95% CI
Cruciani et al 2012	42.9%	0.07 [-0.16, 0.31]	
Hershman et al 2013	52.8%	0.07 [-0.14, 0.28]	
Kraft et al 2012	4.2%	-0.17 [-0.92, 0.57]	
Total (95% CI)	100.0%	0.06 [-0.09, 0.21]	
Heterogeneity: Tau² = 0.00; Chi² = 0.39, df = 2 (P = 0.82); I² = 0%			
Test for overall effect: Z = 0.75 (P = 0.45)			

Favours [L-Carnitine]   Favours [Placebo]

Figure 2. Forest plot of the effect of Carnitine dietary supplement on Cancer-related fatigue. CI = confidence interval; IV = inverse variance.

4. Discussion

Our review identified 12 studies that investigated the use of orally administered carnitine for the treatment of CRF. Despite most (8/12) studies reporting a significant improvement in measures of CRF, most (9/12) studies contain significant limitations that require consideration. Many studies were open-label, single-arm trials which introduces significant performance, selection and detection bias, particularly for fatigue, a self-reported measure that is likely to be susceptible to a placebo response. Some studies either did not analyse or did not find statistical improvements in fatigue when compared to a control or other intervention groups and instead reported improvements in fatigue at the final time point when compared to baseline. The lack of significant improvements compared to a parallel control group further limits the confidence that these improvements are attributed to the intervention alone.

The two largest studies, both randomized controlled trials, reported no significant difference in CRF between intervention and control groups [20,24]. Hershman et al. [20] reported no significant difference in fatigue; however, CRF was a secondary outcome and did not exclusively recruit patients reporting carnitine deficiency or fatigue. The only included study that was sufficiently powered to detect significant differences in fatigue, Cruciani et al. [24], found no effect in any measure of fatigue despite promising results from their earlier studies [27,33]. A possible explanation for these differences is that earlier studies from the same authors recruited carnitine deficient patients only (defined as free carnitine <35 mM/L for males or <25 mM/L for females, or acyl/free carnitine ratio >0.4) which is in contrast to their largest study which recruited patients with moderate to severe fatigue, irrespective of carnitine status [24]. However, an included subgroup analysis of carnitine deficient patients reported no statistically significant differences in CRF despite mean CRF levels in the carnitine group being consistently lower at follow-up time points. The authors noted that the dose used in their study was lower than doses used in studies that have reported improvements in fatigue (1 g versus up to 6 g) [25]. However, there are also studies that have investigated higher doses that have reported no significant improvements [20,22,32].

While the lower doses of carnitine used in some included studies (e.g., 50 mg reported by Iwase et al. [29]) are unlikely to deliver a sufficient dose of absorbable carnitine to provide a therapeutic effect, pharmacokinetic research suggests that higher doses may also be suboptimal [34,35]. Carnitine supplementation has relatively poor oral bioavailability, with 5–16% of carnitine being absorbed after a single dose of 2 g and 6 g of carnitine in healthy participants [34]. Furthermore, plasma concentrations of carnitine are non-linear with one study reporting that doses of 0.5 g, 1 g and 2 g resulted in similar plasma concentrations of carnitine while the 2 g dose resulted in significantly increased plasma concentrations of a proatherogenic metabolite of carnitine, trimethylamine-*N*-oxide [36], indicating that absorption had been saturated and that doses exceeding 2 g may not provide further therapeutic effect [35]. It should be noted, however, that the cited pharmacokinetic studies have all been conducted in healthy participants and the dose of carnitine required to saturate absorption pathways may differ in carnitine deficient populations.

There are multiple risk factors for CRF including but not limited to, inflammation, anaemia and altered neuroendocrine pathways [9]. The lack of control for these potential mechanisms of fatigue in the included studies may have confounded the results. This is partially supported by the positive results of studies that investigated carnitine as part of a multi-ingredient intervention that targeted multiple pathways [25,26,30].

Follow-up periods and patient populations were also inconsistent across studies. Carnitine status fluctuates both during the course of cancer treatment and in response to different chemotherapy regimens [11,12]. For example, doxorubicin is reported to affect carnitine levels to a greater extent than other treatments and Heuberger et al. [37] reported carnitine levels to increase one week after chemotherapy while studies that have measured carnitine status with longer time points have reported a decrease [11,12]. Hence, future studies are required to investigate carnitine fluctuations over the course of chemotherapy treatment and intervention trials may benefit from recruiting homogenous cancer populations.

Future Directions and Clinical Implications

Due to the dearth of clinical studies with low risk of bias, clinical recommendations for the use of carnitine in treating CRF are premature. Only 3 of the 12 studies were suitable for meta-analysis which reduces the conclusions which can be drawn from the analysis. The available evidence indicates carnitine supplementation is unlikely to provide a clinically meaningful benefit for CRF in the chemotherapy cancer-population.

Further research is required to elucidate the safety profile of carnitine in the cancer setting. While the included studies reported carnitine supplementation to be well tolerated, Hershman et al. [20] found symptoms of peripheral neuropathy increased in participants receiving carnitine supplementation, which should be considered before clinical use. Furthermore, carnitine supplementation may increase risk of cardiovascular disease via the increase in proatherogenic microbiota-derived metabolites trimethylamine, trimethylamine-*N*-oxide and γ-butyrobetaine [36] These metabolites have also been shown in animal models to increase concentrations of the carcinogenic compound *N*-nitrosodimethylamine [38]. Therefore, long term carnitine supplementation may increase risk of chronic diseases, particularly at higher doses which provides a greater amount of substrates for these proatherogenic metabolites.

Biases inherent in intervention study designs with high-risk of bias mean it is difficult to determine if the reported adverse events can be attributed solely to carnitine supplementation. Future intervention studies should utilize trial designs with the lowest risk of bias (e.g., randomized controlled trials), implement methods of measuring adherence to intervention (e.g., pill counts and/or serum carnitine), investigate carnitine as a stand-alone intervention and ensure study populations are controlled for aetiology of fatigue and chemotherapy regimens.

5. Conclusions

Of the 12 studies included in this systematic review, eight reported carnitine supplementation to significantly improve measures of cancer-related fatigue. However, due to the significant bias of many included studies, the null findings of the two largest studies and our meta-analysis and the potential increase in peripheral neuropathy, there is currently insufficient evidence to recommend its use in the cancer setting. Future studies should include rigorous study design methods to reduce bias and focus on population subsets with confirmed carnitine deficiency.

Acknowledgments: Publications fees were funded by the Bond University APC Funding Scheme. The authors received no other funding for this publication.

Author Contributions: W.M. and L.T. conceptualized the systematic review, designed and implemented the protocol. R.S.O. and W.M. completed the quality appraisal, J.K. conducted the meta-analysis. All authors contributed to the manuscript development. All authors have read and approved the final version of the manuscript.

Conflicts of Interest: The authors declare no conflict of interest.

References

1. Lawrence, D.P.; Kupelnick, B.; Miller, K.; Devine, D.; Lau, J. Evidence report on the occurrence, assessment and treatment of fatigue in cancer patients. *J. Natl. Cancer Inst. Monogr.* **2004**. [CrossRef] [PubMed]
2. Carelle, N.; Piotto, E.; Bellanger, A.; Germanaud, J.; Thuillier, A.; Khayat, D. Changing patient perceptions of the side effects of cancer chemotherapy. *Cancer* **2002**, *95*, 155–163. [CrossRef] [PubMed]
3. Curt, G.A.; Breitbart, W.; Cella, D.; Groopman, J.E.; Horning, S.J.; Itri, L.M.; Johnson, D.H.; Miaskowski, C.; Scherr, S.L.; Portenoy, R.K.; et al. Impact of cancer-related fatigue on the lives of patients: New findings from the Fatigue Coalition. *Oncologist* **2000**, *5*, 353–360. [CrossRef] [PubMed]
4. Broeckel, J.A.; Jacobsen, P.B.; Horton, J.; Balducci, L.; Lyman, G.H. Characteristics and correlates of fatigue after adjuvant chemotherapy for breast cancer. *J. Clin. Oncol. Off. J. Am. Soc. Clin. Oncol.* **1998**, *16*, 1689–1696. [CrossRef] [PubMed]
5. Curran, S.L.; Beacham, A.O.; Andrykowski, M.A. Ecological momentary assessment of fatigue following breast cancer treatment. *J. Behav. Med.* **2004**, *27*, 425–444. [CrossRef] [PubMed]
6. Groenvold, M.; Petersen, M.A.; Idler, E.; Bjorner, J.B.; Fayers, P.M.; Mouridsen, H.T. Psychological distress and fatigue predicted recurrence and survival in primary breast cancer patients. *Breast Cancer Res. Treat.* **2007**, *105*, 209–219. [CrossRef] [PubMed]
7. Quinten, C.; Maringwa, J.; Gotay, C.C.; Martinelli, F.; Coens, C.; Reeve, B.B.; Flechtner, H.; Greimel, E.; King, M.; Osoba, D.; et al. Patient self-reports of symptoms and clinician ratings as predictors of overall cancer survival. *J. Natl. Cancer Inst.* **2011**, *103*, 1851–1858. [CrossRef] [PubMed]
8. Bower, J.E.; Ganz, P.A.; Desmond, K.A.; Bernaards, C.; Rowland, J.H.; Meyerowitz, B.E.; Belin, T.R. Fatigue in long-term breast carcinoma survivors: A longitudinal investigation. *Cancer* **2006**, *106*, 751–758. [CrossRef] [PubMed]
9. Bower, J.E. Cancer-related fatigue mdash mechanisms, risk factors and treatments. *Nat. Rev. Clin. Oncol.* **2014**, *11*, 597–609. [CrossRef] [PubMed]
10. Winter, S.C.; Szabo-Aczel, S.; Curry, C.J.; Hutchinson, H.T.; Hogue, R.; Shug, A. Plasma carnitine deficiency. Clinical observations in 51 pediatric patients. *Am. J. Dis. Child.* **1987**, *141*, 660–665. [CrossRef] [PubMed]
11. Hockenberry, M.J.; Hooke, M.C.; Gregurich, M.; McCarthy, K. Carnitine plasma levels and fatigue in children/adolescents receiving cisplatin, ifosfamide, or doxorubicin. *J. Pediatr. Hematol. Oncol.* **2009**, *31*, 664–669. [CrossRef] [PubMed]
12. Endo, K.; Tsuji, A.; Kondo, S.; Wakisaka, N.; Murono, S.; Yoshizaki, T. Carnitine is associated with fatigue following chemoradiotherapy for head and neck cancer. *Acta Oto-Laryngol.* **2015**, *135*, 846–852. [CrossRef] [PubMed]
13. Marx, W.; Teleni, L.; Ferguson, M.; Walpole, E.; Isenring, E. The Effect of Chemotherapy on Serum Carnitine Levels and Fatigue in Chemotherapy Naïve Medical Oncology Patients: A Pilot Study. Carnitine, Chemotherapy and Fatigue. *J. Nutr. Disord. Ther.* **2014**. [CrossRef]
14. Mancinelli, A.; D'Iddio, S.; Bisonni, R.; Graziano, F.; Lippe, P.; Calvani, M. Urinary excretion of L-carnitine and its short-chain acetyl-L-carnitine in patients undergoing carboplatin treatment. *Cancer Chemother. Pharmacol.* **2007**, *60*, 19–26. [CrossRef] [PubMed]
15. Marthaler, N.P.; Visarius, T.; Kupfer, A.; Lauterburg, B.H. Increased urinary losses of carnitine during ifosfamide chemotherapy. *Cancer Chemother. Pharmacol.* **1999**, *44*, 170–172. [CrossRef] [PubMed]
16. Ringseis, R.; Keller, J.; Eder, K. Mechanisms underlying the anti-wasting effect of L-carnitine supplementation under pathologic conditions: Evidence from experimental and clinical studies. *Eur. J. Nutr.* **2013**, *52*, 1421–1442. [CrossRef] [PubMed]

17. Moher, D.; Liberati, A.; Tetzlaff, J.; Altman, D.G.; PRISMA Group. Preferred Reporting Items for Systematic Reviews and Meta-Analyses: The PRISMA Statement. *PLoS Med.* **2009**, *6*, e1000097. [CrossRef] [PubMed]
18. DerSimonian, R.; Laird, N. Meta-analysis in clinical trials. *Control. Clin. Trials* **1986**, *7*, 177–188. [CrossRef]
19. Review Manager (RevMan). Available online: http://community.cochrane.org/tools/review-production-tools/revman-5 (accessed on 7 October 2017).
20. Hershman, D.L.; Unger, J.M.; Crew, K.D.; Minasian, L.M.; Awad, D.; Moinpour, C.M.; Hansen, L.; Lew, D.L.; Greenlee, H.; Fehrenbacher, L.; et al. Randomized Double-Blind Placebo-Controlled Trial of Acetyl-l-Carnitine for the Prevention of Taxane-Induced Neuropathy in Women Undergoing Adjuvant Breast Cancer Therapy. *J. Clin. Oncol.* **2013**. [CrossRef] [PubMed]
21. Higgins, J.P.T.; Green, S. *Cochrane Handbook for Systematic Reviews of Interventions*; John Wiley & Sons: Hoboken, NJ, USA, 2011.
22. Kraft, M.; Kraft, K.; Gärtner, S.; Mayerle, J.; Simon, P.; Weber, E.; Schütte, K.; Stieler, J.; Koula-Jenik, H.; Holzhauer, P.; et al. l-Carnitine-supplementation in advanced pancreatic cancer (CARPAN)—A randomized multicentre trial. *Nutr. J.* **2012**, *11*, 52. [CrossRef] [PubMed]
23. Cruciani, R.A.; Dvorkin, E.; Homel, P.; Culliney, B.; Malamud, S.; Lapin, J.; Portenoy, R.K.; Esteban-Cruciani, N. l-carnitine supplementation in patients with advanced cancer and carnitine deficiency: A double-blind, placebo-controlled study. *J. Pain Symptom Manag.* **2009**, *37*, 622–631. [CrossRef] [PubMed]
24. Cruciani, R.A.; Zhang, J.J.; Manola, J.; Cella, D.; Ansari, B.; Fisch, M.J. L-carnitine Supplementation for the Management of Fatigue in Patients With Cancer: An Eastern Cooperative Oncology Group Phase III, Randomized, Double-Blind, Placebo-Controlled Trial. *J. Clin. Oncol.* **2012**, *30*, 3864–3869. [CrossRef] [PubMed]
25. Maccio, A.; Madeddu, C.; Gramignano, G.; Mulas, C.; Floris, C.; Sanna, E.; Cau, M.C.; Panzone, F.; Mantovani, G. A randomized phase III clinical trial of a combined treatment for cachexia in patients with gynaecological cancers: Evaluating the impact on metabolic and inflammatory profiles and quality of life. *Gynecol. Oncol.* **2012**, *124*, 417–425. [CrossRef] [PubMed]
26. Mantovani, G.; Maccio, A.; Madeddu, C.; Serpe, R.; Massa, E.; Dessi, M.; Panzone, F.; Contu, P. Randomized phase III clinical trial of five different arms of treatment in 332 patients with cancer cachexia. *Oncologist* **2010**, *15*, 200–211. [CrossRef] [PubMed]
27. Cruciani, R.A.; Dvorkin, E.; Homel, P.; Malamud, S.; Culliney, B.; Lapin, J.; Portenoy, R.K.; Esteban-Cruciani, N. Safety, tolerability and symptom outcomes associated with L-carnitine supplementation in patients with cancer, fatigue and carnitine deficiency: A phase I/II study. *J. Pain Symptom Manag.* **2006**, *32*, 551–559. [CrossRef] [PubMed]
28. Gramignano, G.; Lusso, M.R.; Madeddu, C.; Massa, E.; Serpe, R.; Deiana, L.; Lamonica, G.; Dessi, M.; Spiga, C.; Astara, G.; et al. Efficacy of L-carnitine administration on fatigue, nutritional status, oxidative stress and related quality of life in 12 advanced cancer patients undergoing anticancer therapy. *Nutrition* **2006**, *22*, 136–145. [CrossRef] [PubMed]
29. Iwase, S.; Kawaguchi, T.; Yotsumoto, D.; Doi, T.; Miyara, K.; Odagiri, H.; Kitamura, K.; Ariyoshi, K.; Miyaji, T.; Ishiki, H.; et al. Efficacy and safety of an amino acid jelly containing coenzyme Q10 and L-carnitine in controlling fatigue in breast cancer patients receiving chemotherapy: A multi-institutional, randomized, exploratory trial (JORTC-CAM01). *Support. Care Cancer Off. J. Multinatl. Assoc. Support. Care Cancer* **2016**, *24*, 637–646. [CrossRef] [PubMed]
30. Madeddu, C.; Dessi, M.; Panzone, F.; Serpe, R.; Antoni, G.; Cau, M.C.; Montaldo, L.; Mela, Q.; Mura, M.; Astara, G.; et al. Randomized phase III clinical trial of a combined treatment with carnitine + celecoxib +/− megestrol acetate for patients with cancer-related anorexia/cachexia syndrome. *Clin. Nutr.* **2012**, *31*, 176–182. [CrossRef] [PubMed]
31. Graziano, F.; Bisonni, R.; Catalano, V.; Silva, R.; Rovidati, S.; Mencarini, E.; Ferraro, B.; Canestrari, F.; Baldelli, A.M.; De Gaetano, A.; et al. Potential role of levocarnitine supplementation for the treatment of chemotherapy-induced fatigue in non-anaemic cancer patients. *Br. J. Cancer* **2002**, *86*, 1854–1857. [CrossRef] [PubMed]
32. Callander, N.; Markovina, S.; Eickhoff, J.; Hutson, P.; Campbell, T.; Hematti, P.; Go, R.; Hegeman, R.; Longo, W.; Williams, E.; et al. Acetyl-l-carnitine (ALCAR) for the prevention of chemotherapy-induced peripheral neuropathy in patients with relapsed or refractory multiple myeloma treated with bortezomib, doxorubicin and low-dose dexamethasone: A study from the Wisconsin Oncology Network. *Cancer Chemother. Pharmacol.* **2014**, *74*, 875–882. [PubMed]

33. Cruciani, R.A.; Zhang, J.; Manola, J.B.; Cella, D.; Ansari, B.; Fisch, M.J. Phase III randomized, placebo-controlled trial of L-carnitine supplementation for fatigue in patients with cancer. *J. Clin. Oncol.* **2009**, *27*, e20532.

34. Harper, P.; Elwin, C.-E.; Cederblad, G. Pharmacokinetics of bolus intravenous and oral doses of L-carnitine in healthy subjects. *Eur. J. Clin. Pharmacol.* **1988**, *35*, 69–75. [CrossRef] [PubMed]

35. Bain, M.A.; Milne, R.W.; Evans, A.M. Disposition and metabolite kinetics of oral L-carnitine in humans. *J. Clin. Pharmacol.* **2006**, *46*, 1163–1170. [CrossRef] [PubMed]

36. Koeth, R.A.; Wang, Z.; Levison, B.S.; Buffa, J.A.; Org, E.; Sheehy, B.T.; Britt, E.B.; Fu, X.; Wu, Y.; Li, L.; et al. Intestinal microbiota metabolism of L-carnitine, a nutrient in red meat, promotes atherosclerosis. *Nat. Med.* **2013**, *19*, 576–585. [CrossRef] [PubMed]

37. Heuberger, W.; Berardi, S.; Jacky, E.; Pey, P.; Krahenbuhl, S. Increased urinary excretion of carnitine in patients treated with cisplatin. *Eur. J. Clin. Pharmacol.* **1998**, *54*, 503–508. [CrossRef] [PubMed]

38. Empl, M.T.; Kammeyer, P.; Ulrich, R.; Joseph, J.F.; Parr, M.K.; Willenberg, I.; Schebb, N.H.; Baumgartner, W.; Rohrdanz, E.; Steffen, C.; et al. The influence of chronic L-carnitine supplementation on the formation of preneoplastic and atherosclerotic lesions in the colon and aorta of male F344 rats. *Arch. Toxicol.* **2015**, *89*, 2079–2087. [CrossRef] [PubMed]

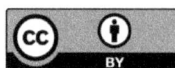

nutrients

Article

Beetroot Juice Supplementation Improves High-Intensity Intermittent Type Exercise Performance in Trained Soccer Players

Jean Nyakayiru [1], Kristin L. Jonvik [1,2], Jorn Trommelen [1], Philippe J. M. Pinckaers [1], Joan M. Senden [1], Luc J. C. van Loon [1,2] and Lex B. Verdijk [1,*]

[1] Department of Human Movement Sciences, NUTRIM School of Nutrition and Translational Research in Metabolism, Maastricht University Medical Centre+, P.O. Box 616, 6200 MD Maastricht, The Netherlands; jean.nyakayiru@maastrichtuniversity.nl (J.N.); kristin.jonvik@maastrichtuniversity.nl (K.L.J.); jorn.trommelen@maastrichtuniversity.nl (J.T.); philippe.pinckaers@maastrichtuniversity.nl (P.J.M.P.); joan.senden@maastrichtuniversity.nl (J.M.S.); l.vanloon@maastrichtuniversity.nl (L.J.C.v.L.)
[2] Institute of Sports and Exercise Studies, HAN University of Applied Sciences, P.O. Box 6960, NL 6503 GL Nijmegen, The Netherlands
*   Correspondence: lex.verdijk@maastrichtuniversity.nl; Tel.: +31-43-3881318

Received: 14 February 2017; Accepted: 18 March 2017; Published: 22 March 2017

Abstract: It has been shown that nitrate supplementation can enhance endurance exercise performance. Recent work suggests that nitrate ingestion can also increase intermittent type exercise performance in recreational athletes. We hypothesized that six days of nitrate supplementation can improve high-intensity intermittent type exercise performance in trained soccer players. Thirty-two male soccer players (age: 23 ± 1 years, height: 181 ± 1 m, weight: 77 ± 1 kg, playing experience: 15.2 ± 0.5 years, playing in the first team of a 2nd or 3rd Dutch amateur league club) participated in this randomized, double-blind cross-over study. All subjects participated in two test days in which high-intensity intermittent running performance was assessed using the Yo-Yo IR1 test. Subjects ingested nitrate-rich (140 mL; ~800 mg nitrate/day; BR) or a nitrate-depleted beetroot juice (PLA) for six subsequent days, with at least eight days of wash-out between trials. The distance covered during the Yo-Yo IR1 was the primary outcome measure, while heart rate (HR) was measured continuously throughout the test, and a single blood and saliva sample were collected just prior to the test. Six days of BR ingestion increased plasma and salivary nitrate and nitrite concentrations in comparison to PLA ($p < 0.001$), and enhanced Yo-Yo IR1 test performance by $3.4 \pm 1.3\%$ (from 1574 ± 47 to 1623 ± 48 m; $p = 0.027$). Mean HR was lower in the BR (172 ± 2) vs. PLA trial (175 ± 2; $p = 0.014$). Six days of BR ingestion effectively improves high-intensity intermittent type exercise performance in trained soccer players.

Keywords: football; nitrate; nitrite; nitric oxide; ergogenic aid

1. Introduction

While nitrate and nitrite were previously considered inert byproducts of the nitric oxide (NO) metabolism, recent insights suggest that (dietary) nitrate can also serve as a precursor for NO through the nitrate -> nitrite -> NO-pathway [1]. Different studies have shown that both plasma nitrate and nitrite concentrations increase following dietary nitrate supplementation in a dose-dependent manner [2,3]. These elevations in plasma concentrations have in turn been associated with improvements in exercise performance, suggesting ergogenic benefits from activation of the nitrate to NO pathway [4–6].

Multiple studies from different laboratories have shown that dietary nitrate ingestion can decrease the oxygen cost of submaximal exercise and increase high-intensity exercise tolerance in recreational athletes [4,7,8]. Furthermore, we have previously shown that nitrate-rich beetroot juice ingestion can not only increase oxygen efficiency during submaximal cycling exercise, but that it can also improve time trial performance in moderately trained cyclists and triathletes [5]. As such, this work, in line with others [6,9], has established a functional benefit of dietary nitrate supplementation on exercise performance.

Most of the earlier work on the ergogenic effects of nitrate supplementation Dutch was focused on endurance type sports, while little attention has been given to high-intensity and/or intermittent type exercise performance. However, recent findings suggest that nitrate might largely convey its effects on exercise performance through type II muscle fibers [10,11]. Ferguson et al. [10] used a rat model to assess the effects of dietary nitrate supplementation on blood flow in vivo during submaximal exercise. The increases in blood flow and vascular conductance in the exercising limbs were primarily observed in fast twitch muscle fibers. In line with these observations, Hernandez et al. [11] reported that dietary nitrate supplementation improves intracellular calcium handling in fast-twitch muscles of mice, which resulted in increased force production. Based on these findings in rodents, it could be suggested that the ergogenic effects of nitrate might be most profound for activities that recruit type II muscle fibers [10,11], i.e., (very) high-intensity exercise bouts of short duration.

Soccer is one of the world's most widely performed team sports and is characterized by players performing multiple bouts of high-intensity running and sprinting throughout the 90 min of a match, during which there is heavy reliance on the contribution of type II muscle fibers [12]. These periods of high-intensity activity are alternated with periods of relative recovery, resulting in an intermittent type intensity profile [12–14]. The Yo-Yo Intermittent recovery test level 1 (Yo-Yo IR1) is an often used measurement tool to simulate these soccer specific activities in a controlled setting, thereby allowing the reliable and feasible assessment of physical performance in soccer players [15]. Indeed, the Yo-Yo IR1 test has been shown to cover aspects of both aerobic as well as anaerobic performance in soccer players, with a strong link towards the ability to perform high-intensity intermittent type exercise throughout a match [12,15]. Using the Yo-Yo IR1, two previous studies described improved high-intensity intermittent type exercise performance following nitrate-rich beetroot juice ingestion in recreationally active team sport players [16,17]. These observations were the first evidence of ergogenic benefits that team sport players (such as soccer players) could have from nitrate ingestion. The earlier of the two studies observed these effects after ingestion of a high nitrate dose (1780 mg, 28.7 mmol) in the 30 h prior to the high-intensity intermittent running test [16]. Although effective, the dosing strategy that was applied in the study strongly deviates from that of current multiday supplementation protocols that have proven effective in endurance athletes [4,5,7]. More in line with current nitrate supplementation regimens, Thompson et al. recently concluded that a five-day nitrate supplementation protocol with a lower daily dose of nitrate was also effective in improving high-intensity intermittent running performance in recreational athletes [17]. Extending on this finding in recreational athletes, we hypothesized that a homogenous group of trained soccer players performing intermittent type exercise would also benefit from nitrate ingestion. Therefore, we assessed the effects of a six-day nitrate-rich beetroot juice supplementation protocol on high-intensity intermittent running performance in a group of trained soccer players.

2. Materials and Methods

2.1. Subjects

A total of 40, first team, male soccer players competing in the 2nd and 3rd Dutch amateur league were recruited to participate in the study. After being informed about the purpose and potential risks of the study, all subjects provided written informed consent. The experimental protocol and procedures were approved by the medical ethical committee of the Maastricht University Medical

Centre, the Netherlands (METC 153006; ClinicalTrials.gov: NCT02436629). Eight subjects failed to complete the study because of injury ($n = 3$), failure to comply with the protocol (dietary/activity standardization procedures; $n = 4$), or due to personal time constraints ($n = 1$). Data of the remaining 32 subjects (age: 23 ± 1 years, height: 181 ± 1 cm, weight: 77 ± 1 kg, BMI: 23.4 ± 0.4 kg/m^2, playing experience: 15.2 ± 0.5 y) was used in the analysis.

2.2. Study Design

This double blind, randomized, placebo-controlled, cross-over study was designed to investigate whether six days of nitrate-rich beetroot juice (BR) supplementation improves intermittent type exercise performance in trained soccer players. Subjects were required to report to the research facility on four occasions, spread over a three-week period. Following a screening session (visit one), subjects visited the research facility ~1 week prior to the first experimental trial to get familiarized with the Yo-Yo intermittent Recovery test level 1 (Yo-Yo IR1) and to receive their supplemental beverages (visit two). No blood or saliva samples were collected during familiarization. The experimental trial days (visits three and four) that followed were each on day six of the nitrate-rich or nitrate-depleted beetroot juice supplementation period, with the last supplemental bolus being ingested 3 h prior to performing the Yo-Yo IR1. Wash-out between the two supplementation periods was at least eight days.

2.3. Supplementation Protocol and Standardization of Physical Activity and Diet

During the two 6-day supplementation periods, subjects ingested 2 × 70 mL/day of beetroot juice. The choice for beetroot juice was largely based on previous observations by us [18], and by others [19], that suggest more pronounced benefits from nitrate ingestion through plant based sources than following sodium nitrate ingestion. The daily 140 mL bolus of nitrate-rich beetroot juice (BR) provided ~800 mg of nitrate (~12.9 mmol), while the beetroot juice placebo (PLA) was similar in taste and appearance but instead was depleted of nitrate (both supplied by Beet It, James White Drinks Ltd., Ipswich, UK). Subjects were instructed to ingest the 2 × 70 mL shots around the same time each day (~5 pm), which was based on the time the final bolus was ingested on day six of supplementation; i.e., 3 h prior to the exercise test. In addition, subjects recorded their activities and dietary intake in the 36 h prior to the first experimental trial, which were then replicated in the 36 h prior to the second trial. Subjects refrained from strenuous physical exercise or labor in the 48 h leading up to the trial days, and did not consume caffeine or alcohol in the 12 h and 24 h prior to each trial, respectively. To prevent any attenuation in the reduction of nitrate to nitrite by commensal bacteria in the oral cavity, subjects refrained from using antibacterial mouthwash/toothpaste and chewing gum during the six-day supplementation periods [20]. No restriction was set for the consumption of nitrate-rich foods. This was done to allow for the determination of the additional effect of dietary nitrate on performance, on top of the normal diet. As has also been done previously [21], on test days, all subjects were provided with a standardized dinner that was consumed ~3.5 h prior to the exercise test. After consumption of this meal and the final supplemental bolus, subjects were only allowed to consume an *ad libitum* amount of water in the hours that followed. The amount of water consumed before and during the first trial was replicated during the second trial.

2.4. Experimental Protocol

On the last day of each supplementation period, subjects reported to the research facility ~2 h after ingesting the last 140 mL bolus of beetroot juice. The trials started with collection of a single antecubital venous blood sample and collection of a saliva sample for determination of pre-exercise nitrate and nitrite concentrations (2.5 h after ingesting the last supplemental bolus). Subjects then filled out a gastrointestinal (GI) tolerance questionnaire to assess GI complaints as a result of supplement ingestion. A heart rate monitor (Zephyr Technology Corporation, Annapolis, MD, USA) was then fitted before subjects performed a standardized 10-min warm-up, after which the Yo-Yo IR1 was performed.

Heart rate was monitored continuously (1 Hz) to calculate mean heart rate throughout the test, as well as peak heart rate reached near the end of the Yo-Yo IR1 (30-s peak heart rate).

The warm-up and the Yo-Yo IR1 were performed indoors in a sports hall, on a 2 by 20 m running lane that was marked by cones, as described previously by Krustrup et al. [15]. The test consisted of repeated 2 × 20 m sprints between a starting, turning, and finishing line at a progressively increasing speed controlled by audio bleeps from an audio system. Between each 2 × 20 min run, subjects had a 10-s active recovery period in an area of 5 × 2 m that was marked by cones behind the start/finishing line. When a subject failed to cross the finish line before the final bleep, a warning was given. When a subject failed to cross the finish line before the bleep for a second time, the final distance covered was registered and represented the end result [15]. Immediately after completing the Yo-Yo IR1, subjects rated their perceived exertion on a Borg 6–20 scale [22].

2.5. Plasma and Saliva Analysis

Blood samples were collected in Lithium-Heparin containing tubes and immediately centrifuged at $1000\times g$ for 5 min, at 4 °C. Aliquots of plasma were frozen in dry-ice after centrifugation, and were stored at −80 °C for subsequent analysis of plasma nitrate and nitrite concentrations. Saliva samples were collected in 2 mL Eppendorf cups and stored at −80 °C until nitrate and nitrite concentrations were determined in both saliva and plasma using chemiluminescence, as described previously [18].

2.6. Statistical Analysis

A sample size of 40 subjects, including a 20% dropout, was calculated with a power of 80% and an alpha of 0.05 (two-sided) to detect a 4.2% difference in the distance covered during the Yo-Yo IR1 between BR and PLA. Performance data from the Yo-Yo IR1, heart rate, and plasma and saliva data were analyzed with a paired samples t-test (BR vs. PLA). Effect size of Yo-Yo IR1 performance was determined using Cohen's d_z statistical calculation for paired samples. Heart rate data of 7 subjects was incomplete (due to technical problems and/or shifting of the chest bands) and was therefore not included in the analysis. Pearson correlation coefficients were calculated to assess whether differences in plasma or saliva nitrate and nitrite concentrations between trials were associated with the difference in Yo-Yo IR1 performance or heart rate variables between BR and PLA. Statistical significance was set at $p < 0.05$, and all data were analyzed using SPSS 21.0 (version 21.0, IBM Corp., Armonk, NY, USA), and are presented as means ± SEM.

3. Results

3.1. Plasma and Saliva Nitrate and Nitrite Concentrations

Ingestion of BR for six subsequent days resulted in elevated nitrate concentrations when compared to PLA, in both plasma (Figure 1A) and saliva (Figure 1C) (both $p < 0.001$). Similarly, nitrite concentrations were higher following BR vs. PLA supplementation in both plasma (632 ± 66 nM vs. 186 ± 13 nM; $p < 0.001$; Figure 1B) and saliva (2882 ± 519 μM vs. 375 ± 54 μM; $p < 0.001$; Figure 1D).

3.2. Yo-Yo IR1 Test

High-intensity intermittent running performance as assessed by the Yo-Yo IR1 significantly improved following BR ingestion (1623 ± 48 m) when compared to PLA (1574 ± 47 m; $p = 0.027$; Figure 2A). The average improvement in distance covered during the test was 3.4 ± 1.3%, with a Cohen's d_z of 0.41. Of the 32 subjects assessed, 18 showed an improved performance during the BR trial vs. the PLA trial (+9 ± 5%), 10 had a slightly worse performance (−5 ± 3%) and 4 showed no difference between trials. Although peak heart rate did not differ between trials ($p = 0.16$; Table 1), average heart rate during the Yo-Yo IR 1 test was lower in the BR trial when compared to PLA ($p = 0.014$; Table 1).

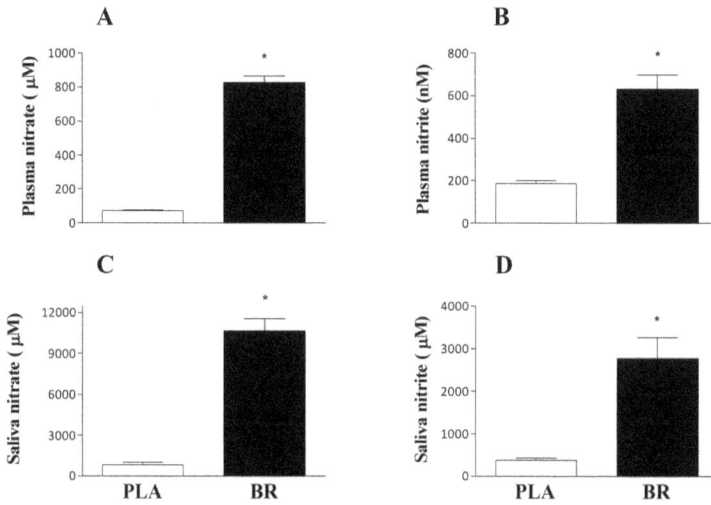

Figure 1. Mean plasma nitrate (**A**) and nitrite (**B**), and saliva nitrate (**C**) and nitrite (**D**) concentrations ~2.5 h after ingestion of the final supplemental bolus for the placebo (PLA) and the six-day nitrate-rich beetroot juice (BR) intervention. Data are means ± SEM ($n = 32$). * BR significantly different from PLA ($p < 0.001$).

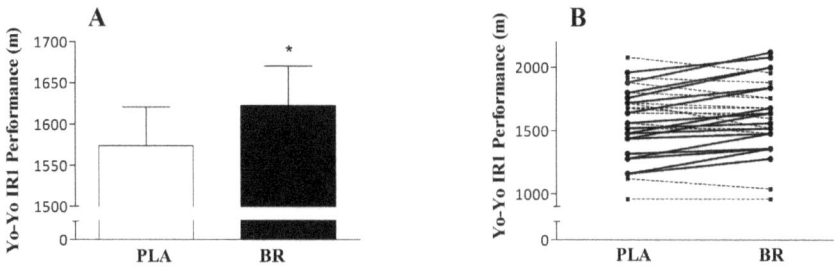

Figure 2. Mean distance covered during the Yo-Yo IR 1 test (**A**), and the individual response (**B**) following 6 days of placebo (PLA) and 6 days of nitrate-rich beetroot juice (BR) ingestion. * Distance covered following BR was significantly greater (3.4%) than that covered following PLA ingestion ($p = 0.027$). Solid lines (-) indicate subjects that showed an improved performance following BR ingestion ($n = 18$). Dashed lines (--) indicate subjects that showed a similar performance ($n = 4$) following BR or PLA ingestion, or subjects that showed a worse ($n = 10$) performance following BR ingestion.

3.3. GI and Borg Score

Subjects tolerated the interventional drinks well and GI discomfort did not differ between interventions. Only two participants reported a bloated stomach during the PLA trial, and one during the BR trial, while flatulence was reported by two participants during the PLA and two participants during the BR trial. Ratings of perceived exertion as determined with the Borg scale were also not different between interventions ($p = 0.23$; Table 1).

Table 1. Heart rate data and Rate of perceived exertion.

Variable	PLA	BR
Mean heart rate (bpm)	175 ± 2	172 ± 2 *
30-sec max heart rate (bpm)	191 ± 1	190 ± 1
RPE (Borg score)	17.6 ± 0.3	17.3 ± 0.4

All values are means ± SEM (n = 25 for HR and n = 32 for RPE). * Significantly different from PLA ($p < 0.05$).

3.4. Correlation Analyses

Despite the substantial elevations in plasma and saliva concentrations following BR ingestion, no significant correlations were found between plasma and saliva nitrate (r = 0.076, p = 0.697) or plasma and saliva nitrite (r = 0.264, p = 0.144) concentrations. In addition, no associations were observed between (differences in) plasma or saliva concentrations on the one hand, and the (differences in) distance covered, or heart rate variables on the other hand (all $r \leq 0.296$; all $p \geq 0.092$).

4. Discussion

The current study demonstrates that six days of nitrate-rich beetroot juice supplementation improves high-intensity intermittent type exercise performance in trained soccer players. The improvements in intermittent type exercise performance were accompanied by a lower mean heart rate during the high-intensity intermittent running test, and were preceded by increases in both plasma and saliva nitrate and nitrite concentrations.

Nitrate related research in the past years has primarily focused on establishing the effects of nitrate supplementation on endurance type exercise performance. While improvements in exercise capacity [4,8,23] and exercise performance [5,6] have indeed been observed in endurance athletes, recent literature suggests possible performance benefits of nitrate ingestion in more high-intensity and intermittent type sports and activities [16,24]. Extending on previous observations in recreationally active team-sport players [17], the present study specifically assessed the effects of a multiday supplementation protocol with nitrate-rich beetroot juice on high-intensity intermittent type exercise performance in a large sample of trained soccer players.

We found that six days of BR supplementation elevated nitrate and nitrite concentrations in both plasma and saliva (Figure 1). The observed 11-fold increase in plasma nitrate and 3-fold increase in plasma nitrite concentrations are in line with previous observations where a similar nitrate dose was administered [18,24]. In addition to the changes in plasma concentrations, the current findings suggest that saliva samples might represent a (less invasive) alternative to assess the postprandial response to beetroot juice ingestion. Salivary nitrate and nitrite concentrations were respectively 13-fold and 7-fold higher following BR ingestion when compared to PLA (Figure 1C,D). However, no correlations were observed between plasma concentrations and saliva concentrations. As such, it seems that saliva samples may be used as a means to assess compliance to nitrate supplementation and to confirm the endogenous reduction of nitrate into nitrite. Nevertheless, analysis of salivary nitrate and nitrite does not seem to represent a valid surrogate for quantitative changes in plasma nitrate or nitrite concentrations.

In addition to changes in nitrate and nitrite concentrations, the six-day BR supplementation protocol also resulted in quantifiable improvements in high-intensity intermittent running performance in the soccer players. We observed a 3.4% increase in intermittent type exercise performance on the Yo-Yo IR1 test (Cohen's d_z: 0.41; Figure 2A). This is in line with a previous report of improvements in high speed running performance in recreationally active team sport players following a multiday BR supplementation regimen [17]. Although the exact mode of action explaining this effect is still unclear, animal studies have shown that nitrate supplementation can increase blood flow [10], and enhance contractile function in type II muscle fibers [11]. There is some suggestion that these adaptations might be responsible for the improved performance observed during high intensity/intermittent type exercise in which type II fibers are heavily recruited [25]. Interestingly, while such cellular changes have been proposed to only occur following a multiday supplementation regimen [10,11,26], two studies from the same laboratory observed improvements in high-intensity intermittent type exercise performance following both an acute high dose BR supplementation protocol (~29 mmol within 36 h; 4.2% improvement) [16], as well as following a five-day BR supplementation approach with a lower daily dose of nitrate (6.4 mmol/day; 3.9% improvement) [17]. The use of a multiday protocol would seem preferred as it likely allows sufficient time for (some of) the suggested cellular adaptations to occur, that might drive the ergogenic effects of nitrate [10,11]. Furthermore, it is believed that trained subjects may require a different nitrate supplementation strategy (i.e., higher dose and/or for a longer period) to elicit beneficial performance effects in comparison to recreational athletes [9,27,28]. The current study therefore assessed the ergogenic effect of a conventional six-day supplementation protocol with BR (12.9 mmol/day nitrate) in a homogenous sample of trained soccer players. Performance on the Yo-Yo IR1 test was on average ~15% higher when compared to the recreational subjects included in the recent study from Thompson et al. [17]. Nonetheless, we observed a 3.4% improvement in high-intensity intermittent running performance, suggesting that a six-day BR supplementation protocol represents a practical and effective regimen for trained soccer players to improve their performance. Clearly, such a performance benefit should be attained without any major negative side effects. In line with previous work [18], only very mild GI discomfort was reported in a few subjects during the current study, supporting the non-adverse use of beetroot juice in relative short-term interventions. Furthermore, as recently reviewed by Bryan and Ivy [29], there is currently no clear indication of adverse health risks accompanying high nitrate intakes for a prolonged period of time. At present, though any potential risks always need to be carefully considered, the established benefits of nitrate, which may be even more pronounced when consuming nitrate through 'natural' nitrate-rich vegetable sources [18,19], seem to outweigh the potential risks [29].

Intriguingly, and in contrast to previous studies in team sport players, we observed that ingestion of BR for six consecutive days also had an effect on heart rate during the high-intensity intermittent running test (Table 1). While no changes were observed in peak heart rate, mean heart rate during the Yo-Yo IR1 was lower following BR ingestion than following PLA ingestion. To the best of our knowledge, the current findings are the first evidence of changes in heart rate following nitrate ingestion in young healthy athletes. Whether the decrease in mean heart rate is related to the improved exercise performance is unclear, as the only available literature describing effects of inorganic nitrate-nitrite on heart rate are from heart failure patients [30,31]. Borlaug and colleagues showed that a nitrite infusion protocol in heart failure patients increased cardiac output during exercise [30]. The observed increase in stroke volume was suggested to be explained by improved contractility of the left ventricle. While it is currently unclear whether nitrate and/or nitrite ingestion can similarly increase cardiac contractility in healthy individuals, such an effect could explain the decrease in heart rate observed in our study; i.e., allowing the same cardiac output with increased stroke volume, but lower heart rate. Interestingly, a recent study in rodents also showed increased cardiac contractility following nitrate ingestion, most likely as a result of enhanced expression of calcium handling proteins [32]. As nitrate ingestion has also been shown to enhance expression of calcium handling proteins in type II skeletal muscle fibers [11], such an explanation would fit with both the observed increase in intermittent type exercise performance, and the lower mean heart rate in the current study.

Although nitrate supplementation increased plasma and saliva nitrate and nitrite concentrations, improved exercise performance, and reduced heart rate, no correlations were observed between any of these parameters. Only a limited number of studies have been able to show correlations between plasma concentrations and subsequent performance benefits [2,17,24,27]. In the present study, only a single sample of saliva and plasma was collected ~30 min prior to the exercise test. It could be suggested that a time point closer to, or even during the exercise test may have revealed a relation between plasma concentrations and changes in performance. Despite the fact that all subjects showed substantially increased plasma and saliva nitrate and nitrite concentrations, not all subjects showed improvements in performance (Figure 2B). It is unclear what the exact explanation is for this lack of effect, although it seems likely that the large day-to-day variability inherent to the Yo-Yo test played a role [33] (Figure 2B). Taking this variability into account, the inclusion of a large sample of trained soccer players allowed us to show a significant and relevant improvement in Yo-Yo IR1 test performance following BR ingestion. Importantly, Yo-Yo IR1 performance has been described to strongly correlate with the ability to perform high speed running and sprinting activities throughout a soccer match [15]. As such, our findings suggest that nitrate supplementation could represent an effective nutritional strategy to improve exercise performance in soccer players, especially towards the end of the match when sprint intensity/frequency has been shown to decrease significantly due to fatigue [34]. Even though in general, day-to-day variation in exercise performance tests combined with small sample sizes make it difficult to study potential ergogenic benefits in highly-trained athletes, future work should be undertaken to establish whether these performance improvements in high-intensity intermittent-type exercise in trained soccer players can also be translated toward the elite level.

5. Conclusions

Based on the present findings in a large sample of trained soccer players, we conclude that six days of nitrate-rich beetroot juice ingestion improves high-intensity intermittent type exercise performance.

Acknowledgments: This study was financially supported by a grant from the Dutch Technology Foundation STW.

Author Contributions: The study was designed by Jean Nyakayiru, Kristin L. Jonvik, Luc J. C. van Loon and Lex B. Verdijk; data were collected and analyzed by Jean Nyakayiru, Jorn Trommelen, Philippe J. M. Pinckaers, and Joan M. Senden; data interpretation and manuscript preparation were undertaken by Jean Nyakayiru, Luc J. C. van Loon, and Lex B. Verdijk. All authors approved the final version of the paper.

Conflicts of Interest: The authors declare no conflict of interest.

References

1. Lundberg, J.O.; Weitzberg, E.; Lundberg, J.M.; Alving, K. Intragastric nitric oxide production in humans: Measurements in expelled air. *Gut* **1994**, *35*, 1543–1546. [CrossRef] [PubMed]
2. Wylie, L.J.; Kelly, J.; Bailey, S.J.; Blackwell, J.R.; Skiba, P.F.; Winyard, P.G.; Jeukendrup, A.E.; Vanhatalo, A.; Jones, A.M. Beetroot juice and exercise: Pharmacodynamic and dose-response relationships. *J. Appl. Physiol.* **2013**, *115*, 325–336. [CrossRef] [PubMed]
3. Hoon, M.W.; Jones, A.M.; Johnson, N.A.; Blackwell, J.R.; Broad, E.M.; Lundy, B.; Rice, A.J.; Burke, L.M. The Effect of Variable Doses of Inorganic Nitrate-Rich Beetroot Juice on Simulated 2000 m Rowing Performance in Trained Athletes. *Int. J. Sports Physiol. Perform.* **2013**, *9*, 615–620. [CrossRef] [PubMed]
4. Bailey, S.J.; Winyard, P.; Vanhatalo, A.; Blackwell, J.R.; Dimenna, F.J.; Wilkerson, D.P.; Tarr, J.; Benjamin, N.; Jones, A.M. Dietary nitrate supplementation reduces the O2 cost of low-intensity exercise and enhances tolerance to high-intensity exercise in humans. *J. Appl. Physiol.* **2009**, *107*, 1144–1155. [CrossRef] [PubMed]
5. Cermak, N.; Gibala, M.; van Loon, L. Nitrate supplementation improves 10 km time trial performance in trained cyclists. *Int. J. Sport Nutr. Exerc. Metab.* **2011**, *22*, 64–71. [CrossRef]
6. Lansley, K.E.; Winyard, P.; Bailey, S.; Vanhatalo, A.; Wilkerson, D.; Blackwell, J.; Gilchrist, M.; Benjamin, N.; Jones, A. Acute dietary nitrate supplementation improves cycling time trial performance. *Med. Sci. Sports Exerc.* **2011**, *43*, 1125–1131. [CrossRef] [PubMed]
7. Larsen, F.J.; Weitzberg, E.; Lundberg, J.O.; Ekblom, B. Effects of dietary nitrate on oxygen cost during exercise. *Acta Physiol. (Oxf.)* **2007**, *191*, 59–66. [CrossRef] [PubMed]
8. Bailey, S.J.; Varnham, R.L.; DiMenna, F.J.; Breese, B.C.; Wylie, L.J.; Jones, A.M. Inorganic nitrate supplementation improves muscle oxygenation, O(2) uptake kinetics, and exercise tolerance at high but not low pedal rates. *J. Appl. Physiol.* **2015**, *118*, 1396–1405. [CrossRef] [PubMed]
9. Porcelli, S.; Ramaglia, M.; Bellistri, G.; Pavei, G.; Pugliese, L.; Montorsi, M.; Rasica, L.; Marzorati, M. Aerobic Fitness Affects the Exercise Performance Responses to Nitrate Supplementation. *Med. Sci. Sports Exerc.* **2015**, *47*, 1643–1651. [CrossRef] [PubMed]

10. Ferguson, S.K.; Hirai, D.M.; Copp, S.W.; Holdsworth, C.T.; Allen, J.D.; Jones, A.M.; Musch, T.I.; Poole, D.C. Impact of dietary nitrate supplementation via beetroot juice on exercising muscle vascular control in rats. *J. Physiol.* **2013**, *591 Pt 2*, 547–557. [CrossRef] [PubMed]

11. Hernandez, A.; Schiffer, T.A.; Ivarsson, N.; Cheng, A.J.; Bruton, J.D.; Lundberg, J.O.; Weitzberg, E.; Westerblad, H. Dietary nitrate increases tetanic [Ca2+]i and contractile force in mouse fast-twitch muscle. *J. Appl. Physiol.* **2012**, *590 Pt 15*, 3575–3583. [CrossRef] [PubMed]

12. Krustrup, P.; Mohr, M.; Steensberg, A.; Bencke, J.; Kjaer, M.; Bangsbo, J. Muscle and blood metabolites during a soccer game: Implications for sprint performance. *Med. Sci. Sports Exerc.* **2006**, *38*, 1165–1174. [CrossRef] [PubMed]

13. Bangsbo, J.; Mohr, M.; Krustrup, P. Physical and metabolic demands of training and match-play in the elite football player. *J. Sports Sci.* **2006**, *24*, 665–674. [CrossRef] [PubMed]

14. Bradley, P.S.; Di Mascio, M.; Peart, D.; Olsen, P.; Sheldon, B. High-intensity activity profiles of elite soccer players at different performance levels. *J. Strength Cond. Res.* **2010**, *24*, 2343–2351. [CrossRef] [PubMed]

15. Krustrup, P.; Mohr, M.; Amstrup, T.; Rysgaard, T.; Johansen, J.; Steensberg, A.; Pedersen, P.K.; Bangsbo, J. The yo-yo intermittent recovery test: physiological response, reliability, and validity. *Med. Sci. Sports Exerc.* **2003**, *35*, 697–705. [CrossRef] [PubMed]

16. Wylie, L.J.; Mohr, M.; Krustrup, P.; Jackman, S.R.; Ermiotadis, G.; Kelly, J.; Black, M.I.; Bailey, S.J.; Vanhatalo, A.; Jones, A.M. Dietary nitrate supplementation improves team sport-specific intense intermittent exercise performance. *Eur. J. Appl. Physiol.* **2013**, *113*, 1673–1684. [CrossRef] [PubMed]

17. Thompson, C.; Vanhatalo, A.; Jell, H.; Fulford, J.; Carter, J.; Nyman, L.; Bailey, S.J.; Jones, A.M. Dietary nitrate supplementation improves sprint and high-intensity intermittent running performance. *Nitric Oxide* **2016**, *61*, 55–61. [CrossRef] [PubMed]

18. Jonvik, K.L.; Nyakayiru, J.; Pinckaers, P.J.; Senden, J.M.; van Loon, L.J.; Verdijk, L.B. Nitrate-Rich Vegetables Increase Plasma Nitrate and Nitrite Concentrations and Lower Blood Pressure in Healthy Adults. *J. Nutr.* **2016**, *146*, 986–993. [CrossRef] [PubMed]

19. Flueck, J.L.; Bogdanova, A.; Mettler, S.; Perret, C. Is beetroot juice more effective than sodium nitrate? The effects of equimolar nitrate dosages of nitrate-rich beetroot juice and sodium nitrate on oxygen consumption during exercise. *Appl. Physiol. Nutr. Metab.* **2016**, *41*, 421–429. [CrossRef] [PubMed]

20. Govoni, M.; Jansson, E.; Weitzberg, E.; Lundberg, J. The increase in plasma nitrite after a dietary nitrate load is markedly attenuated by an antibacterial mouthwash. *Nitric Oxide* **2008**, *19*, 333–337. [CrossRef] [PubMed]

21. Nyakayiru, J.; Jonvik, K.L.; Pinckaers, P.J.; Senden, J.; Van Loon, L.J.; Verdijk, L.B. No Effect of Acute and 6-Day Nitrate Supplementation on VO2 and Time-Trial Performance in Highly-Trained Cyclists. *Int. J. Sport Nutr. Exerc. Metab.* **2016**, *27*, 11–17. [CrossRef] [PubMed]

22. Borg, G.A. Psychophysical bases of perceived exertion. *Med. Sci. Sports Exerc.* **1982**, *14*, 377–381. [CrossRef] [PubMed]

23. Breese, B.C.; McNarry, M.A.; Marwood, S.; Blackwell, J.R.; Bailey, S.J.; Jones, A.M. Beetroot juice supplementation speeds O2 uptake kinetics and improves exercise tolerance during severe-intensity exercise initiated from an elevated baseline. *Am. J. Physiol. Regul. Integr. Comp. Physiol.* **2013**, *305*, R1441–R1450. [CrossRef] [PubMed]

24. Thompson, C.; Wylie, L.J.; Fulford, J.; Kelly, J.; Black, M.I.; McDonagh, S.T.; Jeukendrup, A.E.; Vanhatalo, A.; Jones, A.M. Dietary nitrate improves sprint performance and cognitive function during prolonged intermittent exercise. *Eur. J. Appl. Physiol.* **2015**, *115*, 1825–1834. [CrossRef] [PubMed]

25. Jones, A.M.; Ferguson, S.K.; Bailey, S.J.; Vanhatalo, A.; Poole, D.C. Fiber Type-Specific Effects of Dietary Nitrate. *Exerc. Sport Sci. Rev.* **2016**, *44*, 53–60. [CrossRef] [PubMed]

26. Larsen, F.J.; Schiffer, T.A.; Borniquel, S.; Sahlin, K.; Ekblom, B.; Lundberg, J.O.; Weitzberg, E. Dietary inorganic nitrate improves mitochondrial efficiency in humans. *Cell Metab.* **2011**, *13*, 149–159. [CrossRef] [PubMed]

27. Wilkerson, D.P.; Hayward, G.M.; Bailey, S.J.; Vanhatalo, A.; Blackwell, J.R.; Jones, A.M. Influence of acute dietary nitrate supplementation on 50 mile time trial performance in well-trained cyclists. *Eur. J. Appl. Physiol.* **2012**, *112*, 4127–4134. [CrossRef] [PubMed]

28. Cermak, N.M.; Res, P.; Stinkens, R.; Lundberg, J.O.; Gibala, M.J.; van Loon, L.J. No improvement in endurance performance after a single dose of beetroot juice. *Int. J. Sport Nutr. Exerc. Metab.* **2012**, *22*, 470–478. [CrossRef] [PubMed]

29. Bryan, N.S.; Ivy, J.L. Inorganic nitrite and nitrate: Evidence to support consideration as dietary nutrients. *Nutr. Res.* **2015**, *35*, 643–654. [CrossRef] [PubMed]

30. Borlaug, B.A.; Koepp, K.E.; Melenovsky, V. Sodium Nitrite Improves Exercise Hemodynamics and Ventricular Performance in Heart Failure With Preserved Ejection Fraction. *J. Am. Coll. Cardiol.* **2015**, *66*, 1672–1682. [CrossRef] [PubMed]

31. Zamani, P.; Rawat, D.; Shiva-Kumar, P.; Geraci, S.; Bhuva, R.; Konda, P.; Doulias, P.T.; Ischiropoulos, H.; Townsend, R.R.; Margulies, K.B.; et al. Effect of inorganic nitrate on exercise capacity in heart failure with preserved ejection fraction. *Circulation* **2015**, *131*, 371–380; discussion 380. [CrossRef] [PubMed]

32. Pironti, G.; Ivarsson, N.; Yang, J.; Farinotti, A.B.; Jonsson, W.; Zhang, S.J.; Bas, D.; Svensson, C.I.; Westerblad, H.; Weitzberg, E.; et al. Dietary nitrate improves cardiac contractility via enhanced cellular Ca(2+) signaling. *Basic Res. Cardiol.* **2016**, *111*, 34. [CrossRef] [PubMed]

33. Bangsbo, J.; Iaia, F.M.; Krustrup, P. The Yo-Yo intermittent recovery test: A useful tool for evaluation of physical performance in intermittent sports. *Sports Med.* **2008**, *38*, 37–51. [CrossRef] [PubMed]

34. Bradley, P.S.; Sheldon, W.; Wooster, B.; Olsen, P.; Boanas, P.; Krustrup, P. High-intensity running in English FA Premier League soccer matches. *J. Sports Sci.* **2009**, *27*, 159–168. [CrossRef] [PubMed]

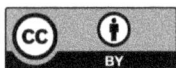

nutrients

Article

Effects of Six-Week *Ginkgo biloba* Supplementation on Aerobic Performance, Blood Pro/Antioxidant Balance, and Serum Brain-Derived Neurotrophic Factor in Physically Active Men

Ewa Sadowska-Krępa [1,*], Barbara Kłapcińska [1], Ilona Pokora [1], Przemysław Domaszewski [2], Katarzyna Kempa [1] and Tomasz Podgórski [3]

[1] Department of Physiological and Medical Sciences, The Jerzy Kukuczka Academy of Physical Education, 40-065 Katowice, Poland; b.klapcinska@awf.katowice.pl (B.K.); i.pokora@awf.katowice.pl (I.P.); k.kempa@awf.katowice.pl (K.K.)

[2] Department of Tourism and Health Promotion, University of Technology, Faculty of Physical Education and Physiotherapy, 45-758 Opole, Poland; domaszewskiprzemek@wp.pl

[3] Department of Biochemistry, Poznan University of Physical Education, 61-871 Poznań, Poland; podgorski@awf.poznan.pl

* Correspondence: e.sadowska-krepa@awf.katowice.pl; Tel.: +48-32-207-54-71

Received: 11 May 2017; Accepted: 24 July 2017; Published: 26 July 2017

Abstract: Extracts of *Ginkgo biloba* leaves, a natural source of flavonoids and polyphenolic compounds, are commonly used as therapeutic agents for the improvement of both cognitive and physiological performance. The present study was aimed to test the effects of a six-week supplementation with 160 mg/day of a standardized extract of *Ginkgo biloba* or a matching placebo on aerobic performance, blood antioxidant capacity, and brain-derived neurotrophic factor (BDNF) level in healthy, physically active young men, randomly allocated to two groups ($n = 9$ each). At baseline, as well as on the day following the treatment, the participants performed an incremental cycling test for the assessment of maximal oxygen uptake. Venous blood samples taken at rest, then immediately post-test and following 1 h of recovery, were analyzed for activities of antioxidant enzymes and plasma concentrations of non-enzymatic antioxidants, total phenolics, uric acid, lipid peroxidation products, ferric reducing ability of plasma (FRAP), and serum brain-derived neurotrophic factor (BDNF). Our results show that six weeks' supplementation with *Ginkgo biloba* extract in physically active young men may provide some marginal improvements in their endurance performance expressed as VO$_2$max and blood antioxidant capacity, as evidenced by specific biomarkers, and elicit somewhat better neuroprotection through increased exercise-induced production of BDNF.

Keywords: dietary supplements; *Ginkgo biloba* extract; antioxidant capacity; BDNF

1. Introduction

Several epidemiological studies have evidenced that high dietary intake of natural polyphenolic compounds synthesized by plants is associated with lower incidence of several chronic diseases associated with increased oxidative stress in humans [1,2]. It should be stressed that dietary flavonoids and other polyphenolic compounds can stimulate the expression of antioxidant enzyme genes and may limit, or even prevent, exercise-induced tissue damage. The most promising health benefits associated with the intake of foods rich in natural polyphenols include a reduced risk of coronary heart disease, and prevention of cancer and some neurodegenerative diseases [1–3]. The discrepancies in findings among several studies suggest that many polyphenols may have also pro-oxidant activities both in vitro and in vivo [4,5]. Although polyphenols are believed to be highly important for human health, they do not meet the classical criteria of essential nutrients because they are not necessary for growth and development. However, as they are essential for reaching the full lifespan, they have been termed "lifespan essential" [6]. Standardized *Ginkgo biloba* extract (EGb) includes over 60 bioactive components, the most important being flavonoids and terpene lactones [7,8]. Due to their potent antioxidant properties, flavonoids, such as quercetin and kaempferol, can directly quench free radicals; however, through induction of cytochrome P450 enzyme system activity, they can also indirectly reduce free radical formation [4,9,10]. However, flavonoid bioavailability is rather low due to their poor absorption. They are not absorbed intact by the intestinal mucosa as, prior to absorption, they undergo enzymatic conversion by the natural flora of the small intestine. The resultant aglycones are absorbed into the blood stream and, along with albumines, are transported to the liver. There, in the presence of phase I and phase II enzymes, they are metabolized to secondary metabolites transported to the tissues or eliminated in bile and urine [3,11]. Maximal concentrations of polyphenols in human plasma is usually reached about 1.5 to 5.5 h after consumption of polyphenol-rich foods [12]. Of note, maximum concentration of quercetin conjugates (the main flavonoids present in ginkgo [13]); in the plasma is reached 9 h after ingestion and its elimination is relatively slow (with a half-life of 24 h), possibly due to its high affinity for plasma albumin. Yet, the elimination half-life period for most flavonoids absorbed in the small intestine is much shorter (1–2 h) [11,14]. Terpene lactones (such as ginkgolides and bilobalide) possess very specific and potent antagonist activity against platelet aggregation factor (PAF). They facilitate blood flow through the cerebrum, dilate the capillary vessels, have protective effects on myelin sheaths, prevent thrombosis, and boost concentration and the learning process [15]. EGb supplementation has been shown to have a neuroprotective effect and capacity to improve cognitive functions by decreasing oxidative stress and increasing the concentration of brain-derived neurotrophic factor (BDNF) [16]. BDNF is a molecular mediator of synaptic plasticity, hence, the BDNF signaling pathway is reduced in many neurodegenerative and psychiatric diseases [17]. Of note, BDNF expression is augmented by physical exercise [18].

Taking into account a growing interest in the use of natural herbal supplements, the aim of this study was to examine the effect of *Ginkgo biloba* supplementation on aerobic performance, blood pro/antioxidant balance, and the level of BDNF in physically active men.

2. Materials and Methods

2.1. Participants

Eighteen healthy (as evidenced by medical certificate), non-smoking male physical education students (aged 20–24 years) volunteered to participate in this study. All individuals were informed about the purpose and nature of the experiment before giving their written consent to participate. The study protocol conformed to the ethical guidelines of the World Medical Association Declaration of Helsinki, was approved by the Institutional Ethics Committee at the Jerzy Kukuczka Academy of Physical Education in Katowice (certificate of approval No. 4/2013). The exclusion criteria were the use of tobacco products, alcohol consumption, and the use of any medicine or dietary supplements during the four weeks prior to the study.

The participants were randomly allocated to two groups: (1) the control placebo group ($n = 9$, PLA); and (2) the study group ($n = 9$, EGb) supplemented with standardized *Ginkgo biloba* extract, in the form of soft gelatinous capsules (Ginkoflav® forte, Olimp Labs, Dębica, Poland) administered at a dose of two capsules once a day after breakfast for six weeks. EGb capsules contained 80 mg of standardized *Ginkgo biloba* extract containing 19.2 mg flavonoid glycosides (24%), 4.8 mg terpene lactones (6%), and additional substances, such as maltodextrin, microcrystalline cellulose, and magnesium stearate. Placebo capsules contained microcrystalline cellulose, magnesium stearate, and maltodextrin instead of Ginkgo plant extract. There were no dropouts from the study and all participants completed the full survey.

2.2. Study Design

All subjects performed an incremental test on a cycle ergometer (Sport Excalibur, Groningen, The Netherlands) while connected to a breath-by-breath gas analyzer (MetaLyzer 3B-R2, Leipzig, Germany) to determine maximal oxygen uptake (VO_2max). After a short warm-up cycling at 20 W, the subjects cycled in stages of 3 min duration starting at a power output of 40 W, increasing progressively by 40 W, and continuing until exhaustion. The students participated in the exercise test twice, i.e., before the start (first trial) and after six weeks of supplementation with EGb or PLA (second trial). In each trial, venous blood samples from the antecubital vein were drawn into tubes without anticoagulant or into the heparinized test tubes at rest, then at 3 min post-test, and again after 1 h of recovery.

2.3. Biochemical Analyses

Samples of venous blood were collected before starting and on the day following the completion of supplementation with EGb or PLA. Fresh whole blood samples were immediately assayed for reduced glutathione (GSH) by a colorimetric method with 5,5′-dithiobis-2-nitrobenzoic acid [19], or collected in test tubes for the separation of serum or plasma. A portion of heparinized blood was centrifuged for 10 min at $1000 \times g$ at 4 °C to separate plasma and erythrocytes that were then washed three times with cold saline (4 °C) and kept frozen at -80 °C (for a period not longer than one month, without repeated freezing and thawing) until analysis for activities of red blood cell antioxidant enzymes, i.e., superoxide dismutase (SOD, EC 1.15.1.1) using the commercially available RANSOD SD125 kit (Randox Laboratories Ltd., Crumlin, UK); glutathione peroxidase (GSH-Px, EC 1.11.1.9) with the commercial RANSEL RS505 kit (Randox Laboratories Ltd., Crumlin, UK), catalase (CAT, EC 1.11.1.6) by the method of Aebi [20], and glutathione reductase (GR, EC 1.6.4.2) according to Glatzle et al. [21]. The activities of all antioxidant enzymes were measured at 37 °C and expressed per 1 g of haemoglobin as assayed by a standard cyanmethemoglobin method using a diagnostic kit No. HG980 (Randox Laboratories Ltd., Crumlin, UK). Fresh plasma samples were assayed for the concentration of uric acid (UA) using diagnostic kits from Randox Laboratories (UA230). The total antioxidant capacity of plasma was assessed using the ferric reducing ability of plasma (FRAP) assay according to Benzie and Strain [22]. Assessment of plasma lipid peroxidation was conducted using the thiobarbituric acid (TBARS) reaction according to Buege and Aust [23]. Plasma concentration of total phenolics was measured by the colorimetric method [24]. The serum level of brain-derived neurotrophic factor (BDNF) was determined by the immunoenzymatic method using a diagnostic RayBioHuman® BDNF ELISA kit No. ELH-BDNF-001 (RayBiotech, Inc., Norcross, GA, USA). Biochemical analyses were performed in our certified laboratory fulfilling the requirements of PN EN-ISO 9001:2009 (certificate No. 129/2015) according to instructions provided by the manufacturers of laboratory tests used in this study.

2.4. Statistical Analysis

Data presented as means ($\pm$SD) were calculated for all variables. A three-way repeated-measures ANOVA with two groups (PLA and EGb) $\times$ two trials (at the start—"First trial"—and the end—"Second trial"—of the experiment) $\times$ three time-points (at rest, 3 min post-test, and post-1 h recovery) as the main factors followed, when appropriate, by the Bonferroni post hoc tests, which were used to test the significance of between group differences. All statistical analyses were computed using Statistica 10.0. software (StatSoft, Tulsa, OK, USA). The level of significance was set at $p < 0.05$.

3. Results

3.1. Subjects

All participants not involved in sports activities other than those scheduled at the faculty were characterized by comparable baseline maximal oxygen uptake (VO_2max) within the range of 40 to 55 mL O_2/min/kg$_{BW}$, rated as average or above average for their age category (18–25 years), thus they may be categorized as active college-aged males. No significant intergroup differences were found in somatic parameters and peak VO_2 values. The basic characteristics of participants are presented in Table 1.

Table 1. Basic characteristics of the participants at pre- and post-treatment stages.

Group	Age (Years)	Height (cm)	Body Weight (kg)	VO$_2$max (mL/min/kg)	
				First Trial	Second Trial
PLA	22.3 ± 1.1	179.7 ± 7.8	79.7 ± 10.8	45.7 ± 5.1	46.1 ± 4.1
EGb	22.5 ± 0.9	182.1 ± 5.9	80.1 ± 6.8	46.2 ± 4.8	48.9 ± 5.8

Note: Data are means $\pm$ SD, PLA: placebo, EGb: *Ginkgo biloba* extract.

3.2. Antioxidant Capacities

The results of biochemical analyses of the studied enzymatic and non-enzymatic antioxidant defense components are presented, respectively, in Figures 1 and 2. The activities of SOD and CAT were not significantly affected by supplementation with *Ginkgo biloba* extract, although SOD activities recorded in both groups at rest and post-exercise were slightly higher compared to the corresponding baseline values. A repeated measures three-way ANOVA revealed a significant trial effect ($F = 4.49$, $p < 0.05$) on SOD. In contrast, GPx activity in both groups was lower in the second compared to the first trial, as evidenced by a significant trial effect ($F = 15.24$, $p < 0.001$), although larger declines were recorded in the EGb group, also revealed by the trial $\times$ group interaction close to significance ($F = 3.84$, $p = 0.07$). There were also significant time-effect ($F = 5.21$, $p < 0.01$) and trial $\times$ group interaction ($F = 5.09$, $p < 0.05$) on GR activity.

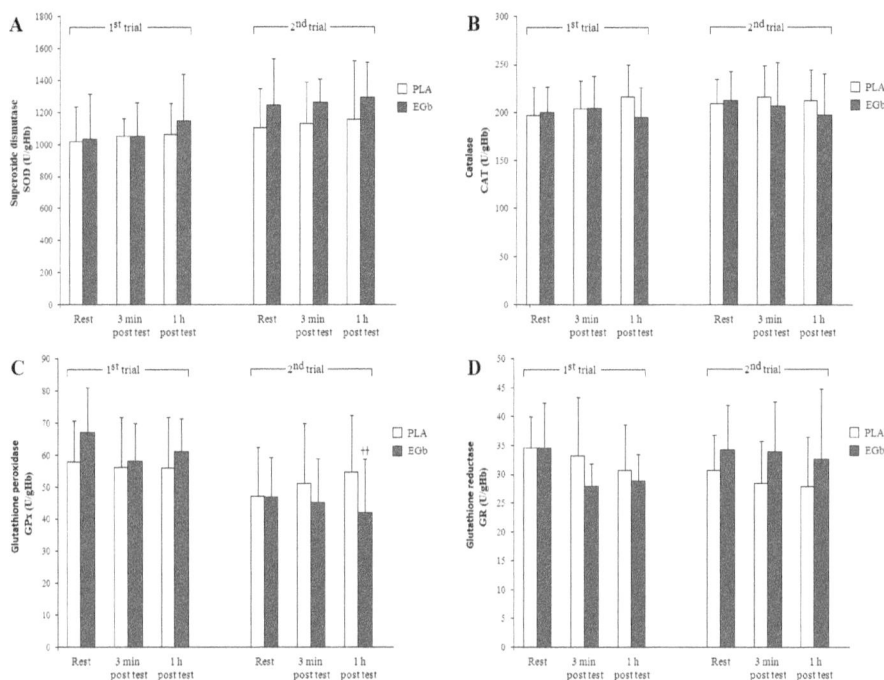

Figure 1. Changes in blood antioxidant enzymes activities in response to dietary supplementation and exercise. Note: Data are means $\pm$ SD; significant differences: †† $p < 0.01$ vs. respective values before treatment. PLA: placebo, EGb: *Ginkgo biloba* extract. SOD: superoxide dismutase (**A**); CAT: catalase (**B**); GPx: glutathione peroxidase (**C**); and GR: glutathione reductase (**D**).

Despite the lack of significant differences between the pre- and post-exercise GSH concentrations, significant trial (F = 11.38, $p < 0.001$) and trial × group interaction effects (F = 4.87, $p < 0.05$) as well as close to significance time-effect (F = 2.64, $p = 0.09$) on GSH were noted (see Figure 2). Supplementation with EGb did not affect the UA level, although in both the placebo (PLA) and EGb-supplemented groups, the exercise test induced marked increases in UA levels at 1 h of recovery compared to the respective resting values, as reflected by the highly significant time-effect (F = 36.77, $p < 0.0001$). Similarly, supplementation with *Ginkgo biloba* extract did not affect the total phenolics level, however, in both groups (PLA and EGb) their content decreased immediately after completion of the graded exercise test compared to resting values. The significant time-effect (F = 39.64, $p < 0.0001$) and close to significance trial × group interaction (F = 3.46, $p = 0.08$) were revealed by three-way ANOVA.

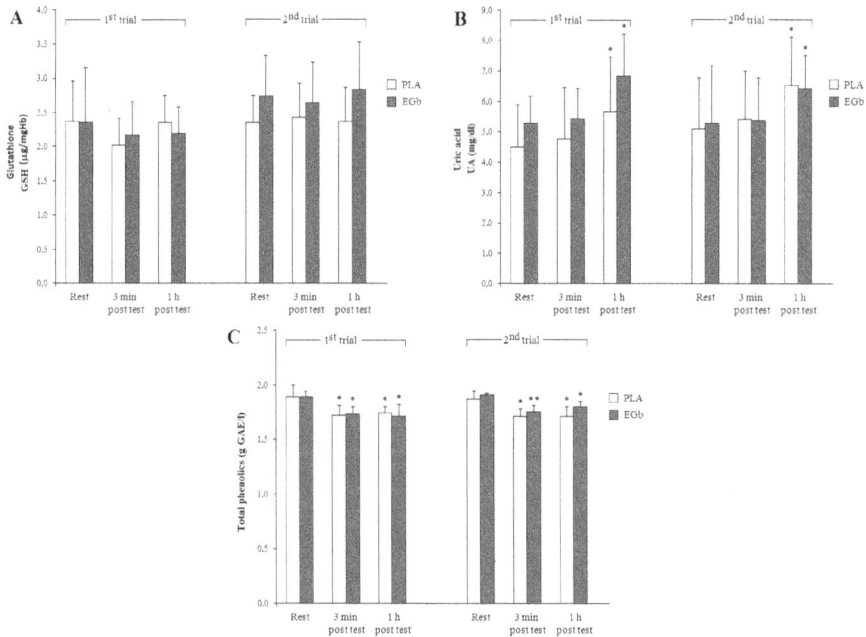

Figure 2. Changes in blood non-enzymatic antioxidants concentrations in response to dietary supplementation and exercise. Note: data are means ± SD; significant differences: * $p < 0.05$, ** $p < 0.001$ vs. resting values. PLA: placebo, EGb: *Ginkgo biloba* extract, GSH: reduced glutathione (**A**); UA: uric acid (**B**); and total phenolics (**C**).

Data regarding antioxidant status evaluated using FRAP assay and lipid peroxidation using the TBARS method, as well as serum BDNF content are presented in Figure 3.

Despite the lack of significant differences between the pre- and post-exercise FRAP levels, a three-way ANOVA revealed significant effects of group (F = 10.37, $p < 0.01$), trial (F = 13.64, $p < 0.001$), and time (F = 16.29, $p < 0.0001$). Increased levels of TBARS, compared to resting values, were recorded immediately after a graded exercise test in both groups, however, significant differences were found only in the PLA group. After a six-week long EGb supplementation, a moderate decrease in resting and post-exercise TBARS levels, compared to respective values recorded in the first trial, was observed. Significant effects of trial (F = 7.08, $p < 0.05$), time (F = 8.03, $p < 0.001$), and a very close to significance trial × time interaction (F = 3.09, $p = 0.06$) on TBARS levels were revealed by three-way ANOVA.

Before and following a six-week PLA or EGb supplementation, a moderate increase in post-exercise serum BDNF compared to resting values was observed, followed by its further decline to basal levels over the recovery. Three-way ANOVA showed significant effects of trial ($F = 5.15$, $p < 0.05$), time ($F = 27.23$, $p < 0.0001$), and trial $\times$ group interaction ($F = 4.57$, $p < 0.05$) on serum BDNF.

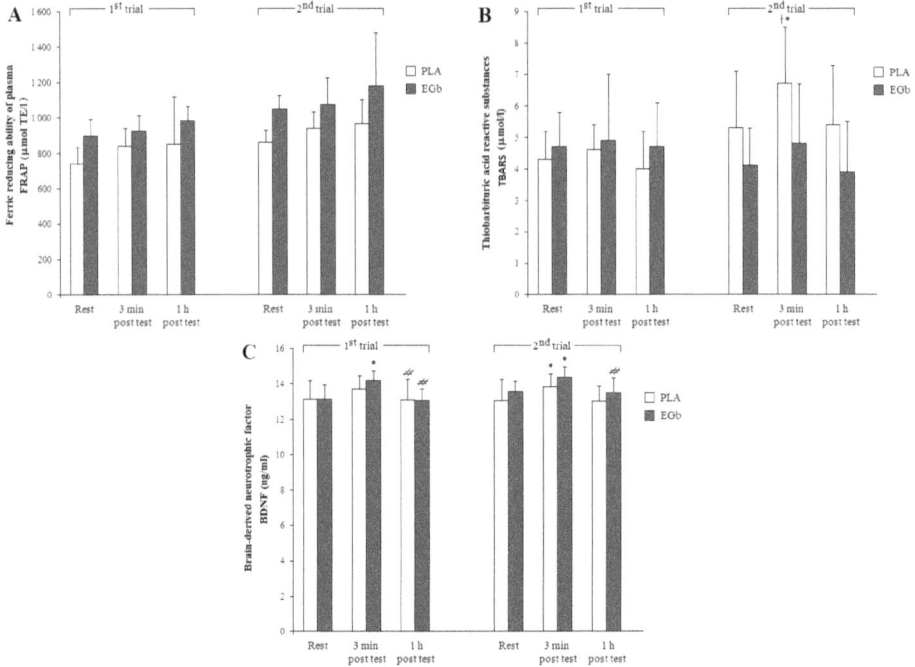

Figure 3. Plasma total blood antioxidant status (FRAP) and lipid peroxidation products (TBARS) level and serum brain-derived neurotrophic factor (BDNF) in response to dietary supplementation and graded exercise. Note: data are means $\pm$ SD; significant differences: * $p < 0.05$ vs. resting values; # $p < 0.05$ vs. values immediately post test; † $p < 0.05$ vs. respective values before treatment. PLA: placebo, EGb: *Ginkgo biloba* extract. FRAP: ferric reducing ability of plasma (**A**); TBARS: thiobarbituric acid reactive substances (**B**); BDNF: brain-derived neurotrophic factor (**C**).

4. Discussion

The main focus of this study was to test whether a six-week supplementation with *Ginkgo biloba* extract would modify aerobic performance, improve blood antioxidant capacity, and enhance BDNF expression in healthy, physically active young men. Previous human studies reported a positive correlation between the increase in endurance capacity (VO_2max) and the consumption of selected herbal supplements rich in polyphenols (i.e., quercetin or epigallocatechin-3-gallate) in healthy, untrained volunteers [25,26]. Flavonoids and terpenes contained in *Ginkgo biloba* extract can stimulate the release of endothelium-derived relaxing factor (EDRF), which may increase muscle tissue blood flow through improved microcirculation and can thus improve aerobic endurance by enhancing muscular energy production [27]. Of note, some improvement of exercise performance evaluated by pain-free walking distance was reported in *Ginkgo biloba*-treated patients with peripheral occlusive arterial disease (POAD) [28], although the efficacy of this treatment is still discussed [29]. Statistically significant, although trivial improvements in VO_2max ranging from 2.3 to 7.5% were reported after five days of supplementation with quercetin (500 to 1000 mg/d) in untrained, active, or moderately-trained individuals with VO_2max levels comparable to those reported in our study [25,30,31]. It seems that the dosage of herbal supplement may be a factor determining aerobic power. Mahady [32] showed that recommended dose of EGb standardized extract to achieve beneficial effects is located in a dose between 40 and 60 mg of EGb 3–4 times daily. In our study, subjects consumed 160 mg of EGb extract once a day for six weeks, which may explain only a marginal (6% vs. 1%) increase in the relative percentage VO$_2$max change (baseline to intervention) scores in individuals receiving, respectively, the EGb or the placebo capsules.

The multifaceted activities of *Ginkgo biloba* extract may also derive from other mechanisms of action, such as their antioxidant potential. Antioxidant effects are connected with a capacity of scavenging reactive oxygen species (ROS) and a possibility of increasing activities of antioxidant enzymes, such as superoxide dismutase (SOD), glutathione peroxidase (GPx), catalase (CAT), and heme-oxygenase-1 by upregulating the expression of antioxidant genes encoding these enzymes [16,33].

First, we decided to evaluate the activities of the main antioxidant enzymes, i.e., SOD, CAT, GPx, and GR, in the blood. Although the statistical analysis did not reveal significant changes in antioxidant enzymes between the first and the second trials, a 20% rise in resting SOD activity was observed after EGb supplementation (reflected by significant trial effect), compared with an 8% increase found in the placebo group. Superoxide dismutase is the most important antioxidant enzyme, as it catalyzes the dismutation reaction resulting in the elimination of superoxide anion radicals, thus preventing the formation of other reactive oxygen species [34]. The product of SOD-catalyzed reaction, hydrogen peroxide, is enzymatically decomposed to water and oxygen by catalase (CAT) and glutathione peroxidase (GPx), the latter with higher affinity to H$_2$O$_2$ than CAT [35]. Since the actions of enzymatic antioxidant defense systems are coordinated, compensatory changes in enzymatic activity might be expected, i.e., a change in the activity of one enzyme may affect the activity of another one. This might particularly concern the competition between GPx and CAT. Our study showed a marginal increase in resting CAT activity and a decrease in GPx in both EGb-supplemented and PLA control groups.

Several non-enzymatic antioxidants were also assessed, including reduced glutathione (GSH), uric acid (UA), and total phenolics. Supplementation with *Ginkgo biloba* extract did not significantly affect concentrations of total phenolics and UA. Only in the case of GSH, which presented slightly higher levels in the second trial (reflected by significant trial effect) in the EGb group, support the previous finding of Moskaug et al. [36], that dietary polyphenols can modulate the expression of the γ-glutamylcysteine synthetase-enzyme involved in GSH synthesis. Of note, significantly higher UA, but lower total phenolics levels, were observed in both groups (EGb and PLA) during the recovery post-graded exercise test. With respect to uric acid, a final product of the degradation of purine nucleosides under conditions of energy stress, when the rate of ATP utilization in skeletal muscle exceeds that of its resynthesis [37], and one of the main antioxidants in human plasma [38], its high levels are characteristic for body fluids, tissues, and cells under severe oxidative stress. As found in our study, neither a six-week EGb supplementation nor a graded exercise test affected the plasma uric acid level recorded immediately post-completion of this test, but in both experimental groups, its significant increase was observed during the recovery period; the main time-effect appeared highly significant. These results are consistent with those reported by Dudzińska et al. [39] and Hellsten-Westing et al. [40], who found that plasma uric acid reached its peak value within an hour after completing a maximal effort, i.e., under the ischemia/reperfusion condition.

It is worth mentioning that the health effects of polyphenols derived from the dietary sources depend on their bioavailability. Importantly, blood samples for biochemical analyses in our study were taken one day after ingesting the last EGb or PLA capsule, which may explain the lack of marked between-group differences in plasma total phenolics levels under resting conditions. We may also refer to the recent report on the dietary intakes estimated for the representative population of Polish adults, in which the calculated daily total polyphenol intake was 989 mg, with phenolic acids and flavonoids as the main contributors [41]. This may explain that the dose contained in *Ginkgo biloba* capsule had little impact on plasma level of total phenolics assessed one day after ingestion of the last EGb capsule. In the present study, independent of the subjects' group and trial, plasma total phenolics were significantly decreased 3 min after completion of the graded exercise test, as reflected by a highly significant time-effect. These results may imply that the plasma polyphenols have been used for scavenging free radicals produced during the exercise test.

It should be stressed, however, that although the antioxidant activity of dietary polyphenols has been well documented in vitro, there is much more doubt about their antioxidant action in vivo. Therefore, considering that polyphenols derived from the diet are present in the circulation and tissues only in low micromolar ranges, it is far more likely that they may activate signaling pathways for the production of cytoprotective enzymes or metabolites [1,10,36,42]. Of note, a major mechanism of action for certain nutritional antioxidant phytochemicals found naturally in plants is the paradoxical oxidative activation of the NF-E2-related factor 2 (Nrf2) signaling pathway, which maintains protective antioxidant enzymes against oxidative damage and nucleophilic components of the antioxidant defense (such as GSH) in a reduced state [5,43]. This presumption is supported by our finding of some increases in SOD activity and GSH content (revealed by significant trial effects: F = 4.49, $p < 0.05$ and F = 11.38, $p < 0.001$, respectively) in EGb-supplemented individuals.

The adverse effects of exercise-induced oxidative stress were evaluated based on lipid peroxidation assessed by TBARS assay. As predicted, the post-exercise rise in lipid peroxidation levels, expressed as TBARS, was recorded in both groups, but apparently lower increases were found in the EGb-supplemented individuals. Our results appear to be similar to those reported by Jówko et al. [44] and Kuo et al. [9], who also found a decrease in post-exercise lipid peroxidation, expressed as malondialdehyde (MDA), following supplementation with natural polyphenol-rich extracts. It is noteworthy that dietary polyphenols may be incorporated into cell membranes, which results in a change in cell structure stability and better protection of cell membranes against lipid peroxidation [4]. The beneficial effect of EGb supplementation on antioxidant capacity was also supported by significant negative correlation between SOD and TBARS (R = −0.57, $p < 0.01$) in EGb-supplemented individuals. When interpreting these data, one should realize that the commonly used levels of TBARS or MDA as markers of lipid peroxidation are now considered somewhat controversial, although they are still usable with cautious interpretation [42].

It is well known that the coordination of antioxidant defense systems presents higher antioxidant potential than a separate antioxidant molecule or antioxidant enzyme. To solve this problem, we evaluated the plasma total antioxidant capacity assessed by the FRAP assay, which provides much more information on free radical scavenging capacity than the concentrations of individual antioxidants [45,46]. Our study revealed a moderate increase in resting and post-exercise FRAP levels after EGb supplementation, reflected by significant effects of group, trial, and time. The observed increases in FRAP levels during recovery may be attributed to a concurrent rise in plasma uric acid, which is the main contributor to total antioxidant capacity expressed as a FRAP value [22,45]. It should be emphasized that only in the EGb-supplemented group was FRAP highly significantly correlated with UA levels (R = 0.83, $p < 0.0001$).

Finally, we have to recall that polyphenols contained in *Ginkgo biloba* extract may provide other health benefits, such as neuroprotection regulated by neurotrophic factors, among which the best studied are nerve growth factor (NGF) and brain-derived neurotrophic factor (BDNF). The effect of regular physical activity on the structure and cognitive functions of the brain has been well documented by experimental and observational studies [47–50]. Regular physical exercise of moderate intensity has a favorable influence on brain vascularization and blood flow, thus improving oxygen and nutrient supply. Physical effort may enhance memory through neurogenesis, changes in the levels of neurotransmitters, and neurotrophic factors, primarily in the brain regions of the hippocampus, cerebral cortex, hypothalamus, and cerebellum [51,52]. Potential synergy between dietary polyphenol consumption and physical activity may also involve signaling pathways regulating different stages of neurogenesis, cell fate, synaptic plasticity, cognitive performance, and blood vessel function [53]. Hence, a combination of active lifestyle and dietary supplements of natural origin seems to be an optimal strategy for improving or maintaining brain function.

Our results have evidenced that a six-week consumption of *Ginkgo biloba* extract did not result in an increase in basal BDNF content. However, during the incremental test to exhaustion, significant increases in serum BDNF concentration immediately post-test and its rapid decline to basal values were observed in both groups (EGb and PLA), although higher post-test BDNF increases were recorded in EGb-supplemented individuals (revealed by significant group × trial interaction). In this context, our data are similar to those reported by Bell et al. [13] and Rojas Vega et al. [54] for male individuals performing a short-duration incremental cycling exercise to exhaustion.

The main limitations of this study were the relatively small number of participants recruited from a population of physically active college-aged males, and the lack of information on their actual food intakes and physical workloads, which limits the generalizability of the research findings to a wider population. Other weakness of this study is that we could not perform more specific and more reliable diagnostic tests for the determination of the plasma total antioxidant capacity and lipid peroxidation.

5. Conclusions

Our results show that six weeks' supplementation with a standardized *Ginkgo biloba* extract in physically active young men may provide some marginal improvements in their endurance performance expressed as VO_2max and blood antioxidant capacity, as evidenced by specific biomarkers (SOD, GSH, UA, FRAP, and TBARS). Moreover, it may provide somewhat better neuroprotection through increased exercise-induced production of BDNF.

Acknowledgments: This study was supported by statutory funds of the Jerzy Kukuczka Academy of Physical Education, Katowice, Poland.

Author Contributions: E.S.K., I.P. and P.D. designed the study. K.K. and T.P. performed the biochemical analyses. E.S.K. performed statistical data analysis. E.S.K. and B.K. collected the literature, wrote the paper. I.P. and T.P. critically reviewed the manuscript. All authors read and approved the final version of the paper.

Conflicts of Interest: The authors declare no conflicts of interest.

References

1. Vauzour, D.; Rodriguez-Mateos, A.; Corona, G.; Oruna-Concha, M.J.; Spencer, J.P.E. Polyphenols and human health: Prevention of disease and mechanisms of action. *Nutrients* **2010**, *2*, 1106–1131. [CrossRef] [PubMed]
2. Willcox, J.K.; Ash, S.L.; Catignani, G.L. Antioxidants and prevention of chronic disease. *Crit. Rev. Food Sci. Nutr.* **2004**, *44*, 275–295. [CrossRef] [PubMed]
3. Middleton, E., Jr.; Kandaswami, C.; Theoharides, T.C. The effects of plant flavonoids on mammalian cells: Implications for inflammation, heart disease, and cancer. *Pharmacol. Rev.* **2000**, *526*, 673–751. [PubMed]
4. Croft, K.D. Dietary polyphenols: Antioxidants or not? *Arch. Biochem. Biophys.* **2016**, *595*, 120–124. [CrossRef] [PubMed]
5. Droy-Lefaix, M.T. Effect of the antioxidant action of Ginkgo biloba extract (EGb 761) on aging and oxidative stress. *Age* **1997**, *29*, 141–148. [CrossRef] [PubMed]
6. Williamson, G.; Holst, B. Dietary reference intake (DRI) value for dietary polyphenols: Are we heading in the right direction? *Br. J. Nutr.* **2008**, *99* (Suppl. 3), S55–S58. [CrossRef] [PubMed]
7. Ude, C.; Schubert-Zsilavecz, M.; Wurglics, M. Ginkgo biloba extracts: A review of the pharmacokinetics of the active ingredients. *Clin. Pharmacokinet.* **2013**, *52*, 727–749. [CrossRef] [PubMed]
8. Mullaicharam, A.R. A review on evidence based practice of Ginkgo biloba in brain health. *Int. J. Pharmaceut. Chem. Anal.* **2013**, *1*, 24–30.
9. Kuo, Y.C.; Lin, J.C.; Bernard, J.R.; Liao, Y.H. Green tea extract supplementation dose not hamper endurance-training adaptation but improves antioxidant capacity in sedentary men. *Appl. Physiol. Nutr. Metab.* **2015**, *40*, 990–996. [CrossRef] [PubMed]
10. Williams, R.J.; Spencer, J.P.E.; Rice-Evans, C. Flavonoids: Antioxidants or signalin g molecules? *Free Radic. Biol. Med.* **2004**, *36*, 838–849. [CrossRef] [PubMed]
11. Williamson, G.; Manach, C. Bioavailability and bioefficacy of polyphenols in humans. II. Review of 93 intervention studies. *Am. J. Clin. Nutr.* **2005**, *81*, 243S–255S. [PubMed]

12. Manach, C.; Williamson, G.; Morand, C.; Scalbert, A.; Rémésy, C. Bioavailability and bioefficacy of polyphenols in humans. I. Review of 97 bioavailability studies. *Am. J. Clin. Nutr.* **2005**, *81*, 230S–242S. [PubMed]

13. Bell, L.; Lamport, J.; Butler, L.T.; Williams, C.M. A review of the cognitive effects observed in humans following acute supplementation with flavonoids, and their associated mechanisms of action. *Nutrients* **2015**, *7*, 10290–10306. [CrossRef] [PubMed]

14. Scalbert, A.; Williamson, G. Dietary intake and bioavailability of polyphenols. *J. Nutr.* **2000**, *130*, 2073S–2085S. [PubMed]

15. DeFeudis, F.V. Bilobalide and neuroprotection. *Pharmacol. Res.* **2002**, *46*, 565–568. [CrossRef]

16. DeFeudis, F.V.; Drieu, K. Ginkgo biloba extract (EGb 761) and CNS functions: Basic studies and clinical applications. *Curr. Drug Targets* **2000**, *1*, 25–58. [CrossRef] [PubMed]

17. Autry, A.E.; Monteggia, L.M. Brain-derived neurotrophic factor and neuropsychiatric disorders. *Pharmacol. Rev.* **2012**, *64*, 238–258. [CrossRef] [PubMed]

18. Cotman, C.W.; Berchtold, N.C.; Christie, L.A. Exercise builds brain health: Key roles of growth factor cascades and inflammation. *Trends Neurosci.* **2007**, *30*, 464–472. [CrossRef] [PubMed]

19. Beutler, E.; Duron, O.; Kelly, B.M. Improved method for the determination of blood glutathione. *J. Lab. Clin. Med.* **1963**, *61*, 882–888. [PubMed]

20. Aebi, H. Catalase in vitro. *Methods Enzymol.* **1984**, *105*, 121–126. [CrossRef] [PubMed]

21. Glatzle, G.; Korner, W.F.; Christeller, S.; Wiss, O. Method for the detection of biochemical riboflavin deficiency stimulation of NADPH2-dependent glutathione reductase from human erythrocytes by FAD in vitro. Investigations on the vitamin B2 status-in healthy people and geriatric patients. *Int. Z. Vitaminforsch.* **1970**, *40*, 166–183. [PubMed]

22. Benzie, I.F.; Strain, J.J. The ferric reducing ability of plasma (FRAP) as a measure of "antioxidant power": The FRAP Assay. *Anal. Biochem.* **1996**, *239*, 70–76. [CrossRef] [PubMed]

23. Buege, J.A.; Aust, S.D. Microsomal lipid peroxidation. *Methods Enzymol.* **1978**, *52*, 302–310. [CrossRef] [PubMed]

24. Singleton, V.L.; Rossi, J.A. Colorimetry of total phenolics with phosphomolybdic-phosphotungstic acid reagents. *Am. J. Enol. Vitic.* **1965**, *16*, 144–158.

25. Davis, J.M.; Carlstedt, C.J.; Chen, S.; Carmichael, M.D.; Murphy, E.A. The dietary flavonoid quercetin increases VO_2max and endurance capacity. *Int. J. Sport Nutr. Exerc. Metab.* **2010**, *20*, 56–62. [CrossRef] [PubMed]

26. Richards, J.C.; Lonac, M.C.; Johnson, T.K.; Schweder, M.M.; Bell, C. Epigallocatechin-3-gallate increases maximal oxygen uptake in adult humans. *Med. Sci. Sports Exerc.* **2010**, *42*, 739–744. [CrossRef] [PubMed]

27. Williams, M. Dietary supplements and sports performance: Herbals. *J. Int. Soc. Sports Nutr.* **2006**, *3*, 1–6. [CrossRef] [PubMed]

28. Peters, H.; Kieser, M.; Hölscher, U. Demonstration of the efficacy of ginkgo biloba special extract EGb 761 on intermittent claudication—A placebo-controlled, double-blind multicenter trial. *Vasa* **1998**, *27*, 106–110. [PubMed]

29. Nicolaï, S.P.A.; Kruidenier, L.M.; Bendermacher, B.L.W.; Prins, M.H.; Stockmans, R.A.; Broos, P.P.H.L.; Teijink, J.A.W. Ginkgo biloba for intermittent claudication. *Cochrane Database Syst. Rev.* **2013**, *6*, CD006888. [CrossRef]

30. Kressler, J.; Millard-Stafford, M.; Warren, G.L. Quercetin and endurance exercise capacity: A systemic review and meta-analysis. *Med. Sci. Sports Exerc.* **2011**, *43*, 2396–2404. [CrossRef] [PubMed]

31. Pelletier, D.M.; Lacerte, G.; Goulet, E.D.B. Effects of quercetin supplementation on endurance performance and maximal oxygen consumption: A meta-analysis. *Int. J. Sport. Nutr. Exerc. Metab.* **2013**, *23*, 73–82. [CrossRef] [PubMed]

32. Mahady, G.B. Ginkgo biloba: A review of quality, safety, and efficacy. *Nutr. Clin. Care* **2001**, *4*, 140–147. [CrossRef]

33. Coimbra, S.; Castro, E.; Rocha-Pereira, P.; Rebelo, I.; Rocha, S.; Santos-Silva, A. The effect of green tea in oxidative stress. *Clin. Nutr.* **2006**, *25*, 790–796. [CrossRef] [PubMed]

34. Abreu, I.A.; Cabelli, D.E. Superoxide dismutases—A review of the metal-associated mechanistic variations. *Biochim. Biophys. Acta* **2010**, *1804*, 263–274. [CrossRef] [PubMed]

35. Arthur, J.R. The glutathione peroxidases. *Cell Mol. Life Sci.* **2000**, *57*, 1825–1835. [CrossRef] [PubMed]

36. Moskaug, J.Ø.; Carlsen, H.; Myhrstad, M.C.W.; Blomhoff, R. Polyphenols and glutathione synthesis regulation. *Am. J. Clin. Nutr.* **2005**, *81*, 277S–283S. [PubMed]

37. Hellsten, Y.; Richter, E.A.; Kiens, B.; Bangsbo, J. AMP deamination and purine exchange in human skeletal muscle during and after intense exercise. *J. Physiol.* **1999**, *520*, 909–920. [CrossRef] [PubMed]

38. De Oliveira, E.P.; Burini, R.C. High plasma uric acid concentration: Causes and consequences. *Diabetol. Metab. Syndr.* **2012**, *4*, 12. [CrossRef] [PubMed]

39. Dudzińska, W.; Lubkowska, A.; Dolegowska, B.; Suska, M.; Janiak, M. Uridine—An indicator of post-exercise uric acid concentration and blood pressure. *Physiol. Res.* **2015**, *64*, 467–477. [PubMed]

40. Hellsten-Westing, Y.; Ekblom, B.; Sjödin, B. The metabolic relation between hypoxanthine and uric acid in man following maximal short-distance running. *Acta Physiol. Scand.* **1989**, *137*, 341–345. [CrossRef] [PubMed]

41. Witkowska, A.M.; Zujko, M.E.; Waśkiewicz, A.; Terlikowska, K.M.; Piotrowski, W. Comparison of various databases for estimation of dietary polyphenol intake in the population of Polish adults. *Nutrients* **2015**, *7*, 9299–9308. [CrossRef] [PubMed]

42. Hollman, P.C.H.; Cassidy, A.; Compe, B.; Heinonen, M.; Richelle, M.; Richling, E.; Serafini, M.; Scalbert, A.; Sies, H.; Vidry, S. The biological relevance of direct antioxidant effects of polyphenols for cardiovascular health in humans is not established. *J. Nutr.* **2011**, *141*, 989S–1009S. [CrossRef] [PubMed]

43. Forman, H.J.; Davies, K.J.A.; Ursini, F. How do nutritional antioxidants really work: Nucleophilic tone and para-hormesis versus free radical scavenging in vivo. *Free Radic. Biol. Med.* **2014**, *66*, 24–35. [CrossRef] [PubMed]

44. Jówko, E.; Długołęcka, B.; Makaruk, B.; Cieśliński, I. The effect of green tea extract supplementation on exercise-induced oxidative stress parameters in male sprinters. *Eur. J. Nutr.* **2015**, *54*, 783–791. [CrossRef] [PubMed]

45. Bartosz, G. Total antioxidant capacity. *Adv. Clin. Chem.* **2003**, *37*, 219–292. [PubMed]

46. Kamińska, J.; Podgórski, T.; Pawlak, M. Variability of selected hematological and biochemical markers in marathon runners. *Trends Sport Sci.* **2015**, *3*, 125–132.

47. Rassmussen, P.; Brassard, P.; Adser, H.; Pedersen, M.V.; Leick, L.; Hart, E.; Secher, N.H.; Pedersen, B.K.; Pilegaard, H. Evidence for a release of brain-derived neurotrophic factor from the brain during exercise. *Exp. Physiol.* **2009**, *94*, 1062–1069. [CrossRef] [PubMed]

48. Erickson, K.I.; Voss, M.V.; Prakash, R.S.; Basak, C.; Szabo, A.; Chaddock, L.; Kim, J.S.; Heo, S.; Alves, H.; White, S.M.; et al. Exercise training increases size of hippocampus and improves memory. *Proc. Natl. Acad. Sci. USA* **2011**, *108*, 3017–3022. [CrossRef] [PubMed]

49. Huang, T.; Larsen, K.T.; Ried-Larsen, M.; Møller, N.C.; Andersen, L.B. The effects of physical activity and exercise on brain-derived neurotrophic factor in healthy humans: A review. *Scand. J. Med. Sci. Sports* **2014**, *24*, 1–10. [CrossRef] [PubMed]

50. Kim, Y.I. The impact of exercise training on basal BDNF in athletic adolescents. *J. Phys. Ther. Sci.* **2016**, *28*, 3056–3069. [CrossRef] [PubMed]

51. Szuhany, K.L.; Bugatti, M.; Otto, M.W. A meta-analytic review of the effects of exercise on brain-derived neurotrophic factor. *J. Psychiatr. Res.* **2015**, *60*, 56–64. [CrossRef] [PubMed]

52. Gomes da Silva, S.; Arida, R.M. Physical activity and brain development. *Expert Rev. Neurother.* **2015**, *15*, 1041–1051. [CrossRef] [PubMed]

53. Spencer, J.P.; Abd El Mohsena, M.M.; Minihanea, A.M.; Mathers, J.C. Biomarkers of the intake of dietary polyphenols: Strengths, limitations and application in nutrition research. *Br. J. Nutr.* **2008**, *99*, 12–22. [CrossRef] [PubMed]

54. Vega, S.R.; Strüder, H.K.; Wahrmann, B.V.; Schmidt, A.; Bloch, W.; Hollmann, W. Acute BDNF and cortisol response to low intensity exercise and following ramp incremental exercise to exhaustion in humans. *Brain Res.* **2006**, *1121*, 59–65. [CrossRef] [PubMed]

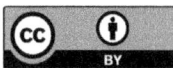

nutrients

MDPI

Article

Effects of Creatine Supplementation on Muscle Strength and Optimal Individual Post-Activation Potentiation Time of the Upper Body in Canoeists

Chia-Chi Wang [1], Shu-Cheng Lin [2], Shu-Ching Hsu [2], Ming-Ta Yang [3] and Kuei-Hui Chan [2,*]

[1] Athletic Department, National Taipei University of Business, Taipei 10051, Taiwan; sunnywang@ntub.edu.tw
[2] Graduate Institute of Athletics and Coaching Science, National Taiwan Sport University, Taoyuan 33301, Taiwan; s0975835@gmail.com (S.-C.L.); jessie800509@gmail.com (S.-C.H.)
[3] Center for General Education, Taipei Medical University, Taipei 10031, Taiwan; yangrugby@gmail.com
*   Correspondence: quenhuen@ntsu.edu.tw; Tel.: +886-3-328-3201 (ext. 2423); Fax: +886-3-328-0619

Received: 29 September 2017; Accepted: 25 October 2017; Published: 27 October 2017

Abstract: Creatine supplementation reduces the impact of muscle fatigue on post-activation potentiation (PAP) of the lower body, but its effects on the upper body remain unknown. This study examined the effects of creatine supplementation on muscle strength, explosive power, and optimal individual PAP time of the upper body during a set of complex training bouts in canoeists. Seventeen male high school canoeists performed a bench row for one repetition at maximum strength and conducted complex training bouts to determine the optimal individual timing of PAP and distance of overhead medicine ball throw before and after the supplementation. Subjects were assigned to a creatine or placebo group, and later consumed 20 g of creatine or carboxymethyl cellulose per day for six days. After supplementation, the maximal strength in the creatine group significantly increased ($p < 0.05$). The optimal individual PAP time in the creatine group was significantly earlier than the pre-supplementation times ($p < 0.05$). There was no significant change in explosive power for either group. Our findings support the notion that creatine supplementation increases maximal strength and shortens the optimal individual PAP time of the upper body in high school athletes, but has no effect on explosive power. Moreover, it was found that the recovery time between a bench row and an overhead medicine ball throw in a complex training bout is an individual phenomenon.

Keywords: complex training; overhead medicine ball throw; bench row

---

1. Introduction

Using ergogenic aids is a strategy or technique that serves to increase performance during exercise, efficiency of exercise, and recovery after exercise in athletes. Creatine (Cr) is one of the most commonly used nutritional ergogenic aids in various athletic populations and was designed to increase exercise-related strength and power for high intensity exercise bouts of short duration (<30 s) [1]. A number of reviews have reported that combined short-term (five–seven days) Cr supplementation (20 g per day) with exercise/training can significantly increase upper and lower body strength, power, and/or work performance during multiple sets of maximal effort muscle contractions [1–4].

The neuromuscular phenomenon of post-activation potentiation (PAP) has been applied in training programmes as a complex training and warm-up activity to increase maximal muscle power and strength in athletes, and this application can positively influence long-term training and acute exercise performance. PAP is commonly defined as the enhanced neuromuscular state observed immediately after a session of heavy resistance exercise (HRE) [5,6]. Three physiological mechanisms behind PAP have been purported to contribute to enhance performances after HRE. The proposed mechanisms include increases in the level of neuromuscular activation, phosphorylation of myosin regulatory light chains, and changes in muscle pennation angle [6]. However, studies have indicated both effective [7–11] and ineffective results [10,12,13] on explosive performance after HRE (three–five repetition maximum (RM) strength). Based on the previous research studies and reviews, it is clear that PAP is influenced by muscle fatigue and is an individualized phenomenon [6,10,14–17].

Previous studies indicated that both muscle fatigue and PAP occur after HRE. Fatigue and PAP have opposing effects on force production and power output in skeletal muscle, hence optimal performance occurs when fatigue has subsided but the potentiated effect still exists [6,14]. Therefore, decreasing muscle fatigue during HRE and recovering faster from muscle fatigue after HRE are important factors for the effectiveness of PAP. Various factors causing fatigue during HRE have been proposed. A decrease in substrate (i.e., adenosine triphosphate (ATP), phosphocreatine (PCr)), an accumulation of metabolic by-products (i.e., lactate, hydrogen ions, and/or inorganic phosphate), and a decreased peak calcium ion concentration in the myoplasm have been associated with fatigue [18]. Previous studies provided compelling evidence suggesting that short-term Cr supplementation (20 g per day for five–seven days) in combination with exercise may augment recovery of skeletal muscle metabolic function and performance [3,19–24]. Positive results were observed in our previous study, in which athletes who consumed 20 g of Cr monohydrate for six days could shorten their optimal individual PAP time from 6.13 min to 4.00 min after a 5-RM half squat, but experienced no effect on peak jump performance [25]. Therefore, Cr supplementation has benefits on reducing fatigue after HRE. However, there has only been a small amount of research investigating the effect of Cr supplementation on the upper body [26,27] and no study has evaluated the effect of Cr supplementation on the optimal individual PAP time, strength, and explosive power of the upper body. Thus, the effects of Cr supplementation on the upper body need to investigated.

Several studies have demonstrated a high degree of lower and upper body power after PAP strategies are used in athletes [6,8,9,11,16,28]. However, to date, the majority of PAP studies have usually concentrated on the use of barbell back squats as an effective means for inducing lower body PAP and have investigated effects on lower body performance, such as jump and sprint performance [10,11]. Relatively little emphasis has been placed on the PAP of the upper body. In fact, 94% of PAP studies investigated the effect of PAP on the lower body, as indicated in a review article [6]. The major exercise used in the study of PAP effects on the upper body is the bench press [16]. Moreover, many studies showed that recovery time between HRE and a subsequent explosive activity should be individualized, because athletes' backgrounds (including muscle fibre type, training experience, and strength level) and the workout structure (type of conditioning activity, intensity of HRE) would affect the PAP response [6,14]. Studies have suggested that the optimal recovery period may vary, including values of 5 min [9], 8 min [16,29], 4–12 min [30], 7–10 min [14], and 8–16 min [31]. However, these studies used the half squat or bench press as the HRE. The bench row is a multi-joint resistance training exercise commonly used in sport disciplines that require upper body pulling, such as canoeing, rowing, and kayaking. A study using different types of exercise to fit different events is necessary to apply the concept of PAP to the upper body.

To the best of the author's knowledge, the effects of Cr supplementation on increasing PAP effects on the upper body have not been investigated. Moreover, the bench row exercise, a common method of upper body training, has not been considered in this context. Therefore, the goal of this study was to examine whether short-term Cr supplementation can attenuate the impact of fatigue on muscle power performance and effectiveness of the optimal individual PAP time between the bench row and a subsequent explosive activity, as well as whether this supplementation can increase upper body strength. It was hypothesized that Cr supplementation would increase upper body strength, increase power performance, and shorten the optimal individual PAP time during a complex training bout, and that the recovery time of the upper body during a complex training movement (bench row and medicine ball throw) would be an individual phenomenon.

2. Experimental Section

2.1. Research Design

To examine the upper body results, the study procedure and method were similar to those of our previous study [25]. Before formal measurements, all subjects visited the laboratory initially to ensure familiarity with the bench row and overhead medicine ball throw (OMBT) technique. Subjects were educated during the familiarization session by a well-trained fitness instructor. The day after the familiarization session, anthropometric indexes and the strength of a one repetition maximum (1-RM) bench row were measured. Two days later, subjects performed two sets of complex training bouts with six 2-min rest intervals by two separated days to determine the individual optimal timing of PAP, and the distance of an OMBT. A double-blind, randomized design was used to assign 17 subjects into a Cr group or a placebo (Pla) group. After six days of high dose Cr or Pla supplementation, the same test procedures performed before supplementation were conducted again to evaluate the effects of Cr supplementation. A low dose of Cr or Pla supplementation was maintained until the end of the study. All familiarization and experimental sessions of this study were performed at the same time (from 10 AM to 2 PM) each day. The study was approved by the Institutional Review Board of the Fu Jen Catholic University, Taiwan.

2.2. Subjects

Seventeen male high school canoeists volunteered to participate in this study. The characteristics of the subjects are described in Table 1. All subjects provided written informed consent before participation. They maintained their basic training programmes and were asked to keep their normal dietary patterns during the experimental period. Subjects were excluded if they had one of the following: (1) injury to an upper limb within the past six months; (2) experience with bench row and OMBT training within the past six months; or (3) use of chronic or daily doses of anti-inflammatory medications or nutritional supplements within the past month.

Table 1. Subject characteristics.

Variable	Cr group (*n* = 8)	Pla group (*n* = 9)
Age (years)	16.75 ± 0.70	16.44 ± 1.13
Height (cm)	169.48 ± 3.61	172.16 ± 3.53
Weight (kg)	65.33 ± 4.65	64.34 ± 7.14
Body fat (%)	14.50 ± 2.58	13.20 ± 2.96

Data are the means ± standard deviation. Cr = creatine; Pla = placebo.

2.3. Supplementation Protocol

After the baseline testing, subjects in the Cr group began consuming 5 g of pure unflavored creatine monohydrate powder (creatine fuel powder; Twinlab, Hauppauge, NY, USA) plus 5 g of dextrose dissolved in 300 mL of water four times (at breakfast, lunch, dinner, and before bedtime) per day for six days. Subjects in the Pla group followed the same protocol but consumed carboxymethyl cellulose (food grade CMC powder, GreenYoung Co., Taichung, Taiwan) instead of Cr. The supplements for both groups were the same colour and taste. For maintenance, subjects ingested single daily doses of 2 g of creatine monohydrate or carboxymethyl cellulose powder plus 2 g dextrose dissolved in 200 mL of water after lunch until the end of the study.

2.4. Prediction of One Repetition Maximum Strength

Prediction of 1-RM strength for the bench row was determined based on the protocol described by Baechle et al. [32]. In brief, subjects jogged for 5 min on a treadmill followed by lower/upper limb light stretching exercises and two light resistance warm-up sets. After 1 min of rest, the subjects were instructed to lie prone on the high bench (Apex B45 adjustable flat bench) and hold a barbell at a load of 87–93% of the predicted 1-RM. On command, the subject raised the bar to the bottom of the bench and then lowered the bar back to full elbow extension. After each successful performance, the load was increased in increments of 8–10% until only one successful repetition could be completed. Four minutes of rest were given between each test. The increase or decrease in the load continued until the subject was able to complete one repetition with the proper exercise technique. Ideally, the subject's 1-RM was measured within five testing sets.

2.5. Optimal Individual PAP Time and Overhead Medicine Ball Throw Test

The OMBT test was selected to evaluate upper body muscular power. Studies have shown that the OMBT test is a valid and reliable test for assessing upper body muscular power and is commonly used for testing upper body power [33–35]. After a low intensity aerobic exercise followed by a light stretching exercise for warm-up, subjects performed two OMBT tests for baseline measurements. During the OMBT test, subjects stood at a line with feet slightly apart, and a 3-kg medicine ball was brought back behind the head, then subjects threw the medicine ball as far forward as possible. The subjects were not allowed to move their feet during the test. Each OMBT was separated by a 5-s rest period. The longest OMBT value was used in the analysis.

After a 5-min rest, subjects executed a set of complex training bouts involving 3-RM bench row exercises to elicit PAP followed by a counterbalanced order of six rest intervals (1, 3, 5, 7, 9, 11 min or 2, 4, 6, 8, 10, 12 min) for two days. The optimal individual PAP time was the rest interval with the maximum delta-values for the throw distance during the complex training bouts minus the baseline values.

2.6. Anthropometric Measurements

All subjects visited the laboratory in the morning for anthropometric measurements including body height (cm), body mass (kg), and body fat percentage (%). Standing body height without shoes or socks was measured to the nearest 0.1 cm with a height meter mounted on a wall. Body mass and body fat percentage were measured by a bioelectrical impedance instrument (InBody 3.0, Biospace, Seoul, Korea) with standard methods used to assess body composition.

2.7. Statistical Analysis

Statistical analyses were performed using SPSS version 19.0 software (SPSS Inc., Chicago, IL, USA). Data are expressed as the means ± standard deviation. An independent sample *t*-test was used to compare the subjects' characteristics between the groups. A mixed design two-way ANOVA (group × time) was used to compare the variables of 1-RM strength, OMBT distance, and optimal individual PAP time. Statistical significance was set at $p < 0.05$.

3. Results

3.1. Subject Characteristics

Subject characteristics for both groups are presented in Table 1. No significant differences were noted for any variable ($p > 0.05$).

3.2. Effects of Cr Supplementation on Maximum Upper Body Muscle Strength and Explosive Power in a Set of Complex Training Bouts

Figure 1 shows the results of a 1-RM strength bench row before and after six days of Cr or Pla supplementation. There was a significant interaction between groups and time. Following supplementation, 1-RM strength in the Cr group significantly increased from 85.63 ± 8.63 kg to 88.12 ± 8.36 kg ($p < 0.05$). However, there were no significant differences in the Pla group or between the Cr and Pla groups ($p > 0.05$). There was no significant change in OMBT distance after the optimal individual PAP time in complex training bouts for either group ($p > 0.05$, Figure 2).

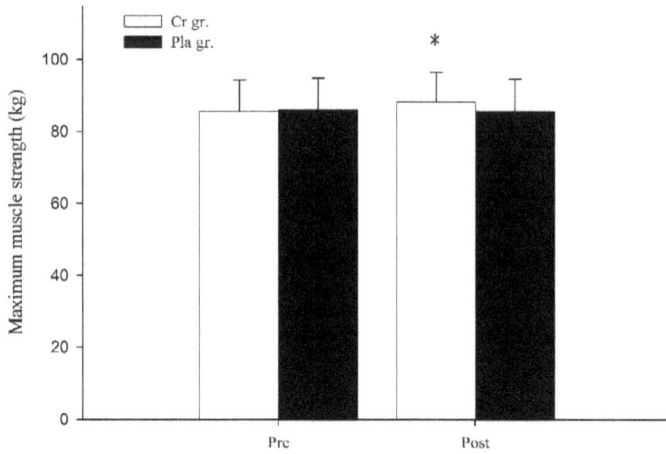

Figure 1. Maximum muscle strength of bench row before and after six days of creatine or placebo supplementation. Data are the means ± standard deviation. Cr gr. = creatine group; Pla gr. = placebo group; Pre = pre-supplementation; Post = post-supplementation. Asterisk (*) indicates a significant difference ($p < 0.05$) from the pre-supplementation value within the group.

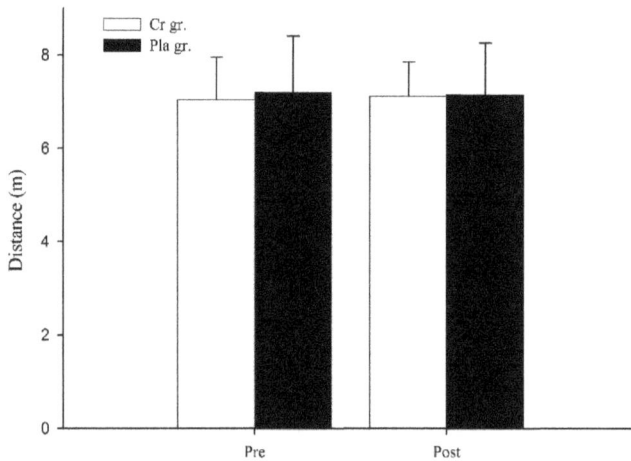

Figure 2. Distance of overhead medicine ball throw after the optimal individual post-activation potentiation (PAP) time in complex training bouts before and after six days of creatine or placebo supplementation. Data are the means ± standard deviation. Cr gr. = creatine group; Pla gr. = placebo group. Pre = pre-supplementation; Post = post-supplementation.

3.3. Optimal Individual PAP Time

Figure 3 shows the optimal individual PAP time points for each individual and illustrates the individual variations in the results. The two groups had their optimal PAP times at different time points. Furthermore, there was a significant interaction between groups and time. After supplementation, the optimal individual PAP time in the Cr group was significantly earlier than it was in that group pre-supplementation from 9.75 ± 2.31 min to 8.12 ± 2.23 min ($p < 0.05$). However, there were no significant differences in the Pla group or between the Cr and Pla groups ($p > 0.05$).

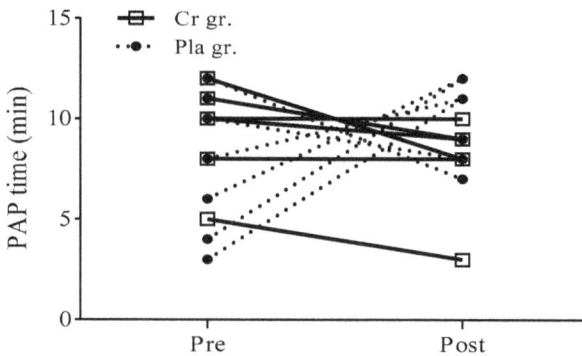

Figure 3. Optimal individual PAP time for each subject following creatine or placebo supplementation. Cr gr. = creatine group; Pla gr. = placebo group; Pre = pre-supplementation; Post = post-supplementation.

4. Discussion

The present study is the first to assess the potential efficacy of short-term Cr supplementation in improving upper body performance in a complex training bout in canoeists. The major findings of this study are that Cr supplementation significantly increased the maximal strength of the bench row and reduced the negative influence of fatigue on the optimal individual PAP time during a set of complex training bouts involving the upper body (3-RM bench row and overhead medicine ball throw). However, this acute benefit could not enhance explosive power during a set of complex training bouts.

The primary and original results of this study indicate that the optimal individual time required to maximize the effect of PAP on the upper body was significantly earlier after Cr supplementation, decreasing from 9.75 min to 8.12 min after supplementation. Based on previous studies, explosive muscle contractions depend on the balance between fatigue and PAP, and fatigue is more dominant in the early stage of recovery [36]. Therefore, it is possible that Cr supplementation caused less fatigue, thereby reducing the diminishing effect of fatigue on the recovery period and allowing the PAP effect to predominate in the early recovery period. Another proposed reason for this result is that Cr supplementation facilitates the reuptake of calcium ions into the sarcoplasmic reticulum [37], thus activating more phosphorylation of myosin regulatory light chains, which is one of the principal mechanisms of PAP [6]. This result was consistent with our previous study [25], in which we observed that Cr supplementation for six days shortened the optimal individual PAP time from 6.13 min to 4.00 min after a 5-RM half squat. In addition, our findings are in agreement with previous studies showing that five days of Cr supplementation (20 g/day) significantly increased the total repetitions performed before fatigue and the total average power output values during repetitive high-power-output exercise bouts involving the upper body [3,23], and increased the time to fatigue during three bouts of submaximal knee extension and isometric handgrip [21]. In theory, Cr supplementation can delay the onset of fatigue during anaerobic exercise by decreasing the contribution of anaerobic glycolysis and then reducing lactate and hydrogen ions accumulation [1]. A meta-analysis revealed the effect of Cr supplementation on performance improvement in high-intensity exercise lasting ≤ 30 s [19]. The present findings suggest that the mechanisms of Cr work to decrease muscle fatigue by increasing the intramuscular concentration of PCr, aiding the rephosphorylation of adenosine diphosphate (ADP) to ATP, reducing pH changes from acidosis by using the hydrogen ions during the creatine kinase reaction and stimulating phosphofructokinase activity. Therefore, there is evidence to support our hypothesis that short-term Cr supplementation has a benefit in attenuating muscle fatigue symptoms and increasing recovery after HRE of the upper body. In addition, our results support previous studies that indicate that the PAP phenomenon is highly individualized. The subjects of our study had their highest PAP performance of complex training involving the upper body within a broad range of rest intervals (3, 4, 5, 6, 8, 10, 11, 12 min), which was consistent with our previous finding [25] that some subjects had the greatest PAP effect at 3–6 min after HRE, whereas this time interval varied for other subjects. Similar findings were observed in studies by Naclerio et al. [38] and Conmyns et al. [15] that indicated that the participants' best performances occurred between 15 s and 12 min. These studies concluded that this result could be attributed to the participants' differing background factors, including training level, strength level, and training experiences. Therefore, the obtained result supports our hypothesis that the optimal individual PAP time for a complex training set consisting of a bench row and medicine ball throw would also be influenced by the individual's background.

Although the optimal individual PAP time was significantly earlier after Cr supplementation, decreasing from 9.75 min to 8.12 min, we observed that the elicited PAP was not sufficient to enhance the peak performance in the OMBT test. This observation is in line with our previous finding, which showed that Cr supplementation did not significantly improve the performance of countermovement jump, despite the fact that the optimal individual PAP time was earlier after supplementation [25]. This result may be explained by the gradual rate of PAP. Previous studies have indicated that the peak PAP is achieved immediately after HRE, but instantly begins to decrease for the remainder of the recovery period. Several studies have assessed the time course of PAP decline after maximal voluntary contraction (MVC) of knee extensors [39–44]. Pääsuke et al. [41] showed that peak twitch was potentiated immediately by 51% after a single 10-s MVC of knee extensors, and there was a sharp decline in potentiation during the first 3 min of recovery, although potentiation was still higher than the pre-MVC value at 5–10 min. This magnitude and time course of PAP decline was similar to those observed in another study, in which twitch potentiation was induced in the knee extensor muscles by a 10-s MVC; the PAP of the twitch peak torque increased by 70.6% immediately but then rapidly declined to +31% at 60 s. Potentiation becomes more gradual over time, resembling an exponential function [39]. Hamada et al. [43] also indicated a greater decline in torque during a 10-s MVC in the elbow extensor compared to the ankle plantarflexor muscles. Similarly, Seize et al. [44] indicated that 6-s maximal dynamic knee extensions elicited significantly increased PAP from 1 to 7 min, and potentiation was still higher than the pre-test value at 7–13 min. Another study also concluded that twitch potentiation in the knee muscles was potentiated within 3–10 min of recovery [42]. Therefore, although Cr supplementation shortened the optimal individual PAP times in our study, the elicited PAP was not sufficient to enhance explosive power, because the peak PAP value had already elapsed.

Additionally, the findings of this study indicated that supplementation with 20 g/day of Cr for six days increased the maximal strength of a bench row. This present finding was consistent with previous studies [2–4], systematic reviews [1], and a meta-analysis [27]. These studies concluded that the potential mechanisms of the acute effect of short-term Cr supplementation (20 g/day for five–seven days) on the maximal upper body strength involves an increase in intramuscular PCr stores, allowing for rapid rephosphorylation of ADP back to ATP to delay the onset of muscular fatigue and improve Ca^{2+} kinetics in the sarcoplasmic reticulum.

5. Conclusions

This study suggests that short-term Cr supplementation in male high school canoeists resulted in improved upper body maximum strength and shortened optimal individual PAP times for training efficiency during a set of complex training bouts involving the upper body. Although short-term Cr supplementation is not enough to improve the explosive power of the upper body, it appears to be an effective supplementation method with respect to efficiency and strength development. Conditioning coaches may apply the results of this study to design proper complex training programs to enhance the performance of specific sports. Moreover, our results support the idea that the PAP phenomenon after a 3-RM bench row is also highly individualized. Further studies could apply the supplement strategy to investigate the effects on the efficiency of long-term complex training involving the upper body and/or lower body for the performance of specific sports.

Acknowledgments: Financial support provided by the Ministry of Sciences and Technology (MOST) of the Executive Yuan, Taiwan under grant No. MOST 104-2410-H-179-007 is gratefully acknowledged.

Author Contributions: Author C.-C.W. carried out the laboratory experiments, analyzed the data, interpreted the results, prepared figures and tables, and prepared the manuscript. Authors S.-C.L., S.-C.H. and M.-T.Y. assisted in the data collection and the discussion of the literature. Author K.-H.C. designed the study, supervised the experimental procedure, and reviewed the entire preparation of the manuscript.

Conflicts of Interest: The authors declare no conflicts of interest.

References

1. Bemben, M.G.; Lamont, H.S. Creatine supplementation and exercise performance: Recent findings. *Sports Med.* **2005**, *35*, 107–125. [CrossRef] [PubMed]
2. Cooper, R.; Naclerio, F.; Allgrove, J.; Jimenez, A. Creatine supplementation with specific view to exercise/sports performance: An update. *J. Int. Soc. Sports Nutr.* **2012**, *9*, 33. [CrossRef] [PubMed]
3. Izquierdo, M.; Ibañez, J.; González-Badillo, J.J.; Gorostiaga, E.M. Effects of creatine supplementation on muscle power, endurance, and sprint performance. *Med. Sci. Sports Exerc.* **2002**, *34*, 332–343. [CrossRef] [PubMed]
4. Bazzucchi, I.; Felici, F.; Sacchetti, M. Effect of short-term creatine supplementation on neuromuscular function. *Med. Sci. Sports Exerc.* **2009**, *41*, 1934–1941. [CrossRef] [PubMed]
5. Docherty, D.; Robbins, D.; Hodgson, M. Complex training revisited: A review of its current status as a viable training approach. *Strength Cond. J.* **2004**, *26*, 52–57. [CrossRef]
6. Tillin, N.A.; Bishop, D. Factors modulating post-activation potentiaiton and its effect on performance of subsequent explosive activities. *Sports Med.* **2009**, *39*, 147–166. [CrossRef] [PubMed]
7. Till, K.A.; Cooke, C. The effects of postactivation potentiation on sprint and jump performance of male academy soccer players. *J. Strength Cond. Res.* **2009**, *23*, 1960–1967. [CrossRef] [PubMed]
8. Rixon, K.P.; Lamont, H.S.; Bemben, M.G. Influence of type of muscle contraction, gender, and lifting experience on postactivation potentiation performance. *J. Strength Cond. Res.* **2007**, *21*, 500–505. [PubMed]
9. Chatzopoulos, D.E.; Michailidis, C.J.; Giannakos, A.K.; Alexiou, K.C.; Patikas, D.A.; Antonopoulos, C.B.; Kotzamanidis, C.M. Postactivation potentiation effects after heavy resistance exercise on running speed. *J. Strength Cond. Res.* **2007**, *21*, 1278–1281. [PubMed]
10. McCann, M.R.; Flanagan, S.P. The effects of exercise selection and rest interval on postactivation potentiation of vertical jump performance. *J. Strength Cond. Res.* **2010**, *24*, 1285–1291. [CrossRef] [PubMed]
11. Esformes, J.I.; Bampouras, T.M. Effect of back squat depth on lower-body postactivation potentiation. *J. Strength Cond. Res.* **2013**, *27*, 2997–3000. [CrossRef] [PubMed]
12. Duthie, G.M.; Young, W.B.; Aitken, D.A. The acute effects of heavy loads on jump squat performance: An evaluation of the complex and contrast methods of power development. *J. Strength Cond. Res.* **2002**, *16*, 530–538. [CrossRef] [PubMed]
13. Hrysomallis, C.; Kidgell, D. Effect of heavy dynamic resistive exercise on acute upper-body power. *J. Strength Cond. Res.* **2001**, *15*, 426–430. [PubMed]
14. Wilson, J.M.; Duncan, N.M.; Marin, P.J.; Brown, L.E.; Loenneke, J.P.; Wilson, S.M.; Jo, E.; Lowery, R.P.; Ugrinowitsch, C. Meta-analysis of postactivation potentiation and power: Effects of conditioning activity, volume, gender, rest periods, and training status. *J. Strength Cond. Res.* **2013**, *27*, 854–859. [CrossRef] [PubMed]
15. Comyns, T.M.; Harrison, A.J.; Hennessy, L.K.; Jensen, R.L. The optimal complex training rest interval for athletes from anaerobic sports. *J. Strength Cond. Res.* **2006**, *20*, 471–476. [PubMed]
16. Evetovich, T.K.; Conley, D.S.; McCawley, P.F. Postactivation potentiation enhances upper- and lower-body athletic performance in collegiate male and female athletes. *J. Strength Cond. Res.* **2015**, *29*, 336–342. [CrossRef] [PubMed]
17. McMahon, S.; Jenkins, D. Factors affecting the rate of phosphocreatine resynthesis following intense exercise. *Sports Med.* **2002**, *32*, 761–784. [CrossRef] [PubMed]
18. Allen, D.G.; Lamb, G.D.; Westerblad, H. Skeletal muscle fatigue: Cellular mechanisms. *Physiol. Rev.* **2008**, *88*, 287–332. [CrossRef] [PubMed]

19. Branch, J.D. Effect of creatine supplementation on body composition and performance: A meta-analysis. *Int. J. Sport Nutr. Exerc. Metab.* **2003**, *13*, 198–226. [CrossRef] [PubMed]

20. Casey, A.; Constantin-Teodosiu, D.; Howell, S.; Hultman, E.; Greenhaff, P.L. Creatine ingestion favorably affects performance and muscle metabolism during maximal exercise in humans. *Am. J. Physiol.* **1996**, *271*, E31–E37. [PubMed]

21. Rahimi, R.; Faraji, H.; Sheikholeslami-Vatani, D.; Vatani, S.D.; Qaderi, M. Creatine supplementation alters the hormonal response to resistance exercise. *Kinesiology* **2010**, *42*, 28–35.

22. Smith, A.E.; Walter, A.A.; Herda, T.J.; Ryan, E.D.; Moon, J.R.; Cramer, J.T.; Stout, J.R. Effects of creatine loading on electromyographic fatigue threshold during cycle ergometry in college-aged women. *J. Int. Soc. Sports Nutr.* **2007**, *4*, 20. [CrossRef] [PubMed]

23. Urbanski, R.L.; Loy, S.F.; Vincent, W.J.; Yaspelkis, B.B., III. Creatine supplementation differentially affects maximal isometric strength and time to fatigue in large and small muscle groups. *Int. J. Sport Nutr.* **1999**, *9*, 136–145. [CrossRef] [PubMed]

24. Zuniga, J.M.; Housh, T.J.; Camic, C.L.; Hendrix, C.R.; Mielke, M.; Johnson, G.O.; Housh, D.J.; Schmidt, R.J. The effects of creatine monohydrate loading on anaerobic performance and one-repetition maximum strength. *J. Strength Cond. Res.* **2012**, *26*, 1651–1656. [CrossRef] [PubMed]

25. Wang, C.C.; Yang, M.T.; Lu, K.H.; Chan, K.H. The effects of creatine supplementation on explosive performance and optimal individual postactivation potentiation time. *Nutrients* **2016**, *8*, 143. [CrossRef] [PubMed]

26. Lanhers, C.; Pereira, B.; Naughton, G.; Trousselard, M.; Lesage, F.X.; Dutheil, F. Creatine supplementation and lower limb strength performance: A systematic review and meta-analyses. *Sports Med.* **2015**, *45*, 1285–1294. [CrossRef] [PubMed]

27. Lanhers, C.; Pereira, B.; Naughton, G.; Trousselard, M.; Lesage, F.X.; Dutheil, F. Creatine supplementation and upper limb strength performance: A systematic review and meta-analysis. *Sports Med.* **2017**, *47*, 163–173. [CrossRef] [PubMed]

28. Robbins, D.W. Postactivation potentiation and its practical applicability: A brief review. *J. Strength Cond. Res.* **2005**, *19*, 453–458. [CrossRef] [PubMed]

29. Kilduff, L.P.; Owen, N.; Bevan, H.; Bennett, M.; Kingsley, M.I.; Cunningham, D. Influence of recovery time on post-activation potentiation in professional rugby players. *J. Sports Sci.* **2008**, *26*, 795–802. [CrossRef] [PubMed]

30. Crewther, B.T.; Kilduff, L.P.; Cook, C.J.; Middleton, M.K.; Bunce, J.P.; Yang, G.Z. The acute potentiating effects of back squats on athlete performance. *J. Strength Cond. Res.* **2011**, *25*, 3319–3325. [CrossRef] [PubMed]

31. Kilduff, L.P.; Bevan, H.R.; Kingsley, M.I.C.; Owen, N.J.; Bennett, M.A.; Bunce, P.J.; Hore, A.M.; Maw, J.R.; Cunningham, D.J. Postactivation potentiation in professional rugby players: Optimal recovery. *J. Strength Cond. Res.* **2007**, *21*, 1134–1138. [CrossRef] [PubMed]

32. Baechle, T.R.; Earle, R.W. *Essentials of Strength Training and Conditioning*, 2nd ed.; Human Kinetics Publishers: Champaign, IL, USA, 2008; pp. 406–413.

33. Gabbett, T.; Georgieff, B. Physiological and anthropometric characteristics of Australian junior national, state, and novice volleyball players. *J. Strength Cond. Res.* **2007**, *21*, 902–908. [PubMed]

34. Viitasalo, J.T. Evaluation of explosive strength for young and adult athlete. *Res. Q. Exerc. Sport* **1988**, *59*, 9–13. [CrossRef]

35. Vossen, J.F.; Kramer, J.F.; Burke, D.G.; Vossen, D.P. Comparison of dynamic push-up training and plyometric push-up training on upper-body power and strength. *J. Strength Cond. Res.* **2000**, *14*, 248–253.

36. Ebben, W.P. Complex training: A brief review. *J. Sports Sci. Med.* **2002**, *1*, 42–46. [PubMed]

37. Murphy, R.M.; Stephenson, D.G.; Lamb, G.D. Effect of creatine on contractile force and sensitivity in mechanically skinned single fibers from rat skeletal muscle. *Am. J. Physiol. Cell Physiol.* **2004**, *287*, C1589–C1595. [CrossRef] [PubMed]

38. Naclerio, F.; Chapman, M.; Larumbe-Zabala, E.; Massey, B.; Neil, A.; Triplett, T.N. Effects of three different conditioning activity volumes on the optimal recovery time for potentiation in college athletes. *J. Strength Cond. Res.* **2015**, *29*, 2579–2585. [CrossRef] [PubMed]

39. Hamada, T.; Sale, D.G.; MacDougall, J.D.; Tarnopolsky, M.A. Postactivation potentiation, fiber type, and twitch contraction time in human knee extensor muscles. *J. Appl. Physiol.* **2000**, *88*, 2131–2137. [PubMed]

40. Requena, B.; Gapeyeva, H.; García, I.; Ereline, J.; Pääsuke, M. Twitch potentiation after voluntary versus electrically induced isometric contractions in human knee extensor muscles. *Eur. J. Appl. Physiol.* **2008**, *104*, 463–472. [CrossRef] [PubMed]

41. Pääsuke, M.; Saapar, L.; Ereline, J.; Gapeyeva, H.; Requena, B.; Oopik, V. Postactivation potentiation of knee extensor muscles in power- and endurance-trained, and untrained women. *Eur. J. Appl. Physiol.* **2007**, *101*, 577–585. [CrossRef] [PubMed]

42. Jubeau, M.; Gondin, J.; Martin, A.; Van Hoecke, J.; Maffiuletti, N.A. Differences in twitch potentiation between voluntary and stimulated quadriceps contractions of equal intensity. *Scand. J. Med. Sci. Sports* **2010**, *20*, e56–e62. [CrossRef] [PubMed]

43. Hamada, T.; Sale, D.G.; Macdougall, J.D. Postactivation potentiation in endurance-trained male athletes. *Med. Sci. Sports Exerc.* **2000**, *32*, 403–411. [CrossRef] [PubMed]

44. Seitz, L.B.; Trajano, G.S.; Dal Maso, F.; Haff, G.G.; Blazevich, A.J. Postactivation potentiation during voluntary contractions after continued knee extensor task-specific practice. *Appl. Physiol. Nutr. Metab.* **2015**, *40*, 230–237. [CrossRef] [PubMed]

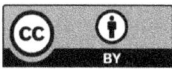

nutrients

MDPI

Article

Stability of Commercially Available Macular Carotenoid Supplements in Oil and Powder Formulations

David Phelan *, Alfonso Prado-Cabreroand John M. Nolan

Nutrition Research Centre Ireland, School of Health Science, Carriganore House, Waterford Institute of Technology, West Campus, Waterford X91 K236, Ireland; APRADO-CABRERO@wit.ie (A.P.-C.); John@ivr.ie (J.M.N.)
* Correspondence: dphelan@wit.ie; Tel.: +35-351-845-505

Received: 8 September 2017; Accepted: 13 October 2017; Published: 17 October 2017

Abstract: We previously identified that the concentration of zeaxanthin in some commercially available carotenoid supplements did not agree with the product's label claim. The conclusion of this previous work was that more quality assurance was needed to guarantee concordance between actual and declared concentrations of these nutrients i.e., lutein (L) zeaxanthin (Z) and *meso*-zeaxanthin (MZ) in commercially available supplements. Since this publication, we performed further analyses using different commercially available macular carotenoid supplements. Three capsules from one batch of eight products were analysed at two different time points. The results have been alarming. All of the powder filled products ($n = 3$) analysed failed to comply with their label claim (L: 19–74%; Z: 57–73%; MZ: 83–97%); however, the oil filled soft gel products ($n = 5$) met or were above their label claim (L: 98–122%; Z: 117–162%; MZ: 97–319%). We also identified that the carotenoid content of the oil filled capsules were stable over time (e.g., L average percentage change: −1.7%), but the powder filled supplements degraded over time (e.g., L average percentage change: −17.2%). These data are consistent with our previous work, and emphasize the importance of using carotenoid interventions in oil based formulas rather than powder filled formulas.

Keywords: macular carotenoid supplementation; lutein; zeaxanthin; *meso*-zeaxanthin; macular pigment

1. Introduction

Three macular carotenoids, lutein (L), zeaxanthin (Z) and *meso*-zeaxanthin (MZ) accumulate in the central retina (macula), where they are collectively known as macular pigment (MP) or the macular carotenoids [1] (See Figure 1).

The macula is the area of the retina which has the highest visual performance in terms of visual acuity i.e., motion detection, colour perception and contrast sensitivity [2]. MP has a distinctive yellow colour due to the presence of the macular carotenoids. MP has short-wavelength (blue) light filtering, antioxidant, and anti-inflammatory properties [3–5]. The filtration of blue light at the macula is believed to enhance visual performance, due to the attenuation of chromatic aberration; veiling luminescence and blue haze [6–8]. Furthermore, MP actively quenches free radicals, and this antioxidant capacity is optimised when all three macular carotenoids are present [9]. L and Z are consumed in a typical diet from sources such as fruits and leafy green vegetables [10,11]. MZ is not present in a typical diet, although it has been detected in shrimp, fish and turtle [12], and also in the liver of frog and quail [13]. More recently MZ has been identified in trout skin and trout flesh [14,15], thereby confirming the presence of this carotenoid in the human food chain [16].

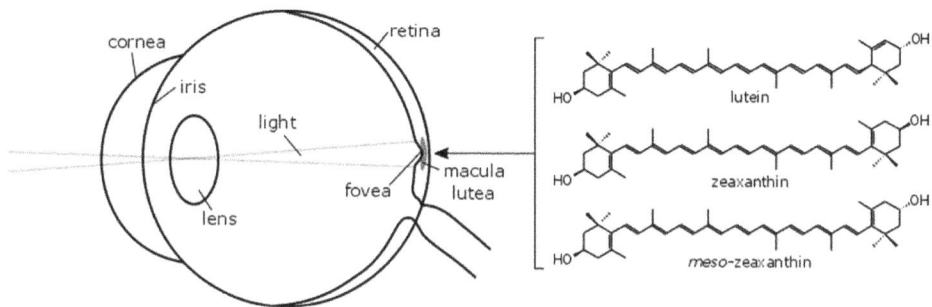

Figure 1. Schematic of the human eye showing the approximate location of the macular pigments and the chemical structure of the carotenoids which comprise macular pigment.

A large number of published studies have tested the efficacy of macular carotenoid supplementation (dietary and food supplementation), on serum and tissue response. The majority of these trials demonstrated a significant response in serum and target tissue (i.e., the retina). This tells us that we are not obtaining optimal amounts of these carotenoids from our standard diet. Hence, and given the known health benefits of these carotenoids for human health (e.g., visual performance and cognitive function) [17], it appears that there is a role for supplementation with these nutrients. For example, we know that supplementation with the macular carotenoids increases MP and enhances visual performance in diseased and non-diseased eyes, and clinical studies have shown that a combination of the macular carotenoids is the best way to achieve this goal [18–26]. Importantly, laboratory studies conducted on commercially available macular carotenoid supplements have shown that the capsule contents do not always comply with the product label claim [27]. A previous publication by our group investigated the concordance between declared and actual concentrations of the macular carotenoids in commercially available formulations [15]. In that study, MZ was present in six of seven products which did not declare MZ on their label. Also, concentrations of Z ranged from 47 to 248% of label claim. This has also been shown by Breithaupt et al. (2005), who reported that half ($n = 14$) of the products they tested did not meet label claim [28]. Therefore, the obvious question to address here is why some commercially available food supplements fail to meet their label claim. In the first instance, it appears that the regulation for food supplements is very weak, and attention to quality and stability has been shown to be neglected [15]. Of note, the Food and Drug Administration (FDA) does not require manufacturers of food supplements to include an expiration date on the label of these products [28].

Also, there are many factors which are known to affect the stability of carotenoid supplements, including product capsule and product matrix. The capsule type will have an impact on the stability of the product. Soft gel capsules are manufactured using a process where the fill and the shell are manufactured in one operation. It is known that the oil will limit oxidation and enhance the stability and therefore shelf life of the carotenoid [29]. Also, the manufacturing process for oil filled soft gels provides an inert environment during manufacturing (i.e., nitrogen blanketing for oxygen sensitive compounds), and a thorough de-aeration of the fill formulation to remove any dissolved air (oxygen) [30]. This process is extremely important for the preservation of these oxygen sensitive compounds [9,31]. In contrast, carotenoid supplements prepared as powder formulations are subject to oxidation, as there is no oil present to prevent direct contact with oxygen. Also, powder filled capsules are prepared simply by filling one side of the capsule with carotenoid and filler, and then pushing the other side to close the capsule. As these powder filled capsules are not fully sealed, the contents are subject to oxidation from the oxygen within the capsule and potentially from oxygen entering the capsule (See Figure 2).

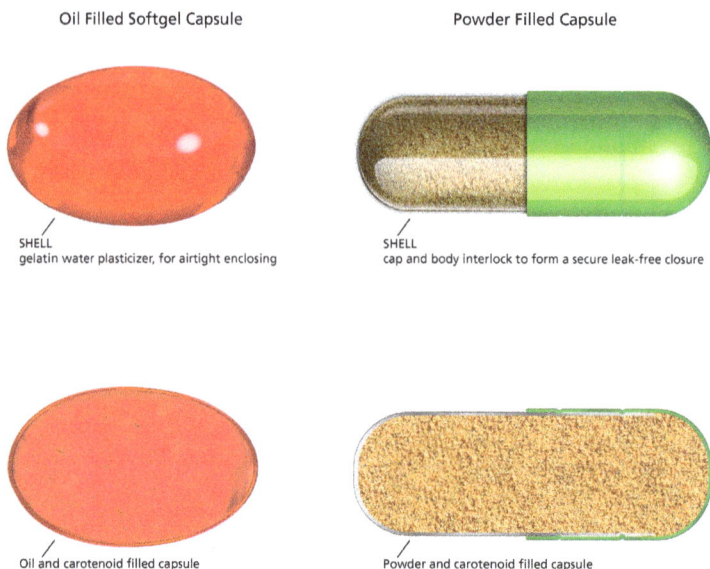

Figure 2. Graphic representation of an oil filled soft gel capsule and a two part powder filled capsule.

The aim of this study was to measure the concentration of L, Z and MZ in commercially available food supplements. This work allowed us to compare concordance to label claim for powder and oil filled carotenoid containing capsules. Also, we assessed the stability of the carotenoid contents of these formulations. This work is important, given the vast amount of carotenoid products available, and given that the regulation for carotenoid products is currently not robust. All the supplements analysed in this study contained carotenoid concentrates in their free form.

2. Materials and Methods

2.1. Supplements Analysed

In this experiment, we analysed two types of commercially available carotenoid supplements, namely oil filled soft gel capsules and powder filled capsules. As we were analyzing commercially available products from a number of manufacturers, it was not possible to align expiration dates to provide a uniform stability study and as such we were limited to analyzing and reanalyzing the products without a uniform time to expiry from date of analysis. The oil filled soft gel capsules analysed included: MacuSave (Zeon healthcare Ltd., Oxfordshire, UK), Doctor's Best (Doctor's Best Inc., San Clemente, CA, USA), Lutigold Extra (Puritans Pride Inc., Oakdale, NY, USA), MacuHealth LMZ[3] (MacuHealth, Birmingham, MI, USA), and MacuShield (Alliance Pharma PLC, Wiltshire, UK).

The powder filled capsules analysed included: MacuSafe (OcuSci, Del Mar, CA, USA), Eye Vitality Plus (Green Valley Hyperion LLC, Lexington, VA, USA) Vision Alive (Holistic Labs Ltd., Hollywood, FL, USA), and MaxiVision (MedOp Health Inc., Oldsmar, FL, USA). The MaxiVision product is a powder filled beadlet formulation. For this formulation, we used a different analytical method, see Section 2.4.

2.2. Macular Carotenoid Standards and Solvents

L standard [(3R,3′R,6′R)-β,ε-Carotene-3,3′-diol] and Z standard (racemic mixture of the three Z enantiomers (3R,3′R)-β,β-Carotene-3,3′-diol, (3S,3′S)-β,β-Carotene-3,3′-diol and (3R,3′S)-β,β-Carotene-3,3′-diol) were supplied by CaroteNature GmbH (Ostermundigen, Switzerland).

The Standard Reference Material (SRM) 968e (fat-soluble vitamins, carotenoids, and cholesterol in human serum) was obtained from NIST (National Institute for Standards and Technology, Gaithersburg, MD, USA). The solvents THF (tetrahydrofuran), hexane and isopropanol, all HPLC grade, were purchased from Sigma-Aldrich (Vale Road, Arklow, Wicklow, Ireland) or Thermo Fisher Scientific (Blanchardstown Corp Pk 2, Ballycoolin, Dublin, Ireland). BHT (butylated hydroxytoluene) was purchased from Sigma-Aldrich.

2.3. Supplement Extraction Method 1: Oil Filled Soft Gel Capsules and Powder Filled Capsules

Sample extraction and preparation were performed under amber light provided by LED lamps installed in our laboratory (Philips BCP473 36xLED-HB/AM 100–277 V) in order to prevent carotenoid isomerization. The antioxidant BHT was added to the extraction solvents to prevent carotenoid degradation. Each supplement was analysed in triplicate i.e., 3 individual capsules were analysed. Single capsules were selected at random and placed in separate 50 mL falcon tubes along with 10 mL of THF. Powder capsules were separated by hand and the contents added to the Falcon tube and an additional 10 mL of THF was added. Oil filled gelatin capsules were pierced with a blade and the contents of the capsule were allowed to mix with the solvent. The blade was washed with 10 mL of THF to reach a final volume of 20 mL. Each tube was vortexed for 10 s, sonicated at 24 °C for 2 min and vortexed again for 10 s, in order to efficiently separate the capsule contents from the shell. The tubes were centrifuged at 4700 rpm at 25 °C without brake to avoid resuspension of the pellet. Dilutions of each tube were then prepared. An aliquot of each dilution was dried in a centrifugal vacuum concentrator (GeneVac MiVac Duo Concentrator, Ipswich, UK) and re-suspended in HPLC mobile phase. The HPLC method is thoroughly described in a previous publication from our group [15]. All products were stored at room temperature in cardboard boxes prior to analysis and between analyses.

2.4. Supplement Extraction Method 2: Beadlet Analysis

Sample extraction and preparation were performed under amber light. The Beadlet products capsule and contents were added to a 50 mL Falcon tube, and then 5 mL of 4% (w/v) ammonium chloride buffer (pH adjusted to 8.6) was added to the capsule contents along with 200 µL of protease K enzyme. Finally 20 mL of THF with 0.1% BHT was added. Each tube was vortexed for 10 s, sonicated for 40 min at 50 °C and then vortexed again for 10 s, in order to efficiently separate the macular carotenoids from the beadlets and other formulation components. The tubes were centrifuged at 4700 rpm at 25 °C without brake to avoid resuspension of the pellet. Dilutions of each tube were then prepared. An aliquot of each dilution was dried in a centrifugal vacuum concentrator and re-suspended in HPLC mobile phase. One capsule only was used for this analysis. This method was adapted from personal communications received from Professor Neal Craft, President of Craft Technologies.

2.5. High Performance Liquid Chromatography

The analytical method to analyse supplements has been previously published by our group [15]. L, Z and MZ were separated and quantified on an Agilent Technologies (Palo Alto, CA, USA) 1260 Series HPLC system equipped with a Diode Array Detector (DAD, G1315C), binary pump, degasser, thermostatically controlled column compartment, thermostatically controlled high-performance autosampler (G1367E) and thermostatically controlled analytical fraction collector. For system control and data processing, the software ChemStation (Agilent Technologies) was used. The standard injection volume was 10 µL. Carotenoid quantification was performed using a Daicel Chiralpak IA-3 column, composed of amylose tris (3,5-dimethylphenylcarbamate) bonded to a 3 µm silica gel (250 × 4.6 mm i.d.; Chiral Technologies Europe, Cedex, France). The column was protected with a guard column containing a guard cartridge with the same chemistry of the column. Isocratic elution was performed with hexane and isopropanol (90:10, v/v) and a flow rate of 0.5 mL min^{-1}. The column temperature was set at 25 °C. The LOQ for L and Z was assessed as the lowest concentration which achieved less than 5% RSD from 9 replicate injections (L = 57.4 pmol, Z = 3.3 pmol) [32].

3. Results

3.1. Oil Filled Soft Gel Capsules

All the oil filled soft gel capsules were in close concordance with their label claim for L (98–122%); however, Z and MZ concentration in these supplements were either close to or consistently higher than label claim (Z: 117–162% and MZ: 97–319%). These data are presented in Tables 1 and 2 as well as Figures 3 and 4. One company, Puritans Pride, who sell the Lutigold Extra supplement, declared Z and MZ on the product label, but did not specify the concentration of these carotenoids.

Table 1. Macular carotenoid concentration of the commercially available supplements analysed.

Supplement Name	Type	Batch Number	Expiry	Time to Expiry at Time of Testing (Months)	Macular Carotenoid (mg/Capsule)	
					Declared	Measured x̄ ± SD
MacuSafe	1	12603	June 2019	28	L→10	1.92 ± 0.09
					Z→2	1.14 ± 0.02
					MZ→12	9.66 ± 0.28
Eye Vitality Plus	1	13577	August 2019	31	L→15	4.35 ± 0.42
					Z→2	1.46 ± 0.06
					MZ→10	8.32 ± 0.59
Vision Alive	1	424951	June 2018	14	L→10	7.38 ± 0.27
					Z→nc	1.24 ± 0.02
					MZ→nc	1.58 ± 0.04
MacuSave	2	3001777	August 2019	35	L→10	11.01 ± 0.13
					Z→2	3.23 ± 0.02
					MZ→10	9.67 ± 0.11
Doctors Best	2	16052523A	December 2019	32	L→20	21.33 ± 1.39
					Z→2	2.35 ± 0.30
					MZ→1	3.19 ± 0.19
Lutigold Extra	2	462536-02	August 2019	27	L→20	19.65 ± 1.02
					Z→nq	2.14 ± 0.15
					MZ→nq	3.05 ± 0.11
MacuHealth	2	C1600284	September 2019	25	L→10	11.32 ± 0.06
					Z→2	2.72 ± 0.18
					MZ→10	12.60 ± 0.26
MacuShield	2	120480	March 2017	4	L→10	12.24 ± 0.41
					Z→2	11.98 ± 0.43
					MZ→10	13.21 ± 0.48
Maxivision *	3	33690818	None	No expiry date on product	L→10	10.82
					Z→2	3.68
					MZ→10	11.19

1 = powder filled capsule 2 = oil filled soft gel gelatin capsule 3 = powder filled beadlet formulation. nc = not claimed on product label n/a = not applicable nq = not quantified on label * Supplement extraction method 2: Beadlet analysis (*n* = 1). The oil filled soft gel capsules analysed included: MacuSave (Zeon healthcare Ltd., Oxfordshire, UK), Doctor's Best (Doctor's Best Inc., San Clemente, CA, USA), Lutigold Extra (Puritans Pride Inc., Oakdale, NY, USA), MacuHealth LMZ³ (MacuHealth, Birmingham, MI, USA), and MacuShield (Alliance Pharma PLC, Wiltshire, UK). The powder filled capsules analysed included: MacuSafe (OcuSci, Del Mar, CA, USA), Eye Vitality Plus (Green Valley Hyperion LLC, Lexington, VA, USA) and Vision Alive (Holistic Labs Ltd., Hollywood, FL, USA). The beadlet formulation analysed was: MaxiVision (MedOp Health Inc., Oldsmar, FL, USA). One capsule of MaxiVision was analysed; the rest of the supplements were analysed in triplicate.

Table 2. Re-analysis of macular carotenoid concentration of the commercially available supplements analysed after storage.

Supplement Name	Storage Time Months	Type	Batch Number	Expiry	Time to Expiry at Time of Testing (Months)	Macular Carotenoid (mg/Capsule)	
						Declared	Measured x̄ ± SD
MacuSafe	5	1	12603	June 2019	23	L→10 Z→2 MZ→12	0.0 ± 0.0 0.0 ± 0.0 0.0 ± 0.0
Eye Vitality Plus	6	1	13577	August 2019	25	L→15 Z→2 MZ→10	0.84 ± 0.02 0.84 ± 0.02 2.00 ± 0.19
Vision Alive	3	1	424951	June 2018	11	L→10 Z→nd MZ→nd	6.48 ± 0.27 1.14 ± 0.05 1.52 ± 0.01
MacuSave	8	2	3001777	August 2019	25	L→10 Z→2 MZ→10	10.39 ± 0.18 3.74 ± 0.17 9.69 ± 0.33
Doctors Best	3	2	16052523A	December 2019	29	L→20 Z→2 MZ→1	21.74 ± 0.65 2.38 ± 0.09 3.09 ± 0.08
Lutigold Extra	2	2	462536-02	August 2019	25	L→20 Z→nq MZ→nq	19.05 ± 0.70 1.99 ± 0.08 2.97 ± 0.06
MacuHealth	5	2	C1600284	March 19	20	L→10 Z→2 MZ→10	11.58 ± 0.39 2.98 ± 0.05 13.21 ± 0.48
MacuShield	3	2	120480	March 2017	1	L→10 Z→2 MZ→10	11.75 ± 0.41 2.15 ± 0.17 12.02 ± 0.27

1 = powder filled capsule 2 = oil filled soft gel gelatin capsule. nd = not detected. Storage time in months is the time between initial analysis and subsequent re-analysis. The oil filled soft gel capsules analysed included: MacuSave (Zeon healthcare Ltd., Oxfordshire, UK), Doctor's Best (Doctor's Best Inc., San Clemente, CA, USA), Lutigold Extra (Puritans Pride Inc., Oakdale, NY, USA), MacuHealth LMZ[3] (MacuHealth, Birmingham, MI, USA), and MacuShield Alliance Pharma PLC (Wiltshire, UK). The powder filled capsules analysed included: MacuSafe (OcuSci, Del Mar, CA, USA), Eye Vitality Plus (Green Valley Hyperion LLC, Lexington, VA, USA) and Vision Alive (Holistic Labs Ltd., Hollywood, FL, USA). All supplements were analysed in triplicate.

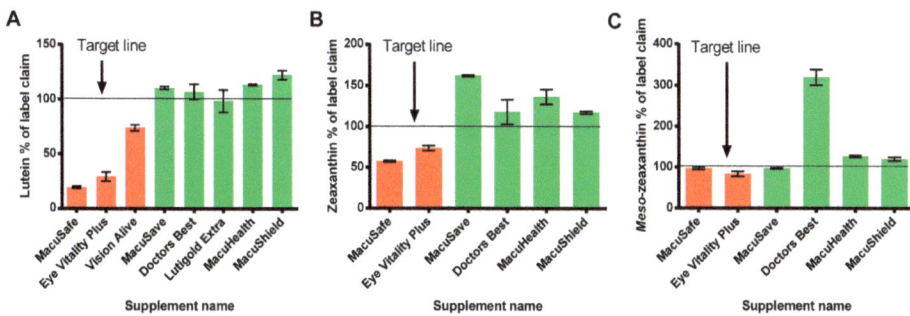

Figure 3. Initial time point analysis illustrating concentration of L (**A**) Z (**B**) and MZ (**C**) expressed as a % of label claim for each product analysed (powder filled capsules are in red, oil filled capsules are in green). Vision Alive and Lutigold products are not shown in (**B**) and (**C**), as these products made no label claim regarding the concentration of Z and MZ. All supplements were analysed in triplicate.

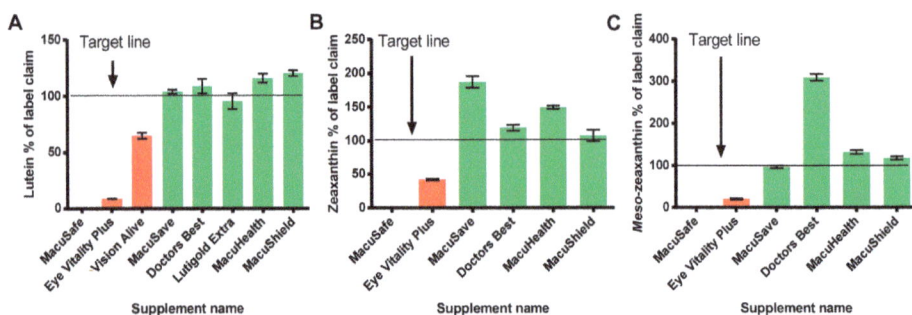

Figure 4. Second time point analysis illustrating concentration of L (**A**) Z (**B**) and MZ (**C**) expressed as a % of label claim for each product analysed (powder filled capsules are in red, oil filled capsules are in green). Vision Alive and Lutigold products are not shown in (**B**) and (**C**) as these products made no label claim regarding the concentration of Z and MZ. All supplements were analysed in triplicate.

3.2. Powder Filled Capsules

For powder filled capsules, none of the products achieved label claim for L (19–74%), Z (57–73%) or MZ (83–97%). These data are presented in Tables 1 and 2 as well as Figures 3 and 4. One company, Holistic labs Ltd. (Hollywood, FL, USA) who sell the Vision Alive supplement did not declare Z or MZ on the product label, but these carotenoids were present in their supplement (albeit in small concentrations).

3.3. Powder Filled Beadlet Capsules

The carotenoid contents of this product (MaxiVision) did meet or were above their label claim amount for L, Z and MZ (108.2%, 184.0% and 111.9% respectively, see Table 1 and Figure 3). However, in order to extract the carotenoids from this formulation, we needed to use a more aggressive extraction technique (see above, Section 2.4).

3.4. Stability of Carotenoid Supplements

To determine if the products were stable over time, we reanalyzed the same batch of each supplement (from the same container) after a number of months (see Table 2). In brief, the oil filled carotenoid supplements yielded similar results to the initial analysis; but the powder filled capsules exhibited a reduction in carotenoid concentration (see Table 2 and Figure 4).

4. Discussion

Our experiment confirms that oil filled carotenoid products match or are above their label claim, whereas powder filled carotenoid products do not meet their label claim. Moreover, we identified that oil filled carotenoid products are stable overtime, but powder filled carotenoid products are not.

One of the powder filled carotenoid products (MacuSafe), which the initial analysis showed was not in agreement with the products label claim (% of label claim: L:19.2%, Z:57.0% and MZ: 96.6%) degraded to 0% carotenoid content for each carotenoid within five months, and therefore patients consuming this product would have received no carotenoid intervention/benefit. Of note, this product was still within its expiry date (Expiry June 2019). Also, the other powder filled products degraded over time, but the oil filled soft gel gelatin capsules were stable over time. The results obtained from this experiment are consistent with previous research performed on commercially available carotenoid supplements [15,27,33]. In these previous studies, a large proportion of the supplements analysed did not meet label claim; also, MZ and Z were present in supplements tested although these nutrients were not listed on the label of the product. As observed previously by our group, this experiment identified a large discrepancy between the amount of Z claimed on the product label (for oil and powder). For example, Prado-Cabrero reported that the Z% of label claim varied between 47 and 248%, and in the current study we report that the Z% of label claim ranged from 57 to 319%. The most likely explanation for the lower than claimed concentrations of the carotenoids in these supplements is due to degradation caused by oxidation. It is known that carotenoids react with oxygen via one of three possible mechanisms: oxidation, electron transfer or hydrogen abstraction [34,35]. Interestingly, this is consistent with our results as in the powder formulations L appeared to be consistently lower than MZ and Z in these products, and also appeared to be less stable over time (from our reanalysis, Table 2). In other words, it appears that L is more susceptible to oxidation than Z and MZ and this finding is consistent with the chemistry of the molecules. In brief, the structure of the Z and MZ carotenoid isomers makes them less sensitive to oxygen due to the presence of a double beta ring, whereas in L the presence of a beta and an epsilon ring appears to make this carotenoid more reactive to oxygen [36].

It is likely that the products that exhibited higher concentrations of L, Z and MZ than their label claim was simply due to the fact that these companies added more than required at formulation stage. This is known to occur in the food supplement industry where companies endeavor to ensure label claim is met, or (in some cases) where accurate measurement of the formulation is not performed.

Of note, only one of the powder filled formulations exhibited good results, but this formulation (MaxiVision) provides the carotenoids in a beadlet. For food supplements, beadlets are typically used to protect sensitive molecules (e.g., carotenoids) from degradation (e.g., from oxygen) [37]. There are a variety of functions and purposes of beadlets. For example, beadlets may provide for the separate containment of ingredients within the dietary supplement to improve the stability of the entrapped ingredients. However, very little is known about the bioavailability of these beadlet carotenoid formulations, and clinical trials in human subjects are needed to provide evidence regarding the efficacy of these formulations. Indeed, even for our analysis the analytical procedure required to extract L, Z and MZ from the beadlets was far more aggressive than that required for the oil filled soft gel capsule or the powder filled carotenoid capsules. In brief, extraction of the carotenoids from the beadlets required high temperature control (50 °C), long sonication times, and the use of digestive enzymes (protease), parameters not required to extract the carotenoids from the oil or powder formulations.

5. Conclusions

The data presented in this study provides important information concerning carotenoid food supplements. We confirm that a number of commerically available carotenoid food supplements do not achieve their label claim. The evidence from this study is that oil filled soft gel capsules are the best way to provide a stable carotenoid supplement for the consumer. At present, clinicians and consumers are not adequately informed via product labelling, and the food supplement industry does not appear to have sufficient regulations in place to protect the consumer from clinically untested, unstable or degraded products. However, it is also important to point out that there are quality and effective carotenoid products on the market, which have scientific evidence to back up their claims of label and efficacy. In other words, it is our view that clinicians and consumers should select macular carotenoid products which have appropriate scientific evidence confirming product stability and efficacy. The current experiment confirms the importance of using carotenoid interventions in oil based formulas, rather than powder filled formulas.

Acknowledgments: The authors wish to acknowledge the Howard Foundation, (Registered UK Charity No. 285822), Iosa (Industrial Orgánica S.A., Monterrey, Nuevo León, Mexico), MacuHealth LLC™ (Birmingham, MI, USA) and Alliance Pharma plc (Chippenham, Wiltshire, UK) for the financial support of this research. The Principal Investigator (JMN) is also funded by the European Research Council (CREST Grant No. 281096).

Author Contributions: David Phelan conceived and designed the experiments, performed the experiments and analyzed the data. David Phelan wrote the paper with Alfonso Prado-Cabrero and John M. Nolan.

Conflicts of Interest: D.P. is a Howard Fellow, and his research program is supported by the Howard Foundation (English Charity reg. number 285822) via a grant from IOSA (Industrial Orgánica S.A., Monterrey, Nuevo León, Mexico), MacuHealth LLC™ (Birmingham, MI, USA) and Alliance Pharma plc (Chippenham, Wiltshire, UK); all of the above organizations have an interest in commercially available supplements containing the macular carotenoids. APC was the previous incumbent of the Howard fellowship within the NRCI but currently has no conflict of interest. JMN does consultancy work for nutraceutical companies as a director of Nutrasight Consultancy Ltd. The sponsors had no involvement in study design, collection, analysis or interpretation of data, in the writing of the manuscript or in the decision to submit the article for publication.

References

1. Hammond, B.R., Jr.; Johnson, E.J.; Russell, R.M.; Krinsky, N.I.; Yeum, K.J.; Edwards, R.B.; Snodderly, D.M. Dietary modification of human macular pigment density. *Investig. Ophthalmol. Vis. Sci.* **1997**, *38*, 1795–1801.
2. Hirsch, J.; Curcio, C.A. The spatial resolution capacity of human foveal retina. *Vis. Res.* **1989**, *29*, 1095–1101. [CrossRef]
3. Naguib, Y.M.A. Antioxidant activities of astaxanthin and related carotenoids. *J. Agric. Food Chem.* **2000**, *48*, 1150–1154. [CrossRef] [PubMed]
4. Snodderly, D.M. Evidence for protection against age-related macular degeneration by carotenoids and antioxidant vitamins. *Am. J. Clin. Nutr.* **1995**, *62*, 1448s–1461s. [PubMed]
5. Snodderly, D.M.; Auran, J.D.; Delori, F.C. The macular pigment. II. Spatial distribution in primate retinas. *Investig. Ophthalmol. Vis. Sci.* **1984**, *25*, 674–685.
6. Bone, R.A.; Landrum, J.T.; Hime, G.W.; Cains, A.; Zamor, J. Stereochemistry of the human macular carotenoids. *Investig. Ophthalmol. Vis. Sci.* **1993**, *34*, 2033–2040.
7. Hammond, B.R., Jr.; Wooten, B.R.; Snodderly, D.M. Preservation of visual sensitivity of older subjects: Association with macular pigment density. *Investig. Ophthalmol. Vis. Sci.* **1998**, *39*, 397–406.
8. Howarth, P.A.; Bradley, A. The longitudinal chromatic aberration of the human eye, and its correction. *Vision Res.* **1986**, *26*, 361–366. [CrossRef] [PubMed]
9. Li, B.; Ahmed, F.; Bernstein, P.S. Studies on the singlet oxygen scavenging mechanism of human macular pigment. *Arch. Biochem. Biophys.* **2010**, *504*, 56–60. [CrossRef] [PubMed]
10. Johnson, E.J.; Maras, J.E.; Rasmussen, H.M.; Tucker, K.L. Intake of lutein and zeaxanthin differ with age, sex, and ethnicity. *J. Am. Diet. Assoc.* **2010**, *110*, 1357–1362. [CrossRef] [PubMed]
11. Nebeling, L.C.; Forman, M.R.; Graubard, B.I.; Snyder, R.A. Changes in carotenoid intake in the United States: The 1987 and 1992 national health interview surveys. *J. Am. Diet. Assoc.* **1997**, *97*, 991–996. [CrossRef]
12. Maoka, T.; Arai, A.; Shimizu, M.; Matsuno, T. The first isolation of enantiomeric and meso-zeaxanthin in nature. *Comp. Biochem. Physiol. B* **1986**, *83*, 121–124. [CrossRef]
13. Khachik, F.; de Moura, F.F.; Zhao, D.Y.; Aebischer, C.P.; Bernstein, P.S. Transformations of selected carotenoids in plasma, liver, and ocular tissues of humans and in nonprimate animal models. *Investig. Ophthalmol. Vis. Sci.* **2002**, *43*, 3383–3392.
14. Nolan, J.M.; Beatty, S.; Meagher, K.A.; Howard, A.N.; Kelly, D.; Thurnham, D.I. Verification of *Meso*-zeaxanthin in fish. *J. Food Process. Technol.* **2014**, *5*, 335. [CrossRef] [PubMed]
15. Prado-Cabrero, A.; Beatty, S.; Howard, A.; Stack, J.; Bettin, P.; Nolan, J.M. Assessment of lutein, zeaxanthin and *Meso*-zeaxanthin concentrations in dietary supplements by chiral high-performance liquid chromatography. *Eur. Food Res. Technol.* **2016**, *242*, 599–608. [CrossRef] [PubMed]
16. Nolan, J.; Meagher, K.; Kashani, S.; Beatty, S. What is meso-zeaxanthin, and where does it come from? *Eye* **2013**, *27*, 899–905. [CrossRef] [PubMed]
17. Bernstein, P.S.; Li, B.; Vachali, P.P.; Gorusupudi, A.; Shyam, R.; Henriksen, B.S.; Nolan, J.M. Lutein, zeaxanthin, and meso-zeaxanthin: The basic and clinical science underlying carotenoid-based nutritional interventions against ocular disease. *Prog. Retin. Eye Res.* **2016**, *50*, 34–66. [CrossRef] [PubMed]
18. Nolan, J.M.; Power, R.; Stringham, J.; Dennison, J.; Stack, J.; Kelly, D.; Moran, R.; Akuffo, K.O.; Corcoran, L.; Beatty, S. Enrichment of macular pigment enhances contrast sensitivity in subjects free of retinal disease: Central retinal enrichment supplementation trials—Report 1. *Investig. Ophthalmol. Vis. Sci.* **2016**, *57*, 3429–3439. [CrossRef] [PubMed]
19. Akuffo, K.; Nolan, J.; Howard, A.; Moran, R.; Stack, J.; Klein, R.; Klein, B.; Meuer, S.; Sabour-Pickett, S.; Thurnham, D.; et al. Sustained supplementation and monitored response with differing carotenoid formulations in early age-related macular degeneration. *Eye* **2015**, *29*, 902–912. [CrossRef] [PubMed]

20. Connolly, E.E.; Beatty, S.; Loughman, J.; Howard, A.N.; Louw, M.S.; Nolan, J.M. Supplementation with all three macular carotenoids: Response, stability, and safety. *Investig. Ophthalmol. Vis. Sci.* **2011**, *52*, 9207–9217. [CrossRef] [PubMed]

21. Connolly, E.E.; Beatty, S.; Thurnham, D.I.; Loughman, J.; Howard, A.N.; Stack, J.; Nolan, J.M. Augmentation of macular pigment following supplementation with all three macular carotenoids: An exploratory study. *Curr. Eye Res.* **2010**, *35*, 335–351. [CrossRef] [PubMed]

22. Ma, L.; Liu, R.; Du, J.H.; Liu, T.; Wu, S.S.; Liu, X.H. Lutein, zeaxanthin and meso-zeaxanthin supplementation associated with macular pigment optical density. *Nutrients* **2016**, *8*, 426. [CrossRef] [PubMed]

23. Meagher, K.A.; Thurnham, D.I.; Beatty, S.; Howard, A.N.; Connolly, E.; Cummins, W.; Nolan, J.M. Serum response to supplemental macular carotenoids in subjects with and without age-related macular degeneration. *Br. J. Nutr.* **2013**, *110*, 289–300. [CrossRef] [PubMed]

24. Nolan, J.M.; Stringham, J.M.; Beatty, S.; Snodderly, D.M. Spatial profile of macular pigment and its relationship to foveal architecture. *Investig. Ophthalmol. Vis. Sci.* **2008**, *49*, 2134–2142. [CrossRef] [PubMed]

25. Thurnham, D.; Nolan, J.; Howard, A.; Beatty, S. Macular response to supplementation with differing xanthophyll formulations in subjects with and without age-related macular degeneration. *Graefes Arch. Clin. Exp. Ophthalmol.* **2015**, *253*, 1231–1243. [CrossRef] [PubMed]

26. Crosby-Nwaobi, R.; Hykin, P.; Peto, T.; Sivaprasad, S. An exploratory study evaluating the effects of macular carotenoid supplementation in various retinal diseases. *Clin. Ophthalmol.* **2016**, *10*, 835–844. [PubMed]

27. Breithaupt, E.D.; Schlatterer, J. Lutein and Zeaxanthin in New Dietary Supplements—Analysis and Quantification. *Eur. Food Res. Technol.* **2005**, *220*, 648–652. [CrossRef]

28. Guidance for Industry: Current Good Manufacturing Practice in Manufacturing, Packaging, Labeling, or Holding Operations for Dietary Supplements; Small Entity Compliance Guide. Available online: https://www.fda.gov/food/guidanceregulation/guidancedocumentsregulatoryinformation/ dietarysupplements/ucm238182.htm (accessed on 31 August 2017).

29. Hu, M.; Jacobsen, C. *Oxidative Stability and Shelf Life of Foods Containing Oils and Fats*; Elsevier Science: Amsterdam, The Netherlands, 2016.

30. Gullapalli, R.P. Soft gelatin capsules (softgels). *J. Pharm. Sci.* **2010**, *99*, 4107–4148. [CrossRef] [PubMed]

31. Shimidzu, N.; Goto, M.; Miki, W. Carotenoids as singlet oxygen quenchers in marine organisms. *Fish. Sci.* **1996**, *62*, 134–137. [CrossRef]

32. Prado-Cabrero, A.; Beatty, S.; Stack, J.; Howard, A.; Nolan, J.M. Quantification of zeaxanthin stereoisomers and lutein in trout flesh using chiral high-performance liquid chromatography-diode array detection. *J. Food Compost. Anal.* **2016**, *50*, 19–22. [CrossRef] [PubMed]

33. Aman, R.; Bayha, S.; Carle, R.; Schieber, A. Determination of carotenoid stereoisomers in commercial dietary supplements by high-performance liquid chromatography. *J. Agric. Food Chem.* **2004**, *52*, 6086–6090. [CrossRef] [PubMed]

34. Britton, G. Structure and properties of carotenoids in relation to function. *FASEB J.* **1995**, *9*, 1551–1558. [PubMed]

35. Boon, C.S.; McClements, D.J.; Weiss, J.; Decker, E.A. Factors influencing the chemical stability of carotenoids in foods. *Crit. Rev. Food Sci. Nutr.* **2010**, *50*, 515–532. [CrossRef] [PubMed]

36. Miller, N.J.; Sampson, J.; Candeias, L.P.; Bramley, P.M.; Rice-Evans, C.A. Antioxidant activities of carotenes and xanthophylls. *FEBS Lett.* **1996**, *384*, 240–242. [CrossRef]

37. Deshpande, J. Stable Beadlets of Lipophilic Nutrients. U.S. Patent 2005/0095301 A1, 5 May 2005.

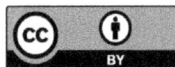

nutrients

MDPI

Article

Short-Term Effects of a Ready-to-Drink Pre-Workout Beverage on Exercise Performance and Recovery

P. Blaise Collins [1], Conrad P. Earnest [1,2], Ryan L. Dalton [1], Ryan J. Sowinski [1], Tyler J. Grubic [1], Christopher J. Favot [1], Adriana M. Coletta [1], Christopher Rasmussen [1], Mike Greenwood [1] and Richard B. Kreider [1,*]

[1] Exercise and Sport Nutrition Lab, Human Clinical Research Facility, Texas A&M University, College Station, TX 77843, USA; blaise_collins@tamu.edu (P.B.C.); conradearnest@exchange.tamu.edu (C.P.E.); ryanldalton@exchange.tamu.edu (R.L.D.); ryansowinski6@gmail.com (R.J.S.); tylergrubic@tamu.edu (T.J.G.); cfavot@tamu.edu (C.J.F.); AMColetta@mdanderson.org (A.M.C.); crasmussen@tamu.edu (C.R.); mgreenwood26@tamu.edu (M.G.)
[2] Nutrabolt, Bryan, 3891 S. Traditions Drive, Bryan, TX 77807, USA
* Correspondence: rbkreider@tamu.edu; Tel.: +1-979-4581498

Received: 5 June 2017; Accepted: 27 July 2017; Published: 1 August 2017

Abstract: In a double-blind, randomized and crossover manner, 25 resistance-trained participants ingested a placebo (PLA) beverage containing 12 g of dextrose and a beverage (RTD) containing caffeine (200 mg), β-alanine (2.1 g), arginine nitrate (1.3 g), niacin (65 mg), folic acid (325 mcg), and Vitamin B12 (45 mcg) for 7-days, separated by a 7–10-day. On day 1 and 6, participants donated a fasting blood sample and completed a side-effects questionnaire (SEQ), hemodynamic challenge test, 1-RM and muscular endurance tests (3×10 repetitions at 70% of 1-RM with the last set to failure on the bench press (BP) and leg press (LP)) followed by ingesting the assigned beverage. After 15 min, participants repeated the hemodynamic test, 1-RM tests, and performed a repetition to fatigue (RtF) test at 70% of 1-RM, followed by completing the SEQ. On day 2 and 7, participants donated a fasting blood sample, completed the SEQ, ingested the assigned beverage, rested 30 min, and performed a 4 km cycling time-trial (TT). Data were analyzed by univariate, multivariate, and repeated measures general linear models (GLM), adjusted for gender and relative caffeine intake. Data are presented as mean change (95% CI). An overall multivariate time $\times$ treatment interaction was observed on strength performance variables ($p = 0.01$). Acute RTD ingestion better maintained LP 1-RM (PLA: -0.285 (-0.49, -0.08); RTD: 0.23 (-0.50, 0.18) kg/kg$_{FFM}$, $p = 0.30$); increased LP RtF (PLA: -2.60 (-6.8, 1.6); RTD: 4.00 (-0.2, 8.2) repetitions, $p = 0.031$); increased BP lifting volume (PLA: 0.001 (-0.13, 0.16); RTD: 0.03 (0.02, 0.04) kg/kg$_{FFM}$, $p = 0.007$); and, increased total lifting volume (PLA: -13.12 (-36.9, 10.5); RTD: 21.06 (-2.7, 44.8) kg/kg$_{FFM}$, $p = 0.046$). Short-term RTD ingestion maintained baseline LP 1-RM (PLA: -0.412 (-0.08, -0.07); RTD: 0.16 (-0.50, 0.18) kg/kg$_{FFM}$, $p = 0.30$); LP RtF (PLA: 0.12 (-3.0, 3.2); RTD: 3.6 (0.5, 6.7) repetitions, $p = 0.116$); and, LP lifting volume (PLA: 3.64 (-8.8, 16.1); RTD: 16.25 (3.8, 28.7) kg/kg$_{FFM}$, $p = 0.157$) to a greater degree than PLA. No significant differences were observed between treatments in cycling TT performance, hemodynamic assessment, fasting blood panels, or self-reported side effects.

Keywords: resistance training; dietary supplement; sport nutrition; ergogenic aid

---

1. Introduction

Ready-to drink (RTD) pre-workout supplements and energy drinks have been purported to improve exercise performance and/or cognitive function [1–3]. These supplements typically contain combinations of various purported ergogenic nutrients including carbohydrate, caffeine, amino acids, creatine, beta-alanine, vasodilators (e.g., nitrates, L-citrulline, L-arginine), nutrients purported to improve concentration (e.g., citicoline), and various vitamins [3–6]. Recent position stands from the International Society of Sports Nutrition (ISSN) concluded that consuming energy drinks primarily containing caffeine and beta alanine can approve acute exercise performance, cognitive function, and/or training adaptations [3,7,8]. More recently, ingestion of nitrates prior to exercise has been reported to improve endurance exercise efficiency and high-intensity exercise performance [9–13]. Consequently, there has been interest in examining the individual and synergistic effects of ingesting pre-workout supplements and/or energy drinks prior to exercise and during training [3,6]. Additionally, to assess the acute and short-term safety of adding these types of supplements to the normal diet, at the absolute doses recommended, as this is the typical way consumers take these supplements. This study examined the use of an RTD version of a market leading pre-workout supplement containing caffeine anhydrous (200 mg), beta-alanine (2.1 g), arginine nitrate (1.3 g), niacin (65 mg), folic acid (325 mcg) and cobalamin (45 mcg) on indices of muscular strength and endurance.

In brief, caffeine has been shown to improve mental acuity, maximal strength, maximal power, and muscular endurance when taken acutely at doses of 3 to 9 mg/kg [7,14–18]. For example, doses as low as 5 mmol of nitrates (310 mg) have been shown to enhance sprint performance and increase time to fatigue [19–21]. β-alanine has been reported to improve strength and endurance performance typically when ingested at doses of 4 to 6 g/day for several weeks [8]. Similarly, L-arginine has been reported to activate the nitric oxide synthase pathway, resulting in vasodilation and enhanced blood flow to working tissues [22]. However, less is known about the combination of arginine and nitrate [23–27]. The rationale of combining these two ingredients is to enhance the bioavailability of L-arginine; hence potentially increasing an overall ergogenic effect [6].

Recent work from our group has demonstrated that combining various combinations of caffeine, nitrate, creatine, and β-alanine as part of a pre-workout powdered drink formula had some positive effects on cognitive and/or exercise performance [28–30]. The aim of this study was to examine the effects of consuming a "ready-to-drink" (RTD) version of a market leading pre-workout supplement. Our primary outcome was the assessment of exercise performance recovery after acute and short-term supplementation, while the secondary outcome was assessment of acute and short-term safety. We hypothesize that the RTD studied would improve resistance-exercise performance recovery and 4 km cycling time-trial (TT) performance without undue alterations in hepatorenal and muscle enzyme function, hemodynamic response to a hemodynamic challenge, or self-reported side effects.

2. Materials and Methods

2.1. Study Overview

Prior to starting the study, approval was obtained from the Texas A&M University Institutional Review Board (#2016-754F). Although not required, we also registered the study with clinicatrials.gov (#NCT03032549). Recreationally active men and women between the ages 18–40 years were recruited to participate in this study through the campus email system as well as posting flyers throughout the university. Participants responding to recruitment advertisements were initially screened by phone to determine general eligibility. Inclusion criteria required that each participant have at least six months of resistance training experience immediately prior to entering the study, inclusive of bench press and leg press or squat training. Participants were excluded from participation if they had a history of treatment for metabolic disease (i.e., diabetes), hypertension, hypotension, thyroid disease, arrhythmias, and/or cardiovascular disease; if they were currently using any prescription medication with the exception of birth control; if they were pregnant, lactating, or planned to become pregnant within the next month; if they had a history of smoking; if they drank excessively (>12 drinks per week); or, if they had a recent history of consuming dietary supplements or energy drinks containing β-alanine or high amounts of caffeine within eight weeks of the start of supplementation.

Figure 1 presents the general study design. Participants meeting initial phone screening conditions were invited to attend a familiarization session. During the familiarization session, participants signed informed consent statements and had a physical exam inclusive of providing their medical history, determination of resting heart rate and blood pressure, and assessment of body composition via dual-energy X-ray absorptiometry (DXA) and bioelectrical impedance (BIA). Once cleared to participate, participants had bench one-repetition maximum (1-RM) determined, performed 3 sets of 10 repetitions on the bench press at 70% of 1-RM, with the last set completed to failure. Participants followed a similar familiarization on the leg press and then rested for 15 min prior to performing a warm-up and a 4 km TT on an electronically-braked cycle ergometer. Participants were then randomized to initiate the study with their respective treatments.

Protocol Overview					
	Baseline			Follow-Up	
Familiarization	Day 1	Day 2	Day 3-5	Day 6	Day 7
Physical Exam	BIA	8-h fasting blood sample		BIA	8-h fasting blood sample
Body Weight	8-h fasting blood sample	Side Effects Questionnaire		8-h fasting blood sample	Side Effects Questionnaire
DXA Body Composition	Side Effects Questionnaire	Ingest Supplement		Side Effects Questionnaire	Ingest Supplement
BIA Body Water	Pre-Ingestion Hemodynamic Tilt Test	Wait 30-min		Pre-Ingestion Hemodynamic Tilt Test	Wait 30-min
Bench Press & Leg Press 1RM and 70% 1RM Test	Pre-Ingestion Initial Strength Testing	4-km Time Trial		Pre-Ingestion Initial Strength Testing	4-km Time Trial
Practice 4 km Cycling Time Trial	Ingest Supplement	Side Effects Questionnaire		Ingest Supplement	Side Effects Questionnaire
Schedule Baseline Testing	Wait 30-min			Wait 30-min	
Randomize to Treatment	Post Ingestion Hemodynamic Tilt Test			Post Ingestion Hemodynamic Tilt Test	
	Post Ingestion Recovery Strength Testing			Post Ingestion Recovery Strength Testing	
	Side Effects Questionnaire			Side Effects Questionnaire	

Figure 1. Protocol Overview.

Baseline testing took place on two days. Day 1 included fasting blood, hemodynamic assessment, and strength testing while Day 2 included the 4 km TT. All fasting blood samples were obtained following an 8 h fast primarily between the hours of 0600–0900. Participants performed a pre-supplementation hemodynamic postural challenge test using a tilt table, performed 1-RM and a muscular endurance test (3 sets of 10 repetitions with the last set to failure) on the bench press and leg press. Participants then ingested their assigned RTD, waited 15 min and were placed in the supine position on the tilt table for 15 min prior to performing the postural hemodynamic challenge test. Participants then repeated the 1-RM test and one-set to failure at 70% of 1-RM on the bench press and leg press to assess recovery. The rationale for this approach was to determine whether ingestion of the RTD would influence exercise capacity after exhaustive exercise and toward the end of a training session. On Day 2, participants ingested the assigned treatment, waited 30 min, performed a standard warm-up, and performed a 4 km cycling TT. Participants continued the supplementation protocol for Days 3 to 5 and then returned to the laboratory for follow-up testing on Day 6 and Day 7 to repeat experiments as described.

2.2. Supplementation Protocol

Participants were instructed to maintain normal training, diet, and caffeine intake habits throughout the study. Participants were assigned in a randomized, double-blind, cross-over manner to a placebo (PLA) beverage containing 6.0 g dextrose and non-caloric sweetener or a beverage (RTD) containing caffeine anhydrous (200 mg), β-alanine (2.1 g), niacin (65 mg), folic acid (325 mcg), Vitamin B12 (45 mcg), arginine nitrate (1.3 g providing about 350 mg of nitrates and 950 mg of arginine). A 7 to 10 days washout period was observed between treatment experiments consistent with prior research on caffeine and nitrates using crossover designs. The beverages were prepared by a third party (South East Bottling and Beverage, Dade City, FL, USA) in 10 oz. of purified water matched for color and flavor in indistinguishable bottles. The nutrient contents of the RTD's were analyzed for contaminants and nutrient content by Century Foods International (Sparta, WI, USA). The pre-packaged bottles were received in boxes containing sealed bottles generically labeled as "Treatment A" and "Treatment B" for double-blind administration. The supplement code was maintained in a sealed envelope and was not disclosed to the researchers until the completion of the study for statistical analysis.

2.3. Test Methodology

2.3.1. Anthropometry & Body Composition

Standardized anthropological testing included assessments for body mass and height on a Healthometer Professional 500KL (Pelstar LLC, Alsip, IL, USA) self-calibrating digital scale with an accuracy of ±0.02 kg. Total body water was determined under standardized conditions using an ImpediMed DF50 bioelectrical impedance analyzer (ImpediMed, San Diego, CA, USA). Whole body bone density and body composition measures (excluding cranium) were determined with a Hologic Discovery W Dual-Energy X-ray Absorptiometer (Hologic Inc., Waltham, MA, USA) equipped with APEX Software (APEX Corporation Software, Pittsburg, PA, USA) by using standardized procedures [31,32]. Mean test-retest reliability studies performed on male athletes in our lab over repeated standardized assessment procedures have demonstrated coefficients of variation for total bone mineral content and total fat free/soft tissue mass of 0.31–0.45% with a mean intraclass correlation of 0.985 [32]. On the day of each test, the equipment was calibrated following the manufacturer's guidelines.

2.3.2. Blood Collection Procedures

Participants provided an 8 h fasted blood sample via venipuncture of an antecubital vein in the forearm in accordance with standard phlebotomy procedures. Approximately 10 mL of whole blood was collected at the beginning of each testing day, in one 7.5 mL BD Vacutainer® serum separation tube (Becton, Dickinson and Company, Franklin Lakes, NJ, USA) and in one 3.5 mL BD Vacutainer® K_2 EDTA tube (Becton, Dickinson and Company, Franklin Lakes, NJ, USA). Both tubes sat at room temperature for 15 min, then the 7.5 mL serum separation tube was centrifuged at 3500-rpm for 10 min using a 4 °C refrigerated bench top ThermoScientific Heraeus MegaFuge 40R Centrifuge (Thermo Electron North America LLC, West Palm Beach, FL, USA). Both tubes were stored at 4 °C for 3 to 4 h prior to analysis or storage. Serum was stored at −80 °C in polypropylene microcentrifuge tubes for later analysis.

2.3.3. Blood Chemistry

Blood serum samples were analyzed for the following: alkaline phosphatase (ALP), aspartate transaminase (AST), alanine transaminase (ALT), creatinine, blood urea nitrogen (BUN), creatine kinase (CK), lactate dehydrogenase (LDH), glucose, total cholesterol, high density lipoprotein (HDL), low density lipoprotein (LDL), and triglycerides (TG) using a Cobas® c111 (Roche Diagnostics, Basel, Switzerland) automated clinical chemistry analyzer. The Cobas® c111 automated clinical chemistry analyzer was calibrated daily per manufacturer guidelines. This analyzer has been known to be valid and reliable in previously published reports [33]. The internal quality control for the Cobas® c111 is performed using two levels of control fluids purchased from the manufacturer to calibrate acceptable standard deviation (SD) and coefficient of variation (C_V) values for all assays. Samples were re-run if the values observed were outside control values and/or clinical norms according to standard procedures. Prior analysis in our lab has yielded test-to-test reliability of a range of CV from 0.4 to 2.4% for low control samples and 0.6–1.9% on high controls. Precision has been found between 0.8 and 2.4% on low controls and 0.5–1.7% on high controls.

2.3.4. Hemodynamic Challenge Test

During the strength testing days (Days 1 and 6) participants had hemodynamic response assessed at two time points, prior to initial strength testing measures and following supplementation. Participants were placed on a standard tilt table in a supine position (Gravity 4000 Inversion Table; City of Industry, CA, USA). After 15 min, blood pressure and heart rate were assessed and recorded. Next, the tilt table was adjusted to vertical where the participant rested for 2 min and the metrics were re-assessed. Participants then performed pre-supplementation muscular strength and endurance tests, ingested the assigned treatment, and rested for 15 min prior to be placing on the tilt table in the supine position for 15 min. Heart rate and blood pressure measurements were then taken prior to and after 2 min of being moved to a vertical position. Mean arterial pressure was calculated as $((2 \times DBP) + SBP)/3$ as an indicator of venous return. Rate pressure product (RPP) was calculated as the product of heart rate times systolic blood pressure and represents an indirect assessment of myocardial oxygen demand. We chose these latter two tests as they represent a more robust response to a cardiovascular challenge compared to heart rate or blood pressure alone. Hemodynamic response was defined as the change in systolic blood pressure, diastolic blood pressure, heart rate, mean arterial pressure and rate pressure product from the supine to upright position.

2.3.5. Self-Reported Side Effects

The side effect questionnaires were completed before and after each testing session to access perceived side effects and monitor compliance with the supplementation protocol. The questionnaires were completed a total of 16 times by each participant over the duration of the study: two times each testing day for four testing days per supplement for two different supplements. Participants were asked to rank the frequency and severity of their symptoms—dizziness, headache, tachycardia, heart skipping or palpitations, shortness of breath, nervousness, blurred vision, and unusual or adverse effects. Participants were asked to rank their perception of symptoms using the following scale: 0 (none), 1 (minimal: 1–2/week), 2 (slight: 3–4/week), 3 (occasional: 5–6/week), 4 (frequent: 7–8/week), or 5 (severe: 9 or more/week).

2.3.6. Strength Testing

Participants performed three warm up sets prior to performing 1-RM attempts (i.e., one set of 10 at 50%, one set of 5 at 70%, and one set of 3 at 90% of anticipated 1-RM). Following the warm-up, participants gradually increased weight between 1-RM attempts until they could not lift the load under their own volition. Following determination of 1-RM, participants performed two sets of 10 repetitions with 2 min rest recovery between sets at the closest bar/leg press weight corresponding to 70% of familiarization session 1-RM. Participants then rested 2 min and performed a third set to failure. After 2 min of rest, participants followed the same procedure to determine leg press 1-RM and leg press muscular endurance. Hand placement on the bench press bar and seat and foot positioning on the leg press were placed in the same position among attempts and testing sessions.

The initial strength tests were performed to pre-fatigue the participant before assessing recovery performance after RTD ingestion. The recovery muscular strength and endurance performance assessment involved performing a 1-RM test and then one set to failure at 70% of the familiarization 1-RM following similar procedures as described above. In this way, the effects of acute RTD ingestion could be assessed on muscular strength and endurance recovery following a standard bout of resistance exercise on Day 1, the effects of 6 days of RTD ingestion could be assessed on initial muscular strength and performance on Day 6, and the effects of acute RTD ingestion on recovery of exhaustive exercise could be assessed after 6 days of supplementation on Day 6. We did not have the participants repeat their performance of 2 sets of 10 repetitions during recovery analysis, as the initial bout of exercise fatigued the participants, it was unlikely participants could complete all 10 repetitions of these sets, and it was unnecessary to assess recovery muscular endurance.

Total 1-RM weight lifted in kg and the number repetitions performed each set using 70% of the familiarization weight (rounded to the nearest 2.27 kg or 5 lbs. that could be put on the bar) were recorded. Total lifting volume was calculated by multiplying the 70% of 1-RM weight lifted times the number of repetitions performed each set and summing the total volume performed for all sets. Total combined lifting volume was calculated by adding the bench press and leg press total lifting volumes. Day to day test reliability of performing this performance test in our lab on resistance-trained participants has yielded a CV of 0.34 and an intraclass correlation coefficient of 0.99 for three sets of bench press total lifting volume and an intraclass correlation coefficient of 0.96 for three sets of leg press total lifting volume.

2.3.7. Time-Trial Performance

Time-trial performance was examined on a magnetically braked cycle ergometer (Lode Sport Excalibur, Groningen, The Netherlands) over a distance of 4 km. Participants were allowed a one minute warm up with a gradually increasing load. At the completion of the warm up, a standardized resistance (4 J/kg/rev) was applied and the participant was instructed to complete the distance in as short a time as able. Upon completion, the participant was instructed to continue at a slow pace to facilitate recovery. Data were recorded as time to completion and average power in Watt.

2.4. Statistical Analysis

Data were analyzed using IBM® SPSS® Version 24 software (IBM Corp., Armonk, NY, USA). The sample size was determined based on the expectation of a five percent improvement in exercise performance and corresponding power of 0.80. The analysis was initiated by inspecting data for missing values using Little's test for data missing completely at random (MCAR). This analysis showed the data were MCAR ($p = 1.0$, <1.5%) and subsequently replaced using a multiple imputation algorithm. Data were then analyzed using univariate, multivariate and repeated measures general linear models (GLM) using gender and relative caffeine intake (mg/kg) as covariates using the following models.

Model 1. The cohort was examined for potential gender-by-treatment effects, finding none. Hence, the data were pooled into one cohort instead of reporting gender data separately.

Model 2. Since menstrual cycle, birth control medications, and other gender-related parameters were not controlled, gender was included as a covariate.

Model 3. Given the weight difference between males and females in the study, we further adjusted our analysis for relative caffeine intake (mg/kg). Herein, we present the results for Model 3 with performance-related data expressed in absolute and relative terms to fat free mass.

Data were also examined for a treatment order effect to confirm that randomization procedures were effective. Least significant difference post hoc comparisons were used to compare between-treatment differences when significant time × treatment interaction effects were observed. Hematological variables were also examined relative to normal clinical limits to examine the frequency of changes in hematology outside of normal, clinical limits from baseline to follow-up using a Chi-square and adjusted residual analyses. This analyses examined the likelihood of excursions outside of clinical limits for each treatment as follows: (1) No change; (2) Normal at Baseline, High at Follow-up; (3) High at Baseline, High at Follow-up; (4) High at Baseline, Normal at Follow-up. Data are reported as mean (SD), mean change from baseline and 95% confidence intervals, and frequency of occurrence according to the chi-square analysis. Data were considered statistically significant when the probability of type I error was 0.05 or less while tendencies towards statistical significance were noted when *p*-levels were $p > 0.05$ to $p < 0.10$.

3. Results

3.1. Participants

Thirty-one individuals initially signed informed consent prior to data collection; however, five individuals dropped out prior to baseline testing due to schedule or personal reasons. Twenty-six participants began the study, with one male dropping out after the first baseline session due to time constraints. Data from a total of 25 participants were included in statistical analysis. Participant demographic data are presented in Table 1. These data demonstrate that the participants were recreationally active resistance-trained individuals and that participants differed based on gender on a number of variables. No time × gender × treatment interactions were observed on variables evaluated or relative caffeine intake effect. Further, the fully adjusted statistical model did not produce a substantial difference to the unadjusted model. Nevertheless, since menstrual cycle and birth control medication was not controlled, results were adjusted via covariate analysis for gender and relative caffeine intake.

Table 1. Baseline Demographics.

Measurement	Male ($n = 12$)	Female ($n = 13$)	Overall ($n = 25$)	
	Mean SD	Mean SD	Mean SD	*p*-Values
Age (year)	23.3 ± 4	24.5 ± 4	23.9 ± 4	0.43
Height (cm)	177 ± 7	166 ± 5	171 ± 8	0.00
Weight (kg)	81.7 ± 13	65.1 ± 8	73.1 ± 13	0.00
Body Mass Index (kg/m^2)	26.0 ± 4	23.7 ± 3	24.8 ± 4	0.12
Body Fat (%)	17.2 ± 6	28.4 ± 6	23.0 ± 8	0.00
Fat Free Mass (kg)	67.1 ± 9	47.8 ± 8	57.1 ± 13	0.00
Bench Press 1RM (kg)	88.3 ± 27	37.9 ± 10	62.1 ± 32	0.00
Bench Press 1RM (kg/kg$_{FFM}$)	1.31 ± 0.4	0.80 ± 0.2	1.05 ± 0.4	0.00
Leg Press 1RM (kg)	455 ± 175	284 ± 89	366 ± 160	0.01
Leg Press 1RM (kg/kg$_{FFM}$)	6.7 ± 2.0	6.0 ± 1.6	6.3 ± 1.8	0.18

Mean data presented as means ± SD. One-way ANOVA *p*-values listed for each variable. PLA: placebo, RTD: ready-to-drink pre-workout supplement, 1RM: one repetition maximum, FFM: fat free mass, kg/kg$_{FFM}$: weight relative to participant fat free mass.

3.2. Performance

Table 2 presents muscular strength and performance results normalized to fat free mass (FFM). Multivariate analysis revealed a significant overall Wilks' Lambda treatment × time interaction effect ($p = 0.01$). Univariate analysis revealed significant treatment × time interactions in bench press ($p = 0.04$) and leg press repetitions to failure ($p = 0.04$) while bench press lifting volume ($p = 0.09$) and total combined lifting volume ($p = 0.09$) tended to interact. Post-hoc analysis revealed that acute RTD ingestion on Day 1 significantly improved recovery bench press muscular endurance to a greater degree than following PLA ingestion. Pair-wise differences were also observed between treatments in Day 1 recovery leg press endurance ($p = 0.01$) and tended to improve leg press lifting volume ($p = 0.054$). No significant differences were observed between groups in follow-up assessments. Similar findings were observed when analyzing absolute performance results. No significant differences were observed among treatments in cycling performance time or average power output expressed in absolute (*W*) or relative (W/kg$_{FFM}$) terms (Table 3).

Table 2. Strength and Muscular Endurance Relative to Fat Free Mass.

Variable	Treatment	Day 1 Pre-Ingestion Mean SD	Day 1 Post Ingestion Mean SD	Day 6 Pre-Ingestion Mean SD	Day 6 Post Ingestion Me SD	Treatment Mean SE		p-Value
BP 1-RM (kg/kgFFM)	PLA	1.02 ± 0.38	0.94 ± 0.36	1.01 ± 0.36	0.97 ± 0.37	0.99 ± 0.06	Time	0.001
	RTD	1.03 ± 0.37	0.99 ± 0.35	1.04 ± 0.35	1.00 ± 0.36	1.02 ± 0.06	Trt	0.72
	Time	1.02 ± 0.37	0.97 ± 0.35 *	1.03 ± 0.35	0.99 ± 0.36 ‡		I	0.23
BP Repetitions to Failure @ 70% 1RM	PLA	9.96 ± 3.23	9.60 ± 3.65	10.13 ± 3.37	12.27 ± 3.22 *	10.5 ± 0.71	Time	0.38
	RTD	10.28 ± 4.37	12.32 ± 5.28 *†	10.30 ± 4.04	13.31 ± 4.86 *	11.6 ± 0.71	Trt	0.27
	Time	10.1 ± 3.81	11.0 ± 4.70	10.2 ± 3.69	12.8 ± 4.12		I	0.04
BP Lifting Volume (kg/kgFFM)	PLA	7.40 ± 3.77	7.46 ± 4.57	7.46 ± 3.73	9.17 ± 4.44	7.87 ± 0.67	Time	0.36
	RTD	7.45 ± 3.75	8.89 ± 4.07	7.48 ± 3.16	9.45 ± 3.54	8.32 ± 0.67	Trt	0.64
	Time	7.43 ± 3.73	8.17 ± 4.34	7.47 ± 3.42	9.31 ± 3.98		I	0.09
LP 1-RM (kg/kgFFM)	PLA	6.70 ± 1.66	6.41 ± 1.58	6.80 ± 1.38	6.38 ± 1.35	6.57 ± 0.26	Time	0.66
	RTD	6.72 ± 1.42	6.74 ± 1.41	6.83 ± 1.29	6.67 ± 1.52	6.74 ± 0.26	Trt	0.66
	Time	6.71 ± 1.53	6.57 ± 1.49	6.81 ± 1.33	6.53 ± 1.43		I	0.04
LP Repetitions to Failure @ 70% 1RM	PLA	21.2 ± 10.8	18.6 ± 8.4	20.8 ± 10.7	20.9 ± 11.0	20.3 ± 1.81	Time	0.78
	RTD	22.4 ± 15.1	26.4 ± 13.0 †	19.8 ± 9.31	25.1 ± 14.1	23.9 ± 1.80	Trt	0.17
	Time	21.8 ± 13.0	22.5 ± 11.6	20.3 ± 9.94	23.0 ± 12.7		I	0.11
LP Lifting Volume (kg/kgFFM)	PLA	94.3 ± 77.9	81.1 ± 44.4	88.3 ± 49.7	91.9 ± 57.9	88.9 ± 10.60	Time	0.75
	RTD	96.6 ± 66.7	116.3 ± 74.9 ‡	90.7 ± 47.6	106.9 ± 55.4	102.6 ± 10.60	Trt	0.37
	Time	95.5 ± 71.8	98.7 ± 63.5	89.5 ± 48.2	99.4 ± 56.6		I	0.11
Combined Lifting Volume (kg/kgFFM)	PLA	101.7 ± 79.0	88.6 ± 46.8	95.8 ± 50.5	101.1 ± 60.2	96.8 ± 10.87	Time	0.76
	RTD	104.1 ± 66.4	125.2 ± 75.5 †	98.2 ± 48.8	116.4 ± 57.3	111.0 ± 10.87	Trt	0.36
	Time	102.9 ± 72.2	106.9 ± 64.9	97.0 ± 49.2	108.8 ± 58.7		I	0.09

Values are means ± standard deviations. Multivariate analysis revealed overall Wilks' Lambda treatment ($p = 0.792$), time ($p = 0.010$), and treatment × time ($p = 0.010$). Greenhouse-Geisser p-levels are reported with univariate analyses for time, treatment, and time × treatment interactions for each variable. * indicates a significant difference from initial measure, † indicates a significant between-treatment difference, and ‡ indicates a statistical trend between-treatments. BP = bench press, LP = leg pres, 1-RM = 1 repetition maximum, R FFM = Fat Free Mass, TBPV = Total Bench Press Volume, TLPV = Total Leg Press Volume, TCLV = Total Combined Lifting Volume, PLA = Placebo, RTD = Ready-to-drink Pre-workout supplement, Trt = Treatment, I = Time × Treatment interaction.

Nutrients **2017**, *9*, 823

Table 3. Time Trial Performance.

Variable	Treatment	Day 2 Mean SD	Day 7 Mean SD	Treatment Mean SE		p-Values
Time (s)	PLA	296 ± 105	284 ± 104	240 ± 11	Time	0.70
	RTD	282 ± 94	276 ± 95	281 ± 11	Trt	0.56
	Time	289 ± 99	280 ± 99		I	0.41
Power (W)	PLA	224 ± 82	242 ± 93	235 ± 10	Time	0.12
	RTD	238 ± 85	246 ± 95	240 ± 10	Trt	0.62
	Time	231 ± 83	244 ± 82		I	0.26
Power (W/kg$_{FFM}$)	PLA	3.87 ± 0.89	4.16 ± 0.94	4.01 ± 0.17	Time	0.26
	RTD	4.17 ± 0.87	4.29 ± 0.98	4.23 ± 0.17	Trt	0.38
	Time	4.02 ± 0.89	4.22 ± 0.95		I	0.25

Values are means ± standard deviations. Multivariate analysis revealed overall Wilks' Lambda treatment ($p = 0.62$), time ($p = 0.036$), and treatment × time ($p = 0.53$). Greenhouse-Geisser p-levels are reported with univariate analyses for time, treatment, and time × treatment interactions for each variable. PLA = Placebo, RTD = Ready-to-drink Pre-workout supplement, FFM = Fat Free Mass, Trt = Treatment, I = Time × Treatment interaction.

Figures 2–5 show mean changes from baseline with 95% CI's for 1-RM, repetitions to failure (RtF), lifting volume, and time-trial performance data, respectively. Acute RTD ingestion tended to maintain BP 1-RM to a greater degree (PLA: −0.071 (−0.09, −0.05); RTD: −0.043 (−0.05, −0.01) kg/kg$_{FFM}$, $p = 0.086$) and maintained leg press 1-RM performance (PLA: −0.285 (−0.49, −0.08); RTD: 0.23 (−0.50, 0.18) kg/kg$_{FFM}$, $p = 0.30$) compared to PLA (Figure 2). After 6 days of supplementation, recovery LP 1-RM significantly decreased in the PLA but not RTD treatment (PLA: −0.412 (−0.08, −0.07); RTD: 0.16 (−0.50, 0.18) kg/kg$_{FFM}$, $p = 0.30$). As noted in Figure 3, recovery RtF on the BP tended to be greater in the RTD versus PLA treatment on Day 1 (PLA: −4.41 (−5.8, −3.0); RTD: −2.59 (−4.0, −1.19) repetitions, $p = 0.072$) while LP RtF was significantly greater than PLA (PLA: −2.60 (−6.8, 1.6); RTD: 4.00 (−0.2, 8.2) repetitions, $p = 0.031$). On Day 6, RtF on the LP was significantly increased above baseline in the RTD group but not PLA (PLA: 0.12 (−3.0, 3.2); RTD: 3.6 (0.5, 6.7) repetitions, $p = 0.116$). Bench press lifting volume (Figure 4) was significantly increased above baseline and was significantly greater than PLA (PLA: 0.001 (−0.13, 0.16); RTD: 0.03 (0.02, 0.04) kg/kg$_{FFM}$, $p = 0.007$) while LP lifting volume tended to be greater (PLA: −13.18 (−36.9, 10.5); RTD: 19.6 (−4.1, 43.3) kg/kg$_{FFM}$, $p = 0.055$) in the RTD treatment on Day 1. On Day 6, LP lifting volume was increased above baseline values in the RTD but not PLA treatment (PLA: 3.64 (−8.8, 16.1); RTD: 16.25 (3.8, 28.7) kg/kg$_{FFM}$, $p = 0.157$). Recovery total lifting volume was significantly greater in the RTD treatment compared to PLA (PLA: −13.12 (−36.9, 10.5); RTD: 21.06 (−2.7, 44.8) kg/kg$_{FFM}$, $p = 0.046$) on Day 1 and was increased above baseline while remaining unchanged with PLA treatment on Day 6 (PLA: 5.35 (−7.4, 18.1); RTD: 18.22 (5.5, 30.9) kg/kg$_{FFM}$, $p = 0.157$). Finally, as seen in Figure 5, cycling performance times and power output improved to a greater degree in the PLA trial from baseline (PLA: −11.48 (−22.3, −1.73); RTD: −5.72 (−15.5, 4.03) s; PLA: 0.289 (0.09, 0.49); RTD: 0.122 (−0.08, 0.32) W/kg$_{FFM}$). However, it should be noted that baseline and follow-up performance times were faster in the RTD trials than the PLA trials (see Table 3) so it cannot be concluded that the RTD promoted an ergolytic effect.

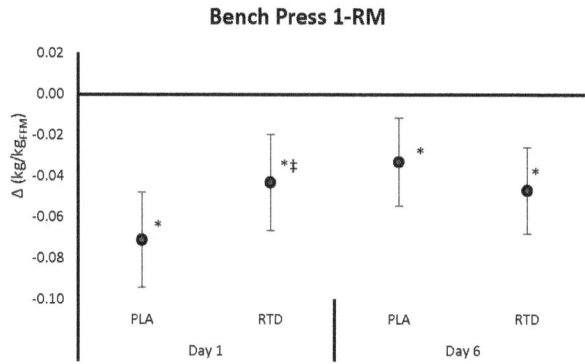

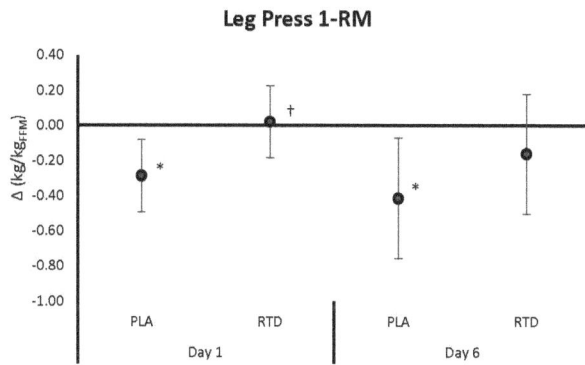

Figure 2. Data present mean change (95% CI) in bench press (Panel **A**) and leg press (Panel **B**) one repetition maximum (1-RM) from baseline. Confidence intervals not crossing zero are statistically significant ($p < 0.05$). * Represents $p < 0.05$ difference from baseline, † represents $p < 0.05$ difference between treatments. ‡ Represents $p < 0.05$ to 0.10 tendency towards significance between treatments.

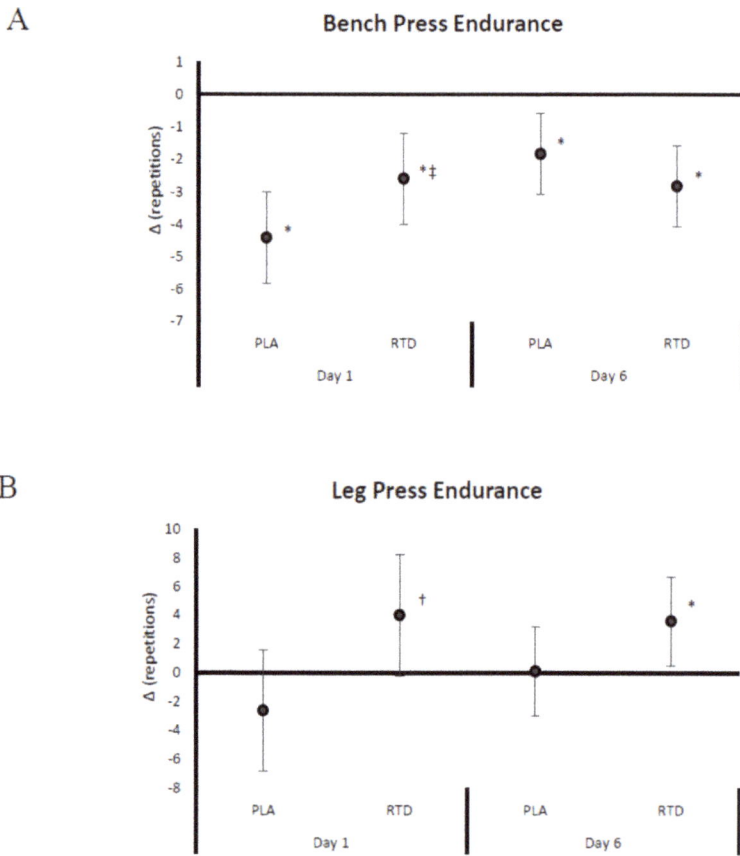

Figure 3. Data present mean change (95% CI) in bench press (**A**); and leg press (**B**) muscular endurance repetitions to failure at 70% of one repetition maximum (1-RM) from baseline. Confidence intervals not crossing zero are statistically significant ($p < 0.05$). * Represents $p < 0.05$ difference from baseline, † represents $p < 0.05$ difference between treatments. ‡ Represents $p > 0.05$ to 0.10 tendency towards significance between treatments.

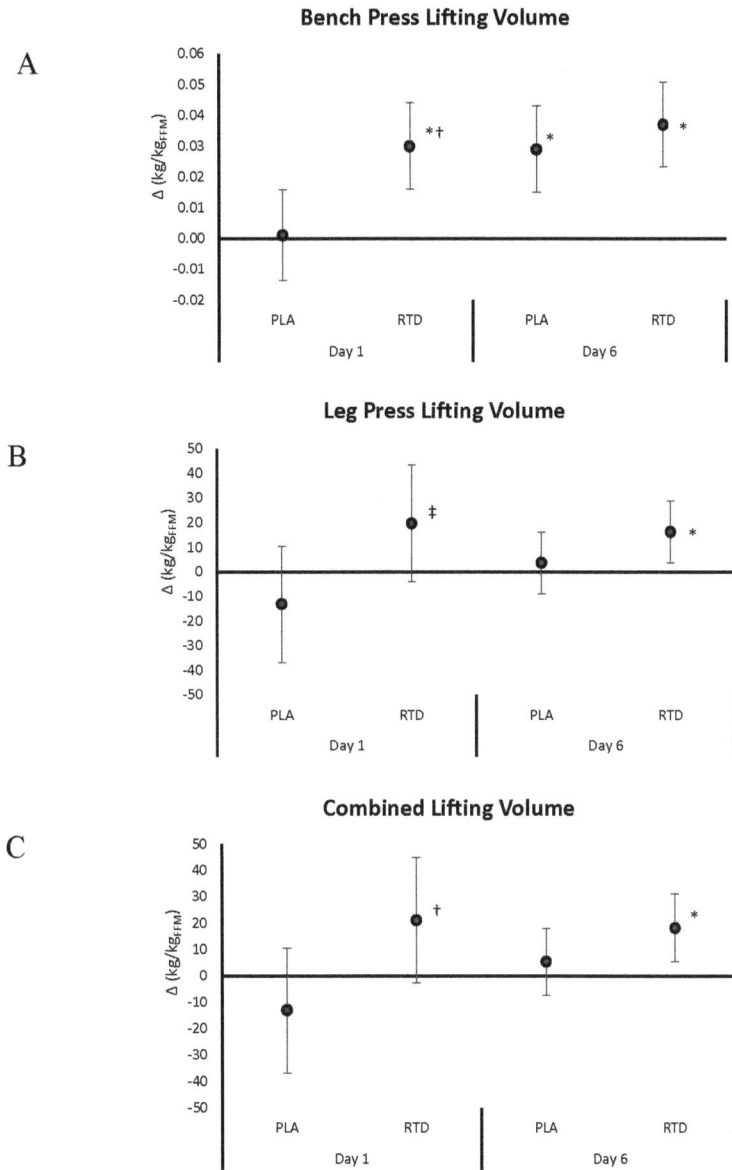

Figure 4. Data present mean change (95% CI) in bench press (**A**); leg press (**B**) and total (combined) lifting volume; (**C**) from baseline. Confidence intervals not crossing zero are statistically significant ($p < 0.05$). * Represents $p < 0.05$ difference from baseline, † represents $p < 0.05$ difference between treatments. ‡ Represents $p > 0.05$ to 0.10 tendency towards significance between treatments.

A

Time Trial Performance

B

Time Trial Performance

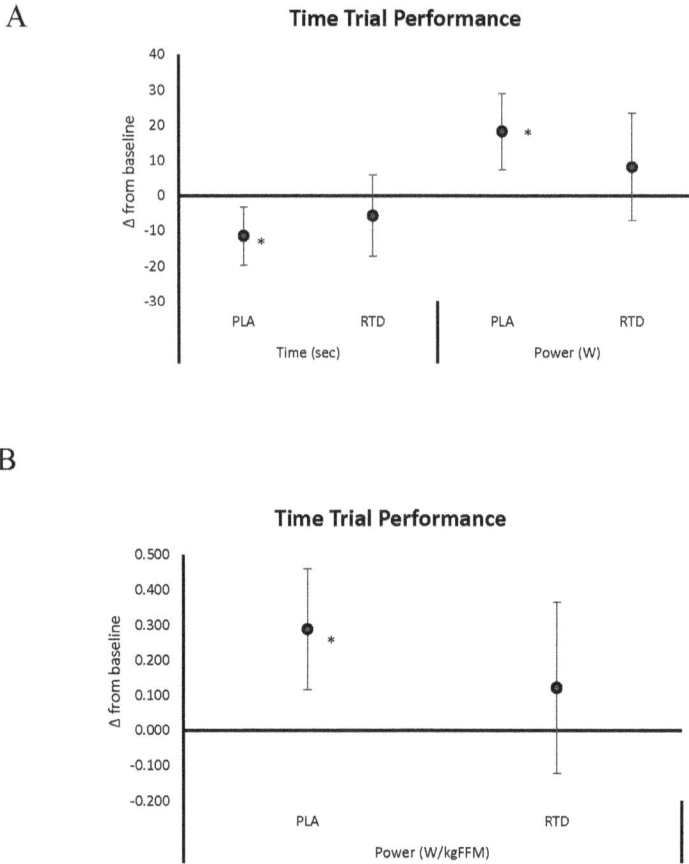

Figure 5. Data present mean change (95% CI) in 4 km time-trial performance from baseline expressed in completion time and absolute power output (**A**); and relative power output (**B**). Confidence intervals not crossing zero are statistically significant ($p < 0.05$). * represents $p < 0.05$ difference from baseline.

3.3. Safety Analysis

Table S1 presents hemodynamic challenge results. Although some time effects were observed as expected when changing postural position, no significant overall multivariate interaction effects ($p = 0.15$) or univariate interaction effects were observed between treatments in HR, SBP, DBP, MAP, or RPP. Blood pressure and heart rate values observed remained low and were well within normal values for apparently healthy younger individuals. Similarly, no overall multivariate or univariate effects were observed among serum or whole blood markers analyzed (Tables S2–S4) or when analyzing the frequency of changes in blood parameters outside of normal clinical ranges (Table S5). Finally, as shown in Tables S6 and S7, no significant differences were observed between treatments in perceived side effects monitored (i.e., headache, dizziness, tachycardia, palpitations, dyspnea, nervousness, or blurred vision).

4. Discussion

The aim of this study was to examine whether acute and/or short-term term ingestion of a commercially available pre-workout RTD beverage would affect workout performance, hemodynamic reactivity, and/or hematological affects during a 7 days intervention period. Overall, there was some evidence of better maintenance of recovery 1-RM and improvement in recovery muscular endurance with acute (Day 1) and short-term (Day 6) RTD supplementation. These findings suggest that acute and/or short-term ingestion of this RTD beverage may provide ergogenic benefit after a short recovery from resistance-training. However, ingestion of this RTD had no effects on 4 km cycling time-trial performance. Additionally, we observed no evidence that acute or short-term ingestion of this RTD negatively affected hemodynamic responses to a standardized hemodynamic challenge, fasting blood makers, or perceived side effects. Based on these findings, we accept our hypotheses that the RTD studied would improve resistance-exercise performance and recovery following pre-exhaustive exercise without undue alterations in hepatorenal and muscle enzyme function, hemodynamic responses to a postural challenge, or self-reported side effects. However, we found no evidence that acute and/or short-term ingestion of this RTD affected 4 km cycling time-trial performance in non-trained cyclists. The following discussion provides additional insight as to results observed.

4.1. Performance

Caffeine is a well-known for improving cognitive and exercise performance [7,16,34]. The general recommendation is that individuals consume between 3–9 mg/kg of caffeine in order to promote ergogenic benefit in terms of exercise [7]. However, a number of studies have reported that ingestion of absolute or relative doses of caffeine in doses less than 200 mg or 3 mg/kg improved exercise performance [7,14,35–40]. Caffeine is a primary ingredient in pre-workout supplements and drinks that have also been reported to enhance cognitive and/or exercise performance [3]. For example, Souza et al. [34] performed a meta-analysis of caffeine-containing energy drinks and reported that consumption of these products promoted significant improvements in muscle strength and endurance (ES = 0.49), endurance performance (ES = 0.53), jumping (ES = 0.29) and sport-specific actions (ES = 0.51), but not in sprinting (ES = 0.14).

In the present study, participants consumed 200 mg of caffeine providing relative caffeine intake of 2.51 ± 0.4 mg/kg for males and 3.1 ± 0.5 mg/kg for the females. While the relative doses of caffeine contained in the RTD studied were slightly less than recommendations, we found that ingesting this RTD prior to exercise (acute) and/or for 6 days (short-term) promoted better maintenance of 1-RM strength and muscle endurance. These findings support our prior reports [28–30] as well as previous studies reporting ergogenic benefits of consuming caffeine containing energy drinks on exercise and/or cognitive performance [14,35–40]. It is possible that since caffeine was ingested with other nutrients, there may be synergistic effects thereby reducing the need to ingest as much caffeine [3]. For example, Souza and colleagues [34] reported that consuming energy drinks with taurine may have a greater impact on efficacy than the caffeine content. While taurine was not contained in the RTD studied in the present study, results provided evidence of some ergogenic benefit. However, not all studies have reported that ingestion of caffeine containing pre-workout supplements improve performance. For example, Hendrix et al. [41] examined the effects of ingesting a pre-workout supplement containing 400 mg of caffeine, 67 mg of capsicum, and 10 mg of bioperine on performance. The researchers found that ingestion of the pre-workout supplement had no effect on bench or leg press 1-RM or time to exhaustion when cycling at 80% of maximal power output.

A number of studies have reported that ingestion of about 300 mg of nitrates prior to exercise can improve exercise performance [6,13,17]. Most of the initial research on nitrate supplementation focused on the impact of nitrates on improving submaximal exercise efficiency [17,18,42,43]. However, there has been more recent interest in examining the effects of nitrate supplementation on high-intensity intermittent exercise performance [9–11,44–48]. These studies generally demonstrate that nitrate supplementation prior to exercise can affect endurance and high-intensity intermittent exercise performance. For this reason, addition of nitrates to pre-workout supplements have also been of interest [9,12,23,28–30,46,49–53]. Results of the present study support prior reports indicating that acute and/or short-term ingestion of supplements containing nitrates prior to exercise can affect muscular strength and/or endurance. However, in contrast to recent findings [9,12,23,29,46,51–53], we did not find that ingesting the RTD containing nitrates prior to exercise enhanced short duration time-trial performance. The contrasting results may be related to greater variability in studying non-trained cyclists, differences in the dosages and/or timing of ingestion of the nitrate containing RTD, or use of arginine nitrate rather than other forms of nitrates.

4.2. Safety

The primary concerns related to ingesting pre-workout supplements containing caffeine and/or nitrates is the potential safety impact on cardiovascular and hemodynamic responses to exercise [3,54–57]. This was the primary reason for testing hemodynamic reactivity prior to and following resistance training exercise, as participants regularly move from a supine to standing position and, as such, could be prone to reactive hypotension accompanying RTD supplementation during exercise. In the present study, we found no evidence that ingestion of the RTD study adversely affects heart rate or blood pressure responses to a standardized postural challenge. Accordingly, we found no evidence to suggest that acute and/or short-term ingestion of this RTD significantly affected the hematological variables studied or the incidence of self-reported side effects. Consequently, the acute and short-term use of this RTD appears to be safe within the dosages and manner it was assessed in the current study. These findings are consistent with our prior studies with supplementation periods as long as 8 weeks [28–30,52], as well as other similar studies [58,59].

4.3. Strengths and Limitations

A strength of our study is that we used a fairly large cohort comprised of men and women who ingested their respective treatments in addition to their normal diet in a randomized double blind, cross-over manner. Additionally, our protocol was vigorous with regard to the number of exercises performed during testing and applicable as typical resistance-training sessions are comprised of multiple sets of multiple exercises. Thus, the design used allowed for a practical assessment of the ability of resistance-trained participants to maintain performance throughout a rigorous workout. A strength of this study was also that we examined a mixed cohort of men and women in a crossover manner. While this does not discount the possibility that gender differences may exist when using a larger or single-gender study protocol, we used gender as a covariate to account for gender differences. Finally, a strength of this study was that we made a concerted effort to examine several parameters associated with safety by examining potential hemodynamic changes accompanying supplementation and exercise as well as a thorough analysis of hepatorenal and muscle enzyme function associated with the supplementation protocol. Assessment of the cardiovascular and hemodynamic responses to a postural challenge represents a similar pattern of movement as would take place during resistance training, as athletes often go from supine to standing positions throughout a workout and may experience orthostatic hypotension. Moreover, another strength of this study was that we extended the traditional reporting schema of most trials to include potential changes out of normal clinical ranges, without adverse consequence.

Potential limitations in our study included the utilization of recommended absolute serving sizes rather than relative doses to body weight or fat-free mass. It is possible that more consistent performance results would have been observed if relative doses were used. However, this is not how these types of supplements are consumed so we decided to use normal serving sizes and control for this limitation by using relative caffeine intake as a covariate in our analysis. Additionally, although we have examined the effects of ingesting pre-workout supplements for up to 8 weeks, this study only assessed the acute and short-term effects. It is possible that the ergogenic benefits may lessen with longer periods of supplementation due to habituation, but research in this arena is limited. However, RTD products are marketed as having an immediate effect on performance without requiring a loading period or alterations in diet, so we feel this design was a practical analysis of how individuals may use this type of supplement. Another potential limitation was that we examined the effects of this RTD on

Nutrients **2017**, *9*, 823

recreationally-active resistance-trained participants. While this population was well-prepared to assess changes in muscular strength and endurance performance, they were not trained cyclists accustomed to performing sprints. Thus, it is conceivable that the lack of effect observed on 4 km cycling time-trial performance may have been affected by a lack of familiarity with cycling, regardless of partaking in a familiarization session. Additional research should examine whether ingestion of this type of RTD may affect sprint and/or high-intensity short-duration sprint performance.

5. Conclusions

Within the limitations of the study, results indicate that the RTD studied provided some ergogenic benefit on recovery from resistance exercise with no apparent side effects observed. However, consumption of this RTD beverage did not affect 4 km cycling TT performance among non-cycling trained participants. Additional research should assess the safety and efficacy of nutrients found in pre-workout supplements so that active individuals can make an informed decision about the whether they should or should not use them during training and/or competition.

Supplementary Materials: The following are available online at www.mdpi.com/2072-6643/9/8/823/s1, Table S1: Hemodynamic Response to Postural Challenge; Table S2: Liver, Kidney, and Muscle Hematological Data; Table S3: Blood Lipids, Macronutrients, and Nitrate data; Table S4: Whole Blood Chemistry; Table S5: Change in blood markers relative to normal clinical limits from Day 1 to Day 7; Table S6: Frequency of Self-Reported Side Effects; Table S7: Severity of Self-Reported Side Effects.

Acknowledgments: We would like to thank all individuals who participated in this study as well as Peter S. Murano (P.S.M), and Aimee G. Reyes for their assistance in this study. This study was supported by Nutrabolt (Bryan, TX, USA) through an unrestricted research grant provided to Texas A & M University. However, the sponsor was not involved in data collection or data entry and there were no restrictions on publication of the data or preparation of this paper. As stated below, competing interests were supervised and managed by a university approved management plan to insure that data were accurately reported.

Author Contributions: P.B.C. served as study coordinator and assisted with data collection, data analysis, and manuscript preparation. R.L.D., R.J.S., T.J.G., and A.M.C. assisted in data collection. C.J.F. assisted in data collection as well as data analysis. C.R. served as lab coordinator and project manager for the study coordinator. C.P.E. served as a scientific liaison to the sponsor, assisted in study design, data analysis and interpretation, and provided comments on the manuscript. However, C.P.E. was not involved in data collection or data entry and there were no restrictions on publication of the data or preparation of this paper. M.G. assisted in study oversight, data, analysis, and manuscript review. R.B.K. obtained the grant, served as study PI and assisted in the design of the study, data analysis, and manuscript preparation. All authors read and approved the final manuscript.

Conflicts of Interest: C.P.E. serves as a paid consultant for Nutrabolt and is a Research Associate in the ESNL. Further, he holds scientific consultancies with Naturally Slim (Dallas, TX, USA) and Catapult Health (Dallas, TX, USA). R.B.K. serves as a university approved scientific advisor for Nutrabolt. P.S.M. served as quality assurance supervisor in accordance to a conflict of interest management plan that was approved by the university's research and compliance office, the internal review board, and office of grants and contracts and monitored by research compliance. Remaining investigators have no competing interests to declare. The results from this study do not constitute endorsement by the authors and/or the institution concerning the nutrients investigated.

References

1. Applegate, E.A.; Grivetti, L.E. Search for the competitive edge: A history of dietary fads and supplements. *J. Nutr.* **1997**, *127*, 869S–873S. [PubMed]
2. Dickinson, A.; Blatman, J.; El-Dash, N.; Franco, J.C. Consumer usage and reasons for using dietary supplements: Report of a series of surveys. *J. Am. Coll. Nutr.* **2014**, *33*, 176–182. [CrossRef] [PubMed]
3. Campbell, B.; Wilborn, C.; La Bounty, P.; Taylor, L.; Nelson, M.T.; Greenwood, M.; Ziegenfuss, T.N.; Lopez, H.L.; Hoffman, J.R.; Stout, J.R.; et al. International society of sports nutrition position stand: Energy drinks. *J. Int. Soc. Sports Nutr.* **2013**, *10*, 1. [CrossRef] [PubMed]
4. Kreider, R.B.; Kalman, D.S.; Antonio, J.; Ziegenfuss, T.N.; Wildman, R.; Collins, R.; Candow, D.G.; Kleiner, S.M.; Almada, A.L.; Lopez, H.L. International society of sports nutrition position stand: Safety and efficacy of creatine supplementation in exercise, sport, and medicine. *J. Int. Soc. Sports Nutr.* **2017**, *14*, 18. [CrossRef] [PubMed]

5. Bruce, S.E.; Werner, K.B.; Preston, B.F.; Baker, L.M. Improvements in concentration, working memory and sustained attention following consumption of a natural citicoline-caffeine beverage. *Int. J. Food Sci. Nutr.* **2014**, *65*, 1003–1007. [CrossRef] [PubMed]

6. Close, G.L.; Hamilton, D.L.; Philp, A.; Burke, L.M.; Morton, J.P. New strategies in sport nutrition to increase exercise performance. *Free Radic. Biol. Med.* **2016**, *98*, 144–158. [CrossRef] [PubMed]

7. Goldstein, E.R.; Ziegenfuss, T.; Kalman, D.; Kreider, R.; Campbell, B.; Wilborn, C.; Taylor, L.; Willoughby, D.; Stout, J.; Graves, B.S.; et al. International society of sports nutrition position stand: Caffeine and performance. *J. Int. Soc. Sports Nutr.* **2010**, *7*, 5. [CrossRef] [PubMed]

8. Trexler, E.T.; Smith-Ryan, A.E.; Stout, J.R.; Hoffman, J.R.; Wilborn, C.D.; Sale, C.; Kreider, R.B.; Jager, R.; Earnest, C.P.; Bannock, L.; et al. International society of sports nutrition position stand: Beta-alanine. *J. Int. Soc. Sports Nutr.* **2015**, *12*, 30. [CrossRef] [PubMed]

9. Thompson, C.; Wylie, L.J.; Blackwell, J.R.; Fulford, J.; Black, M.I.; Kelly, J.; McDonagh, S.T.; Carter, J.; Bailey, S.J.; Vanhatalo, A.; et al. Influence of dietary nitrate supplementation on physiological and muscle metabolic adaptations to sprint interval training. *J. Appl. Physiol.* **2017**, *122*, 642–652. [CrossRef] [PubMed]

10. Shannon, O.M.; Barlow, M.J.; Duckworth, L.; Williams, E.; Wort, G.; Woods, D.; Siervo, M.; O'Hara, J.P. Dietary nitrate supplementation enhances short but not longer duration running time-trial performance. *Eur. J. Appl. Physiol.* **2017**, *117*, 775–785. [CrossRef] [PubMed]

11. Nyakayiru, J.; Jonvik, K.L.; Trommelen, J.; Pinckaers, P.J.; Senden, J.M.; van Loon, L.J.; Verdijk, L.B. Beetroot juice supplementation improves high-intensity intermittent type exercise performance in trained soccer players. *Nutrients* **2017**, *9*, 314. [CrossRef] [PubMed]

12. Muggeridge, D.J.; Sculthorpe, N.; James, P.E.; Easton, C. The effects of dietary nitrate supplementation on the adaptations to sprint interval training in previously untrained males. *J. Sci. Med. Sport* **2017**, *20*, 92–97. [CrossRef] [PubMed]

13. McMahon, N.F.; Leveritt, M.D.; Pavey, T.G. The effect of dietary nitrate supplementation on endurance exercise performance in healthy adults: A systematic review and meta-analysis. *Sports Med.* **2017**, *47*, 735–756. [CrossRef] [PubMed]

14. Spriet, L.L. Exercise and sport performance with low doses of caffeine. *Sports Med.* **2014**, *44*, S175–S184. [CrossRef] [PubMed]

15. Graham, T.E.; Helge, J.W.; MacLean, D.A.; Kiens, B.; Richter, E.A. Caffeine ingestion does not alter carbohydrate or fat metabolism in human skeletal muscle during exercise. *J. Physiol.* **2000**, *529*, 837–847. [CrossRef] [PubMed]

16. Graham, T.E.; Spriet, L.L. Performance and metabolic responses to a high caffeine dose during prolonged exercise. *J. Appl. Physiol.* **1991**, *71*, 2292–2298. [PubMed]

17. Jones, A.M. Influence of dietary nitrate on the physiological determinants of exercise performance: A critical review. *Appl. Physiol. Nutr. Metab.* **2014**, *39*, 1019–1028. [CrossRef] [PubMed]

18. Jones, A.M.; Vanhatalo, A.; Bailey, S.J. Influence of dietary nitrate supplementation on exercise tolerance and performance. *Nestle Nutr. Inst. Workshop Ser.* **2013**, *75*, 27–40. [PubMed]

19. Kelly, J.; Fulford, J.; Vanhatalo, A.; Blackwell, J.R.; French, O.; Bailey, S.J.; Gilchrist, M.; Winyard, P.G.; Jones, A.M. Effects of short-term dietary nitrate supplementation on blood pressure, O_2 uptake kinetics, and muscle and cognitive function in older adults. *Am. J. Physiol.* **2013**, *304*, R73–R83. [CrossRef] [PubMed]

20. Fulford, J.; Winyard, P.G.; Vanhatalo, A.; Bailey, S.J.; Blackwell, J.R.; Jones, A.M. Influence of dietary nitrate supplementation on human skeletal muscle metabolism and force production during maximum voluntary contractions. *Pflügers Arch.* **2013**, *465*, 517–528. [CrossRef] [PubMed]

21. Thompson, K.G.; Turner, L.; Prichard, J.; Dodd, F.; Kennedy, D.O.; Haskell, C.; Blackwell, J.R.; Jones, A.M. Influence of dietary nitrate supplementation on physiological and cognitive responses to incremental cycle exercise. *Respir. Physiol. Neurobiol.* **2014**, *193*, 11–20. [CrossRef] [PubMed]

22. Nishizaki, K.; Ikegami, H.; Tanaka, Y.; Imai, R.; Matsumura, H. Effects of supplementation with a combination of beta-hydroxy-beta-methyl butyrate, L-arginine, and L-glutamine on postoperative recovery of quadriceps muscle strength after total knee arthroplasty. *Asia Pac. J. Clin. Nutr.* **2015**, *24*, 412–420. [PubMed]

23. Sandbakk, S.B.; Sandbakk, O.; Peacock, O.; James, P.; Welde, B.; Stokes, K.; Bohlke, N.; Tjonna, A.E. Effects of acute supplementation of L-arginine and nitrate on endurance and sprint performance in elite athletes. *Nitric Oxide* **2015**, *48*, 10–15. [CrossRef] [PubMed]

24. Keen, J.T.; Levitt, E.L.; Hodges, G.J.; Wong, B.J. Short-term dietary nitrate supplementation augments cutaneous vasodilatation and reduces mean arterial pressure in healthy humans. *Microvasc. Res.* **2015**, *98*, 48–53. [CrossRef] [PubMed]

25. Bondonno, C.P.; Croft, K.D.; Hodgson, J.M. Dietary nitrate, nitric oxide and cardiovascular health. *Crit. Rev. Food Sci. Nutr.* **2015**, *56*, 2036–2052. [CrossRef] [PubMed]

26. Poortmans, J.R.; Gualano, B.; Carpentier, A. Nitrate supplementation and human exercise performance: Too much of a good thing? *Curr. Opin. Clin. Nutr. Metab. Care* **2015**, *18*, 599–604. [CrossRef] [PubMed]

27. Zhao, Y.; Vanhoutte, P.M.; Leung, S.W. Vascular nitric oxide: Beyond enos. *J. Pharmacol. Sci.* **2015**, *129*, 83–94. [CrossRef] [PubMed]

28. Jung, Y.P.; Earnest, C.P.; Koozehchian, M.; Galvan, E.; Dalton, R.; Walker, D.; Rasmussen, C.; Murano, P.S.; Greenwood, M.; Kreider, R.B. Effects of acute ingestion of a pre-workout dietary supplement with and without *p*-synephrine on resting energy expenditure, cognitive function and exercise performance. *J. Int. Soc. Sports Nutr.* **2017**, *14*, 3. [CrossRef] [PubMed]

29. Jung, Y.P.; Earnest, C.P.; Koozehchian, M.; Cho, M.; Barringer, N.; Walker, D.; Rasmussen, C.; Greenwood, M.; Murano, P.S.; Kreider, R.B. Effects of ingesting a pre-workout dietary supplement with and without synephrine for 8 weeks on training adaptations in resistance-trained males. *J. Int. Soc. Sports Nutr.* **2017**, *14*, 1. [CrossRef] [PubMed]

30. Koozehchian, M.S.; Earnest, C.P.; Jung, Y.P.; Collins, P.B.; O'Connor, A.; Dalton, R.; Shin, S.Y.; Sowinski, R.; Rasmussen, C.; Murano, P.S.; et al. Dose response to one week of supplementation of a multi-ingredient preworkout supplement containing caffeine before exercise. *J. Caffeine Res.* **2017**. [CrossRef]

31. Klesges, R.C.; Ward, K.D.; Shelton, M.L.; Applegate, W.B.; Cantler, E.D.; Palmieri, G.M.; Harmon, K.; Davis, J. Changes in bone mineral content in male athletes. Mechanisms of action and intervention effects. *JAMA* **1996**, *276*, 226–230. [CrossRef] [PubMed]

32. Almada, A.; Kreider, R.; Ransom, J.; Rasmussen, C. Comparison of the reliability of repeated whole body dexa scans to repeated spine and hip scans. *J. Bone Miner. Res.* **1999**, *14*, S369.

33. Levers, K.; Dalton, R.; Galvan, E.; O'Connor, A.; Goodenough, C.; Simbo, S.; Mertens-Talcott, S.U.; Rasmussen, C.; Greenwood, M.; Riechman, S.; et al. Effects of powdered montmorency tart cherry supplementation on acute endurance exercise performance in aerobically trained individuals. *J. Int. Soc. Sports Nutr.* **2016**, *13*, 22. [CrossRef] [PubMed]

34. Souza, D.B.; Del Coso, J.; Casonatto, J.; Polito, M.D. Acute effects of caffeine-containing energy drinks on physical performance: A systematic review and meta-analysis. *Eur. J. Nutr.* **2017**, *56*, 13–27. [CrossRef] [PubMed]

35. Pai, K.M.; Kamath, A.; Goel, V. Effect of red bull energy drink on muscle performance: An electromyographic overview. *J. Sports Med. Phys. Fit.* **2015**, *55*, 1459–1465.

36. Astorino, T.A.; Matera, A.J.; Basinger, J.; Evans, M.; Schurman, T.; Marquez, R. Effects of red bull energy drink on repeated sprint performance in women athletes. *Amino Acids* **2012**, *42*, 1803–1808. [CrossRef] [PubMed]

37. Ivy, J.L.; Kammer, L.; Ding, Z.; Wang, B.; Bernard, J.R.; Liao, Y.H.; Hwang, J. Improved cycling time-trial performance after ingestion of a caffeine energy drink. *Int. J. Sport Nutr. Exerc. Metab.* **2009**, *19*, 61–78. [CrossRef] [PubMed]

38. Forbes, S.C.; Candow, D.G.; Little, J.P.; Magnus, C.; Chilibeck, P.D. Effect of red bull energy drink on repeated wingate cycle performance and bench-press muscle endurance. *Int. J. Sport Nutr. Exerc. Metab.* **2007**, *17*, 433–444. [CrossRef] [PubMed]

39. Alford, C.; Cox, H.; Wescott, R. The effects of red bull energy drink on human performance and mood. *Amino Acids* **2001**, *21*, 139–150. [CrossRef] [PubMed]

40. Seidl, R.; Peyrl, A.; Nicham, R.; Hauser, E. A taurine and caffeine-containing drink stimulates cognitive performance and well-being. *Amino Acids* **2000**, *19*, 635–642. [CrossRef] [PubMed]

41. Hendrix, C.R.; Housh, T.J.; Mielke, M.; Zuniga, J.M.; Camic, C.L.; Johnson, G.O.; Schmidt, R.J.; Housh, D.J. Acute effects of a caffeine-containing supplement on bench press and leg extension strength and time to exhaustion during cycle ergometry. *J. Strength Cond. Res.* **2010**, *24*, 859–865. [CrossRef] [PubMed]

42. Jones, A.M.; Bailey, S.J.; Vanhatalo, A. Dietary nitrate and O(2) consumption during exercise. *Med. Sport Sci.* **2012**, *59*, 29–35. [PubMed]

43. Kelly, J.; Vanhatalo, A.; Bailey, S.J.; Wylie, L.J.; Tucker, C.; List, S.; Winyard, P.G.; Jones, A.M. Dietary nitrate supplementation: Effects on plasma nitrite and pulmonary O_2 uptake dynamics during exercise in hypoxia and normoxia. *Am. J. Physiol.* **2014**, *307*, R920–R930. [CrossRef] [PubMed]

44. Rimer, E.G.; Peterson, L.R.; Coggan, A.R.; Martin, J.C. Increase in maximal cycling power with acute dietary nitrate supplementation. *Int. J. Sports Physiol. Perform.* **2016**, *11*, 715–720. [CrossRef] [PubMed]

45. Shannon, O.M.; Duckworth, L.; Barlow, M.J.; Woods, D.; Lara, J.; Siervo, M.; O'Hara, J.P. Dietary nitrate supplementation enhances high-intensity running performance in moderate normobaric hypoxia, independent of aerobic fitness. *Nitric Oxide* **2016**, *59*, 63–70. [CrossRef] [PubMed]

46. Wylie, L.J.; Bailey, S.J.; Kelly, J.; Blackwell, J.R.; Vanhatalo, A.; Jones, A.M. Influence of beetroot juice supplementation on intermittent exercise performance. *Eur. J. Appl. Physiol.* **2016**, *116*, 415–425. [CrossRef] [PubMed]

47. Jo, E.; Fischer, M.; Auslander, A.T.; Beigarten, A.; Daggy, B.; Hansen, K.; Kessler, L.; Osmond, A.; Wang, H.; Wes, R. The effects of multi-day vs. Single pre-exercise nitrate supplement dosing on simulated cycling time-trial performance and skeletal muscle oxygenation. *J. Strength Cond. Res.* **2017**. [CrossRef] [PubMed]

48. McQuillan, J.A.; Dulson, D.K.; Laursen, P.B.; Kilding, A.E. Dietary nitrate fails to improve 1 and 4 km cycling performance in highly trained cyclists. *Int. J. Sport Nutr. Exerc. Metab.* **2017**, *27*, 255–263. [CrossRef] [PubMed]

49. Wylie, L.J.; Mohr, M.; Krustrup, P.; Jackman, S.R.; Ermiotadis, G.; Kelly, J.; Black, M.I.; Bailey, S.J.; Vanhatalo, A.; Jones, A.M. Dietary nitrate supplementation improves team sport-specific intense intermittent exercise performance. *Eur. J. Appl. Physiol.* **2013**, *113*, 1673–1684. [CrossRef] [PubMed]

50. Hoon, M.W.; Jones, A.M.; Johnson, N.A.; Blackwell, J.R.; Broad, E.M.; Lundy, B.; Rice, A.J.; Burke, L.M. The effect of variable doses of inorganic nitrate-rich beetroot juice on simulated 2000-m rowing performance in trained athletes. *Int. J. Sports Physiol. Perform.* **2014**, *9*, 615–620. [CrossRef] [PubMed]

51. De Smet, S.; Van Thienen, R.; Deldicque, L.; James, R.; Sale, C.; Bishop, D.J.; Hespel, P. Nitrate intake promotes shift in muscle fiber type composition during sprint interval training in hypoxia. *Front. Physiol.* **2016**, *7*, 233. [CrossRef] [PubMed]

52. Galvan, E.; Walker, D.K.; Simbo, S.Y.; Dalton, R.; Levers, K.; O'Connor, A.; Goodenough, C.; Barringer, N.D.; Greenwood, M.; Rasmussen, C.; et al. Acute and chronic safety and efficacy of dose dependent creatine nitrate supplementation and exercise performance. *J. Int. Soc. Sports Nutr.* **2016**, *13*, 12. [CrossRef] [PubMed]

53. Porcelli, S.; Pugliese, L.; Rejc, E.; Pavei, G.; Bonato, M.; Montorsi, M.; La Torre, A.; Rasica, L.; Marzorati, M. Effects of a short-term high-nitrate diet on exercise performance. *Nutrients* **2016**, *8*. [CrossRef] [PubMed]

54. Reissig, C.J.; Strain, E.C.; Griffiths, R.R. Caffeinated energy drinks—A growing problem. *Drug Alcohol Depend.* **2009**, *99*, 1–10. [CrossRef] [PubMed]

55. Mora-Rodriguez, R.; Pallares, J.G. Performance outcomes and unwanted side effects associated with energy drinks. *Nutr. Rev.* **2014**, *72*, 108–120. [CrossRef] [PubMed]

56. Higgins, J.P.; Tuttle, T.D.; Higgins, C.L. Energy beverages: Content and safety. *Mayo Clin. Proc.* **2010**, *85*, 1033–1041. [CrossRef] [PubMed]

57. Eudy, A.E.; Gordon, L.L.; Hockaday, B.C.; Lee, D.A.; Lee, V.; Luu, D.; Martinez, C.A.; Ambrose, P.J. Efficacy and safety of ingredients found in preworkout supplements. *Am. J. Health Syst. Pharm.* **2013**, *70*, 577–588. [CrossRef] [PubMed]

58. Joy, J.M.; Lowery, R.P.; Falcone, P.H.; Vogel, R.M.; Mosman, M.M.; Tai, C.Y.; Carson, L.R.; Kimber, D.; Choate, D.; Kim, M.P.; et al. A multi-ingredient, pre-workout supplement is apparently safe in healthy males and females. *Food Nutr. Res.* **2015**, *59*, 27470. [CrossRef] [PubMed]

59. Vogel, R.M.; Joy, J.M.; Falcone, P.H.; Mosman, M.M.; Kim, M.P.; Moon, J.R. Safety of a dose-escalated pre-workout supplement in recreationally active females. *J. Int. Soc. Sports Nutr.* **2015**, *12*, 12. [CrossRef] [PubMed]

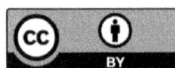

nutrients

MDPI

Article

Effects of Consuming Xylitol on Gut Microbiota and Lipid Metabolism in Mice

Takashi Uebanso *, Saki Kano, Ayumi Yoshimoto, Chisato Naito, Takaaki Shimohata, Kazuaki Mawatari and Akira Takahashi

Department of Preventive Environment and Nutrition, Institute of Biomedical Sciences, Tokushima University Graduate School, 3-18-15, Tokushima 770-8503, Japan; c201302046@tokushima-u.ac.jp (S.K.); sea.by15.koko@gmail.com (A.Y.); chii.cham.0701@gmail.com (C.N.); shimohata@tokushima-u.ac.jp (T.S.); mawatari@tokushima-u.ac.jp (K.M.); akiratak@tokushima-u.ac.jp (A.T.)
* Correspondence: uebanso@tokushima-u.ac.jp; Tel.: +81-88-633-9598; Fax: +81-88-633-7092

Received: 16 June 2017; Accepted: 12 July 2017; Published: 14 July 2017

Abstract: The sugar alcohol xylitol inhibits the growth of some bacterial species including *Streptococcus mutans*. It is used as a food additive to prevent caries. We previously showed that 1.5–4.0 g/kg body weight/day xylitol as part of a high-fat diet (HFD) improved lipid metabolism in rats. However, the effects of lower daily doses of dietary xylitol on gut microbiota and lipid metabolism are unclear. We examined the effect of 40 and 200 mg/kg body weight/day xylitol intake on gut microbiota and lipid metabolism in mice. Bacterial compositions were characterized by denaturing gradient gel electrophoresis and targeted real-time PCR. Luminal metabolites were determined by capillary electrophoresis electrospray ionization time-of-flight mass spectrometry. Plasma lipid parameters and glucose tolerance were examined. Dietary supplementation with low- or medium-dose xylitol (40 or 194 mg/kg body weight/day, respectively) significantly altered the fecal microbiota composition in mice. Relative to mice not fed xylitol, the addition of medium-dose xylitol to a regular and HFD in experimental mice reduced the abundance of fecal *Bacteroidetes phylum* and the genus *Barnesiella*, whereas the abundance of *Firmicutes phylum* and the genus *Prevotella* was increased in mice fed an HFD with medium-dose dietary xylitol. Body composition, hepatic and serum lipid parameters, oral glucose tolerance, and luminal metabolites were unaffected by xylitol consumption. In mice, 40 and 194 mg/kg body weight/day xylitol in the diet induced gradual changes in gut microbiota but not in lipid metabolism.

Keywords: xylitol; triglyceride; cholesterol; *Streptococcus mutans*; denaturing gradient gel electrophoresis (DGGE); capillary electrophoresis–mass spectrometry (CE–MS); caries

1. Introduction

Gut microbiota form many bioactive metabolites from dietary components which can regulate host metabolism [1–5]. For example, an improvement in glucose metabolism induced by dietary fiber is associated with the increased abundance of *Prevotella* [2]. Similarly, some food derivatives and food additives can affect host metabolism after interactions with gut microbiota [1,5].

Xylitol has a caries preventative effect via its capacity to inhibit the growth of *Streptococcus mutans* [6]. Dietary xylitol, metabolized into D-xylulose-5-phosphate, activates the carbohydrate response element binding protein (ChREBP) [7]. We previously reported that dietary xylitol combined with a high-fat diet (HFD) induced hepatic lipogenic gene expression via ChREBP mRNA expression [8]. In this report, we revealed that xylitol can improve HFD-induced hypertriglyceridemia and hypercholesterolemia with cecum enlargement in mice. In another report, the administration of a 2.5–10% xylitol solution reduced serum cholesterol and low density lipoprotein-cholesterol in diabetic mice [9]. Moreover, mice supplemented with 5% xylitol and 0.05%

daidzein in their diet had a lower serum cholesterol versus mice fed a diet containing daidzein alone [10]; xylitol also contributed to the relative reduction of the genera *Bacteroides* and *Clostridium* in gut microbiota. *Clostridium* genus clusters *XI* and *XIVa* participate in the conversion of primary bile acids to secondary bile acids [11]. Cholic acid, one of the primary bile acids, promote cholesterol absorption [12]. Moreover, alteration of the bile acids composition regulates lipid and energy metabolism through the activation of the farnesoid X receptor (FXR) or G-protein-coupled receptors (GPCRs), such as TGR5 [13,14]. On the other hand, the gut microbiota suppress fat accumulation via the short-chain fatty acid production from dietary fiber [15]. Taken together, dietary xylitol is able to improve hyperlipidemia and modify gut microbiota. However, at least 1.5 g/kg body weight/day of dietary xylitol was given in those studies [8–10]. The effects of daily dietary xylitol at relatively lower doses on gut microbiota and lipid metabolism are unclear. Over the past decade, pure xylitol and xylitol comestible products (e.g., gums and candies) have been commercially available to the general public. In addition, some infants are given xylitol tablets for the health of their teeth. Infants can potentially ingest more xylitol, up to 200 mg/kg body weight/day (commercially recommended xylitol tablets), than that of adults. In other reports, 150–300 mg xylitol/kg body weight/day have been used for preventing caries in schoolchildren [16,17]. Because development and expansion of the gut bacterial community occurs relatively slowly during early childhood [18], environmental factors could more strongly affect gut microbes in children than in adults. In the present study, our goal was to estimate the effect of feeding low-dose xylitol on gut microbiota and lipid metabolism in mice from an early stage of life.

2. Materials and Methods

2.1. Animals

Seven-day pregnant female C57Bl/6J mice were purchased from a local breeding colony (Charles River Japan, Yokohama, Japan) and their offspring—male pups only—were used in experiments 1 and 2 of this study. Mice were housed in cages maintained at constant temperature (23 ± 2 °C) and relative humidity (65–75%) with a 12-h light/dark cycle (8:00–20:00). In experiment 1, all three-week-old males were fed the control diet (CD, AIN93G, Oriental Yeast, Osaka, Japan) formulated for rapid growth for 16 weeks, during which time they were divided into three groups as follows: control diet (CD) group, with free access to distilled water (CD, n = 5); low-dose xylitol group, were given xylitol solution of 40 mg/kg body weight/day (CD-LX, n = 5); and a medium-dose xylitol group, were given xylitol solution of 200 mg/kg body weight/day (CD-MX, n = 5). In experiment 2, three-week-old male mice were fed a high-fat diet (HFD32, Japan Crea, Osaka, Japan) for 18 weeks, during which time they were divided into two groups as follows: high-fat diet (HFD) group with free access to distilled water (HFD, n = 5) and an HFD with a medium-dose xylitol group, were given xylitol solution of 200 mg/kg body weight/day (HFD-MX, n = 6). Body weight and fluid intake were measured three or four times weekly. We used to control the xylitol consumption of mice using pair-feeding like method. The xylitol concentration was calculated on the basis of daily fluid intake and body weight; adjustments to the concentration of xylitol in the drinking water were made every 1–2 days to regulate xylitol consumption. In the fecal microbiota transplantation (FMT) experiment, six-week-old male mice were treated with a cocktail of broad spectrum antibiotics (1 g/L ampicillin, neomycin, and metronidazole and 0.5 g/L vancomycin) in their drinking water for three weeks [19]. FMT was performed to transplant gut microbiota from donor mice fed an HFD, with or without xylitol (HFD-MX-FMT and HFD-FMT, respectively) to antibiotic-treated recipient mice as has been reported previously with slight modifications [19]. The transplantation procedure was performed every 3 days, twice per experiment. After an FMT, mice were maintained on HFD for eight weeks. All mice were euthanized; blood was collected in addition to ceca, cecal contents, feces, and liver tissue. The University of Tokushima Animal Use Committee approved the study (T14010), and mice were maintained according to the National Institutes of Health Guide for the Care and Use of Laboratory Animals.

2.2. Oral Glucose Tolerance Test

At week 16, mice fed the HFD and HFD-MX were fasted for 16 h and subsequently administered 2 g glucose/kg body weight orally to test their glucose tolerance. Blood samples taken from the tail vein at indicated times were used to determine plasma glucose concentration (Glucose Pilot, IWAI CHEMICALS COMPANY, Tokyo, Japan).

2.3. Extraction of Genomic DNA and Quantitative PCR

Genomic DNA from fecal and cecal content samples were isolated using the FavorPrep Stool DNA Isolation Mini Kit (FAVORGEN Biotech Corp., Ping-Tung, Taiwan) in accordance with the manufacturer's protocol. The relative abundance of each target's bacterial 16S rRNA gene sequence (see primer sequences in Table 1) was calculated by normalization to the amount of amplified product from all bacteria 16S rRNA gene copy numbers.

Table 1. Oligonucleotide primers.

Primer Name	Sequence (5′–3′)	Reference
Eub338F	ACTCCTACGGGAGGCAGCAG	[20]
Eub518R	ATTACCGCGGCTGCTGG	
HDA1-GC-F	CGCCCGGGGCGCGCCCCGGGCGGGGCGGGGG CACGGGGGGACTCCTACGGGAGGCAGCAGT	[21]
HDA2-R	GTATTACCGCGGCTGCTGGCAC	
Bact934F	GGARCATGTGGTTTAATTCGATGAT	
Bact1060R	AGCTGACGACAACCATGCAG	[22]
Firm934F	GGAGYATGTGGTTTAATTCGAAGCA	
Firm1060R	AGCTGACGACAACCATGCAC	
Prevotella-F	CATGACGTTACCCGCAGAAGAAG	[23]
Prevotella-R	TCCTGCACGCTACTTGGCTG	
mChREBP-F	TCAGCACTTCCACAAGCATC	NM_021455.4
mChREBP-R	GCATTAGCAACAGTGCAGGA	
18sF	AAACGGCTACCACATCCAAG	NR_003278.3
18sR	GGCCTCGAAAGAGTCCTGTA	
mPklr-F	TTGTGCTGACAAAGACTGGC	NM_013631
mPklr-R	CCACGAAGCTTTCCACTTTC	
mFasn-F	TGCCTTCGGTTCAGTCTCTT	NM_007988.3
mFasn-R	GGGCAACTTAAAGGTGGACA	
mScd1-F	CGAGGGTTGGTTGTTGATCT	NM_009127.4
mScd1-R	GCCCATGTCTCTGGTGTTTT	
m II-6-F	CTGATGCTGGTGACAACCAC	NM_031168.2
m II-6-R	TCCACGATTTCCCAGAGAAC	
mTnf-F	AGCCTGTAGCCCACGTCGTA	NM_013693.3
mTnf-R	TCTTTGAGATCCATGCCGTTG	

Eub: Eubacteria (total bacteria), Bact: *Bacteroides*, Firm: *Firmicutes*, ChREBP: Carbohydrate response element binding protein, Pklr: pyruvate kinase liver and red blood cell, Fasn: fatty acid synthase, Scd1: stearoyl-Coenzyme A desaturase 1, Tnf: tumor necrosis factor, II-6: interleukin 6.

2.4. PCR-DGGE Analysis

Denaturing gradient gel electrophoresis (DGGE) was performed as previously described [24] using the DCode^TM Universal Mutation Detection System instrument and model 475 gradient former according to the manufacturer's instructions (Bio-Rad Labs, Hercules, CA, USA). The V2–V3 region of the 16S rRNA genes (positions 339–539 in the *Escherichia coli* gene) of bacteria in gut samples was amplified with the primers HDA1-GC and HDA2. PCR reaction mixtures and the amplification program were the same as described previously [24]. The denaturing gradient was formed with two

8% acrylamide (acrylamide-bis 37.5:1) with denaturing gradients ranging from 20–80% for analysis of the amplified 16S rRNA fragments. The 100% denaturant solution contained 40% (v/v) deionized formamide and 7 M urea. PCR product (40 µL) was mixed with 40 µL dye before loading. Gels were run in 0.5× Tris/Acetate/EDTA buffer at 60 °C for 5.2 h at 180 V, 210 mA, stained with Gel Star (Lonza Japan, Tokyo, Japan) for 30 min, and analyzed by ChemiDoc MP (Bio-Rad, Hercules, CA, USA). Image Lab software, version 5.0 (Bio-Rad) was used for the identification of bands and normalization of band patterns from DGGE gels.

2.5. Determination of Bacterial Strain by Sequence Analysis

Specific bands from DGGE gels were excised for DNA extraction, mashed, and incubated overnight in a diffusion buffer (0.5 M ammonium acetate, 1 mM EDTA, 0.1% SDS, 15 mM magnesium acetate). DNA was purified by the standard ethanol precipitation method. The V2–V3 region of the 16S rRNA genes were amplified by PCR, and purified DNA was used as a template. PCR products were cloned into the pCR2.1-TOPO vector (Invitrogen, Carlsbad, CA, USA), sequenced, and the bacterial genus was identified by BLAST.

2.6. Plasma and Hepatic Lipid Concentrations

Hepatic lipids were extracted and measured as previously described [25]. Plasma and liver triglycerides (TG) and total cholesterol concentration were measured by using Triglyceride-E and Cholesterol-E tests (Wako Pure Chemical Industries, Osaka, Japan), respectively.

2.7. RNA Preparation and Quantitative Reverse Transcriptase PCR

Extraction of total RNA, cDNA synthesis, and real-time PCR analysis were performed as described previously [25]. The relative abundance of each target transcript was calculated by normalization to the amount of amplified product from constitutively expressed β-actin mRNA (see primer sequences in Table 1).

2.8. Metabolome Analysis of Cecum Luminal Content by Capillary Electrophoresis Electrospray Ionization Time-of-Flight Mass Spectrometry

The cecum luminal content was immediately frozen in liquid nitrogen and stored at −80 °C until metabolite extraction. Sample tissues were weighed and completely homogenized in 0.5 mL ice-cold methanol containing 50 µM methionine sulfone and camphor-10-sulfonic acid as internal standards. The homogenates were mixed with 0.5 mL chloroform and 0.2 mL ice-cold Milli-Q water. After centrifugation at 2300× g for 5 min, the supernatant was centrifugally filtrated through 5-kDa cut-off filters (Millipore, Bedford, MA, USA) at 9100× g for 4–5 h to remove proteins. The filtrate was centrifugally concentrated in a vacuum evaporator, dissolved with Milli-Q water, and analyzed by capillary electrophoresis electrospray ionization time-of-flight mass spectrometry (CE-TOFMS).

CE-TOFMS analysis was performed using an Agilent CE system combined with a TOFMS (Agilent Technologies, Palo Alto, CA, USA) as reported by previously [24,26,27]. Each metabolite was identified based on a reference which containing internal standards including 110 metabolites (H3304-1002, Human Metabolome Technology (HMT), Inc., Tsuruoka, Japan) to m/z and migration time, and quantified by peak area.

2.9. Statistical Analyses

Data are expressed as means ± standard errors of the mean (SEM). A significant difference between groups was assessed via an unpaired two-tailed t-test in experiment 2 and FMT experiment. For comparisons among more than three groups, we employed analysis of variance (ANOVA) or the Kruskal-Wallis test in experiment 1. When a significant difference was found by ANOVA or the Kruskal-Wallis test, post hoc analyses were performed using the Tukey-Kramer protected least significant difference test. Concentration-dependent effects were identified via linear regression analysis. Spearman's rank correlation coefficient was used to calculate correlation coefficients between selected variables. Differences were considered significant at $p < 0.05$. Statistical analyses were performed using Mass Profiler Professional and Excel-Toukei 2006 (SSRI, Tokyo, Japan).

3. Results

To elucidate the effect of consuming low-dose xylitol on gut microbiota and lipid metabolism, the mean xylitol dosage administered to mice after weaning was 40 ± 5 mg/kg body weight/day (CD-LX), 194 ± 24 mg/kg body weight/day (CD-MX), and 194 ± 25 mg/kg body weight/day (HFD-MX) (Figure 1A,B). During the treatment periods, body weight, relative epididymal fat weight per body weight, relative liver weight per body weight, and relative cecum weight per body weight were not different between the xylitol-fed groups and the control group of mice in experiment 1 and 2 (Figure 1C,D, and Table 2). The relative amount of total fecal bacteria to fecal DNA displayed a trend towards an increase in the feces of CD-MX mice and was significantly increased in the feces of HFD-MX mice when compared with control mice (Figure 2A,B). In contrast, *Bacteroides*, a phylum of bacteria, was reduced in both MX mice fed a CD or HFD (Figure 2A,B). In addition, the combination of an HFD and ingestion of a medium-dose xylitol solution showed that an increased amount of *Firmicutes phylum*, the *Prevotella genus*, and the relative ratio of *Firmicutes/Bacteroides* and *Prevotella/Bacteroides* than those of HFD fed control mice (Figure 2B,C). To explore in detail the microbiome bacterial composition, we carried out DGGE analysis. We identified five genera, which included two species of *Clostridium* and a *Faecalibaculum* genus which were increased in the MX mice and one from both the *Clostridium* and *Barnesiella genera* which were reduced in the MX mice; different analysis bands were significantly different (Figure 2D–H). Principal component analysis (PCA) allowed us to clearly distinguish among groups based on dietary xylitol exposure, regardless of the control or HFD (Figure 2I,J). Continuous daily consumption of 40 or 194 mg xylitol after weaning induced different populations of gut microbiota in the feces of mice.

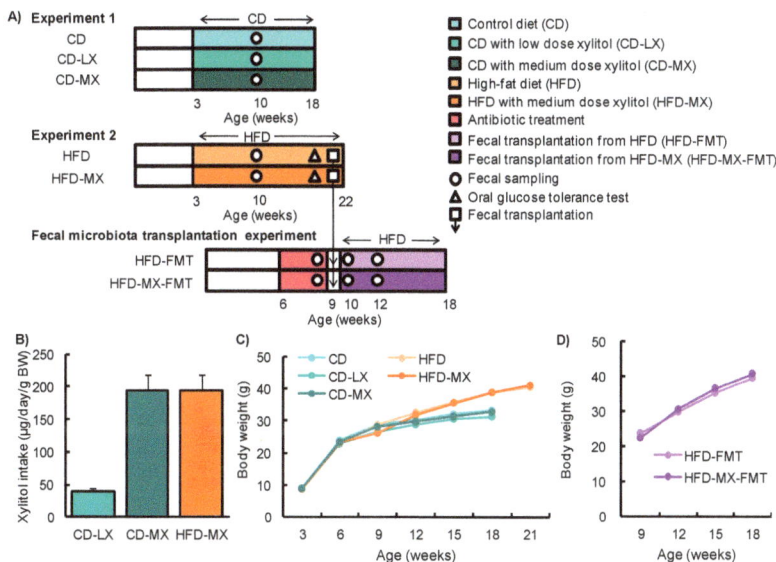

Figure 1. Experimental design and changes in body weight in mice fed xylitol. Study design for experiment 1 and 2 and the fecal transplantation experiment (**A**). Xylitol consumption during experiments (**B**). Changes in body weight (BW) throughout experiment 1 and 2 (**C**) and during the fecal transplantation experiment (**D**). Data represent the mean ± SEM ($n = 5$–6).

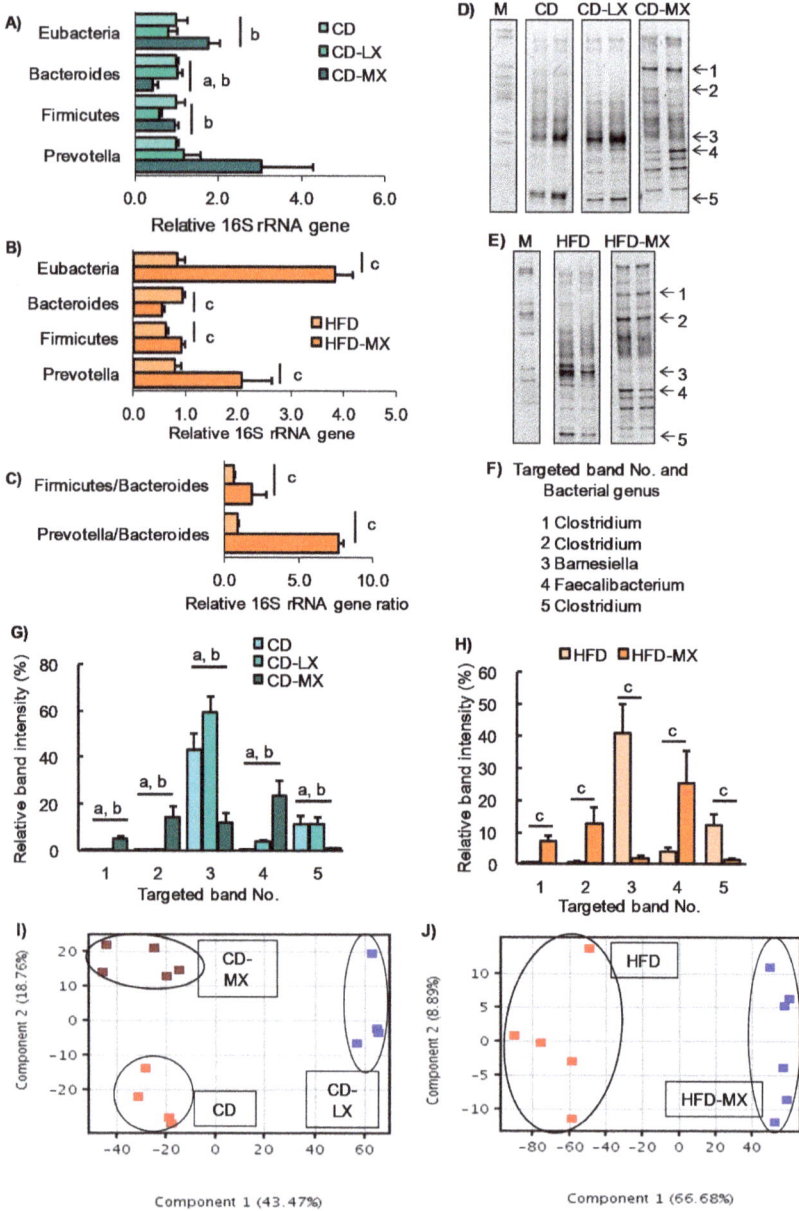

Figure 2. Changes in the fecal microbiota of mice fed xylitol. An abundance of specific bacterial phylum or genus and ratio after seven weeks of xylitol supplementation using specific primer set (Table 1) (**A–C**). Band image of DGGE analysis of DNA from feces after seven weeks of xylitol exposure with CD (**D**) or HFD (**E**). Identified five bacterial genus (No. 1–5) from DGGE band (**F**). Relative band density of identified five bacterial genus from feces after seven weeks of xylitol exposure with CD (**G**) or HFD (**H**). Two-dimensional principal component analysis plot of DGGE band pattern in mice fed xylitol with CD (**I**) or HFD (**J**). Data represent the mean ± SEM (*n* = 5–6). a: $p < 0.05$ between CD and CD-MX. b: $p < 0.05$ between CD-LX and CD-MX. c: $p < 0.05$ between HFD and HFD-MX.

Table 2. Body weight, organ weight, and plasma parameters of mice fed the control diet or the high-fat diet with or without xylitol.

	Diet				
	CD (*n* = 5)	CD-LX (*n* = 5)	CD-MX (*n* = 5)	HFD (*n* = 5)	HFD-MX (*n* = 6)
Final body weight, g	33.4 ± 0.3	31.2 ± 0.5	32.5 ± 0.8	38.5 ± 1.3	40.5 ± 1.3
Visceral fat, g/kg body weight	15.2 ± 1.2	15.8 ± 1.4	19.4 ± 3.8	43.9 ± 4.5	49.1 ± 2.8
Cecum weight, g/kg body weight	17.7 ± 0.9	16.8 ± 1.3	16.3 ± 0.9	8.9 ± 0.8	8.8 ± 1.4
Hepatic parameters					
Liver, g/kg body weight	48.6 ± 0.7	45.1 ± 1.3	43.0 ± 2.3	43.5 ± 3.8	47.6 ± 3.4
Total cholesterol, mmol/liver	7.5 ± 0.8	7.2 ± 0.4	7.1 ± 0.5	21.3 ± 2.8	33.7 ± 7.3
Triglycerides, mmol/liver	8.8 ± 0.8	11.4 ± 1.3	12.0 ± 1.6	56.0 ± 12.3	74.2 ± 9.2
Plasma parameters					
Total cholesterol, mmol/L	2.0 ± 0.1	2.3 ± 0.1	2.0 ± 0.2	3.6 ± 0.7	4.2 ± 0.3
Triglycerides, mmol/L	1.2 ± 0.1	1.5 ± 0.1	1.4 ± 0.3	1.0 ± 0.1	0.8 ± 0.1

Data represent the mean ± SEM (*n* = 5–6).

Our study and others report that a high dose of xylitol improved hyperlipidemia in mice fed an HFD and in diabetic mice [8–10]. To reveal the effect of a low dose of xylitol on lipid metabolism, we investigated cholesterol and triglyceride concentrations in the liver and serum, parameters which were not different among the three groups of mice maintained on the control diet (Table 2). In contrast, an HFD induced hypertriglyceridemia and hypercholesterolemia in the liver, but xylitol supplementation did not ameliorate dyslipidemia (Table 2). We also found that hepatic ChREBP and the expression of its target genes were increased in HFD-MX mice compared with control mice (Figure 3A) as was reported in a previous study [8]. In addition, we investigated glucose tolerance in mice fed an HFD because two reports have shown an abundance of several different species of the genus *Prevotera* that are linked with glucose intolerance or insulin resistance in humans and mice [2,28]. We could not detect any changes in glucose tolerance, as well as the expression of inflammation-related genes, in mice fed the HFD with or without dietary xylitol supplementation (Figure 3A,B).

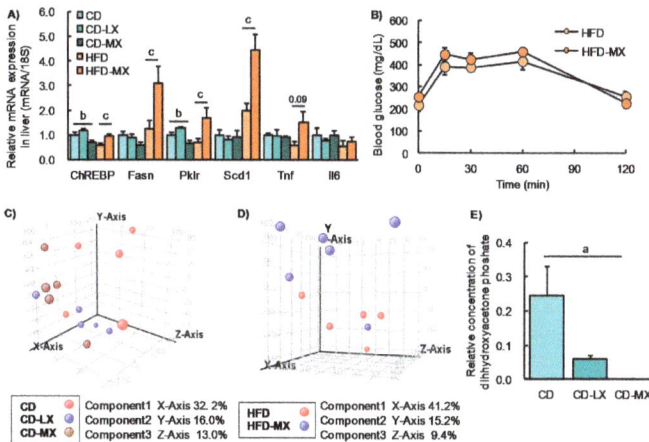

Figure 3. Hepatic gene expression, oral glucose tolerance test, and luminal metabolite in xylitol-fed mice. Relative hepatic gene expression involved in lipid metabolism in mice fed xylitol (**A**). Changes in blood glucose levels during an oral glucose tolerance test (OGTT) in mice fed xylitol with the HFD (**B**). Principle component analysis of 94 luminal metabolites in mice supplemented with xylitol and the CD (**C**) or the HFD (**D**). Changes in relative concentration of luminal dihydroxyacetone phosphate in mice supplemented with xylitol and the CD (**E**). Fasn: fatty acid synthase, Pklr: pyruvate kinase liver and red blood cell. Data represent the mean ± SEM (*n* = 5–6). a: *p* < 0.05 between CD and CD-MX. b: *p* < 0.05 between CD-LX and CD-MX. c: *p* < 0.05 between HFD and HFD-MX.

To further investigate the effects of xylitol intake on luminal metabolites, we conducted a CE-MS analysis. We identified 94 metabolites from a metabolite list provided by HMT. From the PCA plot, we were unable to distinguish any metabolite patterns among the groups of mice in experiment 1 fed the AIN93G diet with or without supplemental dietary xylitol in their drinking water (Figure 3C,D). Only dihydroxyacetone phosphate concentration was different between CD and CD-MX groups. These results suggest that the changes in luminal content microbiota in xylitol supplemented groups had little, if any, effect on overall metabolism.

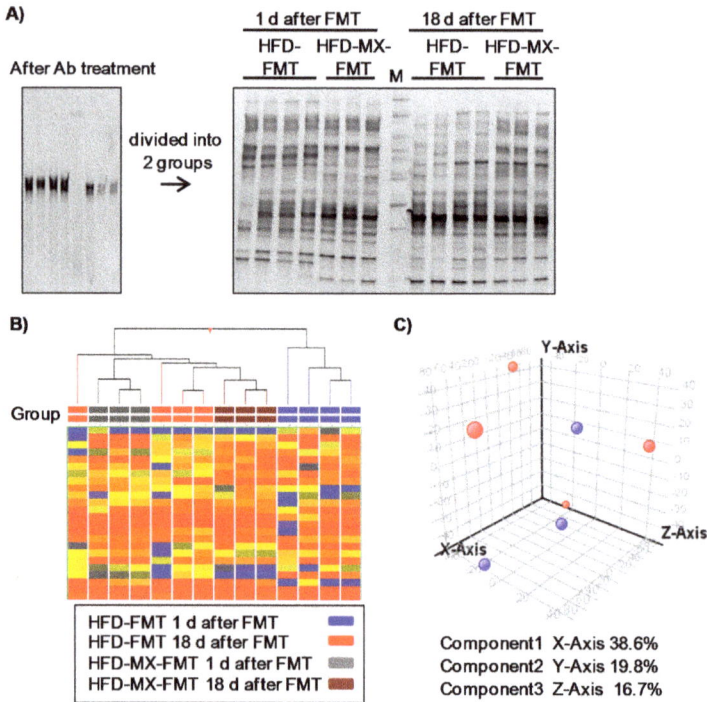

Figure 4. Changes in fecal microbiota and luminal metabolites of recipient mice in fecal transplantation experiment. Fecal transplantations were performed from donor mice fed the HFD with or without xylitol to antibiotic (Ab)-treated recipient mice (HFD-FMT and HFD-MX-FMT). Band patterns (**A**) and hierarchical clustering of band patterns (**B**) in feces 16S V2–V3 rRNA composition in HFD-FMT and HFD-MX-FMT mice. Ab treatment reduced fecal bacteria (left band pattern) and gradual changes in the composition of fecal bacteria in the HFD-FMT and HFD-MX-FMT mice from 1 day after FT to 18 day after FMT. M: Marker. Principle component analysis of luminal metabolites in HFD-FMT (red) and HFD-MX-FMT mice (blue). (**C**). $n = 3$–4.

Finally, we attempted to detect microbiota-dependent effects of xylitol feeding in mice fed an HFD via FMT. One day after the final transplantation, the microbiota was clearly different between the mice that were recipients of feces transplanted from mice fed an HFD (HFD-FMT) and fed an HFD with medium-dose xylitol (HFD-MX-FMT) (Figure 4A,B). These perceptible differences between the two groups disappeared 18 day after the transplantation (Figure 4A,B). No changes in luminal metabolites, body weight, and relative tissue weight between HFD-FMT and HFD-MX-FMT mice were detected (Figure 4C, Table 3). These results indicate that changes in the fecal microbiota of mice fed xylitol are transient and likely continuous xylitol supplementation is necessary to sustain the changes observed. Interestingly, serum cholesterol in the HFD-MX-FMT mice was slightly, but significantly, higher than that of the HFD-FMT mice (Table 3). This suggests that changes in the composition of microbiota induced by dietary xylitol increase serum cholesterol.

Table 3. Body weight, organ weight, and plasma parameters of mice fed the high-fat diet following fecal transplantation from mice fed a high-fat diet with or without xylitol.

	Diet	
	HFD-FMT (*n* = 4)	HFD-MX-FMT (*n* = 3)
Final body weight, g	39.5 ± 2.9	40.8 ± 1.4
Visceral fat, g/kg body weight	55.1 ± 6.3	60.6 ± 8.8
Cecum weight, g/kg body weight	6.6 ± 0.8	8.5 ± 1.2
Hepatic parameters		
Liver, g/kg body weight	44.1 ± 1.8	45.1 ± 6.5
Total cholesterol, mmol/liver	82.3 ± 11.1	101.4 ± 16.7
Triglycerides, mmol/liver	23.8 ± 4.6	31.5 ± 3.6
Plasma parameters		
Total cholesterol, mmol/L	4.9 ± 0.1	5.6 ± 0.3 *
Triglycerides, mmol/L	1.1 ± 0.2	1.0 ± 0.2

Data represent the mean ± SEM (*n* = 5). * Significant differences were observed compared with HFD-FMT ($p < 0.05$).

4. Discussion and Conclusions

In this study, we showed that the administration of xylitol at 40 and 194 mg/kg body weight/day significantly altered gut microbiota in mice. In particular, we noted the relative abundance of the *Bacteroidetes phylum* was reduced in mice in the CD-MX and HFD-MX groups, indicating that xylitol suppressed the growth of some bacterium, including the genus *Barnesiella* in mice fed either CD or HFD. In contrast, the relative abundance of *Firmicutes phylum* and the genus *Prevotella* were increased in the HFD-MX group. Contrary to the significant alteration of microbiota, body composition, lipid parameters, and luminal metabolites were not different between groups, regardless of xylitol consumption.

The improvement of glucose tolerance observed with increased dietary fiber intake is linked with a higher abundance of the genus *Prevotella* [2]. In contrast, the abundance of *Prevotella copri* was positively associated with microbial branched-chain amino acid (BCAA) biosynthesis in the gut and insulin resistance with a soy protein diet which contained a low level of BCAAs [28]. Our present study showed an increased abundance of *Prevotella* and an increase in the *Prevotella/Bacteroidetes* ratio, but no differences were observed in glucose tolerance or luminal BCAA concentrations between the HFD and HFD-MX groups. Because the mice were fed a diet containing casein, which has as the protein source a high BCAA content, we were unable to detect any changes in the luminal BCAA concentrations. These results suggest that changes in the bacterial composition and the supply of dietary components modulates host metabolism in a coordinated manner.

An amount of dietary indigestible fiber and gut microbiota which digest fiber regulates cecum weight [29,30]. In the experiment 1, we used AIN93G as a control diet which contains more fiber (5%) than the HFD which used in experiment 2 (2.9%). In the present study, xylitol feeding did not affect cecum weight, therefore a difference in the amount of dietary fiber might affect cecum weight.

In our study, daily supplemental dietary xylitol of 194 but not 40 mg/kg body weight induced significant changes in microbiota for the genera *Barnesiella*, which was reduced, and *Feacalibaculum*, which was increased. *Barnesiella* and *Feacalibaculum* have been detected in human or mice microbiota [31,32]. *Barnesiella* species have been negatively correlated with the colonization of vancomycin-resistant *Enterococcus faecium* in mice intestines [33] and the relative abundance of the bacterial genera *Faecalibacterium* was significantly decreased in children at risk of asthma [34]. In contrast, dietary xylitol suppressed lipopolysaccharide-induced inflammatory responses in male broiler chickens [35] and has been shown to ameliorate human respiratory syncytial virus infections

Nutrients **2017**, *9*, 756

in mice [36]. Collectively, changes in the fecal microbiota of animals fed xylitol might affect immune responses or colonization of some bacterial species.

Recently, Geidenstam et al. reported that baseline levels of serum xylitol showed an inverse association with a ≥10% weight loss in obese subjects fed low-calorie diet [37]. *Firmicutes phylum* accelerates degradation of food component to supply energy to host, it is, therefore, known as obesity-related bacterial phylum [38]. In our study, the total bacteria/DNA and the relative abundance of *Firmicutes phylum* were increased in the HFD-MX group. Geidenstam and colleague did not examine gut microbiota in their study, human metabolism of xylitol and potential involvement of the gut microbiota could help us to understand the effect of xylitol feeding on human lipid metabolism.

Xylitol metabolized into xylulose-5-phosphate (X-5-P) is synthesized via the pentose phosphate pathway [39] and activates ChREBP through protein phosphatase 2A [40]; this results in its binding to a specific DNA sequence which induces lipogenesis-related genes which increase lipogenesis from carbohydrates [41]. Daily dietary xylitol at exposure levels ranging between 1.5–4.0 g/kg body weight in combination with a HFD showed a trend towards increased expression of hepatic ChREBP mRNA and a reduction in hepatic triglycerides and total cholesterol as reported in a previous study [8]. These findings suggest xylitol has other functions unrelated to the ChREBP pathway. In the present study, we found that an HFD supplemented with 0.2 g/kg body weight/d of dietary xylitol also induced the increased expression of hepatic ChREBP mRNA and but had a tendency to increase hepatic triglycerides and total cholesterol. The differences between the studies may arise from differences in model species, xylitol dose, and diet which used to characterize the effect of xylitol on lipid metabolism. Because plasma triglyceride level was not increased by HFD feeding in this study, another study that uses another diet (e.g., high-fat high-sucrose diet) which strongly induces hypertriglyceridemia will help to understand the effect of xylitol to alter plasma TG levels. Hepatic total cholesterol in HFD-MX-FMT mice was slightly but significantly higher than that of HFD-FMT mice. Taken together, these changes in the gut microbiota induced by dietary xylitol may potentiate the accumulation of cholesterol and upregulation of hepatic ChREBP.

In conclusion, we found that 40 and 194 mg/kg body weight/day of dietary xylitol in mice induced gradual changes in gut microbiota, but did not ameliorate HFD-induced dyslipidemia.

Acknowledgments: This work was financially supported by the Japan Food Chemical Research Foundation Science and JSPS KAKENHI (Grant Numbers JP15H0564710 and JP16K15191, respectively). This study was supported by the Support Center for The Special Mission Center for Metabolome Analysis, School of Medical Nutrition, Faculty of Medicine of Tokushima University and the Support Center for Advanced Medical Sciences, Institute of Biomedical Sciences, and Tokushima University Graduate School provided materials. We gratefully acknowledge the excellent assistance provided by Yumi Harada, Rumiko Masuda, Akiko Uebanso, and staff at the Metabolome Tokumei-Unit in Tokushima University. We also want to thank the staff at the Division for Animal Research Resources and Genetic Engineering Support Center for Advanced Medical Sciences, at the Institute of Biomedical Sciences, Tokushima University Graduate School, for their dedicated mouse husbandry. We wish to express our thanks to Yutaka Taketani (Tokushima University) and Masashi Masuda (Tokushima University) for their kind gifts of some PCR-primers.

Author Contributions: T.U., T.S., K.M. and A.T. designed research; T.U., S.K., C.N. and A.Y. conducted research and analyzed data; T.U. and A.T. wrote paper and had responsibility for final content. All authors read and approved the final manuscript.

Conflicts of Interest: The authors declare no conflict of interest.

References

1. Chassaing, B.; Koren, O.; Goodrich, J.K.; Poole, A.C.; Srinivasan, S.; Ley, R.E.; Gewirtz, A.T. Dietary emulsifiers impact the mouse gut microbiota promoting colitis and metabolic syndrome. *Nature* **2015**, *519*, 92–96. [CrossRef] [PubMed]

2. Kovatcheva-Datchary, P.; Nilsson, A.; Akrami, R.; Lee, Y.S.; De Vadder, F.; Arora, T.; Hallen, A.; Martens, E.; Bjorck, I.; Backhed, F. Dietary fiber-induced improvement in glucose metabolism is associated with increased abundance of prevotella. *Cell Metab.* **2015**, *22*, 971–982. [CrossRef] [PubMed]

3. Meyer, K.A.; Bennett, B.J. Diet and gut microbial function in metabolic and cardiovascular disease risk. *Curr. Dia. Rep.* **2016**, *16*, 93. [CrossRef] [PubMed]

4. Schroeder, B.O.; Backhed, F. Signals from the gut microbiota to distant organs in physiology and disease. *Nat. Med.* **2016**, *22*, 1079–1089. [CrossRef] [PubMed]

5. Suez, J.; Korem, T.; Zeevi, D.; Zilberman-Schapira, G.; Thaiss, C.A.; Maza, O.; Israeli, D.; Zmora, N.; Gilad, S.; Weinberger, A.; et al. Artificial sweeteners induce glucose intolerance by altering the gut microbiota. *Nature* **2014**, *514*, 181–186. [CrossRef] [PubMed]

6. Soderling, E.M.; Ekman, T.C.; Taipale, T.J. Growth inhibition of streptococcus mutans with low xylitol concentrations. *Curr. Microbiol.* **2008**, *56*, 382–385. [CrossRef] [PubMed]

7. Uebanso, T.; Taketani, Y.; Yamamoto, H.; Amo, K.; Ominami, H.; Arai, H.; Takei, Y.; Masuda, M.; Tanimura, A.; Harada, N.; et al. Paradoxical regulation of human FGF21 by both fasting and feeding signals: Is FGF21 a nutritional adaptation factor? *PLoS ONE* **2011**, *6*, e22976. [CrossRef] [PubMed]

8. Amo, K.; Arai, H.; Uebanso, T.; Fukaya, M.; Koganei, M.; Sasaki, H.; Yamamoto, H.; Taketani, Y.; Takeda, E. Effects of xylitol on metabolic parameters and visceral fat accumulation. *J. Clin. Biochem. Nutr.* **2011**, *49*, 1–7. [PubMed]

9. Rahman, M.A.; Islam, M.S. Xylitol improves pancreatic islets morphology to ameliorate type 2 diabetes in rats: A dose response study. *J. Food Sci.* **2014**, *79*, H1436–H1442. [CrossRef] [PubMed]

10. Tamura, M.; Hoshi, C.; Hori, S. Xylitol affects the intestinal microbiota and metabolism of daidzein in adult male mice. *Int. J. Mol. Sci.* **2013**, *14*, 23993–24007. [CrossRef] [PubMed]

11. Ridlon, J.M.; Kang, D.J.; Hylemon, P.B. Bile salt biotransformations by human intestinal bacteria. *J. Lipid Res.* **2006**, *47*, 241–259. [CrossRef] [PubMed]

12. Reynier, M.O.; Montet, J.C.; Gerolami, A.; Marteau, C.; Crotte, C.; Montet, A.M.; Mathieu, S. Comparative effects of cholic, chenodeoxycholic, and ursodeoxycholic acids on micellar solubilization and intestinal absorption of cholesterol. *J. Lipid Res.* **1981**, *22*, 467–473. [PubMed]

13. Jiang, C.; Xie, C.; Lv, Y.; Li, J.; Krausz, K.W.; Shi, J.; Brocker, C.N.; Desai, D.; Amin, S.G.; Bisson, W.H.; et al. Intestine-selective farnesoid *x* receptor inhibition improves obesity-related metabolic dysfunction. *Nat. Commun.* **2015**, *6*, 10166. [CrossRef] [PubMed]

14. Thomas, C.; Gioiello, A.; Noriega, L.; Strehle, A.; Oury, J.; Rizzo, G.; Macchiarulo, A.; Yamamoto, H.; Mataki, C.; Pruzanski, M.; et al. TGR5-mediated bile acid sensing controls glucose homeostasis. *Cell Metab.* **2009**, *10*, 167–177. [CrossRef] [PubMed]

15. Kimura, I.; Ozawa, K.; Inoue, D.; Imamura, T.; Kimura, K.; Maeda, T.; Terasawa, K.; Kashihara, D.; Hirano, K.; Tani, T.; et al. The gut microbiota suppresses insulin-mediated fat accumulation via the short-chain fatty acid receptor GPR43. *Nat. Commun.* **2013**, *4*, 1829. [CrossRef] [PubMed]

16. Campus, G.; Cagetti, M.G.; Sale, S.; Petruzzi, M.; Solinas, G.; Strohmenger, L.; Lingstrom, P. Six months of high-dose xylitol in high-risk caries subjects—A 2-year randomised, clinical trial. *Clin. Oral Investig.* **2013**, *17*, 785–791. [CrossRef] [PubMed]

17. Soderling, E.; ElSalhy, M.; Honkala, E.; Fontana, M.; Flannagan, S.; Eckert, G.; Kokaras, A.; Paster, B.; Tolvanen, M.; Honkala, S. Effects of short-term xylitol gum chewing on the oral microbiome. *Clin. Oral Investig.* **2015**, *19*, 237–244. [CrossRef] [PubMed]

18. Yatsunenko, T.; Rey, F.E.; Manary, M.J.; Trehan, I.; Dominguez-Bello, M.G.; Contreras, M.; Magris, M.; Hidalgo, G.; Baldassano, R.N.; Anokhin, A.P.; et al. Human gut microbiome viewed across age and geography. *Nature* **2012**, *486*, 222–227. [CrossRef] [PubMed]

19. He, B.; Nohara, K.; Ajami, N.J.; Michalek, R.D.; Tian, X.; Wong, M.; Losee-Olson, S.H.; Petrosino, J.F.; Yoo, S.H.; Shimomura, K.; et al. Transmissible microbial and metabolomic remodeling by soluble dietary fiber improves metabolic homeostasis. *Sci. Rep.* **2015**, *5*, 10604. [CrossRef] [PubMed]

20. Fierer, N.; Jackson, J.A.; Vilgalys, R.; Jackson, R.B. Assessment of soil microbial community structure by use of taxon-specific quantitative pcr assays. *Appl. Environ. Microbiol.* **2005**, *71*, 4117–4120. [CrossRef] [PubMed]

21. Tannock, G.W.; Munro, K.; Harmsen, H.J.; Welling, G.W.; Smart, J.; Gopal, P.K. Analysis of the fecal microflora of human subjects consuming a probiotic product containing Lactobacillus rhamnosusDR20. *Appl. Environ. Microbiol.* **2000**, *66*, 2578–2588. [CrossRef] [PubMed]

22. Guo, X.; Xia, X.; Tang, R.; Zhou, J.; Zhao, H.; Wang, K. Development of a real-time pcr method for firmicutes and bacteroidetes in faeces and its application to quantify intestinal population of obese and lean pigs. *Lett. Appl. Microbiol.* **2008**, *47*, 367–373. [CrossRef] [PubMed]

23. Bekele, A.Z.; Koike, S.; Kobayashi, Y. Genetic diversity and diet specificity of ruminal prevotella revealed by 16s rrna gene-based analysis. *FEMS Microbiol. Lett.* **2010**, *305*, 49–57. [CrossRef] [PubMed]
24. Uebanso, T.; Ohnishi, A.; Kitayama, R.; Yoshimoto, A.; Nakahashi, M.; Shimohata, T.; Mawatari, K.; Takahashi, A. Effects of low-dose non-caloric sweetener consumption on gut microbiota in mice. *Nutrients* **2017**, *9*, 560. [CrossRef] [PubMed]
25. Uebanso, T.; Taketani, Y.; Fukaya, M.; Sato, K.; Takei, Y.; Sato, T.; Sawada, N.; Amo, K.; Harada, N.; Arai, H.; et al. Hypocaloric high-protein diet improves fatty liver and hypertriglyceridemia in sucrose-fed obese rats via two pathways. *Am. J. Physiol. Endocrinol. Metab.* **2009**, *297*, E76–E84. [CrossRef] [PubMed]
26. Kami, K.; Fujimori, T.; Sato, H.; Sato, M.; Yamamoto, H.; Ohashi, Y.; Sugiyama, N.; Ishihama, Y.; Onozuka, H.; Ochiai, A.; et al. Metabolomic profiling of lung and prostate tumor tissues by capillary electrophoresis time-of-flight mass spectrometry. *Metabolomics* **2013**, *9*, 444–453. [CrossRef] [PubMed]
27. Ohashi, Y.; Hirayama, A.; Ishikawa, T.; Nakamura, S.; Shimizu, K.; Ueno, Y.; Tomita, M.; Soga, T. Depiction of metabolome changes in histidine-starved Escherichia coli by CE-TOFMS. *Mol. Biosyst.* **2008**, *4*, 135–147. [CrossRef] [PubMed]
28. Pedersen, H.K.; Gudmundsdottir, V.; Nielsen, H.B.; Hyotylainen, T.; Nielsen, T.; Jensen, B.A.; Forslund, K.; Hildebrand, F.; Prifti, E.; Falony, G.; et al. Human gut microbes impact host serum metabolome and insulin sensitivity. *Nature* **2016**, *535*, 376–381. [CrossRef] [PubMed]
29. Cani, P.D.; Neyrinck, A.M.; Maton, N.; Delzenne, N.M. Oligofructose promotes satiety in rats fed a high-fat diet: Involvement of glucagon-like peptide-1. *Obes. Res.* **2005**, *13*, 1000–1007. [CrossRef] [PubMed]
30. Rabot, S.; Membrez, M.; Bruneau, A.; Gerard, P.; Harach, T.; Moser, M.; Raymond, F.; Mansourian, R.; Chou, C.J. Germ-free C57BL/6J mice are resistant to high-fat-diet-induced insulin resistance and have altered cholesterol metabolism. *FASEB J.* **2010**, *24*, 4948–4959. [CrossRef] [PubMed]
31. Lim, S.; Chang, D.H.; Ahn, S.; Kim, B.C. Whole genome sequencing of "faecalibaculum rodentium" ALO17, isolated from C57bl/6J laboratory mouse feces. *Gut Pathog.* **2016**, *8*, 3. [CrossRef] [PubMed]
32. Morotomi, M.; Nagai, F.; Sakon, H.; Tanaka, R. Dialister succinatiphilus sp. nov. and Barnesiella intestinihominis sp. Nov., isolated from human faeces. *Int. J. Syst. Evol. Microbiol.* **2008**, *58*, 2716–2720. [CrossRef] [PubMed]
33. Ubeda, C.; Bucci, V.; Caballero, S.; Djukovic, A.; Toussaint, N.C.; Equinda, M.; Lipuma, L.; Ling, L.; Gobourne, A.; No, D.; et al. Intestinal microbiota containing Barnesiella species cures vancomycin-resistant Enterococcus faecium colonization. *Infect. Immun.* **2013**, *81*, 965–973. [CrossRef] [PubMed]
34. Arrieta, M.C.; Stiemsma, L.T.; Dimitriu, P.A.; Thorson, L.; Russell, S.; Yurist-Doutsch, S.; Kuzeljevic, B.; Gold, M.J.; Britton, H.M.; Lefebvre, D.L.; et al. Early infancy microbial and metabolic alterations affect risk of childhood asthma. *Sci. Transl. Med.* **2015**, *7*, 307ra152. [CrossRef] [PubMed]
35. Takahashi, K.; Onodera, K.; Akiba, Y. Effect of dietary xylitol on growth and inflammatory responses in immune stimulated chickens. *Br. Poult. Sci.* **1999**, *40*, 552–554. [CrossRef] [PubMed]
36. Xu, M.L.; Wi, G.R.; Kim, H.J. Ameliorating effect of dietary xylitol on human respiratory syncytial virus (hRSV) infection. *Biol. Pharm. Bull.* **2016**, *39*, 540–546. [CrossRef] [PubMed]
37. Geidenstam, N.; Al-Majdoub, M.; Ekman, M.; Spegel, P.; Ridderstrale, M. Metabolite profiling of obese individuals before and after a one year weight loss program. *Int. J. Obes.* **2017**, [CrossRef] [PubMed]
38. Khan, M.J.; Gerasimidis, K.; Edwards, C.A.; Shaikh, M.G. Role of gut microbiota in the aetiology of obesity: Proposed mechanisms and review of the literature. *J. Obes.* **2016**, *2016*, 7353642. [CrossRef] [PubMed]
39. Woods, H.F.; Krebs, H.A. Xylitol metabolism in the isolated perfused rat liver. *Biochem. J.* **1973**, *134*, 437–443. [CrossRef] [PubMed]
40. Kabashima, T.; Kawaguchi, T.; Wadzinski, B.E.; Uyeda, K. Xylulose 5-phosphate mediates glucose-induced lipogenesis by xylulose 5-phosphate-activated protein phosphatase in rat liver. *Proc. Natl. Acad. Sci. USA* **2003**, *100*, 5107–5112. [CrossRef] [PubMed]
41. Uyeda, K.; Yamashita, H.; Kawaguchi, T. Carbohydrate responsive element-binding protein (ChREBP): A key regulator of glucose metabolism and fat storage. *Biochem. Pharmacol.* **2002**, *63*, 2075–2080. [CrossRef]

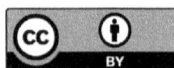

nutrients

MDPI

Article

Dietary Supplement Use during Preconception: The Australian Longitudinal Study on Women's Health

Elle McKenna [1,*], Alexis Hure [2], Anthony Perkins [1] and Ellie Gresham [1]

1   Griffith Health, Griffith University, Southport, QLD 4215, Australia;
    a.perkins@griffith.edu.au (A.P.); ellie.gresham@health.nsw.gov.au (E.G.)
2   School of Medicine and Public Health, The University of Newcastle, Callaghan, NSW 2308, Australia;
    alexis.hure@newcastle.edu.au
*   Correspondence: elle.mckenna@griffithuni.edu.au; Tel.: +61-497-616-462

Received: 29 August 2017; Accepted: 9 October 2017; Published: 13 October 2017

Abstract: Worldwide, dietary supplement use among reproductive aged women is becoming increasingly common. The aim of this study was to investigate dietary supplement use among Australian women during preconception. Self-reported data were collected prospectively for the Australian Longitudinal Study on Women's Health (ALSWH). The sample included 485 women aged 31–36 years, with supplement data, classified as preconception when completing Survey 5 of the ALSWH in 2009. Frequency and contingency tables were calculated and Pearson's chi-square test for associations between demographic variables and supplementation status was performed. Sixty-three per cent of women were taking at least one dietary supplement during preconception. Multiple-micronutrient supplements were the most commonly reported supplement (44%). Supplements containing folic acid and iodine were reported by 51% and 37% of preconception women, respectively. Folic acid (13%), omega-3 fatty acids (11%), vitamin C (7%), B vitamins (4%), iron (3%), and calcium (3%) were the most common single nutrients supplemented during preconception. Women trying to conceive, with no previous children, and born outside Australia were more likely to take dietary supplements. In Australia, dietary supplement use during preconception is relatively high. However, supplementation of recommended nutrients, including folic acid and iodine, could be improved.

Keywords: dietary supplements; preconception; multivitamins; maternal

1. Introduction

Worldwide, women of reproductive age are routinely recommended nutrient supplementation during preconception and pregnancy to reduce their risk of adverse pregnancy and foetal outcomes associated with nutrient deficiencies [1–3]. The effectiveness of folic acid supplementation in the prevention of Neural Tube Defects (NTDs) is well documented [4,5]. The neural tube develops during the first few weeks of pregnancy [6], which is often before a woman recognises she is pregnant and well before her first antenatal care appointment [2]. Following years of voluntary folic acid fortification, mandatory fortification of wheat flour used for bread-making with folic acid was implemented in Australia in September 2009. The prevalence of folic acid deficiency in Australia has reduced, and there has also been a significant decline of 14.4% in the rate of NTDs per 10,000 conceptions, by March 2011 [7,8]. Australian health authorities recommend daily supplementation of folic acid three months before conception and for the first three months of pregnancy, to reduce the risk of NTDs [2,3]. Likewise, mandatory iodine fortification was implemented in Australia in 2009, which required the replacement of non-iodised salt with iodised salt for bread making, with the exception of organic breads. Subsequently, the proportion of females of child-bearing age estimated to have inadequate iodine intakes decreased from 60% to 9% [9]. Daily supplementation of iodine is recommended in Australia three months before conception, as well as for pregnancy and lactation to reduce the risk of iodine deficiency and associated negative impacts on early brain and nervous system development [2,3]. Other nutrients (including iron, omega-3 fatty acids, vitamin D, calcium, and vitamin B12) may be recommended to reproductive aged women with a diagnosed deficiency or inadequate dietary intake [2,3].

Despite supplement use becoming a common practice in Australia, little is known of the national occurrence during preconception, or the demographic characteristics of women who use supplements during this time. There are a limited number of studies on dietary supplement use in Australia during preconception, typically defined as three months before conception, with the prevalence varying considerably (29–67%) [10–13]. The generalizability of the available data is limited with recruitment using convenience sampling from antenatal clinics, and studies collecting data retrospectively (when women are pregnant), increasing the risk of recall bias.

Therefore, the aim of this study was to report on the number of women taking dietary supplements during preconception in Australia using national data from the Australian Longitudinal Study on Women's Health (ALSWH), to explore demographic characteristics and to identify the most common nutrients supplemented by women during preconception.

2. Materials and Methods

2.1. Data Collection

The current study used self-reported data collected prospectively from the ALSWH. The ALSWH recruited 40,393 women in 1996 across three cohorts; those born in 1973–78 (18–23 years), 1946–51 (45–50 years), and 1921–26 (70–75 years), and more recently, a new cohort born in 1989–95 who were first surveyed in 2013 (aged 18–23 years). When the ALSWH began, women were randomly selected from Australia's nationalised health-care system, Medicare, with intentional oversampling in rural and remote areas. Ethical approval was obtained by the Human Research Ethics Committees of the University of Newcastle (H-076-0795) prior to baseline data collection in 1996, with written consent provided by participants. Further details on the ALSWH recruitment and cohort profile have been published elsewhere [14–17].

The present paper examines data from the 1973–78 cohort, who were broadly representative of Australian women the same age at the baseline survey [14]. Paper-based surveys were mailed to participants for Survey 1 in 1996 (*n* = 14,247), Survey 2 in 2000 (*n* = 9688), Survey 3 in 2003 (*n* = 9081), and Survey 4 in 2006 (*n* = 9145). In 2009 (Survey 5, *n* = 8200), 2012 (Survey 6, *n* = 8009), and 2015 (Survey 7, *n* = 7186) participants could opt to complete the survey online or in hard copy. The ALSWH surveys include a broad range of demographic and health behaviour measures, including area of residence, marital status, level of education, parity, smoking status, alcohol use, frequency and intensity of physical activity, weight, height, and income.

2.2. Sample

Women were aged 31 to 36 years at the time of completing Survey 5 in 2009. To derive preconception status, the women's Survey 5 return date and child's date of birth data from subsequent surveys were used. Data management for the ALSWH involves de-identifying participant information, including child dates of birth. All child dates of birth for a particular month are rounded to the 15th of that month. For example, a child date of birth occurring on 1 June would be rounded to 15 June, as would a child date of birth occurring on 30 June. Following the methods of Gresham et al., 'preconception' included women who were 1–6 months before a conception resulting in a birth (i.e., Survey 5 returned 10–15 months before a child's date of birth recorded at a subsequent survey) [18]. Women with a pregnancy resulting in a miscarriage or termination would not have been identified, however, stillbirths may have been included.

2.3. Supplement Data

At Survey 5, women were asked to write down the names of all their medications, vitamins, supplements or herbal therapies they had taken in the last four weeks, with an option to select 'none'. Women were excluded from the present analyses if they (i) were not classified as preconception when completing the survey (n = 7691) or (ii) were classified as preconception with missing supplement data (n = 24).

Women were classified as 'supplementing' if at least one dietary supplement was reported, while women who responded 'none' were classified as 'not supplementing'. Participants were not required to specify the dose or quantity of the supplement consumed, nor did some participants specify the brand. Over-the-counter and prescription supplements were included in this study.

Three stages were used to categorise supplements. The first stage included the World Health Organization (WHO) Anatomical Therapeutic Chemical (ATC) classification system with Defined Daily Dose (DDD). This type of coding categorises drugs into different groups according to the organ or system on which they act and their therapeutic, pharmacological, and chemical properties, in addition to the assumed average maintenance dose per day for the drugs main indication in adults [19]. Further details on the ATC/DDD classification system are available elsewhere [19]. The main active ingredients of the formulation for each original medication and supplement were identified and assigned an ATC code. Other medications, herbal preparations, and tonics were excluded for this analysis.

The second stage of supplement classification used the ATC/DDD system as a framework to generate an extensive list of single nutrient (i.e., folate, iron, calcium), combination nutrients (i.e., iron and folate, iodine, and folate) and multiple micronutrient supplement (MMN) (i.e., three or more micronutrients) categories, without therapeutic doses. The final stage of supplement classification grouped the classifications from the second stage if the supplement category included folic acid, iodine, or iron.

2.4. Other Variables

Women reported their country of birth at Survey 1 (baseline) in 1996. More current demographic characteristics including area of residence, marital status, level of education, parity, smoking status, alcohol use, frequency and intensity of physical activity, weight, height, and income were reported at Survey 5 in 2009. Women were also asked at Survey 5 if they had been diagnosed or treated for 'low iron (iron-deficiency or anaemia)' in the past three years and if they were 'trying to become pregnant'.

2.5. Statistical Analysis

The characteristics of women who were included in the analysis were compared to the remaining 1973-78 ALSWH cohort. The characteristics of women who were classified as preconception and supplementing were compared to women who were preconception and not supplementing. Data were checked for normality using numerical and graphical methods including the Shapiro–Wilk test and histograms. Means and standard deviations were presented for normally distributed continuous variables and groups were compared using two sample t-tests with unequal variance. Proportions were presented for categorical variables, and groups were compared using Pearson chi-square test (X^2) for independence, or in the case of small cell sizes, Fisher's exact test. A p value of ≤ 0.01 was considered statistically significant. All analyses were performed using the statistical software package Stata IC, version 13 (StataCorp, College Station, TX, USA) [20].

3. Results

A total of 485 preconception women were included in the analysis; 6% of all women who completed Survey 5. The selection of cohort participants eligible for inclusion, including the classification of women supplementing (or not) is presented in Figure 1.

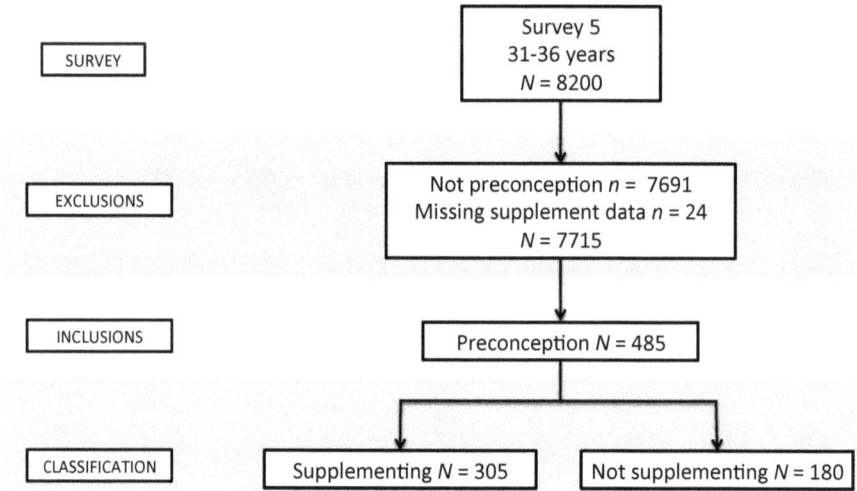

Figure 1. Selection of participants and classification of supplementation status.

Table 1 summarises the baseline characteristics (reported in 1996) of women included in the analysis and for those in the remaining 1973–78 ALSWH cohort. Women included were the same age as those excluded (20.6 and 20.8 years, respectively), with the majority from both groups engaging in high levels of physical activity (34.2% vs. 30.1%). At baseline, women included were more likely to be living in urban areas, be single, have no children, and be less likely to smoke or drink alcohol at risky levels. While there was a similar number of women who attained school or high-school education, more women included in the current analysis reported university education (16.4% vs. 10.9%).

Table 1. Baseline characteristics † for the young cohort of the Australian Longitudinal Study on Women's Health 1973–1978 according to inclusion (*n* = 485) or not in the present study (*n* = 13,762).

Characteristics	Included in the Study N = 485			Not Included in the Study N = 13,762		
	n	Mean	SD	*n*	Mean	SD
Age	485	20.6	1.4	13,762	20.8	1.5
	n	%		*n*	%	
Australian Residence						
Urban	313	64.5		7556	54.9	
Rural	161	33.2		5660	41.1	
Remote	11	2.3		546	4	
Missing	0	-		0	-	
Marital Status						
Married/Defacto	61	12.7		3132	22.9	
Separated/Divorced	1	0.2		128	0.9	
Single	419	87.1		10,431	76.2	
Missing	4	-		66	-	
Parity						
None	475	98.3		12,137	89.7	
One	5	1.1		1023	7.5	
Two or more	3	0.6		374	2.8	
Missing	2	-		228	-	

Table 1. *Cont.*

	Included in the Study N = 485		Not Included in the Study N = 13,762	
Highest educational level				
No formal education	5	1	403	3
School or higher school certificate	323	66.9	9296	67.9
Trade or Diploma	76	15.7	2487	18.2
University or Higher university degree	79	16.4	1497	10.9
Missing	2	-	79	-
Physical activity				
Nil/sedentary	53	11	2085	15.3
Low	141	29.3	3941	28.8
Moderate	123	25.5	3523	25.8
High	165	34.2	4122	30.1
Missing	3	-	91	-
Smoking				
Current smoker	118	25.2	4303	32.7
Non-smoker	350	74.8	8858	67.3
Missing	17	-	601	-
Alcohol Intake				
Non-drinker	31	6.5	1223	9
Low risk/rarely drinks	426	88.9	11,626	85.4
High risk/risky drinker	22	4.6	760	5.6
Missing	6	-	153	-

† Participant characteristics were taken from the baseline survey; SD, Standard Deviation; -, Percent is not calculated for missing values.

Women who reported taking supplements during preconception were more likely to be trying to conceive (48% vs. 23%; $p \leq 0.001$), have no previous children (35% vs. 21%; $p \leq 0.001$), and were born outside of Australia ($p \leq 0.001$) when compared to women who did not supplement (Table 2). There were no statistically significant differences in regards to age, Body Mass Index, education, area of residence, annual household income, marital status, smoking, alcohol intake, or physical activity.

Table 2. Demographic characteristics of women aged 31–36 years in 2009 from the Australian Longitudinal Study on Women's Health who were supplementing and not supplementing during preconception.

	Supplementing N = 305			Not Supplementing N = 180			
Characteristics	*n*	Mean	SD	*n*	Mean	SD	*p* Value
Age	305	33.5	1.4	180	33.5	1.4	0.887
	n	%		*n*	%		
Country of Birth							
Australia	277	91.4		172	96.6		0.009
Outside of Australia	26	8.6		6	3.4		
Missing	2	-		2	-		
Body Mass Index							
Underweight	6	2		3	1.7		0.568
Healthy Weight	183	60.4		98	54.7		
Overweight	76	25.1		49	27.4		
Obese	38	12.5		29	16.2		
Missing	2	-		1	-		

Table 2. *Cont.*

	Supplementing N = 305		Not Supplementing N = 180		
Australian Residence					
Urban	203	67.7	107	62.2	0.179
Rural	90	30	56	32.6	
Remote	7	2.3	9	5.2	
Missing	5	-	8	-	
Marital Status					
Married/Defacto	289	95.1	173	96.1	0.939
Separated/Divorced	8	2.6	3	1.7	
Single	7	2.3	4	2.2	
Missing	1	-	0	-	
Parity					
None	107	36.1	37	20.6	<0.001
One	139	47	85	47.2	
Two or more	50	16.9	58	32.2	
Missing	0	-	0	-	
Highest educational level					
No formal education	2	0.7	2	1.1	0.727
School or higher school certificate	36	12	23	13.1	
Trade or Diploma	62	20.6	30	17.1	
University or higher university degree	201	66.8	120	68.6	
Missing	4	-	5	-	
Annual Household Income					
No income	2	0.7	1	0.6	0.292
$1–$36,999	12	4	5	2.8	
$37,000–$129,999	169	55.8	118	65.9	
$130,000 or more	98	32.3	45	25.1	
Don't know/Don't want to answer	22	7.3	10	5.6	
Missing	2	-	1	-	
Physical activity					
Nil/sedentary	25	8.4	26	14.9	0.138
Low	117	39.5	65	37.4	
Moderate	85	28.7	41	23.6	
High	69	23.3	42	24.1	
Missing	9	-	6	-	
Smoking					
Daily	6	2	11	6.1	0.042
At least weekly (not daily)	3	1	5	2.8	
Less often than weekly	8	2.6	5	2.8	
Not at all	288	94.4	159	88.3	
Missing	0	-	0	-	
Alcohol Intake					
Non-drinker	28	9.2	23	12.8	0.435
Low risk/rarely drinks	260	85.5	148	82.7	
High risk/risky drinker	16	5.3	8	4.5	
Missing	1	-	1	-	
Trying to conceive					
Yes	149	48.4	42	23.5	<0.001
No	159	51.6	137	76.5	
Missing	0	-	1	-	

SD, Standard Deviation; -, Percent is not calculated for missing values.

During preconception, 63% of women (*n* = 305) reported taking at least one dietary supplement. Of those women, 57% (*n* = 173) reported taking only one type of supplement, 28% (*n* = 86) reported taking two types of supplements, and 15% (*n* = 46) reported taking three or more. The highest reported number of supplements taken during preconception was six supplements (*n* = 3).

Table 3 reports the most common types of supplements used by women during preconception. MMN supplements were the most common type of supplement (44%), followed by single nutrient supplements (34% of women reporting). The six most commonly reported single nutrient supplements included folic acid (13%), omega-3 fatty acids (11%), vitamin C (7%), B vitamins (4%), iron (3%), and calcium (3%).

Table 3. Rates of multiple and single micronutrient supplement use among preconception women aged 31–36 years in 2009 from the Australian Longitudinal Study on Women's Health.

	Preconception *N* = 485	
Supplement	*n*	%
Multiple Micronutrient	212	43.7
Single nutrient	167	34.4
Folic acid	62	12.8
Omega-3/Fish oil	52	10.7
Vitamin C	33	6.8
B Vitamins	18	3.7
Iron	15	3.1
Calcium	14	2.9

Participants were able to select multiple supplements, therefore numbers are not mutually exclusive.

Approximately half of the women (51%) reported taking a folic acid-containing supplement, 39% an iron-containing supplement, and approximately a third (37%) an iodine-containing supplement during preconception (Figure 2). Of the women taking an iron-containing supplement, 23% reported an iron deficiency, while the majority (70%) did not report a pre-diagnosed iron deficiency and the remaining had missing data.

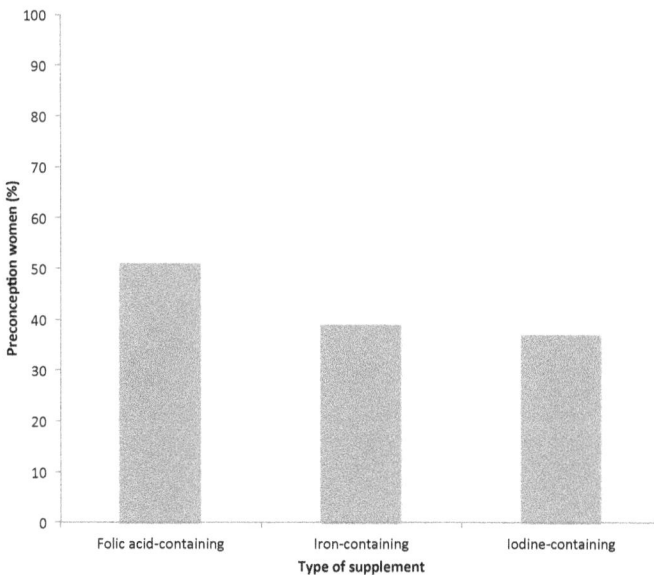

Figure 2. Nutrient-containing dietary supplement use among preconception women aged 31–36 years in 2009 from the Australian Longitudinal Study on Women's Health. Participants were able to select multiple supplements, therefore numbers do not add to 100%. Nutrients from dietary supplements includes nutrients from both multiple micronutrient and single nutrient supplements.

4. Discussion

This study found that just under two thirds (63%) of women aged 31–36 years took one or more dietary supplements during preconception, which broadly captured about one to six months before conception resulting in a live or still-birth. Our study is novel, in that we have analysed data collected prospectively, before the outcome of a planned or unplanned pregnancy was known. Two out of every five women in this study identified that they were 'trying to conceive' in the window we defined as preconception, suggesting that supplementation use is high in women of this age generally, rather than because of recommendations for preconception and pregnancy. In our study, if a woman had given birth preterm, they may have completed the survey as early as eight months prior to conception, which could explain the slightly lower rate (40%) of women who indicated that they were actively 'trying to conceive', compared to the national average (half of all pregnancies are unplanned) [21]. Previous research on contraceptive use and unintended pregnancy in Australia has identified issues of ambiguity and ambivalence around a woman's intentions to fall pregnant, which impacts on a woman's decision to use contraceptives (or not) and the reliability of contraceptives that they use [22]. Women in our study who reported they were not trying to conceive were also less likely to take supplements during preconception, which seems consistent with having some measure of the supplementing behaviours in unplanned pregnancies.

4.1. Interpretation

The high rate of supplementation in our study is similar to the findings of two studies conducted in Australia at large hospitals in major cities [10,11]. Women who were supplementing prior to pregnancy were more often trying to conceive, with no previous children and be born overseas, compared to women not supplementing.

In our study, 13% of women (preconception), reported supplementing with a folic acid-only supplement, increasing to 51% when all folic acid-containing supplements were included. Similar results have been found by other Australian studies reporting on folic acid supplementation; ranging from 27–61% [11,13,23].

Supplementation of iodine was low among women before conception, with approximately a third of women (37%) supplementing with an iodine containing preparation. Our findings are lower than rates reported by a recent study (2016) that collected data from a national online cohort (*n* = 455) and South Australian public maternity hospital cohort (*n* = 402) of pregnant women, where approximately 50% of women reported supplementing with an iodine containing preparation during preconception [11]. This increase may be due to the higher rate of planned pregnancies (74%) reported, in addition to an increasing awareness of supplementation during pregnancy overtime and an increased risk of recall bias associated with retrospective data collection. A higher supplementation rate found by studies in more recent years may be explained by the Australian iodine supplementation recommendations for pregnant women and women considering pregnancy released in 2010 [24], following our supplementation data collection in 2009. Given the low rates of folic acid and iodine supplementation, further research is needed to quantify total oral intake of such nutrients (inclusive of foods containing mandatory fortification of folate and iodine) and whether women are meeting the requirements through diet alone. The barriers to such supplementation, and ongoing education of reproductive aged women about the importance of folic acid and iodine supplementation may be required, if women are not meeting these requirements through diet alone.

Our findings of MMN supplementation among preconception women (44%) is consistent with the findings of a recent study conducted in Sydney where pregnant women were recruited from antenatal clinics at two tertiary teaching hospitals (*n* = 589) [10]. The most frequent MMN supplements reported in our study were among the top market leaders of Australian pregnancy-specific supplements, consistent with other Australian studies' findings [12,25]. These market leader preparations contain a range of nutrients, varying in their dosage of nutrients, and not aligning with the Australian recommendations for supplementation during preconception. One product provides an excess of

300 μg of folic acid and 70 μg of iodine, whilst another provides the recommended amounts for both nutrients [2,3]. These market leader supplements also provide nutrients (including iron, calcium, omega-3 fatty acids, vitamin D, and B vitamins) that are not currently recommended without a confirmed deficiency or low dietary intake, potentially increasing the risk of harm caused by an excessive dietary intake and/or high levels of such nutrients in the body.

Supplementing with iron is not routinely recommended to women in Australia during preconception, due to a lack of evidence for its benefit and increased risk of adverse outcomes during pregnancy [2,26]. Despite the recommendations, our findings show the rate of iron-containing supplementation to be higher than that for iodine-containing (which should be routinely recommended for all women considering pregnancy, during preconception, pregnancy, and lactation). In addition, approximately 70% of women who were supplementing with an iron-containing supplement did not self-report an iron deficiency. There is potential that some of these women were unaware they were low in iron and therefore undiagnosed, however, further research is warranted to determine the potential short and long-term effects of iron supplementation among women without diagnosed deficiencies prior to conception and during pregnancy.

4.2. Implications for Practice and Research

With lower than previously reported rates of folic acid and iodine supplementation during preconception found in this study, alongside the fact that less than half of all pregnancies are being planned, the importance of mandatory fortification of such nutrients to provide adequate reach to the preconception population is highlighted.

General practitioners are generally one of the first health professionals a woman consults to confirm that she is pregnant. This initial consultation would be of no benefit in providing information on dietary supplements during the preconception period, particularly for the reduced risks of NTDs and impaired cognitive development associated with folic acid and iodine supplement use, respectively. However, this consult could be used to identify women with or at risk of nutrient deficiencies, where strategies should be put into place to improve dietary intake and quality during pregnancy, as well as highlighting the importance of at-risk nutrients for subsequent pregnancies.

Further studies are required to quantify total nutrient intake during preconception, while further investigations into supplement use prior to conception and adverse pregnancy and birth outcomes are needed.

4.3. Strengths and Limitations

This study is the first study, worldwide, to report on dietary supplement use during preconception using data collected prospectively. The retention rate for Survey 5 in 2009 was >55% of the initial study sample. Research has shown that women responding at all ALSWH survey waves (Surveys 1–4) are more educated, less likely to smoke and have children than those women responding to some of the surveys. However, while there is a need to consider the potential for bias due to attrition, the identified biases are insufficient to preclude meaningful longitudinal analyses in this cohort of women (1973–1978) [27].

Due to de-identification of participant information, specifically child date of birth data, which is rounded to the 15th day of their birth month, there may be potential for misclassification error according to preconception status using the child's date of birth and survey return date. This would only occur for women who delivered preterm and returned their survey within the number of months they delivered preterm: for example, a woman who delivered at seven months (i.e., 32 weeks gestation) and returned her survey two months preconception, would not have been included in our study, as this survey would fall outside the 10–15 month window. Furthermore, our case definition relies on a date of birth being recorded, so any pregnancy that resulted in a miscarriage or termination would not have been identified, however stillbirth may have been included.

The current study included women aged 31–36 years. In 2009–2010, the median age of women giving birth in Australia was approximately 31 years [28], highlighting that our findings may be broadly generalizable to women of the same age in the Australian population.

Gresham et al. and Hure et al. previously conducted agreement studies of women in the 1973–1978 cohort, demonstrating high agreement ($\geq$87%) between self-reported ALSWH and administrative data for the adverse pregnancy outcomes gestational hypertension, gestational diabetes mellitus, preterm birth, low birth weight [29], and stillbirth [30], offering a high degree of confidence in the accuracy of self-report of women in the ALSWH.

Data on nutrient amounts and frequency of supplementation was unavailable at Survey 5, as women were not asked to provide this information, and as a result total nutrient intakes from dietary supplements and adherence to the recommendations for daily dosage and compliance of supplement regimes were unable to be reported.

Data for this study were collected in 2009, following the development of the Royal Australian and New Zealand Colleague of Obstetricians and Gynaecologists (RANZCOG) 'Vitamin and mineral supplementation and pregnancy' statement in 2008 [3]. Over time, these recommendations have been revised and, in 2011, iodine supplementation was included as a recommendation. During this time there was a reduction in the supplemental dose for folate by 100 µg/day (500 to 400 µg/day), which has not impacted on the reported findings in this study, as supplement intake was not quantified by dosage. Our study found lower rates of iodine supplementation, which may be a result of iodine not being recommended as a standard supplementation for women who were trying to conceive in 2009.

5. Conclusions

The current study is the first study to report on dietary supplement use during preconception in Australia using data collected prospectively from preconception women. The findings suggest that the majority of Australian women take at least one dietary supplement during preconception. Women are frequently taking supplements containing multiple nutrients, of which some of the included nutrients are recommended only to women with diagnosed deficiencies or low dietary intakes. The low supplementation rates of folic acid and iodine warrant further public health interventions to increase awareness of their importance, while further research is needed to determine the role of dietary supplementation during preconception, evaluating short and long term pregnancy outcomes and measuring other factors such as total nutrient intakes and diet quality.

Acknowledgments: The research on which this paper is based was conducted as part of the Australian Longitudinal Study on Women's Health by the University of Queensland and the University of Newcastle. We are grateful to the Australian Government Department of Health for funding and to the women who provided the survey data.

Author Contributions: A.H. and E.G. conceived and designed the study; E.M. analysed the data under the guidance of E.G.; E.M. drafted the manuscript; and all authors critically reviewed and approved the final version of the manuscript for publication.

Conflicts of Interest: The authors declare no conflict of interest.

References

1. World Health Organization. *WHO Recommendations on Antenatal Care for a Positive Pregnancy Experience*; World Health Organization: Geneva, Switzerland, 2016.
2. Australian Health Ministers' Advisory Council. *Clinical Practice Guidelines: Anetnatal Care—Module 1*; Australian Government Department of Health and Ageing: Canberra, Australia, 2012.
3. Womens Health Committee. *Vitamin and Mineral Supplementation and Pregnancy*; The Royal Australian and New Zealand College of Obstetricians and Gynaecologists (RANZCOG): Victoria, Australia, 2015.
4. Czeizel, A.E.; Dudas, I. Prevention of the first occurrence of neural-tube defects by periconceptional vitamin supplementation. *N. Engl. J. Med.* **1992**, *327*, 1832–1835. [CrossRef] [PubMed]

5. De-Regil, L.M.; Pena-Rosas, J.P.; Fernandez-Gaxiola, A.C.; Rayco-Solon, P. Effects and safety of periconceptional oral folate supplementation for preventing birth defects. *Cochrane Database Syst. Rev.* **2015**, CD007950. [CrossRef]

6. Marieb, E.N.; Hoehn, K. *Human Anatomy and Physiology*; Pearson Education Limited: Harlow, UK, 2015.

7. Hilder, L.; National Perinatal Epidemiology and Statistics Unit. *Neural Tube Defects in Australia 2007–2011: Before and after Implementation of the Mandatory Folic Acid Fortification Standard*; University of New South Wales: Sydney, Australia, 2016.

8. Brown, R.D.; Langshaw, M.R.; Uhr, E.J.; Gibson, J.N.; Joshua, D.E. The impact of mandatory fortification of flour with folic acid on the blood folate levels of an Australian population. *Med. J. Aust.* **2011**, *194*, 65–67. [PubMed]

9. Food Standards Australia New Zealand. *Monitoring the Australian Population's Intake of Dietary Iodine before and after Mandatory Fortification*; Food Standards Australia New Zealand: Canberra, Australia, 2016.

10. Shand, A.W.; Walls, M.; Chatterjee, R.; Nassar, N.; Khambalia, A.Z. Dietary vitamin, mineral and herbal supplement use: A cross-sectional survey of before and during pregnancy use in Sydney, Australia. *Aust. N. Z. J. Obstet. Gynaecol.* **2016**, *56*, 154–161. [CrossRef] [PubMed]

11. Malek, L.; Umberger, W.; Makrides, M.; Zhou, S.J. Poor adherence to folic acid and iodine supplement recommendations in preconception and pregnancy: A cross-sectional analysis. *Aust. N. Z. J. Public Health* **2016**, *40*, 424–429. [CrossRef] [PubMed]

12. El-Mani, S.; Charlton, K.E.; Flood, V.; Mullan, J. Limited knowledge about folic acid and iodine nutrition in pregnant women reflected in supplementation practices. *Nutr. Diet.* **2014**, *71*, 236–244. [CrossRef]

13. Lucas, C.J.; Charlton, K.E.; Brown, L.; Brock, E.; Cummins, L. Antenatal shared care: Are pregnant women being adequately informed about iodine and nutritional supplementation? *Aust. N. Z. J. Obstet. Gynaecol.* **2014**, *54*, 515–521. [CrossRef] [PubMed]

14. Brown, W.J.; Bryson, L.; Byles, J.E.; Dobson, A.J.; Lee, C.; Mishra, G.; Schofield, M. Women's health Australia: Recruitment for a national longitudinal cohort study. *Women Health* **1999**, *28*, 23–40. [CrossRef]

15. Lee, C.; Dobson, A.J.; Brown, W.J.; Bryson, L.; Byles, J.; Warner-Smith, P.; Young, A.F. Cohort profile: The Australian longitudinal study on women's health. *Int. J. Epidemiol.* **2005**, *34*, 987–991. [CrossRef] [PubMed]

16. Brown, W.; Lois, B.; Byles, J.; Dobson, A.; Manderson, L.; Schofield, M.; Williams, G. Women's health Australia: Establishment of the australian longitudinal study on women's health. *J. Women Health* **1996**, *5*, 467–472. [CrossRef]

17. Dobson, A.J.; Hockey, R.; Brown, W.J.; Byles, J.E.; Loxton, D.J.; McLaughlin, D.; Tooth, L.R.; Mishra, G.D. Cohort profile update: Australian longitudinal study on women's health. *Int. J. Epidemiol.* **2015**, *44*, 1547a–1547f. [CrossRef] [PubMed]

18. Gresham, E.; Collins, C.E.; Mishra, G.D.; Byles, J.E.; Hure, A.J. Diet quality before or during pregnancy and the relationship with pregnancy and birth outcomes: The Australian longitudinal study on women's health. *Public Health Nutr.* **2016**, *19*, 2975–2983. [CrossRef] [PubMed]

19. WHO Collaborating Centre for Drug Statistics Methodology. *Guidelines for ATC Classification and DDD Assignment 2013*; WHO Collaborating Centre for Drug Statistics Methodology: Oslo, Norway, 2012.

20. StataCorp. *Stata Statistical Software: Release 13*; StataCorp LP: College Station, TX, USA, 2013.

21. Children by Choice Association. *Fact Sheet: Unplanned Pregnancy in Australia*; Children by Choice Association: Brisbane, Australia, 2013.

22. Coombe, J.; Harris, M.L.; Wigginton, B.; Lucke, J.; Loxton, D. Contraceptive use at the time of unintended pregnancy: Findings from the contraceptive use, pregnancy intention and decisions study. *Aust. Fam. Phys.* **2016**, *45*, 842–848.

23. Watson, L.F.; Brown, S.J.; Davey, M.A. Use of periconceptional folic acid supplements in Victoria and New South Wales, Australia. *Aust. N. Z. J. Public Health* **2006**, *30*, 42–49. [CrossRef] [PubMed]

24. National Health and Medical Research Council. *Iodine Supplementation for Pregnant and Breastfeeding Women*; Australian Government: Canberra, Australia, 2010.

25. Conlin, M.L.; MacLennan, A.H.; Broadbent, J.L. Inadequate compliance with periconceptional folic acid supplementation in South Australia. *Aust. N. Z. J. Obstet. Gynaecol.* **2006**, *46*, 528–533. [CrossRef] [PubMed]

26. Pena-Rosas, J.P.; De-Regil, L.M.; Garcia-Casal, M.N.; Dowswell, T. Daily oral iron supplementation during pregnancy. *Cochrane Database Syst. Rev.* **2015**, CD004736. [CrossRef]

27. Powers, J.; Loxton, D. The impact of attrition in an 11-year prospective longitudinal study of younger women. *Ann. Epidemiol.* **2010**, *20*, 318–321. [CrossRef] [PubMed]

28. Australian Bureau of Statistics. *3301.0—Births, Australia, 2015*; Australian Bureau of Statistics: Canberra, Australia, 2016.

29. Gresham, E.; Forder, P.; Chojenta, C.L.; Byles, J.E.; Loxton, D.J.; Hure, A.J. Agreement between self-reported perinatal outcomes and administrative data in New South Wales, Australia. *BMC Pregnancy Childbirth* **2015**, *15*, 161. [CrossRef] [PubMed]

30. Hure, A.J.; Chojenta, C.L.; Powers, J.R.; Byles, J.E.; Loxton, D. Validity and reliability of stillbirth data using linked self-reported and administrative datasets. *J. Epidemiol.* **2015**, *25*, 30–37. [CrossRef] [PubMed]

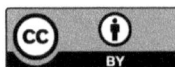

nutrients

MDPI

Article

The Prevalence and Predictors of Dietary Supplement Use in the Australian Population

Stacey K. O'Brien, Eva Malacova, Jill L. Sherriff and Lucinda J. Black *

School of Public Health, Curtin University, Bentley 6102, WA, Australia; stacey.k.obrien@curtin.edu.au (S.K.O.);
eva.malacova@curtin.edu.au (E.M.); j.sherriff@curtin.edu.au (J.L.S.)
* Correspondence: lucinda.black@curtin.edu.au; Tel.: +61-8-9266-2523

Received: 30 August 2017; Accepted: 18 October 2017; Published: 21 October 2017

Abstract: Current dietary supplement use in Australia is not well described. We investigated the prevalence and predictors of supplement use in the Australian population (n = 19,257) using data from the 2014–2015 National Health Survey. We reported the prevalence of supplement use by sex and age group and investigated the independent predictors of supplement use in adults, adolescents, and children using multiple logistic regression models. A total of 43.2% of adults (34.9% of males, 50.3% of females), 20.1% of adolescents (19.7% of males, 20.6% of females), and 23.5% of children (24.4% of males, 22.5% of females) used at least one dietary supplement in the previous two weeks. The most commonly used supplements were multivitamins and/or multiminerals and fish oil preparations. In adults, independent predictors of supplement use included being female, increasing age, being born outside Australia and other main English-speaking countries, having a higher education level, having a healthy BMI compared to those who were obese, being physically active, and being a non-smoker. To our knowledge, this is the first detailed investigation of dietary supplement use in a nationally-representative sample of the Australian population. Future studies investigating the contribution of supplements to overall dietary intakes of vitamins, minerals, and omega-3 fatty acids are warranted.

Keywords: dietary supplements; prevalence; predictors; Australian Health Survey

1. Introduction

Prevalence data on the regular use of dietary supplements by the general population over the last two decades are available for several countries. In the National Health and Nutrition Examination Surveys (NHANES), approximately half of the US adult population aged ≥20 years used at least one dietary supplement in the 30 days before the home interview of each survey since 1999–2000 (mean n per survey = 5423) [1]. This is similar to the Danish age-adjusted data (n = 1923) obtained by 24-h recall in those aged 35–74 years participating in the European Prospective Investigation into Cancer and Nutrition (EPIC) calibration study (1995–2000) [2], but higher than data for all other countries involved (as low as 0.5% for Greece). UK data from the National Diet and Nutrition Survey (NDNS) (September 2008–November 2010, n = 1491) also showed a lower prevalence of supplement use (23% for 19–64 year olds and 39% for those aged >65 years [3]) than NHANES, but this may at least partially reflect the shorter reporting period (4-day food record in the NDNS vs. 30-day recall in NHANES).

The EPIC calibration study used the same question and reporting interval across all eight countries allowing more meaningful comparisons. The wide range of prevalence rates obtained indicates that cultural and/or environmental factors influence the use of dietary supplements [2]. However, the age range of 35–74 years did not allow for the identification of prevalence rates in younger and older age groups, and age has been shown to be one of the main predictors of supplement use [4,5]. Use of dietary supplements is less prevalent in children and adolescents (e.g., 31% of those ≤19 years old, n = 8245 in the NHANES 2007–2010 [6]) and more prevalent in older adults [7].

The general public use dietary supplements for a variety of reasons, including as part of a healthy lifestyle, for assistance with attaining recommended intakes (e.g., calcium and vitamin D) and for management of chronic conditions (e.g., glucosamine) [4,8]. Herbal supplements are also used and concern has been raised regarding potential interactions with medications [8,9]. While the data from serial NHANES indicate that prevalence rates in the US have been constant over the last 20 years, the use of some supplements (e.g., vitamin D) has increased [1], reflecting nutrient concerns of the day. Our focus is to identify which nutrients consumed as supplements need to be included in the determination of total intake; thus, up-to-date and country-specific data on the prevalence of supplement use are required. This study aims to describe the prevalence and predictors of dietary supplement use among Australians of all ages using data from the nationally-representative 2014–2015 National Health Survey (NHS).

2. Materials and Methods

2.1. Study Population

We used questionnaire data from the NHS (n = 19,257), which was conducted between June 2014 and July 2015 across all States and Territories in Australia [10]. Specific methodology of the NHS can be found elsewhere [10,11]. In brief, face-to-face interviews were conducted with a randomly selected adult of the household by trained Australian Bureau of Statistics (ABS) interviewers. For child participants, a parent or guardian answered the questions on behalf of children aged <15 years [11]. Interviews were conducted in the participant's private dwelling in metropolitan and rural areas of Australia [11]. People were excluded from the survey if they were residents of non-private dwellings, such as hotels or boarding schools, or were visitors to a selected dwelling [11]. The interview components of the NHS were conducted under the Census and Statistics Act 1905.

2.2. Identification of Supplement Users

In a face-to-face interview, participants were asked, "What are the names or brands of all the medications, vitamins, minerals or supplements you have taken in the last two weeks?" [10]. Participants were encouraged to have the supplements in front of them, and the name and brand were recorded by the interviewer. For the purposes of the NHS, dietary supplements refer to products defined as Complementary Medicines under the Therapeutic Goods Regulations 1990 [12]. Dietary supplements sold in Australia are regulated by the Therapeutic Goods Administration, which requires them to be listed but not registered (medicines are required to be registered) [12]. Thus, demonstration of efficacy or safety of supplements is not required. It should be noted that products available on international websites are not regulated by the Therapeutic Goods Administration [12]. The Therapeutic Goods Administration advises that consumers do not order dietary supplements over the internet unless the ingredients and legal requirements for importation into Australia are known. However, it is likely that some people obtain their dietary supplements online from international websites. The supplements recorded by the interviewer included those registered with the Therapeutic Goods Administration and those purchased overseas. The ABS categorised supplements into 28 groups (Supplementary Table S1). For the purpose of this study, any participant who reported taking at least one dietary supplement in the previous two weeks was considered a "supplement user".

2.3. Potential Predictors of Supplement Use

Age was provided as a categorical variable and we re-grouped age as follows: ≤9, 10–17, 18–29, 30–49, 50–69, and ≥70 years. We further categorised these groups as adults (≥18 years, n = 14,560), adolescents (10–17 years, n = 1964) and children (≤9 years, n = 2733). Body mass index (BMI; measured weight in kilograms divided by measured height in metres squared) was categorized for adults according to the World Health Organization's cut-off points for underweight, healthy weight, overweight, and obese [13]. For adolescents, cut-off points for BMI categories were assigned using half-yearly sex-and-age specific thresholds as detailed by the International Obesity Task Force [14,15]. We did not assess BMI in children, as BMI is not relevant for those aged <2 years, and our age group included children aged ≤9 years.

State/Territory was assigned for all participants as New South Wales, Victoria, Queensland, South Australia, Western Australia, Tasmania, Northern Territory, and Australian Capital Territory. Region of birth was assigned as Australia, Main English-speaking countries (Canada, Republic of Ireland, New Zealand, South Africa, United Kingdom, United States of America), and Other. As the majority of children were born in Australia and New Zealand, region of birth was assessed only in adults and adolescents.

Educational attainment for adults was defined as none after school, Certificate, Bachelor/Diploma, and postgraduate. Socioeconomic status was described by the Socio-Economic Indexes for Areas (SEIFA) 2011 Index of Relative Socio-Economic Disadvantage (IRSD). This is a general socioeconomic index that summarises a range of information about the economic and social conditions of people and households within an area with scores ranging from low (relatively greater disadvantage in general) to high (relative lack of disadvantage in general) [16]. The SEIFA IRSD was categorised into quintiles.

Physical activity for adults was defined as low, moderate, or high based on the level of physical activity over the past week, incorporating recreation, sport, transport, and fitness [11]. The data items that contributed to this variable were total minutes spent walking for transport in the last week; total minutes walked for fitness, recreation, or sport in last week; total minutes undertaken moderate exercise/physical activity in last week; total minutes undertaken vigorous exercise/physical activity in last week. Physical activity was divided into categories and each had an intensity factor score (e.g., walking for fitness = 3.5, walking for transport = 3.5, moderate exercise/physical activity = 5, and vigorous exercise/physical activity = 7.5). The intensity factor score was multiplied by the duration of physical activity. Varying levels of exercise/physical activity were defined as: low (no exercise to <800); moderate (800 to 1600, or more than 1600 but with less than 1-h vigorous physical activity); high (>1600 and with 1 h or more of vigorous physical activity). Although physical activity information was collected for all participants aged >15 years, we did not investigate physical activity in adolescents, as we did not have data for the entire adolescent group of 10–17 year olds.

Health condition was defined as whether a participant had ever had a long-term health condition, defined as a condition that had lasted, or was expected to last, for at least six months. Common long-term health conditions included asthma, arthritis, cancer, heart and circulatory conditions, diabetes mellitus, kidney disease, osteoporosis, mental or behavioural conditions, along with other less common health conditions [11]. When a participant had a past or present health condition, their health condition was defined as "yes". For adults, smoking was defined as current smoker, past smoker, or never smoked. Self-assessed health in adults was based on how participants felt about their health and was defined as excellent, very good, good, fair, or poor.

2.4. Statistical Analysis

We reported the survey-weighted prevalence of dietary supplement use by sex and age group. The characteristics of the participants were reported for supplement users and non-users among adults, adolescents, and children. All prevalence data were weighted to the Australian population in 2014/2015 [11]. Survey-weighted logistic regression models were used to investigate the independent predictors of supplement use in adults (*n* = 14,560), adolescents (*n* = 1964), and children (*n* = 2733). All models were mutually adjusted for all potential predictors. Potential predictors investigated for all participants were sex, State/Territory, and socioeconomic status. For adults and adolescents, region of birth, BMI category, and health condition were also assessed. We additionally investigated age group, education, physical activity, smoking, and self-assessed health as potential predictors of supplement use in adults. The NHS is based on a stratified, multistage area sample of private households. All households were assigned analytic weights to account for their sampling probability to be included in the survey, and the models accounted for the stratification and clustering of the complex sample design using the Taylor Series Linearization method [11]. All analyses were performed using SAS version 9.4 (SAS Institute, Cary, NC, USA).

3. Results

A total of 43.2% of adults (34.9% of males, 50.3% of females), 20.1% of adolescents (19.7% of males, 20.6% of females), and 23.5% of children (24.4% of males, 22.5% of females) used at least one dietary supplement in the previous two weeks (Figure 1). Characteristics of supplement users vs. non-users are described in Supplementary Tables S2–S4 for adults, adolescents and children, respectively. The maximum number of supplements taken by any individual was 11 among adults, five among adolescents, and seven among children. Among adults, 50.0% of supplement users took more than one supplement in the previous two weeks.

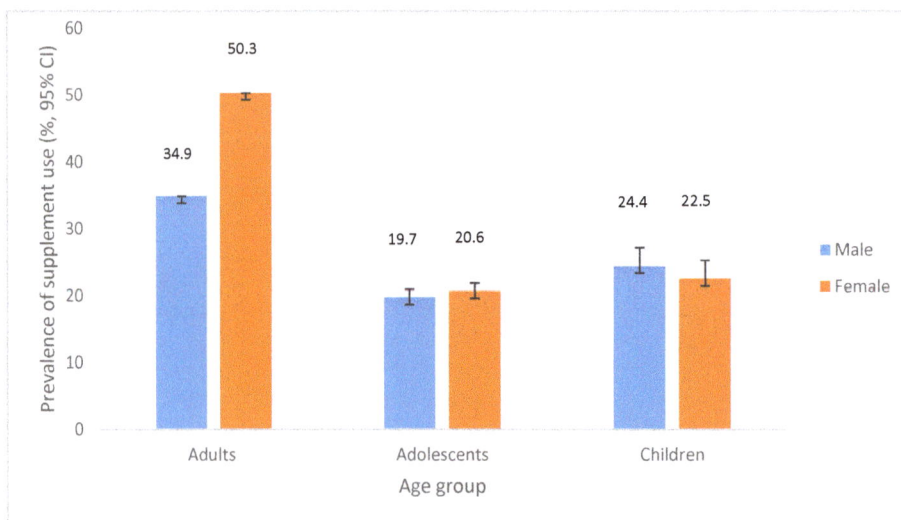

Figure 1. Prevalence (%, 95% CI) of supplement use in the previous two weeks for adults (aged ≥18 years, *n* = 14,560), adolescents (10–17 years, *n* = 1964), and children (≤9 years, *n* = 2733).

In the total population, the most commonly reported dietary supplement type was multivitamin and/or multimineral (without herbal extracts), which was used by 17.5% of the population (males 13.9%, females 20.8%) in the previous two weeks (Supplementary Table S5). A small percentage of the total population (1.5%) used multivitamin and/or multimineral with herbal extracts. Multivitamin and/or multimineral (without herbal extracts) supplement use was most commonly reported in those aged 30–49 years (22.3%; males 17.8%, females 25.8%). A total of 9.2% of the population (males 8.5%, females 9.8%) reported using fish oil preparations (without added nutrients) in the previous two weeks, most commonly in those aged 50–69 years (males 13.2%, females 16.1%).

In adults, significant independent predictors of supplement use were: being female, increasing age, being born outside Australia and other main English-speaking countries, having a higher education level, having a healthy BMI compared to those who were obese, being physically active, and being a non-smoker (Table 1). There were no significant independent predictors of supplement use in adolescents (Table 2). Adolescents in the highest quintile of socioeconomic status and having a health condition had slightly increased odds of supplement use, but the confidence intervals included 1. Being underweight had a reduced odds of supplement use, but its confidence interval also included 1. In children, residing in the Australian Capital Territory and South Australia were associated with slightly decreased odds of supplement use (Table 3). Sex and socioeconomic status were not associated with supplement use in children.

Table 1. Adjusted logistic regression investigating independent predictors of dietary supplement use in Australian adults aged ≥18 years (*n* = 13,539).

	Adjusted OR (95% CI) [1]
Sex (female vs. male)	1.94 (1.78, 2.10)
Age group	
18–29 years	Reference category
30–49 years	1.17 (1.02, 1.34)
50–69 years	1.61 (1.40, 1.85)
≥70 years	1.87 (1.60, 2.19)
Region of birth	
Australia	Reference category
Main English-speaking countries	0.96 (0.85, 1.09)
Other	1.13 (1.01, 1.26)
State/Territory	
New South Wales	Reference category
Victoria	1.01 (0.89, 1.14)
Queensland	1.11 (0.98, 1.25)
South Australia	1.06 (0.93, 1.21)
Western Australia	1.06 (0.92, 1.21)
Tasmania	1.08 (0.94, 1.24)
Northern Territory	0.75 (0.62, 0.91)
Australian Capital Territory	1.10 (0.95, 1.28)
Socioeconomic status	
Lowest quintile	Reference category
Second quintile	1.01 (0.89, 1.15)
Third quintile	1.11 (0.98, 1.27)
Fourth quintile	1.06 (0.93, 1.21)
Highest quintile	1.11 (0.97, 1.28)
Education	
None after school	Reference category
Certificate	1.22 (1.09, 1.37)
Bachelor/Diploma	1.46 (1.32, 1.63)
Postgraduate	1.24 (1.06, 1.45)
BMI category	
Healthy weight	Reference category
Underweight	1.13 (0.80, 1.60)
Overweight	0.94 (0.85, 1.04)
Obese	0.86 (0.77, 0.96)
Physical activity	
Low	Reference category
Moderate	1.12 (1.02, 1.24)
High	1.39 (1.21, 1.60)
Smoking	
Never smoked	Reference category
Past smoker	1.09 (0.99, 1.19)
Current smoker	0.72 (0.63, 0.81)
Self-assessed health	
Poor	Reference category
Fair	1.05 (0.85, 1.29)
Good	1.07 (0.88, 1.30)
Very good	1.05 (0.87, 1.28)
Excellent	0.98 (0.80, 1.21)
Health condition (yes vs. no)	1.07 (0.79, 1.44)

[1] Adjusted for all other variables.

Table 2. Adjusted logistic regression investigating independent predictors of dietary supplement use in Australian adolescents aged 10–17 years (*n* = 1317).

	Adjusted OR (95% CI) [1]
Sex (female vs. male)	1.12 (0.82, 1.53)
Region of birth	
Australia	Reference category
Main English-speaking countries	0.90 (0.44, 1.84)
Other	1.44 (0.82, 2.54)
State/Territory	
New South Wales	Reference category
Victoria	1.10 (0.70, 1.73)
Queensland	0.95 (0.57, 1.57)
South Australia	0.79 (0.45, 1.36)
Western Australia	1.42 (0.87, 2.31)
Tasmania	1.40 (0.83, 2.37)
Northern Territory	0.67 (0.31, 1.45)
Australian Capital Territory	1.15 (0.66, 2.00)
Socioeconomic status	
Lowest quintile	Reference category
Second quintile	1.12 (0.65, 1.95)
Third quintile	1.11 (0.65, 1.91)
Fourth quintile	1.13 (0.66, 1.92)
Highest quintile	1.67 (0.99, 2.82)
BMI category	
Healthy weight	Reference category
Underweight	0.55 (0.25, 1.22)
Overweight	0.73 (0.50, 1.06)
Obese	0.86 (0.47, 1.58)
Health condition (yes vs. no)	1.66 (0.84, 3.29)

[1] Adjusted for all other variables.

Table 3. Adjusted logistic regression investigating independent predictors of dietary supplement use in Australian children aged ≤9 years (*n* = 2733).

	Adjusted OR (95% CI) [1]
Sex (female vs. male)	0.91 (0.74, 1.21)
State/Territory	
New South Wales	Reference category
Victoria	0.98 (0.72, 1.32)
Queensland	0.99 (0.73, 1.34)
South Australia	0.57 (0.39, 0.83)
Western Australia	0.97 (0.70, 1.33)
Tasmania	0.78 (0.53, 1.15)
Northern Territory	0.78 (0.51, 1.19)
Australian Capital Territory	0.47 (0.32, 0.71)
Socioeconomic status	
Lowest quintile	Reference category
Second quintile	1.01 (0.71, 1.43)
Third quintile	0.78 (0.54, 1.12)
Fourth quintile	1.10 (0.78, 1.55)
Highest quintile	1.19 (0.85, 1.68)

[1] Adjusted for all other variables.

4. Discussion

To our knowledge, this study provides the first detailed investigation of dietary supplement use in a nationally representative sample of the Australian population. We found that for adults ≥18 years, the prevalence of supplement use was 43% (35% of males and 50% of females). Interestingly, the values are about twice those obtained in the 1995 Australian National Nutrition Survey, when 15% of adult males and 27% of females reported using dietary supplements in the previous 24 h [17]. However, apart from the 20-year time difference, this immediate reporting period (compared with two weeks in the current study) may have contributed to the lower reported prevalence of supplement use in 1995. The new Australian data are lower than the adult data of 52% (45% males, 58% females) from the NHANES (2011–2012) [1]. These surveys are comparable in that both were conducted over a similar time period, used trained interviewers [1] and referred to a recent but not immediate reporting period (30 days in NHANES vs. two weeks in the current study).

Among adults in the present study, the prevalence of supplement use increased with both age and female sex, a finding that is consistent with other studies [1–4]. The highest prevalence of supplement use was in those aged ≥70 years (40% in males and 58% in females). Australia is a multicultural country with a substantial proportion of the population born overseas in non-English speaking countries, and this analysis shows that adults born outside Australia and other main English-speaking countries are more likely to be supplement users than those born in Australia. Dietary supplement use was much less prevalent in those aged <18 years, with about a quarter of children and adolescents using supplements. These figures are lower than the third of participants aged ≤19 years identified as supplement users in the 2007–2010 NHANES [6]. Both surveys found no sex differences in the prevalence of supplement use among children and adolescents.

Multivitamins and/or multiminerals were the most commonly reported supplements across all participants in our study, which is consistent with other literature [1,5,6,8,18,19]. Fish oil preparations were the second most reported supplement in the present study, particularly in those aged ≥50 years. Prescription omega-3 preparations are also available in Australia, so total use is likely to be higher than that suggested by these data, particularly in the older age groups. The difference in adult male and female supplement use was predominantly explained by the higher use of both multivitamins and/or multiminerals and herbal products by women. While most participants reported using one dietary supplement, many preparations not referred to as multivitamins and/or multiminerals contain more than one nutrient, for example calcium and vitamin D, and fish oil with added nutrients.

Other predictors of supplement use in the Australian population, such as being a previous smoker, being physically active, and having a higher level of education, are consistent with the existing literature, as recently reviewed by Dickinson and MacKay [4]. Overall, the use of dietary supplements associates with aspects of a healthy lifestyle. Other literature investigating supplement use in infants, children and adolescents found that predictors of supplement use included the parents' educational attainment, income and private health insurance coverage [6,18,19], which were not assessed in the current study.

Our study used data from a nationally-representative sample of the Australian population. Collecting dietary supplement use over a two-week period enabled the survey to capture episodic supplement use, typically missed in 24-h recalls [20]. Although supplement use was reported through face-to-face interviews with trained interviewers, and participants were encouraged to have the supplements in front of them, we cannot rule out errors in recording and categorising the supplements.

5. Conclusions

To our knowledge, this is the first detailed investigation of dietary supplement use in a nationally-representative sample of the Australian population. A substantial proportion of the Australian population reported using dietary supplements, with multivitamins and/or multiminerals being the most commonly reported type of supplement. In adults, independent predictors of supplement use included being female, increasing age, being born outside Australia and other main English-speaking countries, being physically active, higher educational attainment, having a healthy BMI compared to those who were obese, and being a non-smoker. Given that the use of multivitamins and/or multiminerals and fish oil preparations is common in the Australian population, future studies investigating the contribution of supplements to overall dietary intakes of vitamins, minerals and omega-3 fatty acids are warranted.

Supplementary Materials: The following are available online at www.mdpi.com/2072-6643/9/10/1154/s1, Supplementary Table S1: Supplement categories, Supplementary Table S2: Characteristics of supplement users and non-users among adults aged ≥18 years participating in the 2014–2015 National Health Survey (*n* = 14,560), Supplementary Table S3: Characteristics of supplement users and non-users among adolescents aged 10–17 years participating in the 2014–2015 National Health Survey (*n* = 1964), Supplementary Table S4: Characteristics of supplement users and non-users among children aged ≤9 years participating in the 2014–2015 National Health Survey (*n* = 2733), Supplementary Table S5: Prevalence of use of different supplement types by participants in the 2014–2015 National Health Survey (*n* = 19,257).

Acknowledgments: L.J.B. was supported by a Curtin University Research Fellowship. The 2014–2015 NHS was conducted by the ABS. We thank Paul Atyeo, Beau Stephen and Barry Tynan of the ABS for their help in using data from the NHS. We gratefully acknowledge the contributions of the NHS participants.

Author Contributions: L.J.B. and J.L.S. designed the research; E.M. analysed the data; S.K.O. and J.L.S. wrote the manuscript; L.J.B., E.M., and J.L.S. contributed to the interpretation of data and critical revision of the manuscript for important intellectual content; L.J.B. had primary responsibility for final content. All authors read and approved the final manuscript.

Conflicts of Interest: The authors declare no conflict of interest.

References

1. Kantor, E.; Rehm, C.; Du, M. Trends in dietary supplement use among US adults from 1999–2012. *JAMA* **2016**, *316*, 1464–1474. [CrossRef] [PubMed]

2. Skeie, G.; Braaten, T.; Hjartåker, A.; Lentjes, M.; Amiano, P.; Jakszyn, P.; Pala, V.; Palanca, A.; Niekerk, E.M.; Verhagen, H.; et al. Use of dietary supplements in the European Prospective Investigation into Cancer and Nutrition calibration study. *Eur. J. Clin. Nutr.* **2009**, *63*, S226. [CrossRef] [PubMed]

3. Department of Health. National Diet and Nutrition Survey: Headline Results from Years 1, 2 and 3 (Combined) of the Rolling Programme September 2008–November 2010. Available online: https://www.gov.uk/government/uploads/system/uploads/attachment_data/file/207707/ndns-y3-executive-summary_final.pdf (accessed on 16 August 2017).

4. Dickinson, A.; Mackay, D. Health habits and other characteristics of dietary supplement users: A review. *Nutr. J.* **2014**, *13*, 2–8. [CrossRef] [PubMed]

5. Bailey, R.L.; Gahche, J.J.; Lentino, C.V.; Dwyer, J.T.; Engel, J.S.; Thomas, P.R.; Betz, J.M.; Sempos, C.T.; Picciano, M.F. Dietary supplement use in the United States, 2003–2006. *J. Nutr.* **2011**, *141*, 261–266. [CrossRef] [PubMed]

6. Bailey, R.; Gahche, J.; Thomas, P.; Dwyer, J. Why children use dietary supplements. *FASEB J.* **2013**, *27*, 242–245. [CrossRef] [PubMed]

7. Gahche, J.J.; Bailey, R.L.; Potischman, N.; Dwyer, J.T. Dietary supplement use was very high among older adults in the United States in 2011–2014. *J. Nutr.* **2017**, *147*, 1968–1976. [CrossRef] [PubMed]

8. Bailey, R.; Gahche, J.; Miller, P.; Thomas, P.; Dwyer, J. Why US adults use dietary supplements. *JAMA Intern. Med.* **2013**, *173*, 355–361. [CrossRef] [PubMed]

9. Yong, P.; Tan, L.; Loh, Y. Consumption of dietary health supplements among hospitalized patients at an acute tertiary hospital. *PharmaNutrition* **2014**, *2*, 135–140. [CrossRef]

10. Australian Bureau of Statistics. National Health Survey 2014-15 Questionnaire. Available online: http://www.ausstats.abs.gov.au/ausstats/subscriber.nsf/0/EFC93ECE5ABE3894CA257F1400133CE1/$File/national%20health%20survey%202014-15%20questionnaire.pdf (accessed on 21 September 2017).

11. Australian Bureau of Statistics. National Health Survey: Users' Guide, 2014-15. Available online: http://www.abs.gov.au/ausstats/abs@.nsf/Lookup/by%20Subject/4363.0~2014-15~Main%20Features~Users%27%20Guide~1 (accessed on 21 September 2017).

12. Therapeutic Goods Administration. An Overview of the Regulation of Complementary Medicines in Australia. Available online: https://www.tga.gov.au/overview-regulation-complementary-medicines-australia (accessed on 19 October 2017).

13. World Health Organization. *Obesity: Preventing and Managing the Global Epidemic*; Report of a WHO Consultation; World Health Organization: Geneva, Switzerland, 2000.

14. Cole, T.J.; Bellizzi, M.C.; Flegal, K.M.; Dietz, W.H. Establishing a standard definition for child overweight and obesity worldwide: International survey. *Br. Med. J.* **2000**, *320*, 1240–1243. [CrossRef]

15. Cole, T.J.; Flegal, K.M.; Nicholls, D.; Jackson, A.A. Body mass index cut offs to define thinness in children and adolescents: International survey. *Br. Med. J.* **2007**, *335*, 194. [CrossRef] [PubMed]

16. Australian Bureau of Statistics. Census of Population and Housing: Socio-Economic Indexes for Areas (Seifa), Australia, 2011. Available online: http://www.abs.gov.au/ausstats/abs@.nsf/Lookup/by%20Subject/2033. 0.55.001~2011~Main%20Features~What%20is%20SEIFA%3f~4 (accessed on 16 August 2017).

17. Australian Bureau of Statistics. National Nutrition Survey Selected Highlights Australia 1995. Available online: http://www.abs.gov.au/ausstats/abs@.nsf/mf/4802.0 (accessed on 16 August 2017).

18. Chen, S.; Binns, C.W.; Maycock, B.; Liu, Y.; Zhang, Y. Prevalence of dietary supplement use in healthy pre-school Chinese children in Australia and China. *Nutrients* **2014**, *6*, 815–828. [CrossRef] [PubMed]

19. Dwyer, J.; Sempos, C.; Bailey, R.; Nahin, R.; Rogers, G.; Jacques, P.; Barnes, P. Prevalence and predictors of children's dietary supplement use: The 2007 national health interview survey. *Am. J. Clin. Nutr.* **2013**, *97*, 1331–1337. [CrossRef] [PubMed]

20. Parnell, W.R.; Wilson, N.C.; Smith, C. Dietary supplements: Prevalence of use in the New Zealand population. *Nutr. Diet.* **2006**, *63*, 199–205. [CrossRef]

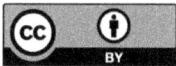

nutrients

MDPI

Article

Dietary Supplement Use among Australian Adults: Findings from the 2011–2012 National Nutrition and Physical Activity Survey

Alissa J. Burnett *, Katherine M. Livingstone , Julie L. Woods and Sarah A. McNaughton

School of Exercise and Nutrition Sciences, Institute for Physical Activity and Nutrition, Deakin University, 221 Burwood Highway, Burwood, VIC 3125, Australia; k.livingstone@deakin.edu.au (K.M.L.); j.woods@deakin.edu.au (J.L.W.); sarah.mcnaughton@deakin.edu.au (S.A.M.)
* Correspondence: ajburnet@deakin.edu.au; Tel.: +61-3-9244-6100

Received: 31 August 2017; Accepted: 8 November 2017; Published: 14 November 2017

Abstract: (1) Background: Supplement use is prevalent worldwide; however, there are limited studies examining the characteristics of people who take supplements in Australia. This study aimed to investigate the demographics, lifestyle habits and health status of supplement users; (2) Methods: Adults aged >19 years (*n* = 4895) were included from the 2011–2012 National Nutrition and Physical Activity Survey (NNPAS). A supplement user was defined as anyone who took one or more supplements on either of two 24-h dietary recalls. Poisson regression was used to estimate the prevalence ratio (PR) of supplement use, according to demographics, lifestyle characteristics and health status of participants; (3) Results: Supplement use was reported by 47% of women and 34% of men, and supplement use was higher among older age groups, among those with higher education levels and from areas reflecting the least socioeconomic disadvantaged. An association was found between blood pressure and supplement use; (4) Conclusions: A substantial proportion of Australians take supplements. Further investigation into the social, psychological and economic determinants that motivate the use of supplements is required, to ensure appropriate use of supplements among Australian adults.

Keywords: supplements; dietary intake; lifestyle

1. Introduction

The use of supplements, which may be defined as multi-vitamins, single vitamins, single minerals, herbal supplements, oil supplements and any other dietary supplementation [1] varies among populations. However, it is highest in countries such as the United States, United Kingdom and Denmark [2], where supplement use is between 35 and 60% of adults [1–5]. On a per capita basis, Australians are some of the world's largest consumers of dietary supplements, with vitamin and mineral sales totaling AUD $646 million in 2013 [3].

The Australian Dietary Guidelines recommend that individuals, with the exception of pregnant women, only take supplements if they are eliminating a food group from their diet [6]. However, many people continue to take supplements. Supplement users may differ from non-users in regard to a range of characteristics. Previous research suggests that supplement users are more likely to be female, older and have a higher educational attainment than non-supplement users [1–5,7]. Supplement use is also higher in people who adopt healthier lifestyle behaviours, such as being more physically active, not smoking and consuming more fruit and vegetables and less alcohol [1,8,9]. Several studies show that less healthy diets are common among supplement non- users, including greater consumption of diets high in fat, low in fibre or low in fruit [8,9].

Just as supplement users have been shown to maintain healthier lifestyle behaviours, individuals who take dietary supplements are more likely to have a better health status [2,8,10] including better self-rated health and fewer cardiovascular risk factors, such as high blood pressure, than non-supplement users.

While supplement users may have more optimal dietary intakes compared to non-supplement users [11], many supplement users have also been found to be exceed the upper recommended intake limit for some vitamins and minerals [11], which is defined as the highest level of individual daily intake that does not pose a threat to health [11]. For example, the Multiethnic Cohort study in the United States reported that, of people who take supplements, 50% of men and 40% of women consumed more than the upper limit for niacin and folate [11].

Studies to date that have characterized supplement users, have lacked detailed dietary records and supplement information, and there has been a paucity of nationally-representative data on supplement use in the Australian population. Given the high prevalence of consumption and the limited understanding of the characteristics of these consumers, this study aimed to examine supplement use within the Australian population. Specifically, the present study aimed to explore the sociodemographic, lifestyle and health status characteristics of supplement users; the dietary intakes of supplement users and the most common types of supplements used among Australian adults.

2. Methods

2.1. Study Design and Participants

This study was a secondary analysis of data collected from adults included in the National Nutrition and Physical Activity Survey 2011–2012 (NNPAS), a component of the Australian Health Survey [12]. The NNPAS collected information from a random sample of private dwellings in both urban and rural areas across all Australia states and territories. A total of 14,363 private dwellings were selected, of which 9519 (77.0%; *n* = 12,153 individuals, 9341 adults >19 years) were fully or adequately responding households to the first interview. Participants completed a household survey, anthropometric measures and dietary intakes were estimated using two 24-h dietary recalls. For the present study, participants were excluded if they were pregnant or lactating, completed only one 24-h dietary recall, or had missing data on outcomes and covariates. The final sample for analysis was 4895. Use of the NNPAS 2011–2012 was approved by the Australian Bureau of Statistics [13] and ethics approval was provided by The Census and Statistics Act 1905 [12].

2.2. Dietary Intake

A 24-h dietary recall collected detailed information on all foods and beverages consumed in a 24-h period, from midnight to midnight. Where possible, the participants were asked to undertake a second 24-h dietary recall, at least eight days after their first recall on a different day of the week. The 24-h dietary recall method was based on the Automated Multiple-Pass Method, developed by The United States Department of Agriculture (USDA), and adapted for use in Australia [14]. The Automated Multiple-Pass Method is divided into five phases: quick list, forgotten foods, time and occasion, detail cycle, and final probe. The information collected included time of consumption, the name of the eating occasion (e.g., lunch), the amount eaten and detailed food descriptions to allow for accurate food coding. Energy (kJ) and nutrient intakes (fat, protein, carbohydrates and fibre (g) and calcium, magnesium, iron, zinc, iodine, selenium, vitamin C, vitamin E (mg), B12 (µg), long chain omega 3 fatty acids, and folate (natural) and folic acid (µg)) were estimated from the 24-h recalls, using the Australian Supplement and Nutrient Database 2011–2013 [15].

Overall, diet quality was assessed using the dietary guideline index (DGI-2013), which is described in detail elsewhere [16–18]. It is calculated using 13 components, with seven of the 13 components assessing the adequacy of the diet (e.g., food variety, vegetables, fruits, cereals, dairy and alternatives, lean meat and alternatives, and fluid intake), and the remaining six components assessing the moderation of dietary intake (e.g., discretionary foods, saturated fat, salt, added sugar and alcohol, and moderate intakes of unsaturated fat). Each component is scored from 0 to 10, to reflect the level of compliance for meeting the Australian dietary guidelines and scores on each component were summed to give the total score. A higher score reflects a better diet quality. This was then categorised into two groups, based on the median (high score or low score).

2.3. Dietary Supplement Use

At the end of the dietary recall, participants were also asked "were dietary supplements, such as vitamins and minerals consumed, and how much?". Participants were asked to report their supplement usage, using the Australian Register of Therapeutic Goods (ARTG) identification number on the supplement container. These were then matched to a list provided by the Therapeutic Goods Administration of over 10,000 dietary supplements registered for sale in Australia. For the purposes of this study, a supplement user was defined as anyone who took one or more supplements during either of the two 24-h dietary recalls.

2.4. Socio-Demographic Measures

Information on respondents' socio-demographics and other characteristics was collected in the household survey. Age (years) was grouped into four categories—19–30, 31–50, 51–70 and 71–85 years—consistent with age groups used in the Australian Nutrient Reference Values [19]. Education was assessed by asking respondents to provide details of their highest education levels, both school and non-school, and categorised as secondary school or less, certificate or diploma, bachelor degree and postgraduate degree. Area-level disadvantage was assessed using the Australian Bureau of Statistics (ABS) Socio-Economic Indexes for Areas (SEIFA), and specifically, the Index of Relative Socio-economic Disadvantage [20], which was compiled from variables such as income, educational attainment, unemployment, and dwellings without motor vehicles [20]. For the present study, this was categorised into quintiles, with the first quintile representing the most disadvantaged group.

2.5. Lifestyle Characteristics

Information on health behaviours was also collected in the household survey. Frequency and duration of moderate and vigorous physical activity in the last week were assessed in the NNPAS, using questions from the Active Australia Survey [21]. Physical activity was measured in relation to Australia's Physical Activity and Sedentary Behaviour Guidelines, which recommend at least 30 min of moderate intensity physical activity on most, preferably all, days [22]. Physical activity included walking for fitness, recreation or sport for at least 10 min, walking continuously to get from place to place for at least 10 min, moderate physical activity/exercise (apart from walking) and vigorous physical activity/exercise. A binary variable was used to estimate whether participants met recommendations of 150 min of physical activity over five or more sessions per week. Sedentary behaviour (min/day) was defined as time spent sitting or lying down for various activities in the last week; participants were asked to record the number of minutes they had spent sitting or lying down on a usual day. Smoking was categorised as current smoker, ex-smoker and never smoked.

Alcohol was assessed by asking respondents to report the number of drinks, alcohol type, size of drinks and brand name of drink they had consumed [23]. The reported quantities were then converted into millilitres of alcohol present in the reported drinks. For the purpose of this study, alcohol intake was then categorised into three categories; no alcohol consumed, one standard drink or less consumed and more than one standard drink consumed. A standard drink was defined as 10 grams of alcohol [6].

Usual fruit and vegetable intake was measured by asking respondents to report the number of serves of fruit and vegetables they ate each day [24]. This was then categorised into whether the participant met the guidelines or not (five serves of vegetables and two serves of fruit per day) [6].

2.6. Health Status Measures

Self-reported health was measured by asking the participants to report their self-perceived health as excellent, very good, good, fair and poor [25]. Fair and poor were grouped together due to a low number of responses. Weight (kg) was measured using digital scales. This was measured during the interview and was voluntary. Body mass index (BMI; kg/m^2) was calculated using Quetelet's metric BMI, which is calculated as weight (kg) divided by height (m^2). This was then categorised into groups: underweight, normal, overweight and obese. Height was measured using a stadiometer. Waist circumference (cm) was measured using a metal tape measure, at the approximate midpoint between the lower margin of the last palpable rib and the top of the iliac crest [26]. This was measured during the interview and was voluntary. Waist circumference was categorised into three groups: no risk, increased risk and substantially increased risk. Blood pressure was measured by the interviewer using an automated blood pressure monitor and was voluntary. Two measurements were taken while participants were sitting down. If there was a significant difference between the two readings (greater than 10 mmHg), a third reading was taken. If there was no significant difference between the two readings, the second reading was recorded [27]. These measurements were then categorised into two groups (<140/90 and >140/90 mmHg). Chronic disease was measured by asking the participants whether they had been diagnosed with either diabetes, heart disease or kidney disease. This was then categorised into two groups (present or absent).

2.7. Statistical Analysis

Data analysis was conducted using Stata 14.2 (Stata Corp., College Station, TX, USA) [28]. Descriptive statistics (frequencies, mean and standard error) were used to describe variables and characteristics of supplement users versus non-users were compared using independent *t*-tests (for continuous variables) and chi square analyses (for categorical variables). Dietary intakes were log transformed for nutrients that were not normally distributed (total zinc, food only vitamin C, total vitamin C, total vitamin E, food only folic acid, total folic acid, food only B12, total B12, food only long chain omega 3 fatty acids and total long chain omega 3 fatty acids). Poisson regression analyses were used to estimate the prevalence ratio (PR) of supplement use (dependent variable), according to demographics, lifestyle characteristics and health status of participants (independent variables). Poisson regression was used to account for robust error variance. Analyses for socio-demographic measures, lifestyle characteristics and self-related health were adjusted for age (continuous) and sex, while health-related characteristics were adjusted for age, sex, education, area level disadvantage, smoking, fruit and vegetable consumption and DGI. Sampling weights were applied to take account of the complex sampling design. For categorical variables, a post hoc analysis was conducted (*F*-test) to test the overall effect of the variable on the dependent variable. Statistical significance was set at *p* < 0.05 for the analysis.

3. Results

Overall, supplement use was reported by 34% of men and 47% of women (Table 1). Supplement use was highest among women, among those aged 71–85 years, those with highest levels of education, those living in areas with the least socio-economic disadvantage, those who met physical activity guidelines and those who met fruit and vegetable guidelines (*p* < 0.05). After adjustment for age (Table 2), the prevalence of supplement use was higher in women and when adjusted for sex, the prevalence of supplement use was higher in older adults (71–85 years). When adjusted for sex and age, the prevalence of supplement use was higher in those in the least area level disadvantaged group, those with higher educational attainment, those who met the guidelines for physical activity (PR 0.79; 95% CI 0.71, 0.88; *p* < 0.001) and fruit and vegetable intakes (PR 0.81; 95% CI 0.68, 0.97; *p* < 0.05), and those with higher DGI scores (PR 1.32; 95% CI 1.20, 1.44; *p* < 0.001). An association was found between being an ex-smoker (PR 1.56; 95% CI 1.31, 1.86; *p* < 0.001) or having never smoked (PR 1.46; 95% CI 1.25, 1.70; *p* < 0.001) and supplement use, when compared with current smokers. No association was found between alcohol intake or sedentary behaviour and supplement use. An inverse association (Table 3) was found between being hypertensive (PR 0.87;

95% CI 0.77, 0.99; p = 0.031) and waist circumference (PR 0.89; 95% CI 0.79, 1.01; p = 0.007) and supplement use. No association was found between BMI, self-assessed health, chronic disease and supplement use.

Table 1. Demographic, lifestyle and health status characteristics of Australian adults in the Australian Health Survey (n = 4895).

Characteristic	All Subjects	Supplement Non-Users	Supplement Users	p-Value [1,2]
Sex n, (%)				<0.001
Male	2340 (47.8)	1547 (66.1)	795 (34.0)	
Female	2555 (52.2)	1365 (53.3)	1195 (46.7)	
Age, years, n, (%)				<0.001
19–30	792 (16.2)	576 (72.7)	216 (27.3)	
31–50	1815 (37.1)	1132 (62.4)	683 (37.6)	
51–70	1648 (33.7)	898 (54.5)	750 (45.5)	
71–85	640 (13.1)	303 (47.3)	337 (52.7)	
Education n, (%)				0.006
Secondary school or less	1813 (37.0)	1146 (63.2)	667 (36.8)	
Certificate or diploma	1714 (35.0)	1022 (59.6)	692 (40.4)	
Bachelor degree	911 (18.6)	520 (57.1)	391 (42.9)	
Postgraduate degree	457 (9.3)	221 (48.4)	236 (51.6)	
Area level disadvantage n, (%)				<0.001
Most disadvantaged (Lowest 20%)	885 (18.1)	569 (64.3)	316 (35.7)	
Second quintile	999 (20.4)	629 (63.0)	370 (37.0)	
Third quintile	941 (19.2)	539 (57.3)	402 (42.7)	
Fourth quintile	889 (18.2)	505 (56.8)	384 (43.2)	
Least disadvantaged (Highest 20%)	1181 (24.1)	667 (56.5)	514 (43.5)	
Physical activity n, (%)				0.005
Met recommended guidelines [3]	2169 (44.3)	1237 (57.0)	932 (43.0)	
Did not meet recommended guidelines	2726 (55.7)	1672 (61.3)	1054 (38.7)	
Sedentary behavior, min [4]	3.31 ± 0.29	3.31 ± 0.29	3.30 ± 0.29	0.889
Smoking n, (%)				<0.001
Current smoker	844 (17.2)	614 (72.8)	230 (27.2)	
Ex-smoker	1663 (34.0)	914 (55.0)	749 (45.0)	
Never smoked	2388 (48.8)	1381 (57.8)	1007 (42.2)	
Alcohol n, (%)				0.691
No alcohol consumed	2570 (52.5)	1542 (60.0)	1028 (40.0)	
One standard drink or less [5]	2234 (45.6)	1303 (58.3)	931 (41.7)	
More than one standard drink	91 (1.9)	64 (70.3)	27 (29.7)	
Fruit and vegetables n, (%)				0.007
Met guidelines [6]	281 (5.7)	132 (47.0)	149 (53.0)	
Did not meet guidelines	4614 (94.3)	2777 (60.2)	1837 (39.8)	
DGI [7] n, (%)				<0.001
Low DGI score	2448 (50.0)	1591 (65.0)	857 (35.0)	
High DGI score	2447 (50.0)	1318 (53.9)	1129 (46.1)	
Self-reported health n, (%)				0.170
Poor/Fair	780 (15.9)	467 (59.9)	313 (40.1)	
Good	1549 (31.6)	920 (59.4)	629 (40.6)	
Very good	1770 (36.2)	1038 (58.6)	732 (41.4)	
Excellent	796 (16.3)	484 (60.8)	312 (39.2)	
Blood pressure n, (%)				0.435
Non-hypertensive	3757 (76.8)	2232 (59.4)	1525 (40.6)	
Hypertensive	1138 (23.3)	677 (59.5)	461 (40.5)	
Chronic disease n, (%)				0.377
Absent	4506 (92.1)	2688 (59.7)	1818 (40.4)	
Present	389 (8.0)	221 (56.8)	168 (43.2)	
Waist circumference, cm				0.472
No risk	1611 (32.9)	976 (60.6)	635 (39.4)	
Increased risk	1156 (23.6)	691 (59.8)	465 (40.2)	
Substantially increased risk	2128 (43.5)	1242 (58.4)	886 (41.6)	
BMI [8], kg/m^2				0.186
Underweight	65 (1.3)	42 (64.6)	23 (35.4)	
Normal	1642 (33.5)	958 (58.3)	684 (41.7)	
Overweight	1820 (37.2)	1069 (58.7)	751 (41.3)	
Obese	1368 (28.0)	840 (61.4)	528 (38.6)	

[1] p-Values comparing supplement users to non-supplement users, determined using chi square for categorical variables; [2] p-Values comparing supplement users to non-supplement users, determined using t-tests for continuous variables; [3] One hundred and fifty min and five sessions a week; [4] Values represent mean and standard error (SE); [5] A standard drink is defined as 10 grams of alcohol; [6] Five serves of vegetables and two serves of fruit per day; [7] Dietary guideline index; [8] Body mass index (BMI; kg/m^2) is calculated as weight (kg) divided by height (m^2).

Table 2. Dietary supplement use (prevalence ratio and 95% confidence intervals) across demographic and lifestyle characteristics in adults from the Australian Health Survey (*n* = 4895).

Characteristic	Crude			Adjusted [1]	
	Supplement User [2]	*p*-Value [3]		Supplement User [2]	*p*-Value [4]
Sex		<0.001			<0.001
Male (reference)	1.00			1.00	
Female	1.26 (1.12, 1.42)			1.24 (1.10, 1.39)	
Age group (years)		<0.001			<0.001
19–30 (reference)	1.00			1.00	
31–50	1.32 (1.06, 1.64)			1.31 (1.05, 1.64)	
51–70	1.55 (1.24, 1.94)			1.54 (1.23, 1.93)	
71–85	1.87 (1.48, 2.36)			1.83 (1.45, 2.31)	
Education		0.006			<0.001
Secondary school or less (reference)	1.00			1.00	
Certificate or diploma	1.16 (0.99, 1.36)			1.25 (1.07, 1.46)	
Bachelor degree	1.28 (1.07, 1.53)			1.43 (1.20, 1.71)	
Postgraduate degree	1.40 (1.14, 1.72)			1.53 (1.25, 1.88)	
Area level disadvantage		<0.001			<0.001
Lowest 20% (reference)	1.00			1.00	
Second quintile	1.18 (0.98, 1.41)			1.22 (1.02, 1.46)	
Third quintile	1.39 (1.13, 1.71)			1.44 (1.20, 1.75)	
Fourth quintile	1.44 (1.20, 1.73)			1.52 (1.28, 1.80)	
Highest 20%	1.49 (1.25, 1.77)			1.57 (1.33, 1.86)	
Physical activity		0.005			<0.001
Met recommended guidelines (reference)	1.00			1.00	
Did not meet recommended guidelines	0.86 (0.77, 0.95)			0.79 (0.71, 0.88)	
Sedentary behaviour (min/day)	0.99 (0.80, 1.21)	0.889		1.12 (0.89, 1.39)	0.330
Smoking		<0.001			<0.001
Current smoker (reference)	1.00			1.00	
Ex-smoker	1.70 (1.43, 2.03)			1.56 (1.31, 1.86)	
Never smoked	1.52 (1.31, 1.77)			1.46 (1.25, 1.70)	
Alcohol		0.676			0.875
No alcohol consumed (reference)	1.00			1.00	
One standard drink or less	1.34 (0.93, 1.16)			1.02 (0.92, 1.14)	
More than one standard drink	0.91 (0.52, 1.58)			0.98 (0.56, 1.72)	
Fruit and vegetables		0.004			0.024
Met guidelines (reference)	1.00			1.00	
Did not meet guidelines	0.75 (0.63, 0.91)			0.81 (0.68, 0.97)	
DGI		<0.001			<0.001
Low DGI score (reference)	1.00			1.00	
High DGI score	1.38 (1.26, 1.52)			1.32 (1.20, 1.44)	
Self-assessed health		0.265			0.053
Poor/Fair (reference)	1.00			1.00	
Good	1.07 (0.91, 1.27)			1.18 (0.99, 1.40)	
Very good	1.13 (0.97, 1.32)			1.26 (1.07, 1.49)	
Excellent	0.96 (0.79, 1.17)			1.10 (0.90, 1.34)	

[1] Poisson regression model adjusted for sex and age; [2] Prevalence ratio (95% CI); [3] *F*-test was conducted to obtain an overall *p*-value for categorical variables; [4] *F*-test was conducted to obtain an overall *p*-value for categorical variables.

The most commonly used supplements were single vitamins (19%), herbal supplements (16%), and multivitamins (16%) (Table 4). The most commonly used supplements used varied by age group, with folic acid being most commonly consumed by the 31–50 year age group, while lipids (e.g., fish oil supplements, fish oil supplements with added nutrients, fish liver oil supplements, evening primrose oil supplements and other lipid supplements grouped together) were most commonly consumed by the 51–70 year age group. Females consumed a higher proportion of multivitamins (62%), single minerals (67%), single vitamins (60%), herbal supplements (63%), iron (62%) and folic acid (59%) than males.

Table 3. Dietary supplement use (prevalence ratio and 95% confidence intervals) across health-related characteristics in adults from the Australian Health Survey (*n* = 4895).

Characteristic	Crude		Adjusted [1]	
	Supplement User [2]	*p*-Value [3]	Supplement User [2]	*p*-Value [4]
Blood pressure		0.443		0.031
Non-hypertensive (reference)	1.00		1.00	
Hypertensive	0.95 (0.85, 1.08)		0.87 (0.77, 0.99)	
Chronic disease		0.372		0.734
Absent (reference)	1.00		1.00	
Present	1.10 (0.89, 1.35)		0.97 (0.79, 1.18)	
Waist Circumference (cm)		0.411		0.007
No risk (reference)	1.00		1.00	
Increased risk	0.97 (0.85, 1.21)		0.89 (0.79, 1.01)	
Substantially increased risk	0.94 (0.84, 1.04)		0.83 (0.75, 0.93)	
BMI (kg/m^2)		0.120		0.081
Underweight (reference)	1.00		1.00	
Normal	1.11 (0.65, 1.89)		0.89 (0.51, 1.55)	
Overweight	1.10 (0.62, 1.96)		0.86 (0.48, 1.54)	
Obese	0.95 (0.58, 1.57)		0.75 (0.45, 1.27)	

[1] Poisson regression model, adjusted for sex, age, education, area level disadvantage, smoking, fruit and vegetable consumption and DGI; [2] Prevalence ratio (95% CI); [3] *F*-test was conducted to obtain an overall *p*-value for categorical variables; [4] *F*-test was conducted to obtain an overall *p*-value for categorical variables.

Table 4. Type of dietary supplements used by age and sex.

	Total	Age					Sex		
	n, (%) [1]	19–30 *n*, (%)	31–50 *n*, (%)	51–70 *n*, (%)	71–85 *n*, (%)	*p*-Value [2]	Males *n*, (%)	Females *n*, (%)	*p*-Value [3]
Multivitamin [4]	1031 (15.2)	133 (12.9)	426 (41.3)	342 (33.2)	130 (12.6)	0.051	395 (38.3)	636 (61.7)	<0.001
Mineral [5]	739 (10.9)	65 (8.8)	221 (29.9)	318 (43.0)	135 (18.3)	<0.001	246 (33.3)	493 (66.7)	<0.001
Vitamins [6]	1230 (18.1)	166 (13.5)	498 (40.5)	413 (33.6)	153 (12.4)	0.693	498 (40.5)	732 (59.5)	0.004
Lipid [7]	998 (14.7)	81 (8.1)	308 (30.9)	436 (43.7)	173 (17.3)	<0.001	407 (40.8)	591 (59.2)	0.019
Herbal [8]	1063 (15.6)	112 (10.5)	367 (34.5)	421 (39.6)	163 (15.3)	0.002	393 (37.0)	670 (63.0)	<0.001
Iron	802 (11.8)	118 (14.7)	341 (42.5)	248 (30.9)	95 (11.9)	0.497	309 (38.5)	493 (61.5)	0.002
Folic acid	932 (13.7)	129 (13.8)	398 (42.7)	297 (31.9)	108 (11.6)	0.181	380 (40.8)	552 (59.2)	0.009

[1] Respondents may have reported using more than one supplement; [2] *p*-Value relates to comparison of age categories and different supplement types, determined using chi square; [3] *p*-Value relates to comparison of sex and different supplement types, determined using chi square; [4] Multivitamin and/or multimineral, multivitamin and/or multimineral, with herbal extracts and multivitamin and/or multimineral containing caffeine; [5] Mineral supplements include calcium supplements, magnesium supplements, zinc supplements, iodine supplements, selenium supplements and other single mineral supplements; [6] Vitamin supplements include vitamin C supplements, vitamin E supplements, folic acid supplements, vitamin D supplements and other single vitamin supplements; [7] Lipid supplements include fish oil supplements, fish oil supplements with added nutrients, fish liver oil supplements, evening primrose oil supplements, long chain omega 3 fatty acid supplements and other lipid supplements; [8] Herbal supplements include all herbal supplements including those containing caffeine, homoeopathic supplements, protein or amino acid supplements, probiotic supplements, propolis or other bee product supplements, glucosamine and/or chondroitin based supplements, coenzyme q10 supplements and other supplements.

When comparing nutrient intakes from food only, supplement users were found to have higher intakes of fibre and most vitamins and minerals (except, zinc and vitamin B12) compared to non-supplement users, although differences were small in many cases (Table 5). Intakes of all vitamins and minerals were higher when the contribution from supplements was added into overall intakes. Intakes of folic acid from food alone were lower among supplements users, but the inclusion of supplement intakes (in the calculation of total intake from food and supplements) reversed the differences. Supplement users were found to be reaching the upper range of the recommended dietary intake (RDI) for magnesium and exceeding the RDI for zinc, vitamin C, vitamin E and B12, when total intakes were considered.

Table 5. Analyses for the association of nutrient intake between dietary supplement users and non-supplement users for adults from the Australian Health Survey (*n* = 4895).

	RDI [3]	Supplement Non-User	Supplement User			
		Food Only Mean ± SD	Food Only Mean ± SD	Food & Supplements Mean ± SD	*p*-Value [1,4]	*p*-Value [2,4]
Energy (kJ)		8489.4 ± 2982.7	8371.5 ± 2842.8	8371.5 ± 2842.8	0.014	0.014
Fat (g)		72.0 ± 32.2	71.0 ± 31.4	71.9 ± 31.5	0.607	0.660
Protein (g)	46–81	89.6 ± 34.2	89.8 ± 33.2	89.9 ± 33.3	0.045	0.035
Carbohydrates (g)		219.6 ± 87.9	215.1 ± 83.7	215.1 ± 83.7	0.802	0.802
Fibre (g)	25–30	21.9 ± 9.7	24.5 ± 10.7	24.5 ± 10.7	<0.001	<0.001
Calcium (mg)	1000–1300	779.0 ± 385.9	817.3 ± 359.8	940.5 ± 425.5	<0.001	<0.001
Magnesium (mg)	310–420	326.0 ± 125.2	352.4 ± 129.1	398.2 ± 163.9	<0.001	<0.001
Iron (mg)	8–18	10.8 ± 4.7	11.3 ± 4.6	13.5 ± 8.0	<0.001	<0.001
Zinc (mg)	8–14	10.8 ± 4.8	11.0 ± 4.8	15.7 ± 9.8	0.107	<0.001
Iodine		169.9 ± 72.8	167.9 ± 72.1	204.5 ± 115.6	0.645	<0.001
Selenium		88.0 ± 42.9	91.7 ± 52.7	99.7 ± 55.5	<0.001	<0.001
Vitamin C (mg)	45	95.4 ± 81.1	111.2 ± 85.4	269.8 ± 598.1	<0.001	<0.001
Vitamin E (mg)	7–10	9.8 ± 5.2	10.9 ± 6.1	28.5 ± 65.6	<0.001	<0.001
Folate (natural) (µg)	400	276.2 ± 124.1	309.7 ± 131.6	309.7 ± 131.6	<0.001	<0.001
Folic acid (µg)		197.9 ± 142.9	173.9 ± 137.8	292.6 ± 226.4	0.001	<0.001
B12 (µg)	2.4	4.5 ± 3.7	4.6 ± 3.3	31.4 ± 114.9	0.252	<0.001
Omega-3		259.7 ± 463.3	304.6 ± 574.0	608.2 ± 869.5	0.065	<0.001

[1] *p*-Value relates to a comparison of supplement non-users' and supplement users' food only intakes, determined using an independent *t*-test; [2] *p*-Value relates to comparison of supplement non-users' and supplement users' total nutrient intakes, determined using an independent *t*-test; [3] Recommended daily intake for adults, according to the National Health and Medical Research Council [29]; [4] Log transformation, performed for total zinc, food only vitamin C, total vitamin C, total vitamin E, food only folic acid, total folic acid, food only B12, total B12, food only long chain omega 3 fatty acids and total long chain omega 3 fatty acids.

4. Discussion

A significant proportion of the Australian population reported supplement use (34% men and 47% women), with supplements users more likely to be female, older, more highly educated and to exhibit healthier lifestyle behaviours and have better health status than supplement non-users. Nutritional supplements are considered complementary medicines within Australia, and undergo less regulation than higher risk products, such as medicines [30]. Therefore, less emphasis is placed on assessing the evidence of the claims being made by the products; these marketing claims may persuade people to consume more dietary supplements [30,31].

Our findings, in relation to the sociodemographic characteristics of supplement users, are consistent with the literature [1,2,4,5,7,9,31–33]. Many previous studies have found that supplement users are more likely to be female, older in age and more highly educated [1,2,4,5,7,9,31–33]. This is reflected within the current study, as the largest percentage of supplement users were older in age. Females have been shown to be more health conscious and therefore may take more dietary supplements to prevent illness [34].

Previous studies have also found that people of a lower socio-economic position are less likely to use supplements, which is reflected within the current study [9,31]. Previous studies have shown that people with a higher socio-economic position are more likely to be more health conscious, which may motivate them to take more dietary supplements [5].

Previous studies suggest that supplement users are more likely to engage in a range of health behaviors and are more likely to meet recommendations for physical activity and fruit and vegetable consumption. Previous research has shown that supplement users are more likely to be physically active [1,2,4,9,35]. The current study found a relationship between supplement use and meeting the physical activity guidelines; however, there was no significant difference found between supplement users and supplement non-users, with regard to sedentary behaviour. It is consistently shown that supplement use is associated with health conscious individuals; however, the lack of association may be due to the inability to modify sedentary behaviour, as much of it occurs in the workplace [36]. Meeting the guidelines for fruit and vegetable consumption was positively associated with dietary supplement use in the present study. This is consistent with previous studies, which found an association between higher consumption of fruit and vegetables and dietary supplement use [2,9,37]. This introduces the question of the need for additional nutritional supplementation in those who already obtain nutrients from a healthy diet, as supplement users' dietary intakes were generally better and met the RDI better than non-supplement takers [2].

The finding that smoking status was associated with supplement use, is consistent with previous research [1,2,5]. The NHANES 1999–2000 found that former smokers and people who have never smoked were more likely to be supplement users than current smokers [1,5]. The NHANES 1999–2000 reported that 61% of former smokers were dietary supplement users, while 52% of people who had never smoked reported using dietary supplements and only 43% of current smokers reported using dietary supplements [1].

Previous research had mixed findings with regard to alcohol consumption and its association with dietary supplement use [1,5,9,35]. Many studies found that people who consume less alcohol were more likely to take supplements [1,5,35]; however, a study from Canada did not find an association between alcohol consumption and dietary supplement use [9]. The current study did not find an association between alcohol consumption and supplement use. These discrepancies may be due to the type of alcohol consumed, as previous studies have found positive associations for wine consumption, but no associations for beer consumption [1,5,38]. Dietary supplement users are more likely to be those who are more health conscious and therefore adopt health behaviours, such as not smoking and consuming less alcohol, which may motivate them to take dietary supplements [39].

Supplement users are also more likely to have a better health status. Previous research has reported varied conclusions in relation to BMI and its relationship to supplement use; however, the current study did not find an association between BMI and supplement use and found an inverse association between waist circumference and supplement use. A study on supplement use in Taiwan, which focused on the use of multivitamin and mineral supplements, calcium, vitamin E and fish oil, found no association between BMI and supplement use [40]. Similarly, NHANES 2007–2008 did not find an association between supplement use and BMI [10]. On the contrary, a study conducted in the United States on herbal supplements found that herbal and specialty supplement users had lower BMIs [37]. Most studies focus on BMI as an indicator of good health status, with regard to supplement use; however, waist circumference has been regarded as a more accurate indicator of metabolic index, with this measure being used when defining metabolic syndrome [41]. The results of a Danish study showed that people who scored lower in the health index—meaning they had lower blood pressure, a lower waist circumference and did not test positive to the urine glucose test—had higher supplement use [2,5]. In line with our findings, a study conducted in the United Kingdom found that people who had a history of high blood pressure were less likely to be taking dietary supplements [2]. Previous studies have reported an association between self-reported health and supplement use; however, the present study did not find this association [2]. The discrepancy may be due to variations in the populations under study, as our study included a wide age range of participants [42].

Supplement users have been shown to have dietary intakes that tend to be healthier, and higher in a range of nutrients, when considering food intake alone, compared to supplement non-users. Supplement users were reported to have a higher fibre consumption from food only compared to supplement non-users, which is consistent with previous research [43,44]. This is reflective of many nutrients, as the diets of those using dietary supplements are higher in nutrients than non-supplement users. Not surprisingly, when the contribution from supplements is taken into account, supplement users have higher vitamin and mineral intakes, compared to supplement non-users. Previous research has suggested that many people are reaching the upper limit for vitamins and minerals, such as niacin, folate, iron and zinc [11]. In the current study, some nutrients intakes may actually be exceeding the

RDI—for example vitamin E, vitamin B12 and zinc—which may result in toxicity [9,45]. It is unclear from the current data how long participants had been consuming the reported supplements, and therefore whether these intakes are higher than the RDI is of concern. Further research focusing on biomarkers of nutritional status may provide insight into understanding the impact of these levels of supplementation.

The strengths of the present study include the nationally-representative data, which make our findings generalizable to the wider population. A limitation to the current study is its cross-sectional design, which did not allow for an investigation of any causal relationships. A further limitation is the differing definitions of supplement users across studies [1,4,5,9,31]. The lack of standardization, in regard to the definition of supplement users, makes it difficult to compare the prevalence between populations. However, despite the methodological differences, similar results, with regard to the demographics, lifestyle habits and health status of supplement users, were identified in a number of studies. Given the widespread use of supplements, further investigation on the social, psychological and economic determinants that motivate the use of supplements is required, to ensure the appropriate use of supplements and to minimise the potential harm which can be caused through excessive use of dietary supplements [32].

5. Conclusions

This study examined supplement use within the Australian population, and found that supplement use was higher among females, older adults, those with higher education levels and among those from areas with the least socioeconomic disadvantage. Supplement users were also more likely to participate in healthier lifestyle behaviours, have underlying diets that were higher in many nutrients and have a more favourable health status, when compared to supplement non-users. Future studies examining the potential beneficial or adverse health effects associated with dietary supplements should adjust for other health behaviors and socio-demographic factors, as these variables may confound the associations attributed to dietary supplement use. Future research should focus on understanding intakes of supplements, including understanding long term intakes and whether they are above recommended levels and understanding the drivers of supplement use, to ensure that there is appropriate use of supplements among Australia adults in the community.

Acknowledgments: S.A.M. is supported by a National Health and Medical Research Council Career Development Fellowship (ID1104636). K.M.L. is supported by an Alfred Deakin Postdoctoral Research Fellowship.

Author Contributions: A.J.B., K.M.L., J.L.W. and S.A.M. contributed to the research design. A.J.B. performed the statistical analysis for the manuscript and drafted the paper. All authors contributed to a critical review of the manuscript during the writing process. All authors approved the final version to be published.

Conflicts of Interest: The authors declare no conflicts of interest.

Abbreviations

SD	standard deviation
NNPAS	National Nutrition and Physical Activity Survey
BMI	body mass index
NHANES	National Health and Nutrition Examination Survey
PR	Prevalence ratios

References

1. Radimer, K.; Bindewald, B.; Hughes, J.; Ervin, B.; Swanson, C.; Picciano, M. Dietary supplement use by US adults: Data from the National Health and Nutrition Examination Survey, 1999–2000. *Am. J. Epidemiol.* **2004**, *160*, 339–349. [CrossRef] [PubMed]

2. Harrison, R.A.; Holt, D.; Pattison, D.J.; Elton, P.J. Are those in need taking dietary supplements? A survey of 21923 adults. *Br. J. Nutr.* **2004**, *91*, 617–623. [CrossRef] [PubMed]

3. Euromonitor International. *Vitamins and Dietary Supplements in Australia*; Euromonitor International: Sydney, Australia, 2013.

4. Yu, X.; Smith, W.; Webb, K.; Mitchell, P.; Leeder, S. Prevalence and predictors of dietary supplement use in an older Australian population. *Aust. J. Nutr. Diet.* **1999**, *56*, 69–75.
5. Kofoed, C.L.F.; Christensen, J.; Dragsted, L.O.; Tjønneland, A.; Roswall1, N. Determinants of dietary supplement use—Healthy individuals use dietary supplements. *Br. J. Nutr.* **2015**, *113*, 1993–2000. [CrossRef] [PubMed]
6. National Health and Medical Research Council. *Australian Dietary Guidelines*; National Health and Medical Research Council: Canberra, Australia, 2013.
7. Bailey, R.; Gahche, J.; Lentino, C.; Dwyer, J.; Engel, J.; Thomas, P.; Betz, J.; Sempos, C.; Picciano, M. Dietary supplement use in the United States, 2003–2006. *J. Nutr.* **2011**, *141*, 261–266. [CrossRef] [PubMed]
8. Sebastian, R.S.; Cleveland, L.E.; Goldman, J.D.; Moshfegh, A.J. Older adults who use vitamin/mineral supplements differ from nonusers in nutrient intake adequacy and dietary attitudes. *J. Am. Diet. Assoc.* **2007**, *107*, 1322–1332. [CrossRef] [PubMed]
9. Guo, X.; Willows, N.; Kuhle, S.; Jhangri, G.; Veugelers, P.J. Use of vitamin and mineral supplements among Canadian adults. *Can. J. Public Health* **2009**, *100*, 357–360. [PubMed]
10. Kennedy, E.T.; Luo, H.Q.; Houser, R.F. Dietary supplement use pattern of U.S. adult population in the 2007–2008 National Health and Nutrition Examination Survey (NHANES). *Ecol. Food Nutr.* **2013**, *52*, 76–84. [CrossRef] [PubMed]
11. Foote, J.; Murphy, S.; Wilkens, L.; Hankin, J.; Henderson, B.; Kolonel, L. Factors associated with dietary supplement use among healthy adults of five ethnicities: The Multiethnic Cohort Study. *Am. J. Epidemiol.* **2003**, *157*, 888–897. [CrossRef] [PubMed]
12. Australian Government. *Census and Statistics Act 1905*; Australian Government: Canberra, Australia, 1905.
13. Australian Bureau of Statistics. *Australian Health Survey: Nutrition and Physical Activity, 2011–2012*; Australian Bureau of Statistics: Canberra, Australia, 2015.
14. United States Department of Agriculture; Agricultural Research Service. Automated Multiple-Pass Method. Available online: https://www.ars.usda.gov/northeast-area/beltsville-md/beltsville-human-nutrition-research-center/food-surveys-research-group/docs/ampm-usda-automated-multiple-pass-method/ (accessed on 23 June 2017).
15. Food Standards Australia New Zealand AUSNUT 2011–13 Food Nutrient Database. Available online: http://www.foodstandards.gov.au/science/monitoringnutrients/ausnut/ausnutdatafiles/Pages/foodnutrient.aspx (accessed on 22 June 2017).
16. Milte, C.M.; Thorpe, M.G.; Crawford, D.; Ball, K.; McNaughton, S.A. Associations of diet quality with health-related quality of life in older Australian men and women. *Exp. Gerontol.* **2015**, *64*, 8–16. [CrossRef] [PubMed]
17. McNaughton, S.A.; Ball, K.; Crawford, D.; Mishra, G.D. An index of diet and eating patterns is a valid measure of diet quality in an Australian population. *J. Nutr.* **2008**, *138*, 86–93. [PubMed]
18. Thorpe, M.G.; Milte, C.; Crawford, D.; McNaughton, S.A. Development of a revised Australian Dietary Guideline Index and its association with key socio-demographic factors, health behaviors and body mass index. *Nutrients* **2016**, *8*, 160. [CrossRef] [PubMed]
19. Australian National Health and Medical Research Council. Nutrient Reference Values for Australia and New Zealand. Available online: https://www.nhmrc.gov.au/guidelines-publications/n35-n36-n37 (accessed on 22 June 2017).
20. Australian Bureau of Statistics. Socio-Economic Indexes for Areas. Available online: http://www.abs.gov.au/websitedbs/censushome.nsf/home/seifa (accessed on 1 September 2015).
21. Australian Institute of Health and Welfare. *The Active Australia Survey: A Guide and Manual for Implementation, Analysis and Reporting*; Australian Institute of Health and Welfare: Canberra, Australia, 2003.
22. Department of Health. Australia's Physical Activity and Sedentary Behaviour Guidelines. Available online: http://www.health.gov.au/internet/main/publishing.nsf/content/health-pubhlth-strateg-phys-act-guidelines (accessed on 28 August 2017).
23. Australian Bureau of Statistics. Alcohol. Available online: http://www.abs.gov.au/ausstats/abs@.nsf/Lookup/9AD599F2C7227404CA257B8D00229E97?opendocument (accessed on 22 June 2017).
24. Australian Bureau of Statistics. 24-h Dietary Recall. Available online: http://www.abs.gov.au/ausstats/abs@.nsf/Lookup/0D6B1FE95EAB8FF3CA257CD2001CA113?opendocument (accessed on 22 June 2017).

25. Australian Bureau of Statistics. Self-Assessed Health Status. Available online: http://www.abs. gov.au/ausstats/abs@.nsf/Lookup/8BFB01655391F7DCCA257B8D00229E88?opendocument (accessed on 22 June 2017).

26. WHO. *STEPwise Approach to Surveillance (STEPS)*; WHO: Geneva, Switzerland, 2008.

27. Australian Bureau of Statistics. Blood Pressure. Available online: http://www.abs.gov.au/ausstats/abs@ .nsf/Lookup/78B3C16892876C2ECA257B8D00229E99?opendocument (accessed on 22 June 2017).

28. StataCorp. *Stata Statistical Software: Release 14.2*; StataCorp LP: College Station, TX, USA, 2015.

29. National Health and Medical Research Council. *Australian Government Recommended Daily Intake for Adults*; National Health and Medical Research Council: Canberra, Australia, 1998.

30. Australian Government. An Overview of the Regulation of Complementary Medicines in Australia. Available online: https://www.tga.gov.au/overview-regulation-complementary-medicines-australia (accessed on 2 October 2017).

31. Chen, S.-Y.; Lin, J.-R.; Chen, T.-H.; Guo, S.-G.; Kao, M.-D.; Pan, W.-H. Dietary supplements usage among elderly Taiwanese during 2005–2008. *Asia Pac. J. Clin. Nutr.* **2011**, *20*, 327–336. [PubMed]

32. Schwab, S.; Heier, M.; Schneider, A.; Fischer, B.; Huth, C.; Peters, A.; Thorand, B. The use of dietary supplements among older persons in Southern Germany—Results from the KORA-age study. *J. Nutr. Health Aging* **2014**, *18*, 510–519. [CrossRef] [PubMed]

33. Waskiewicz, A.; Sygnowska, E.; Broda, G.; Chwojnowska, Z. The use of vitamin supplements among adults in Warsaw: Is there any nutritional benefit? *Rocz. Panstw. Zakl. Hig.* **2014**, *65*, 119–126. [PubMed]

34. Conner, M.; Kirk, S.F.; Cade, J.E.; Barrett, J.H. Why do women use dietary supplements? The use of the theory of planned behaviour to explore beliefs about their use. *Soc. Sci. Med.* **2001**, *52*, 621–633. [CrossRef]

35. Boeing, H.; Bechthold, A.; Bub, A.; Ellinger, S.; Haller, D.; Kroke, A.; Leschik-Bonnet, E.; Müller, M.J.; Oberritter, H.; Schulze, M.; et al. Critical review: vegetables and fruit in the prevention of chronic diseases. *Eur. J. Nutr.* **2012**, *51*, 637–663. [CrossRef] [PubMed]

36. McCrady, S.K.; Levine, J.A. Sedentariness at Work: How Much Do We Really Sit? *Obesity* **2009**, *17*, 2103–2105. [CrossRef] [PubMed]

37. Gunther, S.; Patterson, R.; Kristal, A.; Stratton, K.; White, E. Demographic and Health-Related Correlates of Herbal and Specialty Supplement Use. *J. Am. Diet. Assoc.* **2004**, *104*, 27–34. [CrossRef] [PubMed]

38. Beitz, R.; Mensink, G.B.; Hintzpeter, B.; Fischer, B.; Erbersdobler, H.F. Do users of dietary supplements differ from nonusers in their food consumption? *Eur. J. Epidemiol.* **2004**, *19*, 335–341. [CrossRef] [PubMed]

39. Kirk, S.F.; Cade, J.E.; Barrett, J.H.; Conner, M. Diet and lifestyle characteristics associated with dietary supplement use in women. *Public Health Nutr.* **1999**, *2*, 69–73. [CrossRef] [PubMed]

40. Lin, S.; Lin, Y.; Chuang, Y.; Chang, J.M.C.; Liou, J.; Tsai, A.C. Prevalence and determinants of dietary supplement and non-prescription medicine use by men and women over 53 years old in Taiwan. Results from a population-based cross-sectional survey. *Australas. J. Ageing* **2006**, *25*, 191–197.

41. Zimmet, P.; Magliano, D.; Matsuzawa, Y.; Alberti, G.; Shaw, J. The metabolic syndrome: A global public health problem and a new definition. *J. Atheroscler. Thromb.* **2005**, *12*, 295–300. [CrossRef] [PubMed]

42. Wiltgren, A.R.; Booth, A.O.; Kaur, G.; Cicerale, S.; Lacy, K.E.; Thorpe, M.G.; Keast, R.S.; Riddell, L.J. Micronutrient Supplement Use and Diet Quality in University Students. *Nutrients* **2015**, *7*, 1094–1107. [CrossRef] [PubMed]

43. Saquib, J.; Rock, C.L.; Natarajan, L.; Saquib, N.; Newman, V.A.; Patterson, R.E.; Thomson, C.A.; Al-Delaimy, W.K.; Pierce, J.P. Nutrient intakes from foods and dietary supplements in women at risk for breast cancer recurrence. The Women's Healthy Eating and Living Study Group. *Nutr. Cancer* **1997**, *29*, 133–139.

44. Frank, E.; Bendich, A.; Denniston, M. Use of vitamin-mineral supplements by female physicians in the United States. *Am. J. Clin. Nutr.* **2000**, *72*, 969–975. [PubMed]

45. Marra, M.V.; Wellman, N.S. Multivitamin–Mineral Supplements in the Older Americans Act Nutrition Program: Not a One-Size-Fits-All Quick Fix. *Am. J. Public Health* **2008**, *98*, 1171–1176. [CrossRef] [PubMed]

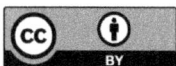

nutrients

MDPI

Article

Risk of Deficiency in Multiple Concurrent Micronutrients in Children and Adults in the United States

Julia K. Bird [1],*, Rachel A. Murphy [2], Eric D. Ciappio [3] and Michael I. McBurney [3]

[1]   Nutrition Innovation Center, Human Nutrition and Health, DSM Nutritional Products,
     Kaiseraugst CH-4303, Switzerland
[2]   School of Population and Public Health, University of British Columbia, Vancouver, BC V6T 1Z3, Canada;
     rachel.murphy@ubc.ca
[3]   Scientific Affairs, DSM Nutritional Products, Parsippany, NJ 07054, USA; eric.ciappio@dsm.com (E.D.C.);
     michael.mcburney@dsm.com (M.I.M.)
*   Correspondence: julia.bird@dsm.com; Tel.: +41-61-815-8522

Received: 12 May 2017; Accepted: 20 June 2017; Published: 24 June 2017

Abstract: Certain population sub-groups in the United States are vulnerable to micronutrient malnutrition. Nationally representative data from the National Health and Nutrition Examination Survey (NHANES) describing the biochemical status of vitamins A, B6, B12, C, D, E, folate, and anemia, were aggregated to determine the overall risk of multiple concurrent deficiencies in U.S. children and adults (n = 15,030) aged >9 years. The prevalence of deficiency risk according to socio-demographic, life-stage, dietary supplement use, and dietary adequacy categories was investigated. Thirty-one percent of the U.S. population was at risk of at least one vitamin deficiency or anemia, with 23%, 6.3%, and 1.7% of the U.S. population at risk of deficiency in 1, 2, or 3–5 vitamins or anemia, respectively. A significantly higher deficiency risk was seen in women (37%), non-Hispanic blacks (55%), individuals from low income households (40%), or without a high school diploma (42%), and underweight (42%) or obese individuals (39%). A deficiency risk was most common in women 19–50 years (41%), and pregnant or breastfeeding women (47%). Dietary supplement non-users had the highest risk of any deficiency (40%), compared to users of full-spectrum multivitamin-multimineral supplements (14%) and other dietary supplement users (28%). Individuals consuming an adequate diet based on the Estimated Average Requirement had a lower risk of any deficiency (16%) than those with an inadequate diet (57%). Nearly one-third of the U.S. population is at risk of deficiency in at least one vitamin, or has anemia.

Keywords: NHANES; nutritional status; deficiency; dietary adequacy; nutritional epidemiology; dietary supplement; multivitamin-mineral

1. Introduction

Numerous sources including the 2015 Dietary Guidelines Advisory Committee Report have highlighted shortfalls in key nutrients within the U.S. population [1,2]. Adequate intakes of micronutrients are essential for supporting the growth and development of children, as well as maintaining overall health across the lifespan. A prolonged, inadequate intake of essential micronutrients results in deficiencies that negatively impact health. Deficiency symptoms include impaired immunity, growth and night blindness from vitamin A deficiency [3], impaired wound healing and bleeding from vitamin C deficiency [4], anemia from iron deficiency [5], and rickets and osteomalacia from vitamin D deficiency [6]. Deficiencies in the B vitamins lead to different types of anemia: folate deficiency leads to megaloblastic anemia, vitamin B6 deficiency results in microcytic anemia, whereas vitamin B12 deficiency causes pernicious anemia, and may result in neurological damage due to impaired myelination [7]. An adequate status of micronutrients in combination is required for many important processes in the body. For example, erythropoiesis requires not only iron, but also folate, vitamin B12, and vitamin A, and dietary vitamin C can improve the absorption of non-heme iron [8]. Sub-clinical deficiency symptoms for many vitamins and minerals are non-specific, and may include fatigue, irritability, aches and pains, decreased immune function, and heart palpitations [4,7].

While estimates of the vitamin and mineral status of the U.S. population have been undertaken for many decades, the initiation of the National Health and Nutrition Examination (NHANES) surveys in the 1970s greatly improved access to representative data on nutrient intakes and deficiencies [9,10]. Cohort studies such as the Framingham Heart Study [11] and the Multiethnic Cohort [12], and large clinical trials [13,14] also provided valuable insights into vitamin intakes and status in certain population groups. The current estimates indicate that vitamin A, vitamin D, vitamin E, folate, vitamin C, calcium, and magnesium are under-consumed relative to the Estimated Average Requirement (EAR), while iron is under-consumed by adolescent and adult females, including those who are pregnant [1]. The Centers for Disease Control and Prevention (CDC) measured biochemical indicators of diet and nutrition in a representative sample of the U.S. population from 2003–2006 [15], and a series publications explores this data in more detail [2,16–20]. From the main report, the deficiency prevalence for each of the vitamins B6, C, and D, and the mineral iron, ranged between 5–10%. The deficiency prevalence estimates were investigated according to ethnicity, age, and gender and showed that women and non-Hispanic Blacks tended to have greater vitamin B6 deficiency, older adults and non-Hispanic Whites had a greater prevalence of vitamin B12 deficiency, men and non-Hispanic Whites had a greater prevalence of vitamin C deficiency, and almost one in three non-Hispanic Blacks had a vitamin D deficiency. However, the report does not examine the prevalence rates in risk groups such as pregnant and breastfeeding women, low-income households, or according to educational status, body mass index (BMI), or measures of dietary intake. A general estimate of the prevalence of multiple concurrent deficiencies was conducted, including a sub-group analysis in a single risk group [2]. This analysis found that although 78% of the U.S. population aged over 6 years was not at risk of deficiency, only 74% of women of childbearing potential (aged 12–49) were not at risk of deficiency, and when iron-deficiency anemia was included, 68% were not at risk of deficiency. The analysis also found that 5.7% of the U.S. population was at risk of two or more vitamin deficiencies. Despite considerable interest in deficiency in single vitamins or minerals, we are not aware of any other estimates of aggregated vitamin or mineral deficiencies in the U.S. population, although some smaller surveys have measured the biochemical status of multiple micronutrients in risk populations in other countries [21–24].

Dietary supplements (DS) can be an important source of vitamins and minerals to prevent inadequate dietary intakes. Approximately half of adults and one third of children report DS use [25–27], primarily in the form of multivitamins with or without minerals. DS users have a lower prevalence of inadequate micronutrient intake among adults [28–30], children, and adolescents [29,31]. In the U.S., DS are used most often to maintain or improve overall health [25,32]. DS are widely used as "nutritional insurance" to cover unintended gaps in dietary intakes [25,33].

Although a commonly used definition of a multivitamin-multimineral supplement is that it contains at least three vitamins and at least one mineral [26], this definition is very broad and captures not only DS intended to be taken every day to fill dietary gaps, but also specialized formulations targeted at specific health benefits such as eye or bone health, or sports supplements. We wanted to investigate whether there was any difference in rates of deficiency when individuals used "full spectrum" multivitamin-multimineral DS (FSMV), which contain all 12 vitamins and the most nutritionally important minerals, i.e., calcium, iron, iodine, magnesium, zinc, selenium, copper, manganese, chromium, and molybdenum. These types of supplements have been used in several long-term clinical trials [34–36], and align more closely with consumer use.

The aims of this study are (1) to determine the risk of deficiency for multiple micronutrients in the U.S., (2) to identify groups with a greater burden of deficiency risk across a broad range of socio-demographic and life span groups, and (3) to determine whether the risk of deficiency differs between DS non-users, DS users, and FSMV users, in the context of dietary adequacy.

2. Materials and Methods

2.1. Description of Dataset

The National Health and Nutrition Examination Survey (NHANES) is a representative survey of the civilian, non-institutionalized U.S. population, and is designed to assess general health and nutritional status. The National Center for Health Statistics Research Ethics Review Board reviewed and approved protocol #98-12 for data collected in the 2003–2004 cycle, and protocol #2005-06 for data collected in the 2005–2006 cycle. NHANES protocols receive ethical review annually, and ongoing changes are submitted through an amendment process [37]. All of the subjects gave their informed consent for inclusion before they participated in the study. The datasets are publicly available from the National Center for Health Statistics. A complex, multistage probability sampling design is used to select a sample representative of the U.S. population, with a subset of participants undergoing biochemical assessments [38].

For our research, we conducted a secondary analysis of 15,030 participants aged 9 years and over for which demographic data were available from the 2003–2004 and 2005–2006 data cycles. These survey years were chosen as they provide the most comprehensive and recent data describing biochemical nutrient status for multiple vitamins and minerals. We included socio-demographic data for age, sex, race/ethnicity, poverty income ratio (PIR, a measure of household income relative to household size), and educational status. Race/ethnicity was used as defined in NHANES (Non-Hispanic White, Non-Hispanic Black, Mexican American; the results for the "Other Hispanic" and "Other Race" categories are not reported due to small sample size). The PIR was categorized as low (<1.85), medium ($\geq$1.85 and <3.5), or high ($\geq$3.5) [18]. Education for adults aged 20 y and over was categorized as "less than high school", "high school graduate", and "some college, or college graduate". The BMI was calculated from height and weight measured during the medical examination, and was categorized as underweight, normal weight, overweight, or obese according to the standard cut-off points for adults aged 20 years and over [18]. Pregnancy status was determined either by self-report or a laboratory test taken during the physical examination. Self-reported current breastfeeding in women 1 year postpartum or less in the reproductive health questionnaire was used to ascertain breastfeeding status. Age, sex, pregnancy status, and breastfeeding status were used to assign participants to Dietary Reference Intake (DRI) categories used by the Institute of Medicine [7].

2.2. Criteria for Determining Biochemical Vitamin and Mineral Status, Biochemical Deficiency Score and Dietary Inadequacy Score

The 2003–2006 NHANES cycles are unique in that they provide comprehensive biochemical measures of micronutrient status for vitamins A, B6, B12, C, D, E, folate, and iron. We used the cut-off points as summarized in Table 1 to identify individuals with biomarker concentrations at risk of deficiency [2]. The cut-offs from the CDC report on biomarkers of nutrient status were used to ascertain the risk of deficiency for vitamins A, B6, B12, folate, C, D, and E [15]. Because the vitamin B6 analysis changed between the 2003–2004 cycle (enzymatic assay) and the 2005–2006 cycle (HPLC method) [39], the data from each cycle are analyzed and reported separately. Vitamin B12 deficiency was defined as either a low serum vitamin B12 (<200 pg/mL) or elevated methylmalonic acid ((MMA); >0.271 μmol/L) [15]. Similarly to the CDC report, any participant with either a low serum folate (<2 ng/mL) or low red blood cell folate (<95 ng/mL) was defined as deficient in folate [15]. Iron deficiency anemia is best determined using a combination of serum ferritin to describe low iron stores, and hemoglobin to determine anemia [40]. However, the serum ferritin test is only available for a limited population within NHANES, namely women of reproductive age and children aged from 1 to 5 years. To assess the entire population, the iron deficiency anemia screening criteria used by the Association of American Family Physicians were used, which uses a combination of low hemoglobin concentrations and a small mean corpuscular volume to detect individuals with anemia who are at risk of iron deficiency anemia [41].

In NHANES, the dietary intake of vitamins and minerals is estimated by two 24 h dietary recalls conducted on non-consecutive days. The mean of two 24 h dietary recalls was used to estimate dietary inadequacy, insufficiency, and excess based on the EAR, Recommended Dietary Allowance (RDA), and Tolerable Upper Limit (TUL), respectively. For each individual, binary categories were created for nutrient status and nutrient intake; a 1 was assigned if the subject's biomarker of nutrient status indicated a risk of deficiency (status), and a 1 when an individual failed to meet his/her age-gender and lifespan specific EAR or RDA for a nutrient, or was above the TUL (intake). When the status or intake for a nutrient was sufficient or adequate, a 0 was assigned. Only subjects with complete data for all biomarkers of nutrient status were used when calculating proportions deficient for multiple deficiencies; other subjects were coded as missing for the summed variable. For the biochemical markers of nutrient status, participants were given a score of 0 to 5 based on the number of vitamins or minerals for which they were below the cut-off for deficiency (no participant was at risk of deficiency for more than five vitamins, or had anemia), and a dietary inadequacy/insufficiency score of 0 to 7 based on the number of micronutrients for which their dietary intake was inadequate/insufficient (Supplementary Tables S1 and S2). Scores describing the risk of multiple deficiencies were aggregated to avoid small cell sizes. Groups were defined as: no deficiency; risk of deficiency in one vitamin, or anemia; risk of deficiency in two vitamins, or anemia; risk of deficiency in three to five vitamins, or anemia for 2-way tables. For 3-way tables, we categorized subjects as either no deficiency; or risk of deficiency in one to five vitamins, or with anemia.

2.3. Selection of Full Spectrum Multivitamin-Multimineral Supplements

The DS used in NHANES 2003–2006 were categorized according to the count of vitamins and minerals in each product. The FSMV category was based on a large cluster of products with a composition that included a broad range of micronutrients, and thus was defined as users of any DS containing ≥12 vitamins and 7 to 16 minerals, as shown in Supplementary Table S3. Based on this definition, participants were classified as DS non-users, FSMV users, and DS users.

2.4. Statistical Methods

All analyses were performed using SAS version 9.3 (SAS Institute Inc., Cary, NC, USA). Statistical significance was set at 0.05, and adjusted by the Bonferroni correction for multiple tests for all sub-group analyses. Procedures that take into account the complex survey design of NHANES were used to produce means and percentages. The Mobile Examination Center sample weight provided by the CDC, adjusted for the 2003–2006 NHANES cycles, was used to create nationally representative estimates for those analyses that did not include dietary analysis, and the Day 2 Dietary sample weights were used for analyses that used the dietary intake datasets. Differences between categorical variables were assessed by comparing confidence intervals with an alpha adjusted by the Bonferroni correction for the number of sub-groups. Significant differences within multiple sub-group categories were marked with superscripts generated according to the method of Dallal [42]. Estimates with a relative standard error greater than 30% were flagged because they lack sufficient precision, as recommended by the CDC [43]. Confidence intervals for proportions were calculated using the SURVEYFREQ procedure, which by default produces Wald (linear) confidence intervals. For confidence intervals of extreme proportions (in our dataset, any confidence interval that included zero as the lower bound), Clopper–Pearson (exact) confidence intervals were computed, as marked in the tables, per the analytical guidelines [43].

Table 1. Deficiency risk criteria and risk of deficiency in individual vitamins or anemia.

Nutritional Biomarker	Deficiency Risk Criteria	Proportion Biochemically Deficient 2003–2004		Proportion Biochemically Deficient 2005–2006		Proportion Biochemically Deficient 2003–2006	
		%	SE	%	SE	%	SE
Vitamin A	Serum retinol <20 µg/dL [15]	0.28	0.65	0.25	0.84	0.26	0.05
Vitamin B6	PLP <20 nmol/L [15]	20*	1.4	11*	0.76	16	0.87
Vitamin B12	Serum vitamin B12 <200 pg/mL or MMA >0.271 µmol/L [15]	7.5*	0.70	2.6*	0.30	5.0	0.44
Folate	Red blood cell folate <95 ng/mL or serum folate <2 ng/mL [15]	0.37	0.10	0.18	0.40	0.27	0.05
Vitamin C	Serum ascorbic acid <0.2 mg/dL [15]	7.5	0.99	4.9	0.59	6.2	0.59
Vitamin D	25-hydroxyvitamin D <12 ng/mL [15]	7.9	1.2	9.8	1.2	8.9	0.83
Vitamin E	Alpha-tocopherol <500 µg/dL [15]	0.75	0.15	0.66	0.09	0.70	0.08
Anemia	Hemoglobin <13 g/dL (men ≥15 years) or <12 (women ≥15 years), adolescents 12–14 years) or <11 g/dL (pregnant women) or <11.5 g/dL (children >12); and mean cell volume <95 fL [40,41]	3.9	0.41	4.6	0.37	4.3	0.28

Data are from NHANES 2003–2006 representative of the U.S. population, aged ≥9 years, based on biochemical indicators of nutrient deficiency. Abbreviations: PLP, pyridoxal-5′-phosphate; MMA, methylmalonic acid; SE, standard error. * Cycles (2003–2004 or 2005–2006) differ significantly p < 0.05.

3. Results

3.1. Individual Biochemical Deficiencies and Insufficient Intakes of Vitamins and Minerals

The most common biochemical deficiency in the U.S. population aged ≥9 years was vitamin B6 (Table 1). The proportion of participants at risk of vitamin B6 deficiency was 20% for the 2003–2004 cycle and 11% for the 2005–2006 cycle. A risk of deficiency in vitamins B12, C, and D was found in 5.0%, 6.2%, and 8.9% of the U.S. population, respectively. Anemia was found in 4.3% of the U.S. population overall. Less than 1% of the population was at risk of deficiency for vitamin A, folate, or vitamin E. Demographic characteristics of the study population and biochemical status are already well described in the literature [15,16,29], therefore these data are presented in Supplementary Tables S4 and S5, respectively.

3.2. Overall Inadequate Biochemical Status According to Demographic Characteristics

The prevalence of deficiency risk in multiple, concurrent vitamins, or anemia, are reported in Table 2. Sixty-nine percent was not at risk of deficiency, and 23%, 6.3%, 1.5%, 0.14%, and 0.053% was at risk of deficiency in one, two, three, four and five vitamins or had anemia, respectively. The prevalence of deficiency risk or anemia was higher in NHANES cycle 2003–2004 than 2005–2006 due to differences in the analytical method used for vitamin B6. Across all demographic, age, and gender groups, a risk of deficiency in a single nutrient or anemia was observed more frequently than multiple concurrent nutrient deficiencies.

The risk of deficiency in 1, 2, or 3–5 vitamins or anemia was higher among females than males ($p < 0.0125$). There were significant differences in deficiency risk by ethnicity: non-Hispanic Whites had the lowest risk whereas non-Hispanic Blacks had the highest risk of deficiency or anemia ($p < 0.0125$). Individuals from low PIR households were more likely to be at risk of deficiency/anemia, compared to the two higher household income categories ($p < 0.0125$). Completing some college or having a college diploma was associated with a lower risk of deficiency in one or two vitamins/anemia compared to participants without a high school diploma ($p < 0.0125$), although there was no significant difference found according to educational attainment for individuals deficient in three or more vitamins.

There was a U-shaped relationship when the deficiency risk was investigated according to BMI. Both underweight and obese individuals had an increased risk of deficiency compared to normal weight and overweight subjects ($p < 0.0125$). Overall, women who were pregnant had a non-significant higher risk of vitamin deficiency or anemia than women of childbearing potential (defined in the NHANES survey as girls aged 8–11 years who had started menstruating, and all girls and women aged 12–59 years who were not pregnant). On the other hand, the extra nutritional demands of lactation did not appear to result in a higher risk of vitamin deficiency or anemia in postpartum women reporting breastfeeding.

3.3. Biochemical Deficiencies across Age and Gender Categories

The overall risk of vitamin deficiency or anemia was investigated according to age, gender, and life stage groups in Table 3. A risk of deficiency/anemia was most frequent in pregnant or breastfeeding females, females aged 19–50 years, and adolescent females 14–18 years. The pattern of low status in certain micronutrients varied by age and gender groups (Table 4), although no significant differences were found for vitamin A and folate ($p < 0.00625$). Male adolescents aged 14–18 years had higher rates of low vitamin E (3.7%) status. Males aged 19–50 years had higher rates of biochemical vitamin C deficiency (8.7%). Females aged 19–50 years were more likely to have a deficient vitamin D status (12%). Vitamin B12 deficiency rates tended to increase with age, with higher rates found in adults aged 51–70 years (6.9%) and 71 years and over (15%) than some younger age groups. The oldest age group (adults 71 years and older) was also more likely to be deficient in vitamin D (9.1%) and have anemia (8.9%). Pregnant and breastfeeding women were more likely to have a deficient status of vitamin B6 (35%) or be anemic (18%). The difference in deficiency prevalence between the 2003–2004 and 2005–2006 vitamin B6 samples appeared to be affected by the age of the subjects and was much more apparent in younger age groups in 2003–2004, and in older age groups in 2005–2006 (results not shown).

Table 2. Risk of multiple vitamin deficiencies and/or anemia according to demographic characteristics.

Characteristic	N	Deficient in 1 *		Deficient in 2 *		Deficient in 3–5 *		Not Deficient	
		%	SE	%	SE	%	SE	%	SE
All participants	13,225	23	0.78	6.3	0.49	1.7	0.18	69	1.2
Cycle									
2003–2004	6600	27	0.82 [a]	7.2	0.64	1.9	0.29	63	1.4 [a]
2005–2006	6625	19	1.1 [b]	5.5	0.68	1.5	0.19	75	1.7 [b]
Sex									
Male	6506	19 [a]	1.1	4.6 [a]	0.39	1.1	0.20	75 [a]	1.4
Female	6719	26 [b]	0.75	8.0 [b]	0.64	2.3	0.29	64 [b]	1.3
Ethnicity [†]									
Mexican American	3195	24 [a]	1.4	5.4 [a]	0.61	1.2 [a]	0.30	69 [a]	2.1
Non-Hispanic White	5647	20 [a]	1.1	5.4 [a]	0.46	1.3 [a]	0.19	73 [a]	1.4
Non-Hispanic Black	3432	36 [b]	1.2	14 [b]	0.81	5.1 [b]	0.37	45 [b]	1.7
PIR (%)									
Low PIR, ≤1.85	5804	27 [a]	0.92	9.8 [a]	0.77	2.8 [a]	0.27	60 [a]	1.4
Medium PIR, >1.85 and ≤3.5	3224	24 [a]	0.91	6.1 [a]	0.80	1.8 [ab]	0.26	68 [b]	1.3
High PIR, >3.5	3570	18 [b]	0.93	3.8 [b]	0.43	0.82 [b]	0.17	77 [c]	1.1
Education [‡]									
Less than high school	2433	27 [a]	1.1	11 [a]	0.84	2.9	0.43	59 [a]	1.6
High school graduate	2105	26 [ab]	1.2	8.0 [ab]	0.91	2.2	0.44	64 [a]	1.5
Some college/college graduate	4043	21 [b]	1.0	5.0 [b]	0.47	1.5	0.23	72 [b]	1.3
BMI [§]									
Underweight	280	23 [ab]	2.6	10	2.4	8.4	1.7	58 [ac]	4.1
Normal weight	2473	23 [ab]	1.2	5.7	0.64	1.5 [ab]	0.25	70 [ab]	1.6
Overweight	2949	21 [a]	0.90	5.4	0.51	0.98 [a]	0.19	73 [b]	1.1
Obese	2891	27 [b]	1.3	9.4	0.88	2.8 [b]	0.33	61 [c]	1.8
Pregnancy status [ǀ]									
Positive	574	33	3.2	14	2.7	4.9	1.3	48	4.8
Negative	4520	27	0.88	7.5	0.72	2.1	0.34	63	1.3
Breastfeeding status [¶]									
Breastfeeding a child	100	21	6.4 **	9.2	3.3 **	3.5	3.3 **	66	8.5
Not breastfeeding	269	35	4.7	15	3.2	3.9	1.6 **	47	4.9

The overall risk of vitamin deficiency or anemia was investigated according to age, gender, and life stage groups in Table 3. A risk of deficiency/anemia was most frequent in pregnant or breastfeeding women. Data are from NHANES 2003–2006 representative of the U.S. population, aged ≥9 years, based on biochemical indicators of nutrient deficiency. Abbreviations: PIR, poverty income ratio. * Risk of deficiency based on vitamins A, B6, B12, C, D, E, folate, or anemia. Different superscripts represent significant differences within demographical categories, p = 0.0125 using, for simplicity, the Bonferroni correction for five comparisons (the maximum number of sub-groups in the demographics categories included) and alpha = 0.05 for the entire table. [†] "Other Hispanic" and "Other race" ethnicity categories not reported due to small sample size. [‡] Education status is restricted to adults aged 20 years and older. [§] Body mass index (BMI) categories are restricted to adults aged 20 years and older. [ǀ] Percentages reflect proportion of women of childbearing potential: menstruating girls aged 8–11 and all women aged 12–59 years. [¶] Percentages reflect proportion of women 0 or 1 years postpartum at the time of the interview. ** Relative standard error >30%.

Table 3. Age, gender, and life stage categories and risk of deficiency.

Age, Gender and Life Stage Category	N	Deficient in 1 *		Deficient in 2 *		Deficient in 3–5 *		Not deficient	
		%	SE	%	SE	%	SE	%	SE
9–13 years, male & female	1734	15 [b]	1.4	1.5 [ab]	0.36	0.06 [a**‡]	0.04	83 [ab]	1.6
14–18 years, male	1242	18 [b]	1.7	2.2 [a]	0.65	0.13 [ab**‡]	0.08	80 [a]	1.9
14–18 years, female	1107	26 [ab]	1.9	5.3 [abc]	0.89	0.98 [abcd]	0.23	68 [bcd]	2.2
19–50 years, male	2442	20 [b]	1.3	3.9 [ab]	0.36	0.70 [abc]	0.23	76 [ab]	1.5
19–50 years, female	2150	30 [a]	1.0	8.5 [cd]	0.89	2.5 [d]	0.43	59 [d]	1.6
51–70 years, male & female	2347	21 [b]	1.2	7.4 [bcd]	0.90	2.0 [cd]	0.27	70 [abc]	1.7
71+ years, male & female	1540	23 [b]	1.0	9.5 [cd]	0.93	3.4 [d]	0.48	64 [cd]	1.7
Pregnant or breastfeeding	683	30 [ab]	3.3	13 [d]	2.2	4.6 [d]	1.5	53 [d]	4.3

Data are from NHANES 2003–2006 representative of the U.S. population, aged ≥9 years, based on biochemical indicators of nutrient deficiency. * Risk of deficiency based on vitamins A, B6, B12, C, D, E, folate, or anemia. Different superscripts represent significant differences between life stage categories, $p < 0.00625$ using Bonferroni correction for eight sub-groups and alpha = 0.05. ** Relative standard error >30%. [‡] Comparison made using Clopper–Pearson (exact) confidence interval.

Table 4. Percentage at risk of deficiency of individual vitamins, or anemia, by age, gender, and life stage categories.

Age, Gender, and Life Stage Category	Serum Retinol <20 µg/dL	PLP <20 nmol/L	Vitamin B12 <200 pg/mL or MMA >0.271 µmol/L	Serum Folate <2 ng/mL or RBC Folate <95 ng/mL	Vitamin C <0.2 mg/dL	Vitamin D <12 ng/mL	Vitamin E <500 µg/dL	Anemia and MCV <95 fL
9–13 years, male & female	0.41 (0.083, 1.2) *‡	9.4 (5.8, 12.9)	1.3 (0.30, 3.5) *‡	0.21 (0.011, 1.0) *‡	1.1 (0.33, 2.6) *‡	4.0 (2.2, 5.8)	1.4 (0.3, 2.5)	1.3 (0.5, 2.2)
14–18 years, male	0.034 (0, 0.53) *‡	5.6 (2.7, 8.4)	2.6 (0.6, 4.5)	0.20 (0.015, 0.85) *‡	3.2 (0.5, 5.8)	7.1 (3.9, 10.3)	3.7 (1.0, 6.3)	0.28 (0.034, 0.97) *‡
14–18 years, female	0.062 (0, 0.64) *‡	16 (11.2, 21.6)	2.2 (0.5, 4.0)	0.33 (0.047, 1.1) *‡	3.6 (0.7, 6.5)	10.6 (5.6, 15.6)	1.3 (0.1, 2.5) *	4.5 (2.2, 6.8)
19–50 years, male	0.20 (0.04, 0.61) *‡	8.1 (5.5, 10.6)	3.0 (1.9, 4.1)	0.25 (0.062, 0.67) *‡	8.7 (5.4, 11.9)	8.0 (5.2, 10.8)	0.5 (0.1, 1.0) *	0.9 (0.4, 1.5)
19–50 years, female	0.28 (0.04, 0.92) *‡	25 (20.3, 29.0)	3.9 (2.4, 5.4)	0.35 (0.074, 0.99) *‡	6.9 (4.3, 9.5)	12 (8.3, 15.3)	0.5 (0.1, 0.8)	6.6 (4.9, 8.3)
51–70 years, male & female	0.19 (0.018, 0.75) *‡	16 (12.6, 19.7)	6.9 (3.7, 10.1)	0.32 (0.076, 0.85) *‡	6.6 (4.0, 9.2)	8.4 (5.3, 11.5)	0.4 (0.1, 0.6)	4.0 (2.7, 5.3)
71+ years, male & female	0.27 (0.025, 1.0) *‡	15 (11.4, 18.8)	15 (10.5, 18.7)	0.10 (0.0020, 0.57) *‡	4.3 (2.3, 6.3)	9.1 (6.7, 11.5)	0.28 (0.047, 0.88) *‡	8.9 (6.2, 11.6)
Pregnant or breastfeeding	1.7 (0.12, 7.0) *‡	35 (25.4, 44.8)	4.5 (2.6, 6.3)	0.21 (0, 1.8) *‡	0.46 (0.047, 1.7) *‡	7.3 (2.0, 12.7)	2.0 (0.12, 8.5) *‡	18 (9.9, 25.3)

Data are from NHANES 2003–2006 representative of the U.S. population, aged ≥9 years, based on biochemical indicators of nutrient deficiency. Values represent percentage at risk of deficiency (99.375% confidence interval). Abbreviations: PLP, pyridoxal-5'-phosphate; MMA, methylmalonic acid; RBC, red blood cell; MCV, mean cell volume. * Relative standard error >30%; ‡ Clopper–Pearson (exact) confidence interval.

3.4. Risk of Vitamin Deficiency or Anemia by Dietary Supplement Use Categories and Age/Gender Groups

Younger age groups reported less frequent use of DS and FSMV than older age groups, and women reported greater use than men (Table 5). Pregnant or breastfeeding women were more likely to use DS than non-pregnant women aged 19–50 years, although the use of FSMV was similar.

DS non-users had the highest risk of deficiency (40%) compared to DS users (28%), whereas users of FSMV had the lowest risk of deficiency (14%, $p < 0.0167$). Similar trends were found in all DRI groups, although the differences did not always reach statistical significance.

3.5. Risk of Vitamin Deficiency According to Dietary Sufficiency Score and Dietary Supplement Use

A low proportion of the U.S. population has an adequate diet. Based on the EAR, 6.4% of the population consumed at least the EAR for each of the vitamins A, B6, B12, C, E, folate, and iron (Supplementary Table S2). Most people did not meet the EAR for vitamin E (89% inadequate), and approximately half the population did not meet the EAR for vitamins A (52% inadequate) and C (48% inadequate; Supplementary Table S1).

A lower dietary inadequacy/insufficiency score and reported DS use were both associated with a lower risk of nutrient deficiencies (Figure 1). For subjects who met their requirements for all of the vitamins and minerals in our analysis (dietary inadequacy score of 0 based on the EAR), 28% of DS non-users, 12% of DS users, and 4.8% of FSMV users were at risk of at least one biochemical deficiency. For subjects with a diet that was highly likely to meet their individual requirements (dietary insufficiency score of 0 based on the RDA), 16% of DS non-users, 6.0% of DS users, and 0.9% of FSMV users were at risk of deficiency for one vitamin or mineral. As the number of dietary inadequacies or insufficiencies increased, the risk of deficiency also increased. In subjects with the poorest diets based on the EAR (dietary inadequacy score of 7), the deficiency risk was 70% in DS non-users, 45% in DS users, and 31% in FSMV users. Based on a dietary insufficiency score derived from the RDA (dietary insufficiency score of 7), the risk of deficiency was 63% in DS non-users, 51% in DS users, and 29% in FSMV users. The proportion of the population with intakes above the Tolerable Upper Limit was low: 1.1%, 0.68%, and 0.31% of the population had excessive intakes of iron, folate, and retinol, respectively, and excessive intakes were not found for the other vitamins (Supplementary Table S2). A sensitivity analysis was conducted to determine whether the length of time taking a dietary supplement, or frequency of taking a dietary supplement over the previous 30 days, had an effect on the deficiency score. While there were general trends towards a lower risk of deficiency when dietary supplements were taken more often in the past 30 days, or for longer than 2 months, the results were not statistically significant (Supplementary Tables S6 and S7).

Table 5. Risk of vitamin deficiency or anemia by type of DS reportedly used by survey respondents, according to age, gender and life stage category.

	Not Taking a DS				Taking a DS but Not an FSMV				Taking an FSMV			
	N	% DS Use *	% Deficient †	SE	N	% DS Use *	% Deficient †	SE	N	% DS Use *	% Deficient †	SE
Entire Dataset	7281	44	40 [a]	1.3	4312	40	28 [b]	1.5	1615	16	14 [c]	0.9
Age, gender and life stage category												
9–13 years, male & female	1321	68	20	1.7	260	20	10	2.5	150	12	18	4.5
14–18 years, male	1007	75	23	2.1	182	20	14	3.9	52	4.8	12	6.0
14–18 years, female	861	69	37 [a]	2.8	194	25	25 [ab]	3.7	50	6.2	13 [b]	6.2
19–50 years, male	1469	52	33 [a]	1.8	740	36	17 [b]	2.1	232	12	7.9 [b]	1.7
19–50 years, female	1138	43	54 [a]	2.0	828	47	35 [b]	2.0	182	10	19 [b]	2.9
51–70 years, male & female	869	30	47 [a]	3.1	957	44	29 [b]	2.0	515	26	13 [c]	1.5
71+ years, male & female	459	25	58 [a]	3.5	731	49	34 [b]	2.2	348	26	17 [c]	2.5
Pregnant or breastfeeding	157	26	55	7.3	420	63	46	4.5	86	11	34	7.4

Data are from NHANES 2003–2006 representative of the U.S. population, aged ≥9 years, based on biochemical indicators of nutrient deficiency. Abbreviations: DS, dietary supplement; FSMV, full-spectrum multivitamin-multimineral supplement containing 12 or more vitamins and 7 to 16 minerals. * Percentage of participants in indicated DS use category, representative of the U.S. population, aged ≥9 years. † Deficiency prevalence, based on vitamins A, B6, B12, C, D, E, folate, or anemia. Different superscripts represent significant differences between DS categories within one category of inadequate status, $p < 0.0167$ using Bonferroni correction for three comparisons and alpha = 0.05.

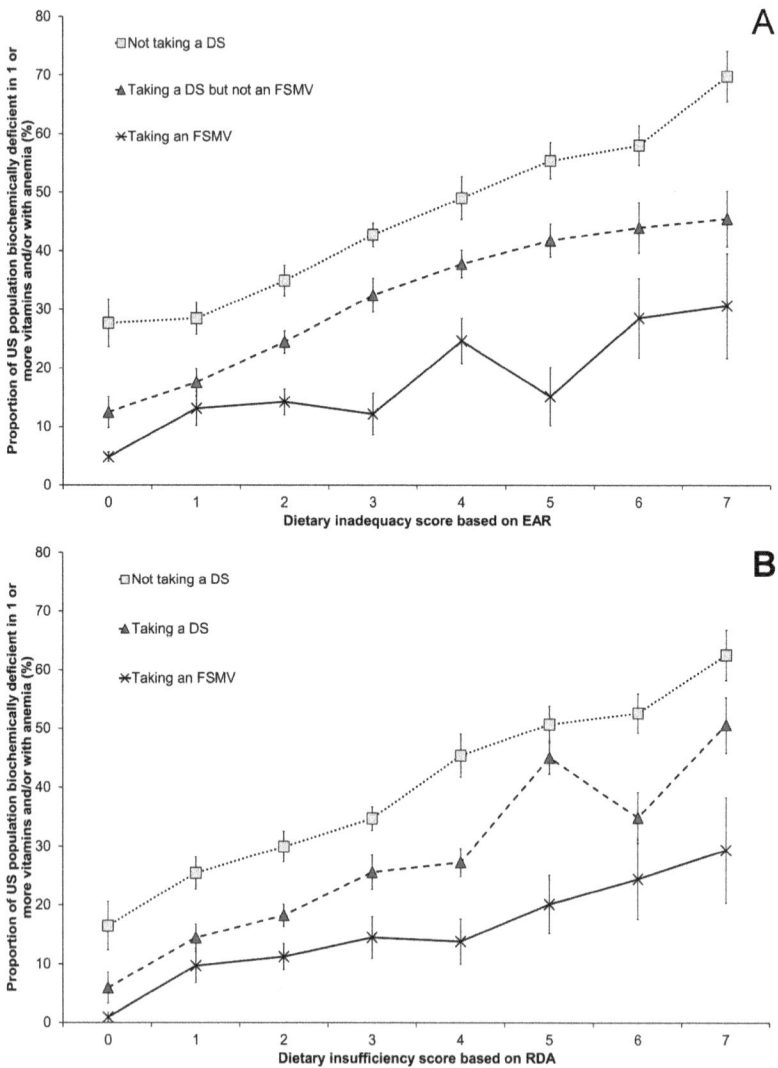

Figure 1. Risk of biochemical vitamin deficiency or anemia, by DS use and dietary vitamin/mineral inadequacy/insufficiency. Dietary inadequacy score reflects the combined number of vitamins and/or minerals for which intake is below the (**A**) Estimated Average Requirement (EAR) or (**B**) Recommended Dietary Allowance (RDA) for vitamins A, B6, B12, C, E, folate, and the mineral iron. Proportions are a percentage of the US population at risk of deficiency in one or more vitamin or with anemia according to biochemical measurements of nutritional status, and error bars reflect the SE. NHANES, National Health and Nutrition Examination Survey; DS, dietary supplement; FSMV, full-spectrum multivitamin-multimineral supplement containing 12 or more vitamins and 7 to 16 minerals.

4. Discussion

Our analysis showed that nearly one third of the U.S. population aged over 9 years is at risk of deficiency in at least one vitamin, or has anemia. Vulnerable groups include females, especially pregnant or breastfeeding females, non-Hispanic Blacks, participants with a low socio-economic status, and underweight and obese individuals. While DS users had a moderately lower risk of deficiency compared to non-users, users of FSMV, in particular, had a much lower deficiency risk. Individuals consuming their EAR or RDA were less likely to be at risk of deficiency, a relationship that was consistent within DS use categories.

Our deficiency risk data for individual vitamins and minerals agree with other NHANES analyses [4,15,16,44–49]. The investigation of multiple concurrent deficiencies conducted using the 2005–2006 cycle of data by Pfeiffer et al. found a lower prevalence of deficiency than our analysis due to differences in rates of deficiencies between survey cycles, our exclusion of young children from the analysis due to uncertainty over appropriate biochemical cut-off values, and differences in the lowest age of children for whom biochemical status was determined between micronutrients. As discussed in more detail below, our use of indicators of iron status for the entire population also had a small impact on the deficiency risk. Our vitamin B6 deficiency estimates agree with Morris et al. [49] for the 2003–2004 data cycle, and with the CDC for the 2005–2006 data cycle [15]. The differences in the prevalence of vitamin B6 deficiency between the 2003–2004 and 2005–2006 cycles reflect changes in analytical methodology.

The CDC reports iron deficiency anemia prevalence based on criteria (hemoglobin and serum ferritin concentrations) that were only available for a limited subset of the population. As we were interested in estimating iron deficiency anemia in the general population, we could only use the less specific blood hemoglobin and mean cell volume measurements. Cogswell et al. provide estimates of the specificity of anemia concentrations to predict iron deficiency anemia in the same survey years as our analysis [50]. In the Cogswell analysis, 6.2% of non-pregnant women aged 12–49 years had anemia, and of this percentage, 76% had iron deficiency anemia. In this population that is at greatest risk of iron deficiency anemia, using the hemoglobin measurement alone results in an overestimation of the prevalence of iron deficiency anemia. It is difficult to predict whether a similar proportion of participants with anemia in other life stage groups have iron deficiency anemia, however it is reasonable to assume a similar ratio. Therefore, our estimations of the prevalence of anemia in the U.S. population are greater than the prevalence of iron deficiency anemia, and it is likely that the actual prevalence of iron deficiency anemia is approximately three quarters of our estimate of 4.3% with anemia.

The finding that women of childbearing age have an elevated risk of vitamin or mineral deficiency has been reported by others [51,52]. In pregnant women, plasma volume expansion may dilute the blood biomarkers of nutrient status, leading to an apparent increase in the risk of deficiency [53,54]. The medical and nutritional significance of plasma volume expansion on markers of nutrient status is unknown. The trend to lower rates of biochemical deficiency in women who breastfeed may relate to higher socio-economic status or better knowledge of nutrition [55]. The markedly higher rates of vitamin D deficiency in non-Hispanic Blacks, found to be 31% in the U.S. population aged 1 year and older for the same survey years and vitamin D cut-off by the CDC [15], is likely to be primarily responsible for the overall greater risk of any deficiency in this racial/ethnic group. In addition, others have found that non-Hispanic blacks are at greater nutritional risk, and this may be due to poorer diets or nutrient intakes [46,56,57]. Inadequate diets found in individuals from lower socio-economic status households [58] may be the cause behind their increased risk of deficiency. Metabolic disturbances related to obesity could be both a cause and a consequence of vitamin deficiency, particularly for vitamins C, B12, folate, and the fat-soluble vitamins, explaining our finding that there was an increased risk of deficiency in obese participants [59].

Given that dietary supplements improve nutrient intakes in general [29], the observation that DS use is associated with a reduced risk of deficiency is consistent with previous observations in the general population, such as has been shown for vitamins B6 [49], B12 [44], and C [4], as well as for folate in pregnant women [45], and for an FSMV in older adults [60]. DS users tend to have a better diet than non-users [31,32,61–63], therefore improvements in nutritional status may be the result of a more nutritious diet rather than DS use. We considered DS use within the context of dietary adequacy/sufficiency and found that a small proportion of participants consuming a diet that met the EAR or RDA still were at risk of deficiency. DS use was associated with a lower risk of deficiency even in well-nourished individuals. FSMV users have a lower risk of deficiency than other DS users, therefore it appears that the type of DS used is important. Individuals who take DS containing a wide range of micronutrients have a lower risk of deficiency, irrespective of the adequacy of their diet.

The strengths of our analysis are that the NHANES dataset is large and well-defined, and therefore can provide a robust cross-sectional analysis of the nutrient status of the U.S. population. Our analysis provides insights into nutrient status across a life cycle, including children, adolescents, and pregnant or breastfeeding women. These population groups are nutritionally vulnerable due to higher demands, and data on their nutritional status and needs should be a priority. We attempted to consider the biochemical markers of nutrient status together with measures of dietary sufficiency.

Nevertheless, our research has some limitations. For pregnant and breastfeeding women, in particular, the sample size is small and may not be nationally representative. The biochemical markers were assessed at a single time point, dietary intakes were based on two 24 h dietary recalls conducted in the period around the time of blood collection, and supplement use was measured over the 30 days prior to the dietary interview. There are uncertainties in using a single biochemical measurement to determine micronutrient status, which should ideally be diagnosed after a physical examination, and a dietary history can be taken to place the laboratory results in perspective. When the "index of individuality"—a measure of the variability of individuals' biochemical measures compared to the population reference interval—is low (<0.6), as it is for folate and vitamins A, B12, and E, our approach is limited to assessing current nutrient status in individuals since it would not be robust enough to detect changes of disease status [64]. Similar analyses of biological variation are lacking for vitamins D, C, and B6.

The biomarkers of nutrient status are affected by inflammation, and this may have affected our results. In the survey years that we analyzed, the vitamins and minerals significantly affected by inflammation (defined as elevated C-reactive protein ≥ 5 mg/L) were serum and red blood cell (RBC) folate, PLP, and vitamins C, D, and E [16]. Depending on the sub-groups' level of inflammation, and the effect of inflammation on each biomarker, the deficiency prevalence in certain sub-groups could be affected [65]. For example, serum PLP is strongly depressed when C-reactive protein is elevated, which could mean that the risk of deficiency is lower than estimated in sub-groups more affected by inflammation, such as women, current smokers, or non-Hispanic Blacks [16,65]. Nevertheless, the application of standard cut-off points provides a snapshot of the prevalence of micronutrient deficiencies among individuals in a nationally representative survey, and represents standard clinical practice in identifying micronutrient deficiencies.

FSMV were defined by the number of vitamins and minerals contained within each product, and not their vitamin or mineral content. It is therefore possible that some FSMV products do not contain all of the vitamins and/or minerals for which biochemical status was assessed. Moreover, supplements may not have been used daily. Even so, as they contained at least 12 vitamins, it is unlikely that there are DS within the FSMV category that do not contain all the vitamins for which biochemical data were available. We limited the number of minerals in the supplement to avoid including unusual formulations containing rare earth metals, and it is possible that some FMSV formulations did not contain iron.

Biochemical deficiency did not correlate well with the dietary intake data for each vitamin. This discrepancy may reflect recall bias known to be a problem with dietary intake methodologies [66]. A further issue relates to the use of a limited number of dietary recall days to assess usual intakes, because they are influenced by the day-to-day variation of the diet and will not accurately reflect long-term usual intakes [5]. Differences seen may also reflect changes in the distribution of nutrient intakes related to biochemical status. This could be related to macro-level shifts in micronutrient sources in a diet, or inherent difficulties in applying the results of small-scale micronutrient depletion–repletion studies used to establish DRIs to heterogeneous populations. Nevertheless, biochemical deficiency rates increased as dietary inadequacy/insufficiency increased, an association that was also consistent in sub-group analyses, lending weight to our findings.

Deficiencies and dietary inadequacies in vitamins and minerals have been found in other well-nourished populations. For example, a low riboflavin status was found in 57% of young UK women [67], intakes were below the estimated average requirement for thiamine (26%), zinc (39%), vitamins B6 (25%), and vitamin B12 (27%) in young Canadian women with mood disorders [68], 17% of New Zealand women in Dunedin had a zinc status indicative of mild deficiency [69], and magnesium status in 18% of Canadian women of South-Asian background was low [70]. Regarding international surveys, intakes of iodine, magnesium, iron, and vitamin D were considered to be a concern in a review of several European countries [71], and over 30% of community-dwelling older adults had intakes of vitamin D, thiamin, riboflavin, calcium, magnesium, and selenium lower than the EAR [72]. Our estimate that nearly one third of U.S. adults is at risk of deficiency in at least one vitamin or has anemia is conservative and does not reflect the full scale of micronutrient deficiencies, as the number of micronutrients analyzed was limited to those with biochemical measures.

Despite evidence that micronutrient intake from the diet is generally higher in those using DS [29,62,63], 14% of FSMV users and 28% of DS users were at risk of deficiency in at least one vitamin or had anemia. Even when FSMV users were consuming a diet that met the EAR or RDA, 4.8% and 0.9% respectively were deficient in at least one vitamin or had anemia. We did not have access to vitamin D intake data; in fact, the dietary contribution of this micronutrient to nutrient status is difficult to determine as cutaneous synthesis is able to provide adequate vitamin D. Due to the way that we selected the FSMV, it is possible that some products do not meet the RDA for all of the vitamins and minerals, and this means that dietary gaps still exist despite FSMV use. The form of vitamin or mineral also affects absorption, which is not always taken into account when DS are being formulated. Nutrient–nutrient interactions can also mean that biochemical deficiency results from the low intake of a nutrient not captured by the NHANES dataset. For example, biochemical riboflavin status, which was not measured within NHANES 2003–2006, can affect iron homeostasis and anemia prevalence [67].

The most common deficiency was vitamin B6. The main symptoms of frank vitamin B6 deficiency include microcytic anemia, convulsions, depression, and confusion [7]. Marginal deficiency is associated with cardiovascular disease, and an elevated risk of Alzheimer's disease [73]. There is a clear, positive correlation between vitamin B6 intake and status [49]. We assume that increasing vitamin B6 intake, particularly for women aged 19–50 years, could reduce the risk of deficiency. There are few studies investigating how to improve the intake of vitamin B6, which is found in all food groups but has few excellent sources, however it seems that increasing the consumption of high-fiber cereals has been able to increase vitamin B6 status [74,75]. Increasing the consumption of organ meats, potatoes and other starchy vegetables, non-citrus fruits, fish, and poultry may also improve vitamin B6 intake and lower the risk of deficiency [5]. Attention to anemia and one of its major causes, poor iron intakes, in adult women, and to anemia and vitamin B12 status in the elderly, could make a significant impact on overall biochemical deficiency rates in the U.S. population. The relatively high rate of vitamin C deficiency found in adult men is most likely related to poor fruit and vegetable intakes [4]. There appear to be gender-based differences in motivators for fruit and vegetable consumption [76–78]. Knowledge of barriers to fruit and vegetable consumption in men, which seem to be related to a lack of interest in a healthy lifestyle and difficulties in food preparation, could be used to design interventions targeting vitamin C intakes and status. Increasing fruit and vegetable consumption may also improve the status of other micronutrients, such as vitamins A and B6 [79]. More consideration should be paid to the risk of vitamin D deficiency in minority populations [80]. Educational interventions to increase vitamin D status may be only marginally effective; food fortification may be more appropriate [81,82]. Our analysis implies that the use of DS, particularly FSMV, is associated with a reduced risk of biochemical deficiency. The low cost of FSMV, typically a few cents per day for generic brands (survey conducted on 6 June 2017 at a major online retailer and a large U.S.-based pharmacy chain, assuming a 200-count adult FSMV), make them an attractive prospect to ensure dietary adequacy.

However, our results are derived from observational research, therefore it is prudent to consume nutritionally-dense foods.

Our finding that nearly one third of the U.S. population is at risk of vitamin deficiency or anemia is a concern, especially since our estimates are likely conservative and do not capture deficiency in all of the essential micronutrients. Yet, the public health significance of this finding is uncertain given that there is no guidance from national or international health organizations regarding acceptable levels of multiple, concurrent deficiencies in populations or their health significance. The identification of risk groups for deficiency such as adult women, non-Hispanic Blacks, and people of lower socio-economic status can help clinicians, dietitians, and public health professionals involved in nutrition interventions to identify deficiencies and tailor nutrition screening and prevention programs to be most effective.

5. Conclusions

The risk of vitamin deficiency or anemia is common in the U.S., and vulnerable groups include women, particularly those of child-bearing age, non-Hispanic Blacks, people of low socio-economic status, underweight and obese individuals, and individuals with poor diets. Adequate dietary intakes and the use of DS, particularly FSMV, are associated with a lower risk of deficiency. Nutrition intervention programs should use an approach targeted at vulnerable groups to reduce the overall burden of poor micronutrient status.

Supplementary Materials: The following are available online at http://www.mdpi.com/2072-6643/9/7/655/s1, Table S1: Proportion of population with Usual Intakes below the EAR, RDA and above the TUL for 6 vitamins and iron in the U.S. population >9 y, from NHANES 2003–2006, Table S2: Dietary inadequacy score in the U.S. population aged ≥9 y, based on NHANES 2003–2006, Table S3: Total counts of vitamins and minerals in dietary supplement products used in NHANES 2003–2006, Table S4: Demographic characteristics in the U.S. population aged ≥9 y from NHANES, 2003–2006, Table S5: Biochemical markers of nutrient status in the U.S. population, aged ≥9 y from NHANES, 2003–2006, Table S6: Risk of deficiency and length of time taking dietary supplements, Table S7: Risk of deficiency and frequency taking dietary supplements over previous 30 days.

Acknowledgments: DSM Nutritional Products supported all authors during the development of the analysis plan, and J.B., E.C. and M.M. were employed by DSM Nutritional Products during data analysis and manuscript writing.

Author Contributions: J.B., R.M., E.C. and M.M. conceived and designed the analysis plan; J.B. analyzed the data; J.B., R.M., E.C. and M.M. wrote the paper.

Conflicts of Interest: At the time that the research plan was conceived and initial data analyses were conducted, all authors were employees of DSM Nutritional Products, a global producer and supplier of vitamins, carotenoids, omega-3 long chain fatty acids and other ingredients to the feed, food, pharmaceutical and personal care industries.

References

1. McGuire, S. Scientific Report of the 2015 Dietary Guidelines Advisory Committee. Washington, DC: US Departments of Agriculture and Health and Human Services, 2015. *Adv. Nutr.* **2016**, *7*, 202–204. [CrossRef] [PubMed]

2. Pfeiffer, C.M.; Sternberg, M.R.; Schleicher, R.L.; Haynes, B.M.; Rybak, M.E.; Pirkle, J.L. The CDC's Second National Report on Biochemical Indicators of Diet and Nutrition in the U.S. Population is a valuable tool for researchers and policy makers. *J. Nutr.* **2013**, *143*, 938S–947S. [CrossRef] [PubMed]

3. Tanumihardjo, S. Biomarkers of vitamin A status: What do they mean. In *Report: Priorities in the Assessment of Vitamin A and Iron Status in Populations, Proceedings of the Priorities in the Assessment of Vitamin A and Iron Status in Populations, Panama City, Panama, 15–19 September 2010*; World Health Organisation: Geneva, Switzerland, 2012; Available online: http://www.who.int/nutrition/publications/micronutrients/background_paper2_report_assessment_vitAandIron_status.pdf (accessed on 22 June 2017).

4. Schleicher, R.L.; Carroll, M.D.; Ford, E.S.; Lacher, D.A. Serum vitamin C and the prevalence of vitamin C deficiency in the United States: 2003–2004 National Health and Nutrition Examination Survey (NHANES). *Am. J. Clin. Nutr.* **2009**, *90*, 1252–1263. [CrossRef] [PubMed]

5. Otten, J.J.; Hellwig, J.P.; Meyers, L.D. *Dietary Reference Intakes: The Essential Guide to Nutrient Requirements*; The National Academies Press: Washington, DC, USA, 2006.

6. Wacker, M.; Holick, M.F. Vitamin D—Effects on skeletal and extraskeletal health and the need for supplementation. *Nutrients* **2013**, *5*, 111–148. [CrossRef] [PubMed]
7. Institute of Medicine Standing Committee on the Scientific Evaluation of Dietary Reference Intakes. *Dietary Reference Intakes for Thiamin, Riboflavin, Niacin, Vitamin B6, Folate, Vitamin B12, Pantothenic Acid, Biotin, and Choline*; National Academies Press (US): Washington, DC, USA, 1998.
8. Lane, D.J.; Richardson, D.R. The active role of vitamin C in mammalian iron metabolism: Much more than just enhanced iron absorption! *Free Radic. Biol. Med.* **2014**, *75*, 69–83. [CrossRef] [PubMed]
9. Kelsay, J.L. A compendium of nutritional status studies and dietary evaluation studies conducted in the United States, 1957–1967. *J. Nutr.* **1969**, *99* (Suppl. 1), 119–166.
10. Yetley, E.; Johnson, C. Nutritional applications of the Health and Nutrition Examination Surveys (HANES). *Annu. Rev. Nutr.* **1987**, *7*, 441–463. [CrossRef] [PubMed]
11. Karakis, I.; Pase, M.P.; Beiser, A.; Booth, S.L.; Jacques, P.F.; Rogers, G.; DeCarli, C.; Vasan, R.S.; Wang, T.J.; Himali, J.J.; et al. Association of Serum Vitamin D with the Risk of Incident Dementia and Subclinical Indices of Brain Aging: The Framingham Heart Study. *J. Alzheimers Dis.* **2016**, *51*, 451–461. [CrossRef] [PubMed]
12. Kolonel, L.N.; Henderson, B.E.; Hankin, J.H.; Nomura, A.M.; Wilkens, L.R.; Pike, M.C.; Stram, D.O.; Monroe, K.R.; Earle, M.E.; Nagamine, F.S. A multiethnic cohort in Hawaii and Los Angeles: Baseline characteristics. *Am. J. Epidemiol.* **2000**, *151*, 346–357. [CrossRef] [PubMed]
13. Bertone-Johnson, E.R.; Powers, S.I.; Spangler, L.; Larson, J.; Michael, Y.L.; Millen, A.E.; Bueche, M.N.; Salmoirago-Blotcher, E.; Wassertheil-Smoller, S.; Brunner, R.L.; et al. Vitamin D supplementation and depression in the women's health initiative calcium and vitamin D trial. *Am. J. Epidemiol.* **2012**, *176*, 1–13. [CrossRef] [PubMed]
14. Wang, L.; Ma, J.; Manson, J.E.; Buring, J.E.; Gaziano, J.M.; Sesso, H.D. A prospective study of plasma vitamin D metabolites, vitamin D receptor gene polymorphisms, and risk of hypertension in men. *Eur. J. Nutr.* **2013**, *52*, 1771–1779. [CrossRef] [PubMed]
15. Centers for Disease Control and Prevention. *Second National Report on Biochemical Indicators of Diet and Nutrition in the U.S. Population*; National Center for Environmental Health: Atlanta, GA, USA, April 2012. Available online: http://www.cdc.gov/nutritionreport/pdf/Nutrition_Book_complete508_final.pdf (accessed on 22 June 2017).
16. Haynes, B.M.; Pfeiffer, C.M.; Sternberg, M.R.; Schleicher, R.L. Selected physiologic variables are weakly to moderately associated with 29 biomarkers of diet and nutrition, NHANES 2003–2006. *J. Nutr.* **2013**, *143*, 1001S–1010S. [CrossRef] [PubMed]
17. Pfeiffer, C.M.; Sternberg, M.R.; Caldwell, K.L.; Pan, Y. Race-ethnicity is related to biomarkers of iron and iodine status after adjusting for sociodemographic and lifestyle variables in NHANES 2003–2006. *J. Nutr.* **2013**, *143*, 977S–985S. [CrossRef] [PubMed]
18. Pfeiffer, C.M.; Sternberg, M.R.; Schleicher, R.L.; Rybak, M.E. Dietary supplement use and smoking are important correlates of biomarkers of water-soluble vitamin status after adjusting for sociodemographic and lifestyle variables in a representative sample of U.S. adults. *J. Nutr.* **2013**, *143*, 957S–965S. [CrossRef] [PubMed]
19. Schleicher, R.L.; Sternberg, M.R.; Pfeiffer, C.M. Race-ethnicity is a strong correlate of circulating fat-soluble nutrient concentrations in a representative sample of the U.S. population. *J. Nutr.* **2013**, *143*, 966S–976S. [CrossRef] [PubMed]
20. Sternberg, M.R.; Schleicher, R.L.; Pfeiffer, C.M. Regression modeling plan for 29 biochemical indicators of diet and nutrition measured in NHANES 2003–2006. *J. Nutr.* **2013**, *143*, 948S–956S. [CrossRef] [PubMed]
21. Anderson, V.P.; Jack, S.; Monchy, D.; Hem, N.; Hok, P.; Bailey, K.B.; Gibson, R.S. Co-existing micronutrient deficiencies among stunted Cambodian infants and toddlers. *Asia Pac. J. Clin. Nutr.* **2008**, *17*, 72–79. [PubMed]
22. Hashizume, M.; Chiba, M.; Shinohara, A.; Iwabuchi, S.; Sasaki, S.; Shimoda, T.; Kunii, O.; Caypil, W.; Dauletbaev, D.; Alnazarova, A. Anaemia, iron deficiency and vitamin A status among school-aged children in rural Kazakhstan. *Public Health Nutr.* **2005**, *8*, 564–571. [CrossRef] [PubMed]
23. Oliveira, C.S.; Sampaio, P.; Muniz, P.T.; Cardoso, M.A. Multiple micronutrients in powder delivered through primary health care reduce iron and vitamin A deficiencies in young Amazonian children. *Public Health Nutr.* **2016**, *19*, 1–9. [CrossRef] [PubMed]

24. Van Nhien, N.; Khan, N.C.; Ninh, N.X.; Van Huan, P.; Hop le, T.; Lam, N.T.; Ota, F.; Yabutani, T.; Hoa, V.Q.; Motonaka, J.; et al. Micronutrient deficiencies and anemia among preschool children in rural Vietnam. *Asia Pac. J. Clin. Nutr.* **2008**, *17*, 48–55. [PubMed]

25. Bailey, R.L.; Gahche, J.J.; Miller, P.E.; Thomas, P.R.; Dwyer, J.T. Why US adults use dietary supplements. *JAMA Intern. Med.* **2013**, *173*, 355–361. [CrossRef] [PubMed]

26. Bailey, R.L.; Gahche, J.J.; Thomas, P.R.; Dwyer, J.T. Why US children use dietary supplements. *Pediatr. Res.* **2013**, *74*, 737–741. [CrossRef] [PubMed]

27. Rock, C.L. Multivitamin-multimineral supplements: Who uses them? *Am. J. Clin. Nutr.* **2007**, *85*, 277S–279S. [PubMed]

28. Bailey, R.L.; Fulgoni, V.L., 3rd; Keast, D.R.; Dwyer, J.T. Examination of vitamin intakes among US adults by dietary supplement use. *J. Acad. Nutr. Diet.* **2012**, *112*, 657–663. [CrossRef] [PubMed]

29. Fulgoni, V.L., 3rd; Keast, D.R.; Bailey, R.L.; Dwyer, J. Foods, fortificants, and supplements: Where do Americans get their nutrients? *J. Nutr.* **2011**, *141*, 1847–1854. [CrossRef] [PubMed]

30. Park, S.Y.; Murphy, S.P.; Martin, C.L.; Kolonel, L.N. Nutrient intake from multivitamin/mineral supplements is similar among users from five ethnic groups: The Multiethnic Cohort Study. *J. Am. Diet. Assoc.* **2008**, *108*, 529–533. [CrossRef] [PubMed]

31. Stang, J.; Story, M.T.; Harnack, L.; Neumark-Sztainer, D. Relationships between vitamin and mineral supplement use, dietary intake, and dietary adequacy among adolescents. *J. Am. Diet. Assoc.* **2000**, *100*, 905–910. [CrossRef]

32. Dickinson, A.; MacKay, D. Health habits and other characteristics of dietary supplement users: A review. *Nutr. J.* **2014**, *13*, 14. [CrossRef] [PubMed]

33. Stewart, P.A.; Hyman, S.L.; Schmidt, B.L.; Macklin, E.A.; Reynolds, A.; Johnson, C.R.; James, S.J.; Manning-Courtney, P. Dietary Supplementation in Children with Autism Spectrum Disorders: Common, Insufficient, and Excessive. *J. Acad. Nutr. Diet.* **2015**, *115*, 1237–1248. [CrossRef] [PubMed]

34. The Age-Related Eye Disease Study (AREDS): Design implications. AREDS report no. 1. *Control Clin. Trials* **1999**, *20*, 573–600.

35. Chew, E.Y.; Clemons, T.; SanGiovanni, J.P.; Danis, R.; Domalpally, A.; McBee, W.; Sperduto, R.; Ferris, F.L. The Age-Related Eye Disease Study 2 (AREDS2): Study design and baseline characteristics (AREDS2 report number 1). *Ophthalmology* **2012**, *119*, 2282–2289. [CrossRef] [PubMed]

36. Gaziano, J.M.; Sesso, H.D.; Christen, W.G.; Bubes, V.; Smith, J.P.; MacFadyen, J.; Schvartz, M.; Manson, J.E.; Glynn, R.J.; Buring, J.E. Multivitamins in the prevention of cancer in men: The Physicians' Health Study II randomized controlled trial. *JAMA* **2012**, *308*, 1871–1880. [CrossRef] [PubMed]

37. Zipf, G.; Chiappa, M.; Porter, K.S.; Ostchega, Y.; Lewis, B.G.; Dostal, J. National health and nutrition examination survey: Plan and operations, 1999–2010. *Vital Health Stat. 1* **2013**, 1–37.

38. National Center for Health Statistics. About the National Health and Nutrition Examination Survey. Available online: http://www.cdc.gov/nchs/nhanes/about_nhanes.htm (accessed on 21 April 2015).

39. Centers for Disease Control and Prevention. 2005–2006 Data Documentation, Codebook, and Frequencies. Vitamin B6 (VIT_B6_D). Analytic notes. Available online: http://www.cdc.gov/nchs/nhanes/nhanes2005-2006/VIT_B6_D.htm#Analytic_Notes (accessed on 10 February 2016).

40. World Health Organization. *Iron Deficiency Anaemia. Assessment, Prevention, and Control. A Guide for Programme Managers*; WHO/NHD/01.3; WHO: Geneva, Switzerland, 2001; Available online: http://whqlibdoc.who.int/hq/2001/WHO_NHD_01.3.pdf (accessed on 22 June 2017).

41. Short, M.W.; Domagalski, J.E. Iron deficiency anemia: Evaluation and management. *Am. Fam. Physician* **2013**, *87*, 98–104. [PubMed]

42. Dallal, G.E. Identifying Similar Groups. Available online: http://www.jerrydallal.com/lhsp/similar_prog.htm (accessed on 29 January 2016).

43. Johnson, C.; Paulose-Ram, R.; Ogden, C.; Carroll, M.; Kruszon-Moran, D.; Dohrmann, S.; Curtin, L. National Health and Nutrition Examination Survey: Analytic guidelines, 1999–2010. *Vital Health Stat.* **2013**, *161*, 1–24.

44. Bailey, R.L.; Carmel, R.; Green, R.; Pfeiffer, C.M.; Cogswell, M.E.; Osterloh, J.D.; Sempos, C.T.; Yetley, E.A. Monitoring of vitamin B-12 nutritional status in the United States by using plasma methylmalonic acid and serum vitamin B-12. *Am. J. Clin. Nutr.* **2011**, *94*, 552–561. [CrossRef] [PubMed]

45. Branum, A.M.; Bailey, R.; Singer, B.J. Dietary supplement use and folate status during pregnancy in the United States. *J. Nutr.* **2013**, *143*, 486–492. [CrossRef] [PubMed]

46. Kant, A.K.; Graubard, B.I. Race-ethnic, family income, and education differentials in nutritional and lipid biomarkers in US children and adolescents: NHANES 2003–2006. *Am. J. Clin. Nutr.* **2012**, *96*, 601–612. [CrossRef] [PubMed]

47. Pfeiffer, C.M.; Hughes, J.P.; Lacher, D.A.; Bailey, R.L.; Berry, R.J.; Zhang, M.; Yetley, E.A.; Rader, J.I.; Sempos, C.T.; Johnson, C.L. Estimation of trends in serum and RBC folate in the U.S. population from pre–to postfortification using assay-adjusted data from the NHANES 1988–2010. *J. Nutr.* **2012**, *142*, 886–893. [CrossRef] [PubMed]

48. Yang, Q.; Cogswell, M.E.; Hamner, H.C.; Carriquiry, A.; Bailey, L.B.; Pfeiffer, C.M.; Berry, R.J. Folic acid source, usual intake, and folate and vitamin B-12 status in US adults: National Health and Nutrition Examination Survey (NHANES) 2003–2006. *Am. J. Clin. Nutr.* **2010**, *91*, 64–72. [CrossRef] [PubMed]

49. Morris, M.S.; Picciano, M.F.; Jacques, P.F.; Selhub, J. Plasma pyridoxal 5'-phosphate in the US population: The National Health and Nutrition Examination Survey, 2003–2004. *Am. J. Clin. Nutr.* **2008**, *87*, 1446–1454. [PubMed]

50. Cogswell, M.E.; Looker, A.C.; Pfeiffer, C.M.; Cook, J.D.; Lacher, D.A.; Beard, J.L.; Lynch, S.R.; Grummer-Strawn, L.M. Assessment of iron deficiency in US preschool children and nonpregnant females of childbearing age: National Health and Nutrition Examination Survey 2003–2006. *Am. J. Clin. Nutr.* **2009**, *89*, 1334–1342. [CrossRef] [PubMed]

51. Hanson, C.; Lyden, E.; Abresch, C.; Anderson-Berry, A. Serum Retinol Concentrations, Race, and Socioeconomic Status in of Women of Childbearing Age in the United States. *Nutrients* **2016**, *8*, 508. [CrossRef] [PubMed]

52. Rai, D.; Bird, J.K.; McBurney, M.I.; Chapman-Novakofski, K.M. Nutritional status as assessed by nutrient intakes and biomarkers among women of childbearing age—Is the burden of nutrient inadequacies growing in America? *Public Health Nutr.* **2014**, *18*, 1–12. [CrossRef] [PubMed]

53. Bodnar, L.M.; Simhan, H.N.; Powers, R.W.; Frank, M.P.; Cooperstein, E.; Roberts, J.M. High prevalence of vitamin D insufficiency in black and white pregnant women residing in the northern United States and their neonates. *J. Nutr.* **2007**, *137*, 447–452. [PubMed]

54. Mathews, F.; Youngman, L.; Neil, A. Maternal circulating nutrient concentrations in pregnancy: Implications for birth and placental weights of term infants. *Am. J. Clin. Nutr.* **2004**, *79*, 103–110. [PubMed]

55. Gibbs, B.G.; Forste, R. Socioeconomic status, infant feeding practices and early childhood obesity. *Pediatr. Obes.* **2014**, *9*, 135–146. [CrossRef] [PubMed]

56. O'Neil, C.E.; Nicklas, T.A.; Keast, D.R.; Fulgoni, V.L. Ethnic disparities among food sources of energy and nutrients of public health concern and nutrients to limit in adults in the United States: NHANES 2003–2006. *Food Nutr. Res.* **2014**, *58*, 15784. [CrossRef] [PubMed]

57. Kirkpatrick, S.I.; Dodd, K.W.; Reedy, J.; Krebs-Smith, S.M. Income and race/ethnicity are associated with adherence to food-based dietary guidance among US adults and children. *J. Acad. Nutr. Diet.* **2012**, *112*, 624.e6–635.e6. [CrossRef] [PubMed]

58. Aggarwal, A.; Monsivais, P.; Cook, A.J.; Drewnowski, A. Positive attitude toward healthy eating predicts higher diet quality at all cost levels of supermarkets. *J. Acad. Nutr. Diet.* **2014**, *114*, 266–272. [CrossRef] [PubMed]

59. Valdes, S.T.; Tostes, M.D.; Anunciacao, P.C.; da Silva, B.P.; Sant'Ana, H.M. Association between Vitamin Deficiency and Metabolic Disorders Related to Obesity. *Crit. Rev. Food Sci. Nutr.* **2016**, *57*, 3332–3343. [CrossRef] [PubMed]

60. Harris, E.; Macpherson, H.; Pipingas, A. Improved blood biomarkers but no cognitive effects from 16 weeks of multivitamin supplementation in healthy older adults. *Nutrients* **2015**, *7*, 3796–3812. [CrossRef] [PubMed]

61. Kofoed, C.L.; Christensen, J.; Dragsted, L.O.; Tjonneland, A.; Roswall, N. Determinants of dietary supplement use—Healthy individuals use dietary supplements. *Br. J. Nutr.* **2015**, *113*, 1993–2000. [CrossRef] [PubMed]

62. Murphy, S.P.; White, K.K.; Park, S.Y.; Sharma, S. Multivitamin-multimineral supplements' effect on total nutrient intake. *Am. J. Clin. Nutr.* **2007**, *85*, 280S–284S. [PubMed]

63. Sebastian, R.S.; Cleveland, L.E.; Goldman, J.D.; Moshfegh, A.J. Older adults who use vitamin/mineral supplements differ from nonusers in nutrient intake adequacy and dietary attitudes. *J. Am. Diet. Assoc.* **2007**, *107*, 1322–1332. [CrossRef] [PubMed]

64. Lacher, D.A.; Hughes, J.P.; Carroll, M.D. Estimate of biological variation of laboratory analytes based on the third national health and nutrition examination survey. *Clin. Chem.* **2005**, *51*, 450–452. [CrossRef] [PubMed]

65. Ong, K.L.; Allison, M.A.; Cheung, B.M.; Wu, B.J.; Barter, P.J.; Rye, K.A. Trends in C-reactive protein levels in US adults from 1999 to 2010. *Am. J. Epidemiol.* **2013**, *177*, 1430–1442. [CrossRef] [PubMed]

66. Dhurandhar, N.V.; Schoeller, D.; Brown, A.W.; Heymsfield, S.B.; Thomas, D.; Sorensen, T.I.A.; Speakman, J.R.; Jeansonne, M.; Allison, D.B.; Energy Balance Measurement Working Group. Energy balance measurement: When something is not better than nothing. *Int. J. Obes. (Lond.)* **2015**, *39*, 1109–1113. [CrossRef] [PubMed]

67. Powers, H.J.; Hill, M.H.; Mushtaq, S.; Dainty, J.R.; Majsak-Newman, G.; Williams, E.A. Correcting a marginal riboflavin deficiency improves hematologic status in young women in the United Kingdom (RIBOFEM). *Am. J. Clin. Nutr.* **2011**, *93*, 1274–1284. [CrossRef] [PubMed]

68. Davison, K.M.; Kaplan, B.J. Vitamin and mineral intakes in adults with mood disorders: Comparisons to nutrition standards and associations with sociodemographic and clinical variables. *J. Am. Coll. Nutr.* **2011**, *30*, 547–558. [CrossRef] [PubMed]

69. Gibson, R.S.; Heath, A.L.; Limbaga, M.L.; Prosser, N.; Skeaff, C.M. Are changes in food consumption patterns associated with lower biochemical zinc status among women from Dunedin, New Zealand? *Br. J. Nutr.* **2001**, *86*, 71–80. [CrossRef] [PubMed]

70. Bertinato, J.; Wu Xiao, C.; Ratnayake, W.M.; Fernandez, L.; Lavergne, C.; Wood, C.; Swist, E. Lower serum magnesium concentration is associated with diabetes, insulin resistance, and obesity in South Asian and white Canadian women but not men. *Food Nutr. Res.* **2015**, *59*, 25974. [CrossRef] [PubMed]

71. Mensink, G.B.; Fletcher, R.; Gurinovic, M.; Huybrechts, I.; Lafay, L.; Serra-Majem, L.; Szponar, L.; Tetens, I.; Verkaik-Kloosterman, J.; Baka, A.; et al. Mapping low intake of micronutrients across Europe. *Br. J. Nutr.* **2013**, *110*, 755–773. [CrossRef] [PubMed]

72. ter Borg, S.; Verlaan, S.; Hemsworth, J.; Mijnarends, D.M.; Schols, J.M.; Luiking, Y.C.; de Groot, L.C. Micronutrient intakes and potential inadequacies of community-dwelling older adults: A systematic review. *Br. J. Nutr.* **2015**, *113*, 1195–1206. [CrossRef] [PubMed]

73. Lamers, Y.; O'Rourke, B.; Gilbert, L.R.; Keeling, C.; Matthews, D.E.; Stacpoole, P.W.; Gregory, J.F., 3rd. Vitamin B-6 restriction tends to reduce the red blood cell glutathione synthesis rate without affecting red blood cell or plasma glutathione concentrations in healthy men and women. *Am. J. Clin. Nutr.* **2009**, *90*, 336–343. [CrossRef] [PubMed]

74. Melanson, K.J.; Angelopoulos, T.J.; Nguyen, V.T.; Martini, M.; Zukley, L.; Lowndes, J.; Dube, T.J.; Fiutem, J.J.; Yount, B.W.; Rippe, J.M. Consumption of whole-grain cereals during weight loss: Effects on dietary quality, dietary fiber, magnesium, vitamin B-6, and obesity. *J. Am. Diet. Assoc.* **2006**, *106*, 1380–1388. [CrossRef] [PubMed]

75. Rodriguez-Rodriguez, E.; Lopez-Sobaler, A.M.; Navarro, A.R.; Bermejo, L.M.; Ortega, R.M.; Andres, P. Vitamin B6 status improves in overweight/obese women following a hypocaloric diet rich in breakfast cereals, and may help in maintaining fat-free mass. *Int. J. Obes. (Lond.)* **2008**, *32*, 1552–1558. [CrossRef] [PubMed]

76. Baker, A.H.; Wardle, J. Sex differences in fruit and vegetable intake in older adults. *Appetite* **2003**, *40*, 269–275. [CrossRef]

77. Naughton, P.; McCarthy, S.N.; McCarthy, M.B. The creation of a healthy eating motivation score and its association with food choice and physical activity in a cross sectional sample of Irish adults. *Int. J. Behav. Nutr. Phys. Act.* **2015**, *12*, 74. [CrossRef] [PubMed]

78. O'Hara, B.J.; Phongsavan, P.; Venugopal, K.; Bauman, A.E. Characteristics of participants in Australia's Get Healthy telephone-based lifestyle information and coaching service: Reaching disadvantaged communities and those most at need. *Health Educ. Res.* **2011**, *26*, 1097–1106. [CrossRef] [PubMed]

79. Polidori, M.C.; Carrillo, J.C.; Verde, P.E.; Sies, H.; Siegrist, J.; Stahl, W. Plasma micronutrient status is improved after a 3-month dietary intervention with 5 daily portions of fruits and vegetables: Implications for optimal antioxidant levels. *Nutr. J.* **2009**, *8*, 10. [CrossRef] [PubMed]

80. Taksler, G.B.; Cutler, D.M.; Giovannucci, E.; Keating, N.L. Vitamin D deficiency in minority populations. *Public Health Nutr.* **2015**, *18*, 379–391. [CrossRef] [PubMed]

Nutrients **2017**, *9*, 655

81. Ethgen, O.; Hiligsmann, M.; Burlet, N.; Reginster, J.Y. Public health impact and cost-effectiveness of dairy products supplemented with vitamin D in prevention of osteoporotic fractures. *Arch. Public Health* **2015**, *73*, 48. [CrossRef] [PubMed]

82. Fuleihan Gel, H.; Bouillon, R.; Clarke, B.; Chakhtoura, M.; Cooper, C.; McClung, M.; Singh, R.J. Serum 25-Hydroxyvitamin D Levels: Variability, Knowledge Gaps, and the Concept of a Desirable Range. *J. Bone Miner. Res.* **2015**, *30*, 1119–1133. [CrossRef] [PubMed]

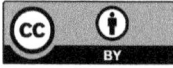

nutrients

Discussion

Considerations for Secondary Prevention of Nutritional Deficiencies in High-Risk Groups in High-Income Countries

Maaike J. Bruins *, Julia K. Bird, Claude P. Aebischer and Manfred Eggersdorfer

DSM Nutritional Products, Wurmisweg 576, Kaiseraugst CH-4303, Switzerland; julia.bird@DSM.com (J.K.B.); claude-p.aebischer@DSM.com (C.P.A.); manfred.eggersdorfer@DSM.com (M.E.)
* Correspondence: maaike.bruins@DSM.com; Tel.: +41-61815-8761

Received: 6 September 2017; Accepted: 28 December 2017; Published: 5 January 2018

Abstract: Surveys in high-income countries show that inadequacies and deficiencies can be common for some nutrients, particularly in vulnerable subgroups of the population. Inadequate intakes, high requirements for rapid growth and development, or age- or disease-related impairments in nutrient intake, digestion, absorption, or increased nutrient losses can lead to micronutrient deficiencies. The consequent subclinical conditions are difficult to recognize if not screened for and often go unnoticed. Nutrient deficiencies can be persistent despite primary nutrition interventions that are aimed at improving dietary intakes. Secondary prevention that targets groups at high risk of inadequacy or deficiency, such as in the primary care setting, can be a useful complementary approach to address persistent nutritional gaps. However, this strategy is often underestimated and overlooked as potentially cost-effective means to prevent future health care costs and to improve the health and quality of life of individuals. In this paper, the authors discuss key appraisal criteria to consider when evaluating the benefits and disadvantages of a secondary prevention of nutrient deficiencies through screening.

Keywords: nutrient inadequacies and deficiencies; nutritional supplements; biomarkers; nutrition screening; public health; cost-effectiveness

---

1. Introduction

Primary prevention in the nutrition setting aims to control risk factors in the general population, such as the dissemination of dietary recommendations to improve nutritional knowledge and enable behavior change [1]. There is a widespread use of primary public health strategies, such as the development and promotion of consumer-based dietary guidelines to improve overall dietary quality in many countries [2–4]. Despite this, survey data in high-income economies show a moderate burden of nutrient deficiencies and dietary inadequacies for several vitamins and minerals, both in vulnerable population groups and in the overall population [5–8]. A complementary secondary prevention strategy attempts to identify individuals with nutrient deficiencies, with a focus on high-risk population groups [1]. Secondary prevention detects individuals at risk of disease through screening and other forms of risk appraisal [1]. Secondary prevention should always complement existing programs that are aimed at improving public health along the continuum of disease risk from the well population to managed chronic disease [1].

The objective of this paper is to discuss key appraisal criteria to consider when evaluating the benefits and disadvantages of a secondary prevention of nutrient deficiencies through screening.

2. Nutrient Inadequacies and Deficiencies

There are a number of interacting factors that can contribute to marginal or low nutrient status, including poor dietary quantity or quality, increased requirements, increased metabolic losses, or impaired gastrointestinal digestion or absorption [9]. The long-term consumption of poor dietary quantity (e.g., due to loss of appetite) or quality (e.g., restrictive, unbalanced, or low-nutrient dense diets [10,11]) increase the risk of poor nutritional status, particularly in individuals with increased needs or losses. Meeting the daily nutrient requirements from the diet is particularly challenging at certain life cycle stages; during pregnancy and lactation [12], infancy and childhood [13], and adolescence [14], nutritional needs for rapid growth and development are significantly increased. In older age groups, many changes, including physical, physiological, and psychosocial factors make it more difficult for nutritional needs to be met, leading to shortfalls in nutrients [15]. In critically ill patients with injury or infectious disease, hypermetabolism is often seen, which is associated with losses and low status of nitrogen, vitamins, and minerals [16,17]. Other factors that contribute to the increased risk for nutritional deficiencies include impaired nutrient absorption capacity (e.g., in gastrointestinal disorders, such as inflammatory bowel disease or coeliac disease, or impaired vitamin B12 absorption in the elderly [18]), poor nutrient bioavailability (e.g., low absorption of iron and zinc from plant-based diets [19]), low bioconversion (e.g., low bioconversion of provitamin A carotenoids from plant-based diets into vitamin A [20]). Other factors that can increase the risk of specific nutrient deficiencies include for instance the use of some medication [21] or genetic polymorphisms [22].

The initial stages of marginal nutrient deficiency are often overlooked, as they may remain asymptomatic for a long time or present with generalized signs and symptoms that may not be recognized by the health care professional [23]. When unrecognized, subclinical symptoms can progress into more severe clinical deficiency states [24,25]. For example, vitamin B12 and folate deficiency can both present as megaloblastic anemia, symptoms of which include weakness and fatigue, neurological effects, such as numbness and tingling in the hands and feet, and poor memory. Vitamin B12 deficiency is a particular problem in older adults who are less able to absorb the vitamin, as well as vegetarians and vegans who consume little vitamin B12 from animal foods [25]. Low folate status in pregnant women is rated as a risk factor for neural tube defects in offspring and poor pregnancy outcomes [25], yet blood levels that are required to prevent neural tube defects are much higher than needed to prevent folate deficiency [26]. Iron deficiency anemia can lead to tiredness, weakness, a weakened immune system, and impaired memory [24,25]. Iron deficiency anemia is common in women with heavy menstrual bleeding, pregnant women, infants and young children, vegetarians and vegans, and people with gastrointestinal disorders. A low vitamin D status has little outward signs initially, but leads to bone pain, muscle weakness, and eventually increased fracture rates if left untreated [24,25]. Vitamin D deficiency is prevalent worldwide, and risk groups include older adults, postmenopausal women, people with dark skin, breastfed infants, and people with gastrointestinal malabsorption conditions [25].

3. Public Health Problem of Inadequate Intakes and Deficiencies of Nutrients

Surveys show that, even in high-income countries, nutrient intakes fail to meet requirements for many people, and overall nutrient status is too low for several essential nutrients [27]. Particularly in vulnerable population groups, specific nutrient inadequacies and deficiencies can present a public health issue [27]. Nutrient deficiencies not only have short-term implications for health and quality of life, but also, long-term consequences for intellectual development and economic productivity [28]. Nevertheless, relatively few efforts have been undertaken in high-income countries to estimate the potential public health benefits and cost savings of overcoming nutrient deficiencies of public health concern.

Population groups at particular risk of nutrient deficiencies include women of childbearing age, especially pregnant and lactating women [29–33], infants and toddlers [34,35], children [33,36], adolescents [31], older adults [33,34,37], obese individuals [38], and the critically ill [17]. Based on representative data from the National Health and Nutrition Examination Survey (NHANES), the US Office of Disease Prevention and Health Promotion classified vitamins A, C, D, E, and folate, calcium, and magnesium as "nutrients of concern" that may pose a substantial public health concern in the general US population [29]. The risk of single or multiple, concurrent micronutrient deficiencies in children and adults based on NHANES data was recently estimated at 31% [33]. We present a quantitative assessment of the burden of poor nutritional intake and status in Figures 1–5 to illustrate the risk of deficiency in a high-income country. Figures 1–4 show the proportion of inadequate nutrient intakes in the US population for macronutrients, water-soluble vitamins, fat-soluble vitamins, and minerals, respectively, as estimated using a Usual Intake distribution calculated according to the National Cancer Institute Method [39]. Figure 5 shows biochemical nutrient deficiencies in the US population, as calculated using the NHANES 2003–2006 dataset. The method and ethics approval are described in [33]. Briefly, the proportion individuals not meeting established cut-points for deficiency for the US population aged nine years or more was calculated, taking the complex sample design into account, and weighted to be representative. Figures 1–4 show that vitamins A, folate, B9, C, D, E, K, magnesium, calcium, potassium, fiber, and long chain omega-3 polyunsaturated fatty acids, are under-consumed compared to the Estimated Average Requirement (EAR). Figure 5 shows a prevalence of over 6% for anemia and vitamin B6, B12, C, and D deficiency, in several sub-population groups for each micronutrient.

	Protein		Fiber		18:3 PUFA	
	Male	Female	Male	Female	Male	Female
1-3 years	2%	2%	98%	98%	30%	31%
4-8 years	2%	2%	98%	98%	34%	33%
9-13 years	2%	2%	98%	98%	49%	38%
14-18 years	2%	2%	98%	98%	64%	43%
19-30 years	2%	2%	98%	98%	44%	31%
31-50 years	2%	2%	98%	94%	42%	31%
51-70 years	2%	5%	98%	83%	42%	25%
71+ years	2%	11%	98%	89%	70%	46%
Pregnant women				92%		45%

Figure 1. Proportion of inadequate macronutrient intakes by age, gender and life stage categories based on percentage of the US population with intakes below the Estimated Average Requirement (EAR) (protein) or adequate intake (fiber, 18:3 PUFA). From National Health and Nutrition Examination Survey (NHANES) 2007–2010). Inadequate intakes: black: >80%, red: 40–80%, yellow: 20–40%, and green: <20% below EAR or adequate intake.

	Thiamin		Riboflavin		Niacin		Vitamin B6		Folate		Vitamin B12		Vitamin C	
	Male	Female	Male	Female	Male	Female	Male	Female	Male	Female	Male	Female	Male	Female
1-3 years	2%	2%	2%	2%	2%	2%	2%	2%	2%	2%	2%	2%	2%	2%
4-8 years	2%	2%	2%	2%	2%	2%	2%	2%	2%	2%	2%	2%	2%	2%
9-13 years	2%	2%	2%	2%	2%	2%	2%	2%	2%	2%	2%	2%	2%	2%
14-18 years	2%	11%	2%	4%	2%	2%	2%	10%	6%	20%	2%	7%	39%	35%
19-30 years	3%	7%	3%	3%	2%	2%	2%	9%	2%	12%	2%	4%	42%	44%
31-50 years	2%	8%	2%	2%	2%	2%	2%	12%	4%	17%	2%	3%	46%	46%
51-70 years	2%	8%	2%	2%	2%	2%	11%	25%	6%	18%	2%	6%	47%	35%
71+ years	7%	13%	2%	4%	2%	8%	19%	33%	11%	25%	2%	8%	49%	42%
Pregnant women		4%		5%		2%		24%		29%		3%		29%

Figure 2. Proportion of inadequate intakes of water-soluble vitamins by age, gender and life stage categories based on percentage of the US population with intakes below the EAR. From NHANES 2007–2010). Inadequate intakes: black: >80%, red: 40–80%, yellow: 20–40%, and green: <20% below EAR.

Nutrients **2018**, 10, 47

	Vitamin A		Vitamin D		Vitamin E		Vitamin K	
	Male	Female	Male	Female	Male	Female	Male	Female
1-3 years	2%	2%	76%	78%	73%	83%	37%	35%
4-8 years	2%	3%	92%	97%	67%	68%	67%	75%
9-13 years	15%	24%	91%	98%	87%	93%	67%	66%
14-18 years	49%	53%	86%	98%	98%	98%	72%	81%
19-30 years	57%	53%	92%	98%	86%	98%	85%	71%
31-50 years	49%	45%	91%	98%	82%	94%	72%	62%
51-70 years	49%	37%	91%	97%	87%	91%	68%	47%
71+ years	42%	37%	93%	98%	90%	98%	81%	61%
Pregnant women		26%		90%		94%		46%

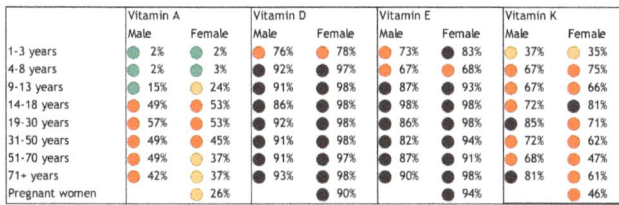

Figure 3. Proportion of inadequate intakes of fat-soluble vitamins by age, gender and life stage categories based on percentage of the US population with intakes below the EAR (vitamins A, D, and E) or adequate intake (vitamin K). From NHANES 2007–2010). Inadequate intakes: black: >80%, red: 40–80%, yellow: 20–40%, and green: <20% below EAR or adequate intake.

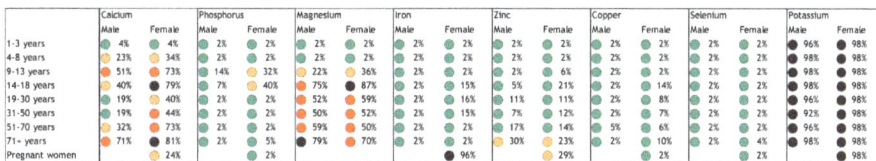

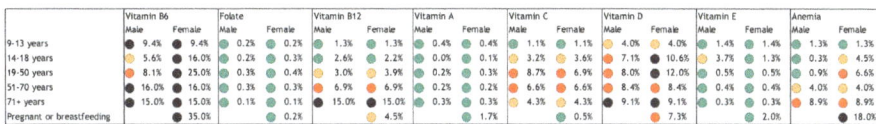

	Calcium		Phosphorus		Magnesium		Iron		Zinc		Copper		Selenium		Potassium	
	Male	Female	Male	Female	Male	Female	Male	Female	Male	Female	Male	Female	Male	Female	Male	Female
1-3 years	4%	4%	2%	2%	2%	2%	2%	2%	2%	2%	2%	2%	2%	2%	96%	98%
4-8 years	23%	34%	2%	2%	2%	2%	2%	2%	2%	2%	2%	2%	2%	2%	98%	98%
9-13 years	51%	73%	14%	32%	22%	36%	2%	2%	2%	6%	2%	2%	2%	2%	98%	98%
14-18 years	40%	79%	7%	40%	75%	87%	2%	15%	5%	21%	2%	14%	2%	2%	98%	98%
19-30 years	19%	40%	2%	2%	52%	59%	2%	16%	11%	11%	2%	8%	2%	2%	96%	98%
31-50 years	19%	44%	2%	2%	50%	52%	2%	15%	7%	12%	2%	7%	2%	2%	92%	98%
51-70 years	32%	73%	2%	2%	59%	50%	2%	2%	17%	14%	5%	6%	2%	2%	96%	98%
71+ years	71%	81%	2%	5%	79%	70%	2%	2%	30%	23%	2%	10%	2%	4%	98%	98%
Pregnant women		24%		2%				96%		29%		2%		2%		98%

Figure 4. Proportion of inadequate intakes of minerals by age, gender and life stage categories based on percentage of the US population with intakes below the EAR (calcium, phosphorus, magnesium, iron, zinc, copper, selenium) or adequate intake (potassium). From NHANES 2007–2010). Inadequate intakes: black: >80%, red: 40–80%, yellow: 20–40%, and green: <20% below EAR or adequate intake.

	Vitamin B6		Folate		Vitamin B12		Vitamin A		Vitamin C		Vitamin D		Vitamin E		Anemia	
	Male	Female	Male	Female	Male	Female	Male	Female	Male	Female	Male	Female	Male	Female	Male	Female
9-13 years	9.4%	9.4%	0.2%	0.2%	1.3%	1.3%	0.4%	0.4%	1.1%	1.1%	4.0%	4.0%	1.4%	1.4%	1.3%	1.3%
14-18 years	5.6%	16.0%	0.2%	0.3%	2.6%	2.2%	0.0%	0.1%	3.2%	3.6%	7.1%	10.6%	3.7%	1.3%	0.3%	4.5%
19-50 years	8.1%	25.0%	0.3%	0.4%	3.0%	3.9%	0.2%	0.3%	8.7%	6.9%	8.0%	12.0%	0.5%	0.5%	0.9%	6.6%
51-70 years	16.0%	16.0%	0.3%	0.3%	6.9%	6.9%	0.2%	0.2%	6.6%	6.6%	8.4%	8.4%	0.4%	0.4%	4.0%	4.0%
71+ years	15.0%	15.0%	0.1%	0.1%	15.0%	15.0%	0.3%	0.3%	4.3%	4.3%	9.1%	9.1%	0.3%	0.3%	8.9%	8.9%
Pregnant or breastfeeding		35.0%		0.2%		4.5%		1.7%		0.5%		7.3%		2.0%		18.0%

Figure 5. Risk of deficiency by age, gender and life stage categories for individual vitamins or anemia, based on percentage of the population aged >9 years with biomarkers below the deficiency cut-off values (vitamin B6, folate, B12, A, C, D, E, and anemia; pyridoxal 5'-phosphate <20 nmol/L; serum folate <2 ng/mL or red blood cell folate <95 ng/mL; vitamin B12 <200 pg/mL or methylmalonic acid >0.271 μmol/L; serum retinol <20 μg/dL; vitamin C <0.2 mg/dL; 25-hydroxyvitamin D <12 ng/mL; α-Tocopherol <500 μg/dL; mean corpuscular volume <95 fL, respectively). Deficient status: black: >9%, red: 6–9%, yellow: 3–6%, and green: <3% below the cut-off value for deficiency. Based on NHANES data 2003–2006.

In other high-income regions, surveys demonstrate that certain macronutrient, vitamin, and mineral deficiencies can be prevalent. For instance, in Arabian Gulf countries, despite year-long sunshine, vitamin D deficiency remains a critical health concern increasing from childhood through adolescence [40,41]. The spectrum of micronutrient deficiencies in Europe and Central Asia and their public health consequences have recently been published by the Food and Agriculture Organization of the United Nations (FAO) [42]. The data show that even in high-income countries like Germany, Austria, France, and UK, iron deficiency anemia (>10%) and zinc deficiency (>4%) are still highly prevalent, and the related disease burden in terms of Disability-Adjusted Life Years (DALYs) is substantial, responsible for 268 DALYs per 100,000 population in the whole Europe and Central Asia region. The recent Global Burden of Disease study demonstrates that unbalanced diets (both over- and under-consumption) contribute considerably to the global disease burden [42,43]. Lack of dietary fiber, seafood long-chain omega-3 polyunsaturated fatty acids, and calcium are among the leading food and nutrient risk factors contributing to the global burden of disease in high-income economies [43].

4. Common Approaches to Prevent Nutrient Inadequacies and Deficiencies

Policy makers are increasingly aware of the public burden and associated costs of under- and over-nutrition. This has resulted in various public health strategies to improve lifestyles and dietary choices, and prevent nutrient deficiencies considered of public health concern. Primary prevention measures taken to ensure more appropriate nutrient intakes in the population often include (1) education programs to encourage healthier and more nutritious food choices; (2) food-based approaches that increase the availability or affordability of nutrient-rich foods; and, (3) national policies to fortify commonly-eaten foods [44].

Encouraging appropriate intakes of healthy nutrient-rich and balanced diets is generally the preferred strategy for meeting nutrient needs, if possible. This can be effective in improving nutrient status, whilst improving overall dietary quality. A recent review of diets quality, demonstrated that increasing unhealthy patterns are outpacing increases in healthy patterns in most world regions particularly in high-income countries [45]. These findings emphasize the continued need for primary prevention strategies to address suboptimal diet quality, both by encouraging consumption of nutritious foods and discouraging consumption of unhealthy foods.

Nutrition surveys in high-income countries have identified that some of the shortfall nutrients continue to persist (see paragraph 3). To address the problem of persistent nutrient inadequacies and deficiencies, policy makers can consider a "secondary prevention strategy" complementary to a population-based primary prevention approach. Secondary prevention involves selecting population subgroups at risk of nutrient deficiencies, in order to administer additional nutritional support to those at greatest need, for example, dietetic services, dietary supplementation, or another approach. Secondary prevention programs, like the US Women's Special Supplemental Food Program for Women, Infants, and Children (WIC), which attempt to address nutrition-related problems in multiple subgroups of the population at risk using a multiple-service integrated food- or education-based approach can be more complex to implement [46]. Another more targeted secondary prevention approach seeks to prevent specific nutrient deficiencies in subgroups at high risk, through screening and targeted intervention at first point of contact with the health care professional.

In most high-income health care economies, health care expenditure is largely directed towards inpatient and outpatient care, and medical goods (mainly pharmaceuticals). For instance, in the US, only 6% is spent on public health and prevention services [47]. Despite evidence that preventive strategies in general practice, such as lifestyle interventions and screening for diabetes could have a large impact on population health, they remain underutilized in Australia [48]. The US Centers for Disease Control and Prevention (CDC) also emphasize that chronic disease conditions are often less expensive to treat when they are detected early and still preventable, recommending that the population should have access to affordable preventative services [49]. The CDC have developed a Diabetes Prevention Impact Toolkit to help employers, insurers, and health departments to calculate the costs and benefits of national diet and physical activity change programs [49]. For secondary nutrition and dietary preventions strategies, the benefits in terms of higher quality of life, less hospitalization, health care costs, and increased productivity are less-well investigated.

Access to dietitian services in primary care for those at risk of diet-related nutrient inadequacies is largely underutilized in most countries [50]. Yet, in an increasing number of countries, preventative health checks are offered as secondary prevention to identify individuals at risk of disease. For instance, screening for cardiovascular risk factors, such as dyslipidemia, have been effective in reducing the overall burden of cardiovascular disease [51]. Screening tests for nutrient inadequacies and deficiencies in asymptomatic individuals are generally not covered by insurance plans. However, some tests are becoming more common as part of an annual health check-up or routine testing in risk groups (e.g., iron deficiency anemia in pregnant women, vitamin D in people at risk, or vitamin B12 status in older adults [52–56]). Nevertheless, nutrient deficiencies are often still recognized and are treated in an unnecessarily late stage, despite the availability of biomarkers allowing the early detection and management of nutritional inadequacies and deficiencies before the onset of symptoms. More focus on implementing evidence-based nutrition strategies complementary to public health approaches would prevent unnecessary nutrient inadequacies and deficiencies in vulnerable groups.

5. Criteria Determining Cost-Effectiveness

A health economic assessment is necessary to judge whether dietary advice and managing nutrient deficiencies in high-risk groups can be cost-effective, and to come to possible recommendations. Few cost-effectiveness assessments have been performed in the national context. at-risk group. Whether providing nutrition services, including dietary advice and if indicated supplemental nutrients, to groups at risk in the primary care setting can be cost-effective depends on multiple factors, as outlined below.

5.1. Public Health and Economic Consequences

First, the public health and economic consequences of nutrient inadequacies and deficiencies are the primary consideration for developing health care policy. The prevalence of nutrient inadequacies or low status is indicative of the public health problem, but the severity of clinical health consequences determines the actual burden of disease. In short, a cost-utility analysis using DALY or Quality Adjusted Life Year (QALY) as an outcome measure is recommended [57]. The analysis should be performed within a timeframe that is long enough to capture the period when the main health effects and costs arise. Sensitivity analysis is also recommended to assess the influence of central assumptions and uncertainty. Preventing nutrient deficiencies in the early years, from conception to five years of age, can be expected to have important effects on lifelong health, physical and mental performance, quality of life, and work capacity, and it is important to consider intergenerational effects [58,59].

5.2. Evidence Base Supporting Improved Health Outcomes, Discomfort and Risks

Second, in order to be cost-effective, provision of dietary services or dietary supplements to at-risk groups should lead to the expected improved health outcomes. The compromised health consequences from essential micro- and macro-nutrient inadequacies and deficiencies are generally well described (see paragraph 2). Although the reversal of nutrient deficiencies through re-supplementation can be expected to exert health benefits for the deficient individual, high-quality evidence from randomized controlled trials is not always available. The baseline nutrient status of the population and dose-response effects of nutrient re-supplementation should be considered where available. Effects of nutrient interventions in several high-quality studies can be inconsistent [60]. Unexplained inconsistency of nutritional effects in several high-quality studies may suggest underlying interactions that are yet unknown. Responsiveness to nutrients may be determined by possible gene-nutrient [60,61], nutrient-nutrient [62], or nutrient-drug [63,64] interactions. Guideline development for nutrition recommendation is often driven by requirements for high-quality evidence from randomized controlled intervention trials, even though the adverse health consequences of their deficiencies are well-known. An example of high-quality evidence approved by the European Food Safety Authorities is based on a several meta-analyses that suggest the beneficial effect of daily vitamin D supplementation in combination with calcium on the reduced the risk of falling [65].

Dietary supplements (tablets, capsules, liquids, powders) may be recommended in conjunction with a dietary advice if the needs for specific nutrients are difficult to be met by a food-based approach alone. No risks are associated with dietary modification. Dietary supplements are expected to be safe when taken under supervision of a health care professional, and under the conditions recommended, i.e. not exceeding the daily safe upper intake level (UL). A UL has been established for several of the vitamins and minerals by various regulatory bodies, below which intakes are likely to pose no risk of adverse effects.

For some of the nutrients, the health consequences of long-term high intakes in subgroups of the population remain debated. For instance, there is a large body of literature demonstrating the efficacy of maternal folic acid intake in preventing birth defects [66]. Nevertheless, some findings in literature link very low and very high folic acid intakes to increased cancer risk [66]. Two authoritative bodies that recently evaluated the possible risks from high folic acid intakes, concluded that evidence for adverse effects of high folic acid intake was not conclusive, but recommended further research to identify whether subgroups (e.g., with preexisting neoplasia or specific genetics) might be at an increased risk [66]. Beta-carotene became the subject of controversy when two studies reported that high β-carotene intake for several years was associated with higher risk of lung cancer in smokers [67,68], particularly in those who were lacking glutathione-S transferase 1 and 2 due to genetic variation [67]. Nevertheless, other large studies did not show such an effect [69].

Examples of adverse nutrient-drug and nutrient-nutrient interactions include high calcium intake that may adversely affect absorption and efficacy of certain antibiotics [70] or the absorption of dietary iron [71]. Examples of beneficial nutrient-nutrient interactions include the enhancing effect of vitamin C intake on iron absorption [62]. As long as these positive or negative effects of nutrients in special groups of the population are not well-established, their formal incorporation into a cost-benefit assessment remains difficult.

In rare cases, for instance, when efficacy of oral supplements is limited by malabsorption or intolerance, nutrients can be administrated by intravenous administration. Iron doses that are recommended for the prevention of iron deficiency may cause gastrointestinal when exceeding the UL, particularly when poorly absorbable iron forms are given [72]. Intravenous iron infusion is reserved for severe anemia or in the case of intolerance or unresponsiveness to oral therapy [73]. For vitamin B12, an initial intramuscular injection followed by oral supplements can be recommended if absorption is poor [74]. However, the associated higher costs of intravenous infusion or intramuscular injection might limit widespread use of these administration forms [75].

Inconveniences and discomfort involved in biomarker-based screening for deficiencies need to be considered. Blood drawing by venipuncture may cause local pain, bruising, and in rare cases, infection. Minimal or non-invasive methods using finger prick, urine- and saliva-based biomarkers that can be performed directly by the individuals may increase acceptance. The benefits of preventing nutrient deficiency-related clinical symptoms are generally expected to prevail over the minor discomforts of screening.

5.3. Availability of an Accurate Test

A prerequisite to screen individuals at-risk for specific nutrient inadequacies or deficiencies is the availability of a suitable test that has sufficient sensitivity and specificity. For many, but not all, vitamins and minerals, blood-, urine-, and saliva-based biomarkers of status exist, requiring minimally invasive sampling [76]. These biomarkers can detect specific nutrient deficiencies in an early stage before symptoms occur. Sensitive methodologies exist that measure omega-3 polyunsaturated fatty acid status requiring blood draw [77], while finger-prick blood tests are available in some countries. For protein status, no single routine and reliable indicator can be recommended at this time. Inexpensive, less accurate, and/or less predictive biomarkers can also be used in an initial screening, and if indicated, followed by more robust accurate and predictive tests to come to a final diagnosis. Examples include an initial hemoglobin test, followed by a serum ferritin test to accurately diagnose iron deficiency anemia [78], or qualitative lateral flow assays for vitamin D3 to test threshold levels [79].

Numerous screening tools have been developed to identify elderly or patients at risk of calorie or protein malnutrition. These tools have the disadvantage that they only detect overt signs of general malnutrition in a late stage, while specific nutrient deficiencies may go unnoticed [80]. Biomarkers indicative of general malnutrition that were found to be useful in older adults included BMI, hemoglobin, and total cholesterol [81]. Other possibilities include the use of validated dietary questionnaires to assess the risk of inadequate intake of (specific) nutrients [82]. However, dietary questionnaires are generally not sensitive and time consuming [83].

"Point-of-care" tests complying with regulatory requirements to diagnose and monitor nutrient inadequacies and deficiencies are expected to become increasingly specific and sensitive in the future. Gold standard testing and procedures for diagnosis, age- and gender-specific ranges, and cut-off levels to define deficiency are needed, although consensus is often lacking. Fast response times and low costs improve the likelihood that physicians and patients accept testing and immediate clinical decisions and guidance policies are met. Time and resource constraints by primary health-care professionals are the main barriers to perform nutrition screening and monitoring in general practice [84], and the actual uptake of a test strongly depends on its convenience for patient and physician. Monitoring to assess improvement in nutrient status or intake may be appropriate in patients with symptomatic deficiency, patients with malabsorption, or when poor adherence is suspected.

5.4. Adoption and Adherence

Third, the effectiveness of an intervention in primary health care strongly depends on its awareness and adoption among health care practitioners; i.e., the proportion aware of the nutrition problem, and the proportion of risk populations testing for deficiency, receiving dietary counseling, and being prescribed a nutrient regimen if indicated [85,86]. A small study showed that health care providers usually do not follow the testing recommendations for vitamin B12 deficiency [87]. Furthermore, the proportion of individuals adhering to the prescribed regimen, or, if applicable, willing to pay out-of-pocket non-reimbursed regimens also determines the effectiveness of secondary prevention [85,86].

Adherence rates can be expected to be lower for preventative therapies than for treatments. For example, folic acid supplementation of pregnant women can be a cost-effective means to prevent debilitating neural tube defects in infants [88], yet program effectiveness strongly depends on women taking folic acid in the critical peri-conceptual period when the supplements are effective in reducing risk of neural tube defects. Cost of food is a primary determinant of food choice and the higher nutrient-dense foods, which are associated with higher prices may reduce adherence [89]. The costs of various dietary supplement forms are generally low but can result in different adherence rates; tablets and capsules are generally shelf-stable over a longer time, provide a fixed dose, and their convenience is likely to maintain compliance. Powders and liquids may be an option, particularly for children, who may have difficulty swallowing tablets or capsules, but powders need to be mixed with food making them less convenient, and sometimes their taste may reduce compliance.

5.5. Costs and Cost Savings

Finally, the expected total direct and indirect costs and cost-savings of a secondary prevention strategy should be considered. Direct expenses involve the costs of diagnostic testing, costs of a dietitian consult, and costs of a dietary supplement regimen. Costs of screening tests vary widely, but as an example, a vitamin D deficiency test can cost on average $50. Costs of dietary consultation vary globally, but are generally low (e.g., about $100–$200 in the US). Nutritional counselling aimed at overnutrition was shown to be potentially cost-effective in various settings [90,91]. Nutrition strategies aimed at preventing deficiencies have not been assessed for their costs and benefits. Dietary supplements vary in their price; vitamin and mineral supplements can cost as little as a few cents per serving, whereas, for instance, costs of protein, omega-3 long-chain fatty acids, or fiber supplements can range from $0.20 to $1.20.

Potential direct cost savings include reduced medical care expenses and indirect costs savings involve gains in work productivity resulting from overcoming the deficiency-related health problems.

Figure 6 shows a checklist of criteria to be considered when assessing the cost-effectiveness of addressing nutrient inadequacies and deficiencies in a secondary prevention program. In a first step, the benefits of overcoming nutrient deficiencies can be balanced against possible constraints and disadvantages in a qualitative manner. Subsequently, the cost-effectiveness of preventing nutrient inadequacies and deficiencies can be evaluated by quantifying net cost savings and the public health impact. It is recommended that health benefits, disadvantages, and cost-effectiveness be evaluated for different scenarios (e.g., different uptake rates).

5.6. Evidence Gaps in Evaluating Secondary Nutrition Strategies

There are several challenges inherent to coming to recommendations for secondary nutrition strategies targeted at subgroups of biggest concern. The main problem is that data needed to come to recommendations of an intended program may be hampered by a lack of certainty, quality, or completeness.

For example, Rukuni et al. [92] systematically analyzed all the risks and benefits of screening and iron treatment of pregnant women in general practice in the UK to reduce iron deficiency anemia. In this review, several major gaps in the evidence were identified in relation to several criteria, for instance, insufficient evidence from high quality randomized controlled trials that early detection is effective in reducing morbidity and mortality, and robust evaluations of the cost-effectiveness of screening programs for iron deficiency anemia.

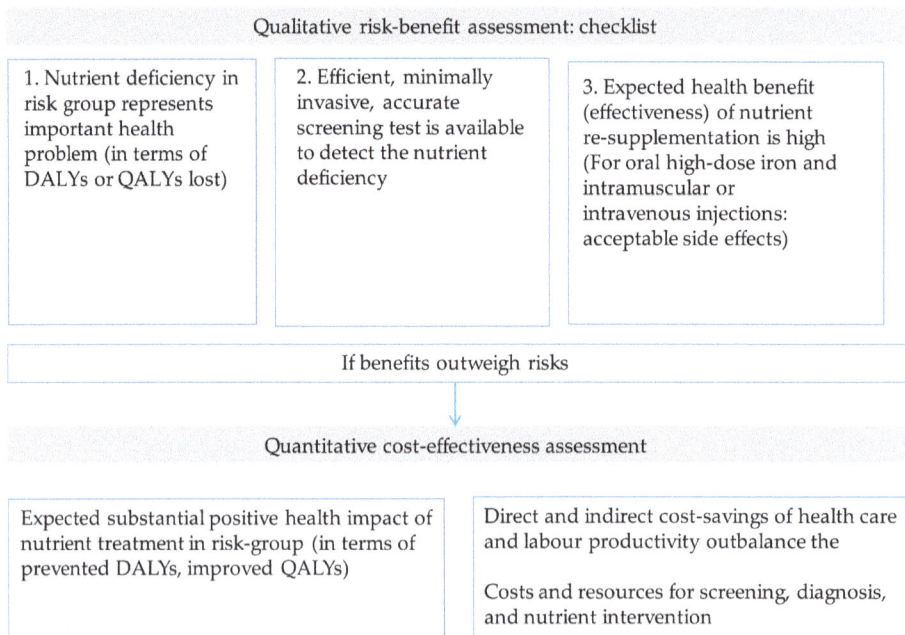

Figure 6. Initial qualitative risk-benefit assessment and subsequent quantitative cost-effectiveness analysis of nutrient supplementation of high-risk groups.

The effects of uncertainties can be assessed in health-economic modelling. The UK National Institute for Health and Care Excellence (NICE) modelled different scenarios for the UK, when comparing supplementation of populations at risk of vitamin D deficiency (pregnant and breastfeeding women, children aged under five, and over 65 years of age), either supplied universally to all at risk, or preceded by deficiency screening [86]. The outcomes strongly depended on several criteria, all affected by a degree of uncertainty; the prevalence of symptomatic vitamin D deficiency at baseline and after the intervention; adoption of the vitamin D recommendation among health professional and patients; the health outcomes expected in each scenario; the cost of testing for vitamin D deficiency; the cost of vitamin D supplements; and, the costs of treating symptomatic vitamin D deficiency. Under the assumed scenario, the results showed that testing to identify the deficient people is likely to cost more than universal vitamin D supplementation of the entire at-risk population without prior testing. A disadvantage of the latter is the unnecessary exposure of adequate individuals to unnecessary high intakes.

As the results of the cost-effectiveness analysis depends on the reliability of the data that it is based on, it is worthwhile to quantify uncertainties in base assumptions using sensitivity analyses.

6. Discussion

A risk-benefit balance followed by a more thorough cost-effectiveness assessment will allow for well-balanced recommendations for addressing nutrition deficiencies of major public health concern in a secondary prevention strategy. Some of the input variables dealing with uncertainty include the rate of adoption of nutrition guidelines among program implementers, as well as adherence of individuals to prescribed nutritional therapy. Moreover, high-quality evidence for the benefits of reducing nutrient deficiencies in at-risk groups is urgently needed to allow for appropriate cost-effectiveness analysis of screening for nutrient deficiencies. To judge the total evidence supporting cost-effective nutrition interventions can be challenging and requires certain estimates and assumptions to be embedded into the cost-effectiveness assessment. Nevertheless, uncertainty in inputs can be analyzed and should not prevent the implementation of a cost-effectiveness assessment.

The various inconsistent recommendations for nutrient management developed by different organizations may be a barrier to effective implementation of a secondary nutrition prevention strategy. Governments should drive policy consensus on guidelines. A more profound problem is the limited access to nutrition services in primary health care: time or expertise of primary health care professionals to counsel individuals on nutrition, access to and collaboration with dietitians or nutritionists, continuous monitoring, and evaluation of the individuals that are at risk, all affect the effectiveness of nutrition interventions. Rapid point-of-care tests are increasingly being administered by trained staff and health care professionals in pharmacies, hospitals, and clinics [93]. In the meantime, increasing the awareness among conscious consumers about the potential link between certain nutrient inadequacies and deficiencies and adverse health outcomes has resulted in an increase in the rate of self-testing [94]. Moreover, the emerging use of self-diagnostic tests by consumers [95] suggests that consumers are becoming more active in diagnosing and managing their own health. In the future, personalized nutritional recommendations based on individuals' genetic testing will further contribute to this. Ultimately, consumer-driven personalized management of nutrient deficiencies based on testing is likely to develop more rapidly than the implementation of targeted prevention strategies via the health care system.

7. Conclusions

National survey data show that adequate nutrient intakes and sufficient status may be difficult to achieve across all age and gender groups. Primary prevention strategies to avoid nutrient deficiencies are often not sufficient in certain subgroups of the population. Screening those at highest risk, followed by targeted nutrition services, is often underestimated and overlooked as a potentially cost-effective intervention to prevent clinical deficiencies. Whether a secondary nutrition prevention approach could be cost-effective or even cost-saving over the medium to long term, depends on various criteria. Some degree of uncertainty is inherent in such health economic evaluation. If a biomarker test is used for screening, the availability of an affordable, predictive, and efficient test of nutrient status in the at-risk population is important in view of the time and resource constraints general practitioners are facing. The success of guidelines to prevent and control nutrient deficiencies in vulnerable population groups strongly depends on the extent that health care professionals are informed, engaged, and implementing them, and individuals adhere to them. To come to recommendations to improve the nutrient supply to those at risk of being deficient requires a balance of the disadvantages and benefits, and a cost-effectiveness assessment.

Author Contributions: M.J.B., J.K.B., C.P.A. and M.E. wrote the paper.

Conflicts of Interest: The authors are employed by DSM Nutritional Products, a manufacturer of vitamins and supplier to the food, dietary supplement, and pharmaceutical industries. There were no other conflicts of interest.

Funding: The authors reported no funding received for this study.

References

1. Boyle, M.A.; Holben, D.H. *Community Nutrition in Action: An Entrepreneurial Approach*, 5th ed.; Wadsworth: Belmont, CA, USA, 2010.
2. Herring, D.; Chang, S.; Bard, S.; Gavey, E. Five years of myplate-looking back and what's ahead. *J. Acad. Nutr. Diet.* **2016**, *116*, 1069–1071. [CrossRef] [PubMed]
3. Montagnese, C.; Santarpia, L.; Iavarone, F.; Strangio, F.; Caldara, A.R.; Silvestri, E.; Contaldo, F.; Pasanisi, F. North and south american countries food-based dietary guidelines: A comparison. *Nutrition* **2017**, *42*, 51–63. [CrossRef] [PubMed]
4. Montagnese, C.; Santarpia, L.; Buonifacio, M.; Nardelli, A.; Caldara, A.R.; Silvestri, E.; Contaldo, F.; Pasanisi, F. European food-based dietary guidelines: A comparison and update. *Nutrition* **2015**, *31*, 908–915. [CrossRef] [PubMed]
5. Pfeiffer, C.M.; Sternberg, M.R.; Schleicher, R.L.; Haynes, B.M.; Rybak, M.E.; Pirkle, J.L. The CDC's second national report on biochemical indicators of diet and nutrition in the U.S. Population is a valuable tool for researchers and policy makers. *J. Nutr.* **2013**, *143*, 938S–947S. [CrossRef] [PubMed]
6. Spiro, A.; Buttriss, J.L. Vitamin D: An overview of vitamin D status and intake in Europe. *Nutr. Bull.* **2014**, *39*, 322–350. [CrossRef] [PubMed]
7. Troesch, B.; Hoeft, B.; McBurney, M.; Eggersdorfer, M.; Weber, P. Dietary surveys indicate vitamin intakes below recommendations are common in representative western countries. *Br. J. Nutr.* **2012**, *108*, 692–698. [CrossRef] [PubMed]
8. Diethelm, K.; Huybrechts, I.; Moreno, L.; De Henauw, S.; Manios, Y.; Beghin, L.; Gonzalez-Gross, M.; Le Donne, C.; Cuenca-Garcia, M.; Castillo, M.J.; et al. Nutrient intake of european adolescents: Results of the helena (healthy lifestyle in Europe by nutrition in adolescence) study. *Public Health Nutr.* **2014**, *17*, 486–497. [CrossRef] [PubMed]
9. Herbert, V. The five possible causes of all nutrient deficiency: Illustrated by deficiencies of vitamin B12 and folic acid. *Aust. N. Z. J. Med.* **1972**, *2*, 69–77. [CrossRef] [PubMed]
10. Serra-Majem, L.; Ribas, L.; Perez-Rodrigo, C.; Garcia-Closas, R.; Pena-Quintana, L.; Aranceta, J. Determinants of nutrient intake among children and adolescents: Results from the enkid study. *Ann. Nutr. Metab.* **2002**, *46* (Suppl. 1), 31–38. [CrossRef] [PubMed]
11. Cordain, L.; Eaton, S.B.; Sebastian, A.; Mann, N.; Lindeberg, S.; Watkins, B.A.; O'Keefe, J.H.; Brand-Miller, J. Origins and evolution of the western diet: Health implications for the 21st century. *Am. J. Clin. Nutr.* **2005**, *81*, 341–354. [PubMed]
12. Marangoni, F.; Cetin, I.; Verduci, E.; Canzone, G.; Giovannini, M.; Scollo, P.; Corsello, G.; Poli, A. Maternal diet and nutrient requirements in pregnancy and breastfeeding. An Italian consensus document. *Nutrients* **2016**, *8*, 629. [CrossRef] [PubMed]
13. Dewey, K.G. The challenge of meeting nutrient needs of infants and young children during the period of complementary feeding: An evolutionary perspective. *J. Nutr.* **2013**, *143*, 2050–2054. [CrossRef] [PubMed]
14. Story, M.; Hermanson, J. Nutrient needs during adolescence and pregnancy: A practical reference guide. In *Nutrient Needs during Adolescence and Pregnancy*; Story, M., Stang, J., Eds.; Center for Leadership, Education, and Training in Maternal and Child Nutrition, University of Minnesota: Minneapolis, MN, USA, 2000; Chapter 5.
15. Leslie, W.; Hankey, C. Aging, nutritional status and health. *Healthcare* **2015**, *3*, 648–658. [CrossRef] [PubMed]
16. Mehta, N.M.; Duggan, C.P. Nutritional deficiencies during critical illness. *Pediatr. Clin. N. Am.* **2009**, *56*, 1143–1160. [CrossRef] [PubMed]
17. Berger, M.M.; Chiolero, R.L. Key vitamins and trace elements in the critically ill. *Nestle Nutr. Workshop Ser. Clin. Perform. Program.* **2003**, *8*, 99–111, discussion 111–117. [PubMed]
18. Wong, C.W. Vitamin B12 deficiency in the elderly: Is it worth screening? *Hong Kong Med. J.* **2015**, *21*, 155–164. [PubMed]

19. Hurrell, R.; Egli, I. Iron bioavailability and dietary reference values. *Am. J. Clin. Nutr.* **2010**, *91*, 1461S–1467S. [CrossRef] [PubMed]

20. West, C.E.; Eilander, A.; van Lieshout, M. Consequences of revised estimates of carotenoid bioefficacy for dietary control of vitamin A deficiency in developing countries. *J. Nutr.* **2002**, *132*, 2920S–2926S. [PubMed]

21. Reilly, W.; Ilich, J.Z. Prescription drugs and nutrient depletion: How much is known? *Adv. Nutr.* **2017**, *8*, 23.

22. Stover, P.J. Influence of human genetic variation on nutritional requirements. *Am. J. Clin. Nutr.* **2006**, *83*, 436S–442S. [PubMed]

23. Suskind, D.L. Nutritional deficiencies during normal growth. *Pediatr. Clin. N. Am.* **2009**, *56*, 1035–1053. [CrossRef] [PubMed]

24. Weininger, J. Nutritional Disease: Nutrient Deficiencies. Available online: https://www.britannica.com/science/nutritional-disease (accessed on 2 January 2018).

25. National Institutes of Health (NIH), Office of Dietary Supplement. Dietary Supplement Fact Sheets. Available online: https://ods.od.nih.gov/factsheets/ (accessed on 2 January 2018).

26. Tinker, S.C.; Hamner, H.C.; Qi, Y.P.; Crider, K.S. U.S. Women of childbearing age who are at possible increased risk of a neural tube defect-affected pregnancy due to suboptimal red blood cell folate concentrations, national health and nutrition examination survey 2007 to 2012. *Birth Defects Res. Part A Clin. Mol. Teratol.* **2015**, *103*, 517–526. [CrossRef] [PubMed]

27. Peter, S.; Eggersdorfer, M.; van Asselt, D.; Buskens, E.; Detzel, P.; Freijer, K.; Koletzko, B.; Kraemer, K.; Kuipers, F.; Neufeld, L.; et al. Selected nutrients and their implications for health and disease across the lifespan: A roadmap. *Nutrients* **2014**, *6*, 6076–6094. [CrossRef] [PubMed]

28. Darnton-Hill, I.; Webb, P.; Harvey, P.W.; Hunt, J.M.; Dalmiya, N.; Chopra, M.; Ball, M.J.; Bloem, M.W.; de Benoist, B. Micronutrient deficiencies and gender: Social and economic costs. *Am. J. Clin. Nutr.* **2005**, *81*, 1198S–1205S. [PubMed]

29. Departments of Agriculture and Health and Human Services. Part D. Chapter 1: Food and nutrient intakes, and health: Current status and trends. In *Scientific Report of the 2015 Dietary Guidelines Advisory Committee*; Departments of Agriculture and Health and Human Services: Washington, DC, USA, 2015.

30. Marvin-Dowle, K.; Burley, V.J.; Soltani, H. Nutrient intakes and nutritional biomarkers in pregnant adolescents: A systematic review of studies in developed countries. *BMC Pregnancy Childbirth* **2016**, *16*, 268. [CrossRef] [PubMed]

31. Blumfield, M.L.; Hure, A.J.; Macdonald-Wicks, L.; Smith, R.; Collins, C.E. A systematic review and meta-analysis of micronutrient intakes during pregnancy in developed countries. *Nutr. Rev.* **2013**, *71*, 118–132. [CrossRef] [PubMed]

32. Gernand, A.D.; Schulze, K.J.; Stewart, C.P.; West, K.P., Jr.; Christian, P. Micronutrient deficiencies in pregnancy worldwide: Health effects and prevention. *Nat. Rev. Endocrinol.* **2016**, *12*, 274–289. [CrossRef] [PubMed]

33. Bird, J.K.; Murphy, R.A.; Ciappio, E.D.; McBurney, M.I. Risk of deficiency in multiple concurrent micronutrients in children and adults in the united states. *Nutrients* **2017**, *9*, 655. [CrossRef] [PubMed]

34. Hilger, J.; Goerig, T.; Weber, P.; Hoeft, B.; Eggersdorfer, M.; Carvalho, N.C.; Goldberger, U.; Hoffmann, K. Micronutrient intake in healthy toddlers: A multinational perspective. *Nutrients* **2015**, *7*, 6938–6955. [CrossRef] [PubMed]

35. Akkermans, M.D.; Eussen, S.R.; van der Horst-Graat, J.M.; van Elburg, R.M.; van Goudoever, J.B.; Brus, F. A micronutrient-fortified young-child formula improves the iron and vitamin D status of healthy young European children: A randomized, double-blind controlled trial. *Am. J. Clin. Nutr.* **2017**, *105*, 391. [CrossRef] [PubMed]

36. Kaganov, B.; Caroli, M.; Mazur, A.; Singhal, A.; Vania, A. Suboptimal micronutrient intake among children in Europe. *Nutrients* **2015**, *7*, 3524–3535. [CrossRef] [PubMed]

37. Forrest, K.Y.; Stuhldreher, W.L. Prevalence and correlates of vitamin D deficiency in US adults. *Nutr. Res.* **2011**, *31*, 48–54. [CrossRef] [PubMed]

38. Tussing-Humphreys, L.; Van Nguyen, T.Q. Adipose tissue and adipokines in health and disease, nutrition and health. In *Obesity and Micronutrient Deficiencies*; Fantuzzi, G., Mazzone, T., Eds.; Springer: New York, NY, USA, 2014.

39. Food Surveys Research Group; Beltsville Human Nutrition Research Center; Agricultural Research Service, U.S. Department of Agriculture (USDA ARS). What We Eat in America, NHANES 2007–2010, Individuals 1 Year and over (Excluding Breast-Fed Children and Pregnant or Lactating Females), Dietary Intake Data. Available online: https://www.cdc.gov/nchs/nhanes/wweia.htm (accessed on 2 January 2018).

40. Hwalla, N.; Al Dhaheri, A.S.; Radwan, H.; Alfawaz, H.A.; Fouda, M.A.; Al-Daghri, N.M.; Zaghloul, S.; Blumberg, J.B. The prevalence of micronutrient deficiencies and inadequacies in the middle east and approaches to interventions. *Nutrients* **2017**, *9*, 229. [CrossRef] [PubMed]

41. Mohammed, E.M.A. Multiple sclerosis is prominent in the gulf states: Review. *Pathogenesis* **2016**, *3*, 19–38. [CrossRef]

42. Food and Agriculture Organization of the United Nations (FAO). *Regional Overview of Food Insecurity: Europe and Central Asia*; FAO: Budapest, Hungary, 2017.

43. Global Burden of Disease (GBD) 2013 Risk Factors Collaborators. Global, regional, and national comparative risk assessment of 79 behavioural, environmental and occupational, and metabolic risks or clusters of risks, 1990–2015: A systematic analysis for the global burden of disease study 2015. *Lancet* **2016**, *388*, 1659–1724.

44. World Health Organization (WHO). *Iron Deficiency Anaemia Assessment, Prevention and Control: A Guide for Programme Managers*; WHO: Geneva, Switzerland, 2001.

45. Imamura, F.; Micha, R.; Khatibzadeh, S.; Fahimi, S.; Shi, P.; Powles, J.; Mozaffarian, D.; Global Burden of Diseases Nutrition and Chronic Diseases Expert Group (NutriCoDE). Dietary quality among men and women in 187 countries in 1990 and 2010: A systematic assessment. *Lancet Glob. Health* **2015**, *3*, e132–e142. [CrossRef]

46. United States Department of Agriculture (USDA), Food and Nutrition Service. In *Women, Infants and Children (WIC). About WIC—How WIC Helps*. Available online: https://www.fns.usda.gov/wic/about-wic-how-wic-helps (accessed on 2 January 2018).

47. Organisation for Economic Co-operation and Development (OECD). *Health at a Glance 2015: OECD Indicators*; OECD: Paris, France, 2015.

48. The Royal Australian College of General Practitioners (RACGP). *Guidelines for Preventive Activities in General Practice*, 9th ed.; RACGP: Melbourne, Australia, 2016.

49. Centers for Disease Control and Prevention (CDC). Available online: https://www.cdc.gov/ (accessed on 2 January 2018).

50. Segal, L.; Opie, R.S. A nutrition strategy to reduce the burden of diet related disease: Access to dietician services must complement population health approaches. *Front. Pharmacol.* **2015**, *6*, 160. [CrossRef] [PubMed]

51. Ford, E.S.; Capewell, S. Proportion of the decline in cardiovascular mortality disease due to prevention versus treatment: Public health versus clinical care. *Annu. Rev. Public Health* **2011**, *32*, 5–22. [CrossRef] [PubMed]

52. Langan, R.C.; Zawistoski, K.J. Update on vitamin B12 deficiency. *Am. Fam. Physician* **2011**, *83*, 1425–1430. [PubMed]

53. Holick, M.F.; Binkley, N.C.; Bischoff-Ferrari, H.A.; Gordon, C.M.; Hanley, D.A.; Heaney, R.P.; Murad, M.H.; Weaver, C.M.; Endocrine, S. Evaluation, treatment, and prevention of vitamin D deficiency: An endocrine society clinical practice guideline. *J. Clin. Endocrinol. Metab.* **2011**, *96*, 1911–1930. [CrossRef] [PubMed]

54. Short, M.W.; Domagalski, J.E. Iron deficiency anemia: Evaluation and management. *Am. Fam. Physician* **2013**, *87*, 98–104. [PubMed]

55. Eck, L.M. Should family physicians routinely screen for vitamin D deficiency? Yes: Targeted screening in at-risk populations is prudent. *Am. Fam. Physician* **2013**, *87*, od1. [PubMed]

56. Lachner, C.; Martin, C.; John, D.; Nekkalapu, S.; Sasan, A.; Steinle, N.; Regenold, W.T. Older adult psychiatric inpatients with non-cognitive disorders should be screened for vitamin B12 deficiency. *J. Nutr. Health Aging* **2014**, *18*, 209–212. [CrossRef] [PubMed]

57. Prüss-Üstün, A.; Campbell-Lendrum, D.; Corvalán, C.; Woodward, A. *The Global Burden of Disease Concept*; WHO Environmental Burden of Disease Series; World Health Organization (WHO): Geneva, Switzerland, 2003; Volume 1.

58. The Royal Children's Hospital Melbourne, Centre for Community Child Health. *Early Childhood and the Lifecourse*; Policy brief No 1. 2006. Available online: https://rch.org.au/ccch/policybrief (accessed on 2 January 2018).

59. Bartley, K.A.; Underwood, B.A.; Deckelbaum, R.J. A life cycle micronutrient perspective for women's health. *Am. J. Clin. Nutr.* **2005**, *81*, 1188S–1193S. [PubMed]
60. Ferguson, L.R.; Eck, P.; Simopoulos, A.P.; Gillies, P.J.; Vanden Heuvel, J.P. Section 1: Examples of some key nutrient-gene interactions. In *Nutrigenomics and Nutrigenetics in Functional Foods and Personalized Nutrition*; Ferguson, L.R., Ed.; CRC Press: Boca Raton, FL, USA, 2016; pp. 3–118.
61. Murphy, M.M.; Fernandez-Ballart, J.D. Homocysteine in pregnancy. *Adv. Clin. Chem.* **2011**, *53*, 105–137.
62. Teucher, B.; Olivares, M.; Cori, H. Enhancers of iron absorption: Ascorbic acid and other organic acids. *Int. J. Vitam. Nutr. Res.* **2004**, *74*, 403–419. [CrossRef] [PubMed]
63. Anadón, A.; Martínez-Larrañaga, M.R.; Ares, I.; Aránzazu Martínez, M. Interactions between nutraceuticals/nutrients and therapeutic drugs. In *Nutraceuticals, Efficacy, Safety and Toxicity*; Gupta, R.C., Ed.; Academic Press: Hopkinsville, KY, USA, 2016; pp. 855–874.
64. Sultan, S.; Jahangir, A. Drug–nutrient interactions in the elderly. In *Molecular Basis of Nutrition and Aging*, 2nd ed.; Malavolta, M., Mocchegiani, E., Eds.; Academic Press: San Diego, CA, USA, 2016; pp. 73–107.
65. European Food Safety Authority (EFSA). Vitamin D and risk of falling. *EFSA J.* **2011**, *9*, 2382.
66. Field, M.S.; Stover, P.J. Safety of folic acid. *Ann. N. Y. Acad. Sci.* **2017**. [CrossRef] [PubMed]
67. Alpha-Tocopherol, Beta Carotene Cancer Prevention Study Group. The effect of vitamin E and beta carotene on the incidence of lung cancer and other cancers in male smokers. *N. Engl. J. Med.* **1994**, *330*, 1029–1035.
68. Omenn, G.S.; Goodman, G.E.; Thornquist, M.D.; Balmes, J.; Cullen, M.R.; Glass, A.; Keogh, J.P.; Meyskens, F.L., Jr.; Valanis, B.; Williams, J.H., Jr.; et al. Risk factors for lung cancer and for intervention effects in caret, the beta-carotene and retinol efficacy trial. *J. Natl. Cancer Inst.* **1996**, *88*, 1550–1559. [CrossRef] [PubMed]
69. Hennekens, C.H.; Buring, J.E.; Manson, J.E.; Stampfer, M.; Rosner, B.; Cook, N.R.; Belanger, C.; LaMotte, F.; Gaziano, J.M.; Ridker, P.M.; et al. Lack of effect of long-term supplementation with beta carotene on the incidence of malignant neoplasms and cardiovascular disease. *N. Engl. J. Med.* **1996**, *334*, 1145–1149. [CrossRef] [PubMed]
70. Bushra, R.; Aslam, N.; Khan, A.Y. Food-drug interactions. *Oman Med. J.* **2011**, *26*, 77–83. [CrossRef] [PubMed]
71. Lonnerdal, B. Calcium and iron absorption–mechanisms and public health relevance. *Int. J. Vitam. Nutr. Res.* **2010**, *80*, 293–299. [CrossRef] [PubMed]
72. Santiago, P. Ferrous versus ferric oral iron formulations for the treatment of iron deficiency: A clinical overview. *Sci. World J.* **2012**, *2012*, 846824. [CrossRef] [PubMed]
73. Wong, L.; Smith, S.; Gilstrop, M.; Derman, R.; Auerbach, S.; London, N.; Lenowitz, S.; Bahrain, H.; McClintock, J.; Auerbach, M. Safety and efficacy of rapid (1000 mg in 1 h) intravenous iron dextran for treatment of maternal iron deficient anemia of pregnancy. *Am. J. Hematol.* **2016**, *91*, 590–593. [CrossRef] [PubMed]
74. Lin, J.; Kelsberg, G.; Safranek, S. Clinical inquiry: Is high-dose oral B12 a safe and effective alternative to a B12 injection? *J. Fam. Pract.* **2012**, *61*, 162–163. [PubMed]
75. Masucci, L.; Goeree, R. Vitamin B12 intramuscular injections versus oral supplements: A budget impact analysis. *Ont. Health Technol. Assess. Ser.* **2013**, *13*, 1–24. [PubMed]
76. Lee, R.D.; Nieman, D.C. *Nutritional Assessment*, 6th ed.; McGraw Hill Higher Education: New York, NY, USA, 2010.
77. Klingler, M.; Koletzko, B. Novel methodologies for assessing omega-3 fatty acid status—A systematic review. *Br. J. Nutr.* **2012**, *107* (Suppl. 2), S53–S63. [CrossRef] [PubMed]
78. Goddard, A.F.; James, M.W.; McIntyre, A.S.; Scott, B.B.; British Society of Gastroenterology. Guidelines for the management of iron deficiency anaemia. *Gut* **2011**, *60*, 1309–1316. [CrossRef] [PubMed]
79. Vemulapati, S.; Rey, E.; O'Dell, D.; Mehta, S.; Erickson, D. A quantitative point-of-need assay for the assessment of vitamin D3 deficiency. *Sci. Rep.* **2017**, *7*, 14142. [CrossRef] [PubMed]
80. McDonagh, M.; Blazina, I.; Dana, T.; Cantor, A.; Bougatsos, C. *Routine Iron Supplementation and Screening for Iron Deficiency Anemia in Children Ages 6 to 24 Months: A Systematic Review to Update the U.S. Preventive Services Task Force Recommendation*; Agency for Healthcare Research and Quality: Rockville, MD, USA, 2015.
81. Zhang, Z.; Pereira, S.L.; Luo, M.; Matheson, E.M. Evaluation of blood biomarkers associated with risk of malnutrition in older adults: A systematic review and meta-analysis. *Nutrients* **2017**, *9*, 829. [CrossRef] [PubMed]

82. National Cancer Institute (NIH). Epidemiology and Genomics Research Program: Register of Validated Short Dietary Assessment Instruments. Available online: https://epi.grants.cancer.gov/diet/shortreg/register.php (accessed on 2 January 2018).

83. Asaad, G.; Sadegian, M.; Lau, R.; Xu, Y.; Soria-Contreras, D.C.; Bell, R.C.; Chan, C.B. The reliability and validity of the perceived dietary adherence questionnaire for people with type 2 diabetes. *Nutrients* **2015**, *7*, 5484–5496. [CrossRef] [PubMed]

84. Hamirudin, A.H.; Charlton, K.; Walton, K.; Bonney, A.; Albert, G.; Hodgkins, A.; Potter, J.; Milosavljevic, M.; Dalley, A. 'We are all time poor'. Is routine nutrition screening of older patients feasible? *Aust. Fam. Physician* **2013**, *42*, 321–326. [PubMed]

85. Lubloy, A. Factors affecting the uptake of new medicines: A systematic literature review. *BMC Health Serv. Res.* **2014**, *14*, 469. [CrossRef] [PubMed]

86. National Institute for Health and Care Excellence (NICE). An Economic Evaluation of Interventions to Improve the Uptake of Vitamin D Supplements in England and Wales. Available online: https://www.nice.org.uk/guidance/ph56/documents/economic-evaluation-report2 (accessed on 2 January 2018).

87. Berg, R.L.; Shaw, G.R. Laboratory evaluation for vitamin B12 deficiency: The case for cascade testing. *Clin Med. Res.* **2013**, *11*, 7–15. [CrossRef] [PubMed]

88. Yi, Y.; Lindemann, M.; Colligs, A.; Snowball, C. Economic burden of neural tube defects and impact of prevention with folic acid: A literature review. *Eur. J. Pediatr.* **2011**, *170*, 1391–1400. [CrossRef] [PubMed]

89. Albuquerque, G.; Moreira, P.; Rosáriode, R.; Araújoa, A.; Teixeira, V.H.; Lopes, O.; Moreirag, A.; Padrãoa, P. Adherence to the mediterranean diet in children: Is it associated with economic cost? *Porto Biomed. J.* **2017**, *2*, 115–119. [CrossRef]

90. Lammers, M.; Kok, L. *Cost-Benefit Analysis of Dietary Treatment*; Dutch Association of Dietitians: Amsterdam, The Netherlands, 2012.

91. Dalziel, K.; Segal, L. Time to give nutrition interventions a higher profile: Cost-effectiveness of 10 nutrition interventions. *Health Promot. Int.* **2007**, *22*, 271–283. [CrossRef] [PubMed]

92. Rukuni, R.; Knight, M.; Murphy, M.F.; Roberts, D.; Stanworth, S.J. Screening for iron deficiency and iron deficiency anaemia in pregnancy: A structured review and gap analysis against UK national screening criteria. *BMC Pregnancy Childbirth* **2015**, *15*, 269. [CrossRef] [PubMed]

93. Gubbins, P.O.; Klepser, M.E.; Dering-Anderson, A.M.; Bauer, K.A.; Darin, K.M.; Klepser, S.; Matthias, K.R.; Scarsi, K. Point-of-care testing for infectious diseases: Opportunities, barriers, and considerations in community pharmacy. *J. Am. Pharm. Assoc. (2003)* **2014**, *54*, 163–171. [CrossRef] [PubMed]

94. Tapley, A.; Magin, P.; Morgan, S.; Henderson, K.; Scott, J.; Thomson, A.; Spike, N.; McArthur, L.; van Driel, M.; McElduff, P.; et al. Test ordering in an evidence free zone: Rates and associations of australian general practice trainees' vitamin D test ordering. *J. Eval. Clin. Pract.* **2015**, *21*, 1151–1156. [CrossRef] [PubMed]

95. Hynes, V. The trend toward self-diagnosis. *Can. Med. Assoc. J. CMAJ* **2013**, *185*, E149–E150. [CrossRef] [PubMed]

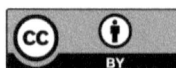

MDPI

St. Alban-Anlage 66

4052 Basel, Switzerland

Tel. +41 61 683 77 34

Fax +41 61 302 89 18

http://www.mdpi.com

Nutrients Editorial Office

E-mail: nutrients@mdpi.com

http://www.mdpi.com/journal/nutrients